Ramamurthy's
Decision Making in Pain Management
An Algorithmic Approach

Ramamurthy's
Decision Making in Pain Management
An Algorithmic Approach

Third Edition

Editors

Ameet Nagpal MD MS MEd
Clinical Assistant Professor
Department of Anesthesiology
Medical Director
UT Medicine Pain Consultants
UT Health San Antonio, San Antonio, TX, USA

Miles Day MD DABA FIPP DABIPP
Traweek-Racz Endowed Professor in Pain Research
Medical Director, The Pain Center at Grace Clinic
Pain Medicine Fellowship Director, Texas Tech University HSC, Lubbock, TX, USA

Maxim S Eckmann MD
Director, Anesthesiology Pain Medicine
Program Director, Pain Medicine Fellowship
Associate Professor
Department of Anesthesiology
UT Health San Antonio, San Antonio, TX, USA

Brian T Boies MD
Clinical Assistant Professor
Department of Anesthesiology, UT Health San Antonio, San Antonio, TX, USA

Larry C Driver MD
Professor
Department of Pain Medicine
Division of Anesthesiology and Critical Care
The University of Texas MD Anderson Cancer Center, Houston, TX, USA

Foreword

Kenneth D Candido

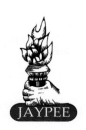

The Health Sciences Publisher
New Delhi | London | Panama

Jaypee Brothers Medical Publishers (P) Ltd.

Headquarters
Jaypee Brothers Medical Publishers (P) Ltd
4838/24, Ansari Road, Daryaganj
New Delhi 110 002, India
Phone: +91-11-43574357
Fax: +91-11-43574314
E-mail: jaypee@jaypeebrothers.com

Overseas Offices

J.P. Medical Ltd
83, Victoria Street, London
SW1H 0HW (UK)
Phone: +44-20 3170 8910
Fax: +44 (0)20 3008 6180
E-mail: info@jpmedpub.com

Jaypee Brothers Medical Publishers (P) Ltd
17/1-B, Babar Road, Block-B, Shaymali
Mohammadpur, Dhaka-1207
Bangladesh
Mobile: +08801912003485
E-mail: jaypeedhaka@gmail.com

Jaypee-Highlights Medical Publishers Inc
City of Knowledge, Bld. 235, 2nd Floor, Clayton
Panama City, Panama
Phone: +1 507-301-0496
Fax: +1 507-301-0499
E-mail: cservice@jphmedical.com

Jaypee Brothers Medical Publishers (P) Ltd
Bhotahity, Kathmandu, Nepal
Phone: +977-9741283608
E-mail: kathmandu@jaypeebrothers.com

Website: www.jaypeebrothers.com
Website: www.jaypeedigital.com

Ramamurthy's Decision Making in Pain Management: An Algorithmic Approach

Third Edition: **2018**
ISBN: 978-93-86261-45-8
Printed at Sanat Printers

Dedicated to

Dr Somayaji Ramamurthy, the Editor of the first two editions of this work. "Rama"—as he is known by his family and friends—pioneered the idea of teaching Pain Medicine/Management as a fellowship discipline. It is not an exaggeration to say it is likely that Rama trained more physicians in the field of Pain Medicine than any other physician in American history. Without his guidance, thousands of patients with chronic pain would have gone untreated. We owe him a debt of gratitude that we will never be able to repay. From this edition forward, the Decision Making in Pain Management series will carry his name eponymously.

– The Editors

CONTRIBUTORS

Adam S Tenforde MD
Assistant Professor
Department of Physical Medicine and
Rehabilitation
Harvard University
Charlestown, MA, USA

Ahmed R Haque MD
Assistant Professor
Department of Anesthesiology and
Pain Medicine
University of Vermont College of
Medicine
Burlington, VT, USA

Aimee A McAnally MD
Texas Pain Relief Group
Fort Worth, TX, USA

Alan B Swearingen MD
Department of Anesthesiology
Pain Medicine Fellow
UT Health San Antonio
San Antonio, TX, USA

Albert H Vu DO
Attending Physician
Cedar Hill Pain and Rehabilitation
Cedar Hill, TX, USA

Alexander Bautista MD
Assistant Professor
Department of Anesthesiology and
Pain Medicine
University of Oklahoma Health
Sciences Center
Oklahoma City, OK, USA

Ameet Nagpal MD MS MEd
Clinical Assistant Professor
Department of Anesthesiology
Medical Director
UT Medicine Pain Consultants
UT Health San Antonio
San Antonio, TX, USA

Andrea L King MD
Anesthesiologist
US Anesthesia Partners
Dallas, TX, USA

Andrew Rubens MD
Pain Medicine Fellow
Department of Anesthesiology Critical
Care and Pain Medicine
Beth Israel Deaconess Medical Center,
Harvard University
Boston, MA, USA

Andrew T Feldman MD
Physician Fellow
Department of Pain Management
San Antonio Uniformed Services
Health Education Consortium
Fort Sam Houston, TX, USA

Anish A Mirchandani DO
Resident Physician
Department of Physical Medicine and
Rehabilitation
New York-Presbyterian Hospital
New York, NY, USA

Ankur B Patel DO
Pain Fellow
Department of Anesthesiology
Texas Tech University
Lubbock, TX, USA

Anton Y Jorgensen MD
Orthopedic Spine Surgeon
Department of Orthopedic Surgery
San Antonio Military Medical Center
San Antonio, TX, USA

Ashley E Sanford PhD
Postdoctoral Fellow (APA Accredited)
Department of Veteran's Affairs
Michael E DeBakey VA Medical Center
Houston, TX, USA

Austin Horrocks DO
Resident
Department of Anesthesiology
UT Health San Antonio
San Antonio, TX, USA

Baker Mitchell MD
Assistant Professor
Department of Anesthesiology
UT Health San Antonio
San Antonio, TX, USA

Ben Marshall DO
Resident Physician
Department of Physical Medicine and
Rehabilitation
Northwestern University School of
Medicine/RIC
Chicago, IL, USA

Benjamin M Keizer PhD
Rehabilitation Psychologist
Center for the Intrepid
Brooke Army Medical Center
Fort Sam Houston, TX, USA

Benjamin J Wallisch DO
Associate Professor
Medical Director of Anesthesiology
Department of Anesthesiology
UT Health San Antonio
San Antonio, TX, USA

Brandon J Goff DO
Assistant Professor
Department of Physical Medicine and
Rehabilitation
Uniformed Services University of
Health Sciences
Bethesda, MD, USA

Brian J Mugleston MEd
UT Health San Antonio
San Antonio, TX, USA

Brian C Joves MD
Interventional Physiatry and Pain
Management
Spine and Nerve Diagnostic Center
Sacramento, CA, USA

Brian S McClure DO
Fellow
Department of Anesthesiology and
Pain Management
Texas Tech University Health Sciences
Center
Lubbock, TX, USA

Brian T Boies MD
Clinical Assistant Professor
Department of Anesthesiology
UT Health San Antonio
San Antonio, TX, USA

Brittany Bickelhaupt MD
Department of Rehabilitation
UT Health San Antonio
San Antonio, TX, USA

Cameron T Nick MD
Capt, MC, USAF
CA-2, SAUSHEC Anesthesiology
San Antonio, TX, USA

Carlos A Pino MD
Associate Professor
Department of Anesthesiology and
Center for Pain Medicine
University of Vermont College of
Medicine
Burlington, VT, USA

Casey M Meizinger MD
Resident Physician
Department of Physical Medicine and
Rehabilitation
Stanford University
Palo Alto, CA, USA

Charles A Odonkor MD MA
Resident Fellow Council Chair
Association of Academic Physiatrists
(AAP)
Resident Physician
Department of Physical Medicine and
Rehabilitation
The Johns Hopkins University School of
Medicine
Baltimore, MD, USA

Charles E Bryant MD
Major, Medical Corps, US Army
Anesthesiologist (60N)/
Interventional Pain Management
Carl R Darnall Army Medical Center
Fort Hood, TX, USA

Christopher Warner MD
Clinical Radiology of Oklahoma
Spine Fracture Institute
Edmond, OK, USA

Christina C Moore MD
Resident Physician
Department of Anesthesia and Critical
Care
University of Chicago
Chicago, IL, USA

Christina Nguyen DO MS
Department of Physical Medicine and
Rehabilitation
UT Health San Antonio
San Antonio, TX, USA

Cindy A McGeary PhD ABPP
Assistant Professor
Department of Psychiatry
UT Health San Antonio
San Antonio, TX, USA

Clayton W Adams MD
Department of Anesthesiology and
Pain Medicine
Texas Tech University Health Sciences
Center
Lubbock, TX, USA

Clinton M Thome MD
Anesthesiology/Pain Medicine
Idaho Pain Clinic
Sandpoint, ID, USA

Craig DiTommaso MD
Medical Director of Inpatient
Rehabilitation
Department of Physical Medicine and
Rehabilitation
Baylor College of Medicine
Houston, TX, USA

Daniel Levin MD
Resident
Department of Anesthesia and Critical
Care
University of Chicago Medical Center
Chicago, IL, USA

Daniel T Jones MD
Anesthesiologist
Community Anesthesia Associates
Indianapolis, IN, USA

David J Kennedy MD
Clinical Associate Professor
Division of Physical Medicine and
Rehabilitation
Department of Orthopedics
Stanford University
Palo Alto, CA, USA

Dean H Hommer MD
Assistant Professor
Department of Physical Medicine and
Rehabilitation
Uniformed Services University of the
Health Sciences
Bethesda, MD, USA

Deena R Liles MD
Associate Professor
Department of Anesthesiology
University of Texas Health
Science Center
San Antonio, TX, USA

Donald D McGeary PhD ABPP
Associate Professor
Department of Psychiatry
University of Texas Health
Science Center
San Antonio, TX, USA

Douglas P Beall MD
Clinical Radiology of Oklahoma
Spine Fracture Institute
Edmond, OK, USA

Edward M Lopez Jr MD
Assistant Professor
Department of Anesthesiology
Uniformed Services University of the
Health Sciences
Fort Sam Houston, TX, USA

Edward K Pang DO
Attending Physician
Department of Physical Medicine and
Rehabilitation
UCLA/VA Greater Los Angeles
Healthcare System
Los Angeles, CA, USA

Emily Davies PharmD CPE
Clinical Pharmacy Specialist—Pain and
Palliative Medicine
Department of Pain Management
San Antonio Military Medical Center
Fort Sam Houston, TX, USA

Enrique Galang MD
Assistant Professor
Department of Physical Medicine and
Rehabilitation
UNC Spine Center
University of North Carolina
Chapel Hill, NC, USA

Eric Leung MD
Assistant Professor
Department of Physical Medicine and
Rehabilitation
Hofstra Northwell School of Medicine
Long Island, NY, USA

Esther M Benedetti MD FIPP
Associate Clinical Professor
Department of Anesthesia
University of Miami
Miami, FL, USA

George C Chang Chien DO
Medical Director of Pain Management
Ventura County Medical Center
Ventura, CA, USA

George Kum-Nji MD FAAPM&R
Major, Medical Corps, US Army
Department of Pain Management
Brooke Army Medical Center (BAMC)
San Antonio, TX, USA

Golnaz Nouri DO
Physical Medicine and Rehabilitation
PGY3 Resident
UT Health San Antonio
San Antonio, TX, USA

Gregory P Kraus MD
Assistant Professor
Department of Anesthesia
Uniformed Services University of the
Health Sciences
Bethesda, MD, USA

Houman Khakpour MD
Assistant Professor
Department of Medicine, Division of
Cardiology
University of California
Los Angeles, CA, USA

Huzefa S Talib BDS FFDRCSI FICOI
DICOI
Clinical Assistant Professor
Department of Oral and Maxillofacial
Surgery
New York University
New York, NY, USA

Jaclyn H Bonder MD
Assistant Professor
Weill Cornell Medical College
New York City, NY, USA

Jacob E Fehl MD
Academic Chief Resident
Department of Physical Medicine and
Rehabilitation
UT Health San Antonio
San Antonio, TX, USA

James McKenny MD MBA
Resident PGY-4
Department of Anesthesiology
UT Health San Antonio
San Antonio, TX, USA

James D Wirthlin MD
Flight Surgeon
Department of Flight and Operational
Medicine
Mountain Home Air Force Base
Hospital
Mountain Home AFB, ID, USA

James Wolf MD
Clinical Instructor
Department of Anesthesiology
University of Vermont Medical Center
Burlington, VT, USA

Jason Chen DO MS
Assistant Professor
Department of Physical Medicine and
Rehabilitation
McGovern Medical School at UT
Health, University of Texas Health
Science Center
Houston, TX, USA

Jennifer J Bartlett DO
Anesthesiology Resident
Department of Anesthesia
Naval Medical Center Portsmouth
Portsmouth, VA, USA

Jeremy R Jones MD
Assistant Professor
Department of Anesthesiology and
Pain Management
Texas Tech University
Health Science Center
Lubbock, TX, USA

John P McCallin MD FAAPMR
Major, Medical Corps, US Army
Chief, Physical Medicine and
Rehabilitation Service
Medical Director, Functional
Restoration Program
Department of Pain Management
San Antonio Military Medical Center
Assistant Professor
Department of Physical Medicine and
Rehabilitation
Uniformed Services University of the
Health Sciences
San Antonio, TX, USA

Jonathan A Benfield DO
Resident
Department of Rehabilitative Medicine
University of Texas Health Science
Center San Antonio
San Antonio, TX, USA

Joseph G William DO MPH
Physical Medicine and Rehabilitation
The University of Texas at Austin
Dell Medical School
Austin, TX, USA

Joshua E Levin MD
Clinical Assistant Professor
Division of Physical Medicine and
Rehabilitation
Department of Orthopedics
Stanford University
Palo Alto, CA, USA

Justin Averna DO
Resident Physician
Department of Physical Medicine and
Rehabilitation
Temple University Hospital
Philadelphia, PA, USA

Karina J Bouffard MD
MPH Attending Physician
Department of Pain Medicine
Rehabilitation Institute of Chicago
Chicago, IL, USA

Karl Lautenschlager MD
Major, Medical Corps, US Army
Anesthesiologist and Pain Management
Specialist
Medical Director
Interventional Pain
Management Center
San Antonio Military Medical Center
San Antonio, TX, USA

Katherine M Slogic MD
Clinical Fellow—Pediatric Anesthesia
Department of Anesthesiology
Boston Children's Hospital
Boston, MA, USA

Katrina M von Kriegenbergh MD
Pain Medicine Fellow
Department of Anesthesiology
Texas Tech University Health Sciences
Center
Lubbock, TX, USA

Kenneth D Candido MD
Professor of Clinical Anesthesiology-
University of Illinois
Clinical Professor of Surgery-University
of Illinosis
Chairman
Department of Anesthesiology
Advocate Illinois Masonic Medical
Center
Chicago, IL, USA

Kenneth J Naylor MD
Anesthesia Pain Medicine Fellow
Physical Medicine and Rehabilitation
Northwestern University, Feinberg
School of Medicine
Evanston, IL, USA

Kevin B Guthmiller MD
Major(P), Medical Corps, US Army
Department of Pain Management
Brooke Army Medical Center (BAMC)
Associate Program Director
Pain Medicine Fellowship
Assistant Professor of Anesthesiology
Uniformed Services University
San Antonio, TX, USA

Kristen S Wells MD
Department of Anesthesiology
UT Health Science Center San Antonio
San Antonio, TX, USA

Kun Zhang MD PhD
Instructor
Department of Anesthesiology
UT Health San Antonio
San Antonio, TX, USA

Larry C Driver MD
Professor
Department of Pain Medicine
Division of Anesthesiology and
Critical Care
The University of Texas
MD Anderson Cancer Center
Houston, TX, USA

Lisa Huynh MD
Clinical Assistant Professor
Physical Medicine and Rehabilitation
Department of Orthopedics
Stanford University
Redwood City, CA, USA

Magdalena Anitescu MD PhD
Associate Professor
Chief, Section of Pain Management
Director, Pain Medicine Fellowship
Program
Department of Anesthesia and
Critical Care
University of Chicago Medicine
Chicago, IL, USA

Maged M Mina MD
Adjunct Assistant Professor
Department of Anesthesiology
UT Health San Antonio
San Antonio, TX, USA

Manuel F Mas MD
Assistant Professor
Department of Physical Medicine and
Rehabilitation
The University of Texas
Health Science Center
McGovern Medical School
Houston, TX, USA

Marcy Rosen MD FACOG
Attending Physician
Northeast OB/GYN
San Antonio, TX, USA

Margaux M Salas PhD
Pain Neuroscientist
Department of Pain Management
Brooke Army Medical Center
JBSA Fort Sam Houston, TX, USA

Marina Mina BS
Student
San Antonio, TX, USA

Mary Caldwell DO
Resident Physician
Department of Physical Medicine and
Rehabilitation
Northwestern University Feinberg
School of Medicine
Chicago, IL, USA

Maunak V Rana MD
Associate Professor
Department of Anesthesiology
University of Chicago Medical Center
Chicago, IL, USA

Maxim S Eckmann MD
Director, Anesthesiology Pain Medicine
Program Director
Pain Medicine Fellowship
Associate Professor
Department of Anesthesiology
UT Health San Antonio
San Antonio, TX, USA

Michael C Bowman DO
Resident
Department of Anesthesiology
UT Health San Antonio
San Antonio, TX, USA

Michael Fredericson MD
Professor
Department of Orthopedic Surgery
Pain Medicine and Rehabilitation
Stanford University
Redwood City, CA, USA

Michael Saulino MD PhD
Assistant Professor
Department of Rehabilitation Medicine
Thomas Jefferson University
Philadelphia, PA, USA

Miles Day MD DABA FIPP DABIPP
Traweek-Racz Endowed Professor in
Pain Research
Medical Director, The Pain Center at
Grace Clinic
Pain Medicine Fellowship Director
Texas Tech University HSC
Lubbock, TX, USA

Mohammad A Issa MD
Resident Physician
Department of Physical Medicine and
Rehabilitation
Baylor College of Medicine
Houston, TX, USA

Monica Verduzco-Gutierrez MD
Assistant Professor
Department of Physical Medicine and
Rehabilitation
University of Texas
Health Science Center
Houston, TX, USA

Monika Y Patel MD
Assistant Professor
Department of Anesthesiology
Division of Pain Medicine
University of Florida
Jacksonville, FL, USA

Nicolas Rios MD
Resident
Department of Anesthesiology
UT Health San Antonio
San Antonio, TX, USA

Nikola Dragojlovic DO
Brain Injury Medicine Fellow
Department of Physical Medicine and
Rehabilitation
University of Texas
Health Science Center
Houston, TX, USA

Paolo C Mimbella MD MSc
Academic Chief Resident
Department of Physical Medicine and
Rehabilitation
University of Texas
Houston, TX, USA

Paul E Hilliard MD
Assistant Professor
Department of Anesthesiology
University of Michigan
Ann Arbor, MI, USA

Peggy Y Kim MD MS MBA
Assistant Professor
Department of Anesthesiology
University of Wisconsin Madison
Madison, WI, USA

Ram D Phull DDS
Clinical Assistant Professor
Department of Oral Pathology
Radiology and Oral Medicine and
Orofacial Pain
New York University College of
Dentistry
Director
TMD Clinic
Hospital of Joint Diseases
New York City, NY, USA

Ratan Banik MD PhD
Assistant Professor
Department of Anesthesiology
University of Minnesota
Minneapolis, MN, USA

Ratna Bhavaraju-Sanka MD
Assistant Professor
Department of Neurology
UT Health San Antonio
San Antonio, TX, USA

Rebecca Ovsiowitz MD
Assistant Clinical Professor of Medicine
UCLA
Department of Medicine/Physical
Medicine and Rehabilitation
University California Los Angeles/WLA
VAMC
Los Angeles, CA, USA

Richard S Thorsted MD
Anesthesiology Resident
Department of Anesthesiology
SAUSHEC Anesthesia Program
Fort Sam Houston, TX, USA

Rituparna Das MD
Assistant Professor
Department of Neurology
Baylor College of Medicine
Houston, TX, USA

Rudy Garza III MD
Assistant Professor
Department of Anesthesiology
UT Health San Antonio
San Antonio, TX, USA

Sameer Soliman MD
Faculty
Department of Anesthesiology
UT Health San Antonio
San Antonio, TX, USA

Samir Patel DO
Assistant Professor/Clinical
Department of Anesthesiology/Pain
Medicine
UT Health San Antonio
San Antonio, TX, USA

Sanjog S Pangarkar MD
Associate Clinical Professor
Department of Medicine
University of California
Los Angeles, CA, USA

Sarah Eisen Ellis MD
Pain Management of Middle Tennessee
Clarksville, TN, USA

Sarah Hwang MD
Assistant Professor of Clinical Physical
Medicine and Rehabilitation
Department of Physical Medicine and
Rehabilitation
University of Missouri
Columbia, MO, USA

Sergio Souza MD
Department of Pain Management
San Antonio Military Medical Center
(SAMMC)
Fort Sam Houston, TX, USA

Shaan Sudhakaran MD
Anesthesiology Resident
Department of Anesthesia and
Critical Care
University of Chicago
Chicago, IL, USA

Shiraz Yazdani MD
Pain Medicine Physician
Lubbock Spine Institute
Lubbock, TX, USA

Shuchita Garg MD
Clinical Assistant Professor
Department of Anesthesia and Chronic
Pain
University of Cincinnati
Cincinnati, OH, USA

Siddarth Thakur MD
Fellow and Instructor—Research
Faculty
Department of Pain Medicine
The University of Texas MD Anderson
Cancer Center
Houston, TX, USA

Siddharth S Arora DO MS
Resident Physician
Neurological Institute and Department
of Pain Management
Cleveland Clinic
Cleveland, OH, USA

Somayaji Ramamurthy MD
Professor (Retired)
Department of Anesthesiology
UT Health San Antonio
San Antonio, TX, USA

Steven J Durning MD
Anesthesiology Resident
Department of Anesthesia
San Antonio Military Medical Center
Fort Sam Houston, TX, USA

Steven M Prust MD
Department of Anesthesiology
UT Health San Antonio
San Antonio, TX, USA

**Tejinder Singh Swaran
Singh** MBBS MD FRCA
Clinical Assistant Professor
Department of Anesthesia and Pain
Medicine
University of Iowa Hospitals and
Clinics
Iowa City, IA, USA

Teresa M Kusper DO MBS
Resident Physician
Department of Anesthesiology
Advocate Illinois Masonic Medical
Center
Chicago, IL, USA

Thomas Chai MD
Assistant Professor
Department of Pain Medicine
University of Texas MD Anderson
Cancer Center
Houston, TX, USA

Thomas L Spain JR MD MPH
Associate Professor
Department of Anesthesiology and
Pain Management
The University of Texas Southwestern
Medical Center
Dallas, TX, USA

Trevor V Walker MD
Resident Instructor
Department of Anesthesiology
Texas Tech Health Sciences Center
Lubbock, TX, USA

Tristan T Lai MD
Assistant Professor
Department of Anesthesia
Uniformed Services University of the
Health Sciences
Bethesda, MD, USA

Troy J Bushman DO
Resident Physician
Department of Physical Medicine and
Rehabilitation
University of Utah
Salt Lake City, UT, USA

Tyler C Roe DO
Resident
Department of Anesthesiology
UT Health San Antonio
San Antonio, TX, USA

Veena Graff MD MS
Assistant Professor
Department of Anesthesiology and
Critical Care
University of Pennsylvania Perelman
School of Medicine
Philadelphia, PA, USA

Viktor Bartanusz MD
Associate Professor
Department of Clinical Neuroscience
Centre Hospitalier Universitaire
Vaudois, Lausanne, Switzerland

William J Kroski DO
Staff Physician
Department of Rehabilitation
Walter Reed National Military
Medical Center
Bethesda, MD, USA

The inspiration for the 3rd edition of this innovative and essential reference work on pain management is Professor Somayaji Ramamurthy, who was my mentor and role model in pain, and who, like me, had his beginnings under the watchful eye of Professor Alon P Winnie at the Cook County Hospital in Chicago. Rama, as Dr Winnie would call him, completed one of the very first pain fellowships in the United States in 1971, long before the American Board of Medical Specialties even recognized the value of pain management fellowships and prior to any formal designation by the American Board of Anesthesiology to certify these pioneer aficionados who were intent on dedicating their lives to the eradication of pain. Rama remained alongside Dr Winnie until 1977 and became an Associate Professor of Anesthesiology at the University of Illinois Hospital when Alon P Winnie was named Chair of the Department. Together they formed a dynamic duo whose collaborations were among the most important in American pain medicine and whose influence extended far beyond the generations of pain fellows each respectively trained. Dr Winnie would routinely state that Ramamurthy was the brightest star, I have ever been affiliated with and his departure (to Texas) was the greatest loss, I have ever had to experience in my professional life. Together they authored 17 original peer-reviewed manuscripts, many of which are considered world anesthesia and pain management classics even now, some 45 years after publication. For example, they were the first to describe the use of a pneumatic tourniquet for intravenous regional anesthesia (Bier Block), the first to describe the use of glycopyrrolate as a substitute for atropine, the first to describe intradural and extradural corticosteroid use for managing sciatic nerve pain, the first to describe an anterior lumbar plexus technique (3-in-1 block) for lower extremity surgery, the first to describe a cervical plexus block using a single-injection technique, the first to use doxapram to reverse acute respiratory depression in the operating room, and the first to publish the clinical effectiveness of ropivacaine for brachial plexus blocks, among many other unique contributions. Indeed, the world of regional anesthesia and acute and chronic pain management were forever changed by these two juggernauts.

Rama would go on to create a dynamic Division of Pain Medicine at the University of Texas Health Science Center at San Antonio, where his imprint was felt over four decades as the Medical Director and Program Director. Rama worked tirelessly to author close to 90 total peer-refereed journal articles and editorials, nine textbooks, almost 80 textbook chapters, and to provide numerous original continuing medical education seminars and lectures worldwide. His contributions are legendary, and just as importantly, he trained dozens of physician champions who have carried forth his message and who preached his many indispensable lessons to current generations of pain practitioners. Several of these champions, including Drs Maxim S Eckmann, Brian T Boies, and Ameet Nagpal, continue his legacy and are among the major editors and contributors of this most recent iteration of the decision making textbook. As is often the case in major reference works such as this, a collaboration among noted authorities is a fundamental key to success. In that regard, the additions of other contributing editors Drs Miles Day and Larry C Driver provide an essential element from other great Texas programs to make this truly a work of diverse thinkers and leaders in pain decision making. And, just as the influence of Professor Ramamurthy has been a key factor in the evolution of the San Antonio contributors, Professor Gabor B Racz has been a mentor to Dr Miles Day, as Professor Philip R Bromage has been to Dr Larry C Driver. So, this reference work is in reality a culmination of some of the world's greatest pioneers in pain management, either by proxy or else as a first-generation work of science.

We, the readers of this work, are truly privileged to be possessors of this insightful, thoughtful, and creative project. The imprint of Dr Ramamurthy, the great visionary of the original concept, is unmistakable. Dr Thomas Edell, a former trainee of Rama, who retired about four years before him, summarized Dr Ramamurthy's influence, perhaps the most coherently in his own retirement speech:

"If the world was filled with pain physicians like Dr Ramamurthy, pain would become a nearly extinct disease like polio."

Though a lofty vision, Dr Ramamurthy did embody the best in ethical treatment and endless pursuit of knowledge.

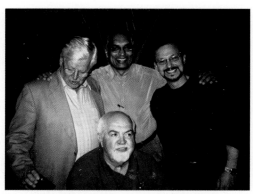

Professor Ramamurthy surrounded by, from left-to-right, Dr Gabor B Racz,
Dr Kenneth D Candido, Professor Alon P Winnie

Dr Ramamurthy, however, was very humble in his own assessment of his career. He has often stated that he did not achieve very much and expressed disappointment that he did not achieve more. Nothing could be further from the truth, and while his humility is genuine and refreshing, it falls far short of describing an icon in the world of pain management, a man who walked among giants but whose own footprints matched theirs in every possible way. This work is a testimonial to his ongoing influence in the domains of pain management and the critical role that decision making plays in first doing no harm, while secondly doing the most good.

Kenneth D Candido MD
Professor of Clinical Anesthesiology-UIC
Clinical Professor of Surgery-UIC
Chairman
Department of Anesthesiology
Advocate Illinois Masonic Medical Center
Chicago, IL, USA

PREFACE

Many clinicians, especially pain medicine physicians, have reiterated the usefulness of the algorithmic approach to the evaluation and treatment of pain which was outlined in the first two editions of *Decision Making in Pain Management: An Algorithmic Approach*.

There have been great advances in the concepts, approaches, treatment options, and technology in pain medicine, which necessitate significant revision in order to make the book more relevant to the present-day practitioner.

This book is not meant to replace in-depth, highly referenced textbooks in pain medicine. It may, nevertheless, be a valuable supplement, providing pain clinicians with a logical, concise, stepwise approach to the identification, diagnosis, and management of various acute or chronic pain conditions or syndromes.

I have maintained the multidisciplinary approach with input from various specialists. Many chapters have been added to reflect the advances in pain medicine. Specifically, novel procedures such as vertebral augmentation and regenerative medicine techniques have been addressed. As well, I have attempted to attend to the growing concern regarding the international opioid epidemic by adding an entire section on the use of opioids to our work. In areas of controversy, the chapters may reflect the preferences of the individual author.

I would like to thank all of the contributors for bringing a multidisciplinary approach, and thus making this book unique. My special thanks to Dr Nagpal for his tireless efforts as the corresponding editor.

I would like to thank Joe Rusko, Bridget Meyer, Nedup Denka, and Angima Shree for their assistance in the completion of this book and for their tireless efforts on behalf of M/s Jaypee Brothers Medical Publishers (P) Ltd, New Delhi, India. In regards to my particular institution, I would like to thank the Chairman, Department of Anesthesiology, University of Texas Health Science Center, Texas, USA, Dr Andrews, for his commitment to our success. We also want to thank Betsy Turner for her dedication to this project.

I must also thank Drs Maxim S Eckmann, Brian T Boies, Miles Day, and Larry C Driver, for their editorial contributions. Finally, I must thank Misty Blaze, our Editorial Assistant, for her incredible and often times Herculean efforts to make sure that the manuscripts were completed and edited to the best of everyone's abilities and for her editorial prowess.

Somayaji Ramamurthy

ACKNOWLEDGMENTS

We would like to thank the editorial team at M/s Jaypee Brothers Medical Publishers (P) Ltd, New Delhi, India (Joe Rusko, Bridget Meyer and Angima Shree), for their assistance in the completion of this book and for their tireless efforts on behalf of M/s Jaypee Brothers Medical Publishers (P) Ltd, New Delhi, India. We also want to thank Betsy Turner for her dedication to this project.

Finally and perhaps most importantly, we must thank Misty Blaze, our Editorial Assistant. Her incredible work is the sole reason that the book was able to be completed. Her tireless efforts at wrangling contributor agreements, editing first submissions, first proofs, second proofs, and sometimes even third proofs, were invaluable and immeasurable. There is no amount of words that can express our gratitude for her dedication to our project.

ACKNOWLEDGMENTS

CONTENTS

SECTION 1   Evaluation
Maxim S Eckmann

SECTION **2** Acute Pain

Maxim S Eckmann

SECTION **3** Chronic Pain Syndromes

Brian T Boies

SECTION 4 Cancer Pain

Brian T Boies

SECTION 5 Head and Neck Pain

Ameet Nagpal

SECTION **6**

Thoracic Pain

Larry C Driver

SECTION **7**

Low Back Pain

Ameet Nagpal

SECTION **8** # Upper Extremity Pain
Miles Day

SECTION **9** # Lower Extremity Pain
Miles Day

SECTION **10** # Pediatric Pain
Miles Day

SECTION **11** # Pharmacology
Ameet Nagpal

SECTION **12** # Opioid Pharmacology
Larry C Driver

SECTION **13** Noninterventional Therapeutic Modalities

Miles Day

SECTION **14** Interventional Therapeutic Modalities

Larry C Driver

SECTION **15** **Other Topics**

Brian T Boies

SECTION 1

Evaluation

Maxim S Eckmann

CHAPTER 1

Initial Management of Acute Pain

Wallisch BJ, Bowman MC

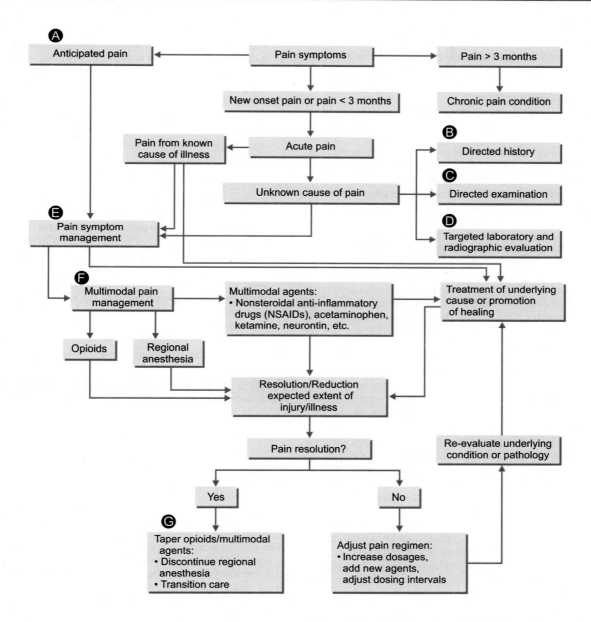

Pain is defined as an unpleasant sensory and emotional experience arising from actual or potential tissue damage or described in terms of such damage. Acute pain lasts less than 3 months and is typically associated with the normal, predicted physiologic response to an adverse chemical, thermal, or mechanical stimulus. Acute pain is usually the result of surgery, trauma, or acute illness and is expected to resolve as part of the normal healing process. Adequate identifica-

tion and treatment of the underlying insult will help alleviate acute pain. Moreover, prompt treatment of acute pain and pain generators can decrease the risks of complications, decrease hospital length of stay, increase patient satisfaction and potentially stop the development of a chronic pain condition.

A *Anticipation:* Patients are at risk of developing difficult to control acute pain if they are undergoing a known invasive or painful procedure, have a prior history of poorly controlled acute pain, are on opioids or other medications for a pre-existing pain condition, or have a coexisting substance abuse disorder. Moreover, failure to recognize and plan for those who are at most risk for developing acute pain can lead to untreated or undertreated acute pain and all its negative consequences. After identifying those at risk for acute pain, you can establish a plan for baseline pain management as well as a plan for breakthrough pain management. Pain management plans should match the expected duration and intensity of the pain as well as appropriate tapering of therapy that follows the anticipated dissipation of symptoms. While controversial, pre-emptive analgesia with regional analgesia has been shown to decrease intraoperative opioid use which can act to decrease central pain sensitization and the development of chronic pain.

B *History*: A detailed pain history should be elicited as well as past experiences with different classes of pain medications. Sensitivity or "allergy" to opioids demands a detailed understanding as cross sensitivity and differences in patient metabolism may have significant implications on treatment effectiveness. Every effort should be made to quantify the degree and severity of pain on a standardized scale, such as visual analog scale (VAS), numeric rating scale (NRS), or Wong-Baker FACES scale. They can help establish pre-existing pain, baseline pain, be used as a trigger for escalating pain therapy, and be used to help establish treatment goals. In the patients who cannot communicate, the clinician should be vigilant for sources of painful insults in combination with nonverbal and physiologic cues. The character, quality, alleviating and aggravating factors and course of the acute pain compliant should be carefully considered during the history and examination. Neuropathic versus nociceptive and somatic versus visceral pain can often be differentiated; these features can guide management.

C *Examination*: A focused physical examination can help establish referred pain versus a localized source. Radiating pain or pain in a specific dermatome suggests the need for examination of the central nervous system. Examination may reveal dynamic pain versus static pain and may guide the utility of pharmacologic agents or prompt the need of a specific intervention. Structural pain, such as musculoskeletal pain, may be recreated with specific movements or maneuvers while the specific locations and responses to degree of stimulation may be more nuanced with abdominal or other visceral pain. Exquisite pain stimulation on examination may help establish an unexpected infection or source of inflammation.

D *Tests*: Laboratory tests and radiographic studies may be needed when the diagnosis is unknown or when there is uncertainty about severity of pathology. Radiographic studies may also be useful to guide therapy, for example, in spine-related pain. Clinical correlation must ultimately guide therapy as there are high numbers of radiographically significant abnormalities that are not the actual source of a patient's pain.

E *Treatment*: Treatment should be aimed at both pain symptom alleviation and targeting of the underlying condition. Whenever possible, multimodal analgesia—the use of two or more analgesic medications—should be employed so as to treat multiple pain receptors and decrease the side effects of a single medication. Multimodal analgesia may provide pharmacologic synergy and allow for reduced doses of individual agents.

F *Multimodal Analgesia:* Multimodal analgesia regimens can include opioids, nonsteroidal anti-inflammatory drugs (NSAIDs), acetaminophen, N-methyl-D-aspartic acid (NMDA) agonists and antineuropathic agents (e.g. gabapentin/pregabalin). Opioids are typically employed as part of a balanced pain regimen for moderate to severe pain. While opioids can be effective for short-term noncancer pain relief, it is incumbent on the provider to initiate a risk mitigation strategy at the initiation of treatment with the goal of directed opioid tapering. Opioids may be delivered as per os (PO) interval regimens, nurse delivered intravenous (IV) regimens or IV patient controlled regimens. No matter the route of delivery, careful attention must be directed to side effects such as respiratory depression, constipation, and somnolence. When appropriate, regional techniques including single shot and continuous peripheral nerve blocks, epidural catheters, and other direct anesthetic delivery methods can reduce opioid consumption and improve recovery times.

G *Resolution:* As the underlying injury or illness resolves, so should the patient's acute pain symptoms. Tapering of medications and discontinuation of regional anesthesia should follow with the reduction symptoms with the goal to return patient to his or her baseline. If pain symptoms persist beyond the expected time period of the underlying pathology (especially > 3 months) or if the reported pain is higher than expected, the patient should be re-evaluated for a new problem or possible development of a chronic pain syndrome. Escalation of medication doses and addition of other agents should occur within the framework of a planned de-escalation in a transitional care model that optimizes continuity of care.

SUGGESTED READING

American Society of Anesthesiologists Task Force on Acute Pain Management. Practice guidelines for acute pain management in the perioperative setting: an updated report by the American Society of Anesthesiologists Task Force on Acute Pain Management. Anesthesiology. 2012;116(2):248-73.

Carr DB, Goudas LC. Acute pain. Lancet. 1999;353:2051-8.

Herr K, Spratt KF, Garand L, et al. Evaluation of the Iowa pain thermometer and other selected pain intensity scales in younger and older adult cohorts using controlled clinical pain: a preliminary study. Pain Med. 2007;8:585-600.

Joshi GP, Ogunnaike BO. Consequences of inadequate postoperative pain relief and chronic persistent postoperative pain. Anesthesiol Clin North America. 2005;23:21-36.

Katz J, Weinrib A, Fashler SR, et al. The Toronto General Hospital Transitional Pain Service: development and implementation of a multidisciplinary program to prevent chronic postsurgical pain. J Pain Res. 2015;8:695-702.

Nett MP. Postoperative pain management. Orthopedics. 2010;33(9 Suppl):23-6.

Richebé P, Rivat C, Liu SS. Perioperative or postoperative nerve block for preventive analgesia: should we care about the timing of our regional anesthesia? Anesth Analg. 2013;116(5):969-70.

Roth W, Kling J, Gockel I, et al. Dissatisfaction with post-operative pain management—a prospective analysis of 1071 patients. Acute Pain. 2005;7:75-83.

CHAPTER 2

Evaluation of the Chronic Pain Patient

Guthmiller KB, Bryant CE, Fehl JE

Initial Screening Evaluation
- Review pertinent past medical history, social history, current medications, allergies, prior treatments or therapies
- Review any available diagnostics tests [imaging, electromyography (EMG)/nerve conduction studies, etc.] and lab results
- Pain/functional/mood disorder scales and risk assessment scales if indicated

History
- OPQRST
- Medications, smoking
- Comorbid psychological history
- Medical history
- History of illicit substances
- Disability/Litigation

Physical Examination
- Appearance/Inspection/Gait
- Focused neurological examination
- Focused musculoskeletal examination
- Provocative maneuvers vs nonorganic symptoms

Imaging and Diagnostic Tests
- *Bony abnormality*: X-ray/computed tomography (CT)
- EMG for suspected neuropathy
- *Inflammation:* Contrast magnetic resonance imaging (MRI)/Scintigraphy
- MRI for disk/soft tissue

Laboratory Testing
- Complete blood count (CBC)
- Metabolic profile
- Urine drug testing
- Coagulation profile
- Erythrocyte sedimentation rate (ESR)/C-reactive protein (CRP)
- Electrocardiography (ECG)

Specialist Pharmacological Evaluation
- Consider consult with clinical pharmacist if concern for polypharmacy or if patient already on chronic opioid therapy
- Coordination of anti-thrombotic therapy bridging with hematologist or cardiologist in planning of interventions

Specialist Psychological Evaluation
- Refer to pain psychology/behavioral health if significant psychosocial stressors present
- Utilize preprocedure psychological evaluation to assess outcome potential
- Employ concurrent cognitive behavioral therapy if indicated
- Concurrent psychiatric pharmacotherapy if indicated

Comprehensive Multidisciplinary Model
- Emphasize active (not passive) treatment modalities
- Refer patient to physical therapy (PT) if inadequate initial trial and encourage exercise program
- Consider nutrition consult or smoking cessation if appropriate
- Consider other adjunctive treatments such as chiropractor, acupuncture, or massage
- Emphasize role is to improve function
- Utilize diagnostic procedures if it will change management
- Targeted interventional therapy for subacute pain conditions of spine, joints, muscles, nerves or as analgesia to augment PT and exercise

The initial evaluation of the chronic pain patient is challenging when executed in comprehensive fashion, as there are frequently strong accompanying behavioral, emotional, social, and cognitive components. Such knowledge is conducive to a focused conversation and will instill confidence in the patient that the provider is prepared and competent. Reviewing (and scoring) intake screening forms should precede the history and physical examination. This integration of information from several sources will help the evaluating provider begin to develop an accurate diagnosis and tailored treatment plan that may include nonpharmacologic, pharmacologic, or interventional pain therapy.

A *Initial Screening Evaluation:* Prior to the appointment, the provider should review the patient's medical records, including any imaging, laboratory results, diagnostic tests, current and prior medications, procedures/surgeries performed, and adjunctive treatment modalities attempted and to what degree. Scales and questionnaires may facilitate the patient's description of their pain and give the healthcare provider further insight into the patient's experience. Several validated patient self-assessment tools exist. Some scales such as the Defense and Veterans Pain Rating Scale (DVPRS; recently validated in a 2015 study by Nassif, et al.) inquire about the impact pain has on a patient's activity, sleep, mood, and stress. Intake forms may also ask patients to outline any prior treatments or therapies for their pain, as well as current or previous pharmacologic management. It is worth noting that patients who use greater than 50 mg oral morphine equivalents (OMEs) daily may be at increased risk for adverse medication events. The American Society of Interventional Pain Physicians (ASIPP) published Opioid Guidelines in 2012 and described the Screener and Opioid Assessment for Patients with Pain-Revised (SOAPP-R) as having a reasonably high-quality deviation which may be used in conjunction with clinical assessment, and suggested in general that opioid assessment screening tools be used jointly with other measures to guide and monitor therapy. The Opioid Risk Tool (ORT) is another such tool that attempts to risk-stratify patients for opioid abuse. The Brief Pain Inventory (BPI; available online) and BPI-sf (short form; available online) are used to evaluate pain severity and impact on daily functioning. The SF-36 (short form-36 health survey; available online) is a widely utilized set of quality-of-life measures that span several domains and is administered to assess patient disability. Because the SF-36 can take several minutes, shorter variants (SF-12 and SF-8) are available. Screening for psychiatric issues, suicidal/homicidal ideations, sleep disturbances, substance abuse potential or history, and disability may clarify the patient's overall pain experience and allow the healthcare provider to recognize potential barriers to improvement.

B *History:* Listening carefully to the patient's description of their pain complaint(s) is essential in generating a differential diagnosis. The mnemonic OPQRST (**O**nset, **P**rovoking/palliative factors, **Q**uality/character, **R**egion/radiation, **S**everity/intensity, and **T**emporal nature)

is a helpful tool in this regard. Concerning quality/character, one should determine whether the patient's pain is nociceptive (somatic or visceral), inflammatory, neuropathic, or mixed in nature. In addition to the OPQRST, it is imperative to elucidate the total duration of pain, how it has evolved over time, and how it limits function. Further, one should explore the perception of suffering by the patient and seek to understand coexisting psychosocial, legal, or economic implications. If the pain is widespread or involves several muscles or joints, additional questioning to uncover a systemic rheumatologic or neurologic condition is reasonable. Ideally, good characterization of the patient's pain complaint(s) will allow the practitioner to better focus the upcoming physical examination as well as formulate a respectable differential diagnosis and treatment plan. Prescribed medications (with degree of compliance), allergies, tobacco and alcohol use, and history of illicit substances should be determined. Additionally, it is important to assess sleep quality, degree of physical activity, stimulant and supplement use, history of addiction, current or previous psychological/psychiatric treatment, occupation, education, family situation, and efficacy of current and previous treatments for the chronic pain condition. Nonorganic pain symptoms and behaviors, unusual family dynamics, and the presence of pending lawsuits or disability claims should prompt the evaluating provider to search for clues that may indicate the possibility of primary or secondary gain. A review of systems (ROS) screens for possible systemic illnesses that a patient may not immediately otherwise report.

C *Physical Examination:* The provider should complete a focused physical examination, which begins as soon as he or she walks into the patient's examination room. Appearance, mood, activity, and interaction with family members or other caregivers can give clues to pain behaviors. While talking with the patient, the provider should observe changes in the patient's positioning, as this may reveal patient discomfort or conversely, that the patient may be distracted from their pain. A basic physical examination includes a regional assessment of each area including visual inspection (atrophy, asymmetry, or other visible abnormalities), palpation of soft tissues and bony prominences, range of motion, and neurological evaluation (sensory, motor, reflexes, gait). Additionally, providers should familiarize themselves with special testing for each region. Provocative maneuvers must be carefully applied and interpreted for concordance without leading the patient. Throughout the performance of the physical examination, the healthcare provider should be vigilant in monitoring for findings that are inconsistent with the patient's history, other examination findings, imaging/diagnostic studies, or unacknowledged observations made by other providers or support staff, all of which may support a nonorganic pain origin.

D *Imaging and Other Diagnostic Tests:* Appropriate radiologic imaging can help correlate clinical pain symptoms to musculoskeletal or neurological pathology.

Plain radiographs can rule out fractures, tumors, hardware failure, or dynamic instability. Magnetic resonance imaging (MRI) may provide further information about soft tissue pathology. Computed tomography (CT) may be helpful in looking for fractures or in patients whom MRI is contraindicated. A nuclear medicine scan can identify areas of pathologic scintigraphic uptake consistent with reactive changes or inflammation. It is important to remember that imaging studies may reveal significant abnormalities in otherwise asymptomatic patients. Electromyography (EMG) and nerve conduction studies (NCS) can classify subacute to chronic nerve injuries but are usually unrevealing of specific pathology when symptoms are mild or intermittent and when physical examination findings are absent.

E *Laboratory Testing*: Laboratory tests may be indicated for a variety of reasons. First, when the history or physical examination suggests a rheumatologic or neurologic condition, a laboratory test may confirm or refute a working diagnosis. Second, as thrombocytopenia, coagulopathy, and poor renal or hepatic function are relative contraindications to many interventional procedures and medications, the evaluating provider may wish to screen with a complete blood count (CBC), renal function panel, and coagulation assay. Third, the presence of an infection or inflammatory condition will be noted with an elevated erythrocyte sedimentation rate (ESR), C-reactive protein (CRP), and/or CBC. Finally, some medications may warrant periodic laboratory monitoring. Urine drug testing (UDT) should arguably be the standard of care for patients who are receiving controlled substances, as the literature demonstrates that a discrepancy frequently exists between prescribed medications and medication regimen adherence. A UDT that can identify all medications prescribed to the patient (not just controlled or illicit substances) is especially useful to test for compliance, and an astute practitioner will very carefully determine when the patient last utilized each medication and compare it to the results of the UDT. Electrocardiography (EKG) may screen for conditions like prolonged QT syndrome for which some medications may be relatively contraindicated (e.g. methadone).

F *Specialist Pharmacological Evaluation:* Consultation with a clinical pharmacist may be particularly helpful in optimizing medical management in patients who are exposed to polypharmacy or who require close follow-up for any number of medication-related reasons.

G *Specialist Psychological Evaluation:* Chronic pain patients frequently harbor psychosocial factors that contribute negatively to pain behavior and serve as barriers to improvement. Patients may benefit from working closely with a behavioral health provider specializing in pain management. A pain psychologist can identify psychological aspects that underpin the patient's ongoing pain state, provide much-needed education, assess for and manage realistic expectations, gauge the need for referral to a psychiatrist, and teach several strategies for mitigating pain.

H *Comprehensive Multidisciplinary Model:* A multidisciplinary team is probably best suited to evaluate the complex chronic pain patient who has undergone several different treatment modalities with providers in various settings and still exhibits high pain scores, low function, and significant psychological distress. Although there are many ways to structure such a model, one paradigm involves having a new patient evaluated by several specialty providers (e.g. pain physician, psychologist, physical therapist, clinical pharmacist, and surgeon) in back-to-back appointments in a single day with subsequent discussion and consensus on a treatment plan. Physical therapy and home exercise plans reduce deconditioning, hypersensitivity, and fear-avoidance behavior. Interventional pain therapy, e.g. epidural steroid injections, may be indicated in the symptomatic management of subacute spine, joint, muscle, and peripheral nerve pain, or may be incorporated as an analgesic plan to reduce hypersensitivity in a comprehensive chronic pain management plan.

SUGGESTED READING

Bohnert AB, Valenstein M, Bair MJ, et al. Association between opioid prescribing patterns and opioid overdose-related deaths. JAMA. 2011;305(13):1315-21.

Borenstein DG, O'Mara JW Jr, Boden SD, et al. The value of magnetic resonance imaging of the lumbar spine to predict low-back pain in asymptomatic subjects: a seven-year follow-up study. J Bone Joint Surg Am. 2001;83-A(9):1306-11.

Edwards RR, Berde CB. Pain assessment. In: Benzon H, Fishman S, Raja S, Cohen S, Liu S (Eds). Essentials of Pain Medicine, 3rd edition. Philadelphia: Elsevier Saunders; 2011.

Fishman SM, Ballantyne JC, Rathmell JP. Bonica's Management of Pain, 4th edition. Philadelphia, PA: Lippincott Williams & Wilkins; 2010.

Manchikanti L, Abdi S, Atluri S, et al. American Society of Interventional Pain Physicians (ASIPP) guidelines for responsible opioid prescribing in chronic non-cancer pain: Part I – evidence assessment. Pain Physician. 2012;15:S1-65.

Nassif TH, Hull A, Holliday SB, et al. Concurrent validity of the Defense and Veterans Pain Rating Scale in VA outpatients. Pain Med. 2015;16(11):2152-61.

Urman RD, Vadivelu N. Pocket Pain Medicine. Philadelphia, PA: Lippincott Williams & Wilkins; 2011.

Warfield CA, Bajwa ZH. Principles and Practice of Pain Medicine, 2nd edition. New York, NY: McGraw-Hill; 2004.

Webster LR. The role of urine drug testing in chronic pain management: 2013 Update. [online] Available from *http://painmedicinenews.com/download/UDT_PMNSE2013_WM.pdf*. [Accessed January, 2017].

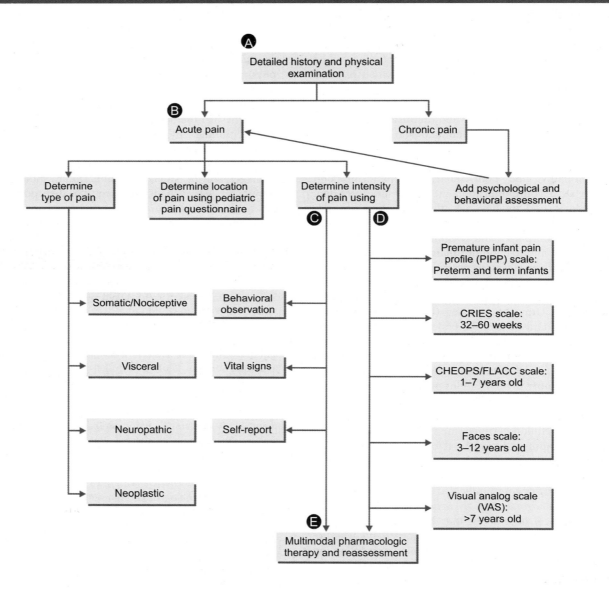

Evaluating pediatric pain is much more difficult to assess than that of an adult, leading to untreated or undertreated pain with negative effects on quality of life. This results in social, economic and emotional consequences for both the child and the parents. Pain can involve both peripheral and central pathways accompanied by emotional factors and could be (1) somatic, (2) visceral, (3) neuropathic, or (4) neoplastic. Pain perception starts around the third trimester with different perception related to the maturity of the central nervous system. Hence, exposure to pain in early stages of life

could be detrimental, leading to changes in the social and emotional aspects.

Ⓐ Clear documentation on the assessment of pain and the methodology used should be taken into consideration, along with cognitive abilities and psychosocial aspects of these children. Different methods are used with no gold standard. Evaluation of pain in children should be done routinely using appropriate pain assessment tools mostly done by the nursing staff in a hospital setting (who are usually first to address pain) followed by parents,

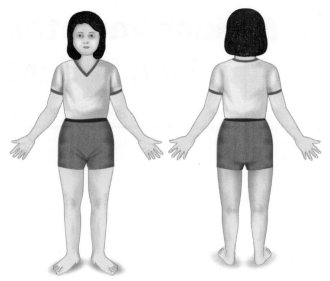

Fig. 1: Pediatric pain questionnaire

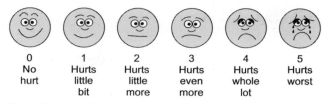

| 0 | 1 | 2 | 3 | 4 | 5 |
| No hurt | Hurts little bit | Hurts little more | Hurts even more | Hurts whole lot | Hurts worst |

Fig. 2: Faces scale

and then physicians. Adequate education on assessment tools, documentation of methods used, treatment options given, threshold of pain level to therapy given, and response to treatment and side effects should be documented with clear communications between all medical staff.

B Acute pain, including postprocedural and postoperative, should be assessed using appropriate tools routinely. However, chronic pediatric pain (with or without acute pain), mostly seen as outpatient, has a different scope of assessment. Identifying the location and type of the pain helps to determine etiology using a pediatric pain questionnaire **(Fig. 1)**, where the child can color the area of the body involved.

C There are three principal methods of assessing pain *intensity* in children:
1. *Behavioral/Observation*: The child is observed for a few minutes and a number is chosen that matches their behavior observing body language, facial expressions, and sleep-wake patterns, but needs additional sources, such as feedback from parents or caregivers to exclude other forms of stress such as hunger or anxiety.
2. *Biological measures*: Relies on vitals.
3. *Self-report*: Child can adequately express their pain which is the gold standard.

D For children who are unable to self-report, Behavioral and Biological scales can be used in conjunction with combined scales, like the Objective Pain Scale and the Comfort Scale used to assess procedural and post-operative pain.
1. *For preterm and term infants*: Premature infant pain profile (PIPP) is composed of seven indicators: gestational age, behavioral state before painful stimulus, change in heart rate during painful stimulus, change in oxygen saturations during painful stimulus, brow bulge during painful stimulus, eye squeeze during painful stimulus, and nasolabial furrow during painful stimulus.

2. *From 32 weeks to 60 weeks*: CRIES scale is an acronym for crying, requires oxygen, increased vital signs, expression, and sleep.
3. *From 2 months to 7 years*: FLACC scale is an acronym for face, legs, activity, cry, and consolability.
4. *From 1 year to 7 years*: The Children's Hospital of Eastern Ontario Pain Scale (CHEOPS) contains six parameters including cry, facial, verbal, torso, touch, and legs.
5. *From 3 years to 18 years of ages*:
   • *Simple descriptive scale*: Uses descriptive words to describe the intensity of the pain
   • *Numeric scale*: Uses a straight line from 0 to 10, with 0 being no pain and 10 being the worst pain, and the patients choose the number that best fits the intensity of their pain
   • *Faces scale (**Fig. 2**)*: Six faces with varying expressions ranging from happy to crying
   • *Poker chip scales*, where the child's pain is represented in the amount of poker chips used.
6. *Cognitively impaired children*: Noncommunicating child pain checklist—postoperative version is recommended.

E *Multimodal Therapy:* Once pain is assessed, the 2012 WHO guidelines recommend a two-step approach, where step one is mild pain treated with acetaminophen and nonsteroidal anti-inflammatory drugs (NSAIDs) followed by step two for moderate to severe pain requiring adding an opioid such as codeine or morphine. Adjuvant medications can be added at any step such as anticonvulsants. Pain should be assessed before, during, and after treatment using the same scale, so that there is a baseline threshold and a way to make sure the treatment is working. There should be guidelines set-up in the hospital for the nurses to be aware of what treatment should be administered depending on the level of pain the patient is in.

ACKNOWLEDGMENTS

For their great efforts in collecting and reviewing the research and data: Eman Mina, Eirene Rophael, Marina Mina, Cyril Mina.

SUGGESTED READING

Chiaretti A, Pierri F, Valentini P, et al. Current practice and recent advances in pediatric pain management. Eur Rev Med Pharmacol Sci. 2013;17 (Suppl 1):112-26.

Mazur A, Winnicki IR, Szczepański T. Pain management in children. Ann Agric Environ Med. 2013;Special Issue 1:28-34.

Wong D, Baker C. Pain in children: comparison of assessment scales. Pediatric Nursing. 1988;14(1):9-17.

Evaluation of the Geriatric Pain Patient

Boies BT, Horrocks A

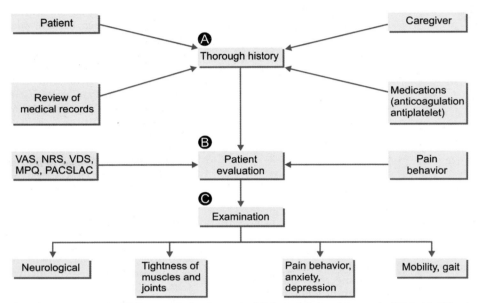

VAS, visual analog scale; NRS, numerical rating scale; VDS, verbal descriptor scale; MPQ, McGill pain questionnaire; PACSLAC, Pain Assessment Checklist for Seniors with Limited Ability to Communicate

In 2010, 13% of the population was considered to be of old age, as defined by one being 65 years of age or older. By 2030, that population is estimated to expand to over 20%. The prevalence of pain is estimated from 50% to 75% in this population, with women having a higher prevalence than men. However, pain in the elderly is undertreated because of misconceptions such as that the elderly are "expected to have pain" or they are "too ill and too sensitive to medications" and cannot be safely treated. This is further compounded by patient reluctance to "burden" family with their pain complaints, and decreasing ability to clearly express themselves secondary to short-term memory problems, the onset of dementia, and the debilitating effects of numerous medications being taken for various systemic illnesses. However, poorly controlled pain can negatively impact many aspects of a patient's life, including their activity level, cognition, and mood, all of which can lead to further worsening of the plethora of concurrent medical issues in this population.

A A thorough history and complete review of the medical records, including all medications the patient is taking and has previously tried, is important because elderly patients have significant concurrent illnesses requiring numerous medications. Because of debility, short-term memory problems, and associated dementia, it is essential to obtain complete information. This frequently requires obtaining the information from the caregivers regarding the medications, activities of daily living, history of falls, and pain behavior. Frequently, patients are not aware of anticoagulant and antiplatelet medications they are taking. This can lead to serious problems secondary to drug interactions or following invasive procedures.

B The pain evaluation can be extremely difficult because of poor eyesight, impaired hearing, debility, memory problems, and dementia. There are various pain scales available for use today. The verbal descriptor scale (VDS) appears to be the easiest test to complete and the most informative; it requires the patients to describe their pain from "no pain" to "worst pain possible." A combination of the visual analog scale (VAS) (marking perceived pain level on a 10 cm line between "zero pain" and "worst pain possible"), numerical rating scale (NRS) (correlating pain on a 0 to 10 scale with 10 being the most severe), and the VDS, however, is likely to yield information that is more complete. These tests require short yes or no answers and are more likely to be understood by the elderly patient. The McGill pain questionnaire (MPQ) is a more comprehensive test on which patients select words from each of

20 sections that best describes their pain. Point values are assigned to each word, and a cumulative score is then calculated. The MPQ may not be as reliable in populations with low reading comprehension. The short form MPQ is also available and is a shorter, less time-consuming version of the MPQ. In patients with significant dementia, observation of the pain behavior and information gathered from the caregivers is essential when evaluating the patient's pain. This information can be used to complete the Pain Assessment in Advanced Dementia (PAINAD) or Pain Assessment Checklist for Seniors with Limited Ability to Communicate (PACSLAC) checklist which attempts to quantify pain in seniors with limited ability to communicate by evaluating factors such as facial expression, body movement, and mood. Additionally, pain diaries may be critical to document reliably the responses to medications and procedures. Results from all pain scales should be used in conjunction with, and not as a substitute for, a detailed history and physical examination.

C In addition to a thorough neurologic examination, it is essential to evaluate for significant deconditioning, decreased joint motion, and muscle tightness. A multidisciplinary examination is useful for evaluating gait (get up and go test), mobility, the need for assistance (cane, walker, wheelchair), the activities of daily living, and pain behavior. The Katz Index of Independence in Activities of Daily Living (Katz ADL) is a tool that can be used to evaluate adequacy in performance of basic daily functions such as bathing and feeding. Significant anxiety and depression are common and require thorough evaluation and treatment to control pain adequately.

SUGGESTED READING

Abdulla A, Adams N, Bone M, et al. Guidance on the management of pain in older people. Age Ageing. 2013;42 (Suppl 1):il-57.

Hawker GA, Mian S, Kendzerska T, et al. Measures of adult pain. Arthritis Care Res. 2011;63.S11:240-52.

Herr K, Spratt KF, Garand L, et al. Evaluation of the Iowa pain thermometer and other selected pain intensity scales in younger and older adult cohorts using controlled clinical pain: a preliminary study. Pain Med. 2007;8(7):585-600.

Rastogi R, Meek B. Management of chronic pain in elderly, frail patients: finding a suitable, personalized method of control. Clin Interv Aging. 2013;8:37-46.

Zwakhalen SM, Hamers JP, Abu-Saad HH, et al. Pain in elderly people with severe dementia: a systematic review of behavioural pain assessment tools. BMC Geriatr. 2006;6:3.

CHAPTER 5

Evaluation and Preparation for Regional Anesthesia

Wallisch BJ, Rios N

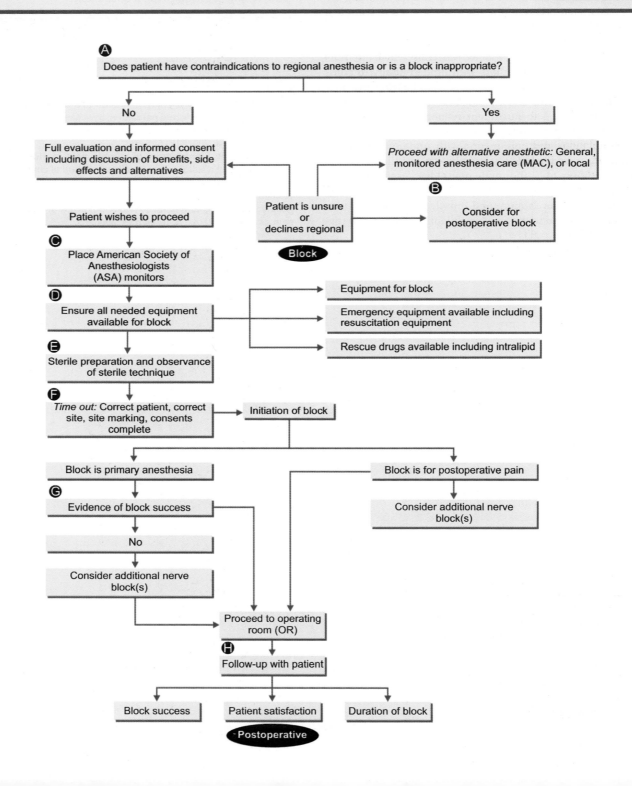

A Does patient have contraindications to regional anesthesia or is a block inappropriate?

- No
  - Full evaluation and informed consent including discussion of benefits, side effects and alternatives
    - Patient wishes to proceed
    - **C** Place American Society of Anesthesiologists (ASA) monitors
    - **D** Ensure all needed equipment available for block
      - Equipment for block
      - Emergency equipment available including resuscitation equipment
      - Rescue drugs available including intralipid
    - **E** Sterile preparation and observance of sterile technique
    - **F** *Time out:* Correct patient, correct site, site marking, consents complete
      - Initiation of block
        - Block is primary anesthesia
          - **G** Evidence of block success
            - No
              - Consider additional nerve block(s)
        - Block is for postoperative pain
          - Consider additional nerve block(s)
      - Proceed to operating room (OR)
        - **H** Follow-up with patient
          - Block success
          - Patient satisfaction
          - Duration of block
          - **Postoperative**

- Yes
  - *Proceed with alternative anesthetic:* General, monitored anesthesia care (MAC), or local
    - **B** Consider for postoperative block

Patient is unsure or declines regional

Block

Successful performance of regional anesthesia is dependent on matching an appropriate patient with the best regional anesthetic for their procedure. Patients should undergo full evaluation and an informed written consent. Full consent requires a discussion of the risks, benefits and alternatives to the procedure as well as any expected side effects of the block. The expected length of pain relief or anesthesia should also be discussed. Patient refusal remains one of the main contraindications to any elective procedure. Proper psychological preparation improves the patient and practitioner experience as well as screen for candidates who might have difficulty. Special attention should be directed toward use, cessation, and resumption of anticoagulants or antiplatelet agents in the setting of regional anesthesia. Generally, neuraxial techniques should be avoided in the presence of full systemic anticoagulation. Peripheral blocks in the patient taking antiplatelet agents or systemic anticoagulation require a case-by-case approach that balances the risk of bleeding and feasibility of compression in the event of a hematoma against the benefits of the procedure. Consensus guidelines, such as those from the American Society of Regional Anesthesia and Pain Medicine, are available to assist decision making. Planning for postprocedure resumption of anticoagulation should be made in coordination with surgical services or other consultants.

A *Decision to Use Regional Anesthesia:* It is in the best interest of the process that surgeons are fully educated about the benefits of regional anesthesia as well as its limits and expected side effects. Regional anesthesia can cause changes in surgical workflow and if the benefits are not immediately apparent, this can be perceived to be inefficient or detrimental to patient care. Numerous studies have demonstrated improved patient experience and functional outcome and a well-designed regional anesthesia process can reap efficiency benefits in both anesthesia control times and postanesthesia care unit (PACU) times. A procedure done entirely under regional block has the added benefit of minimal induction time, no emergence time and often phase one recovery bypass. In order to reap those benefits however, the evaluation, consent, and procedure must be performed efficiently and with enough time to set-up prior to surgical incision. It is imperative that the process is seen in the context of an overall decrease in anesthesia control time rather than a preoperative delay.

B *Postoperative Blocks:* Postoperative analgesic blocks are an option in the case of patient indecision, uncertainty of the invasiveness of procedure, or emergency cases. Every effort should be made to discuss the procedure and obtain an informed consent prior to administration of sedatives or general anesthesia. While postoperative blocks potentially miss the opportunity for pre-emptive analgesia, they can make a significant impact in reducing postoperative opioid use and promote faster recovery times and shorten PACU stays.

C *Sedation and Monitors:* When the patient has been satisfactorily evaluated, consented for anesthesia, and operating room (OR) readiness is confirmed (including surgical consent, laterality and site marking, and nursing evaluation), the patient is ready for the procedure. All patients should have standard American Society of Anesthesiologists (ASA) monitoring—especially continuous heart rate monitor—to detect inadvertent intravascular injection or development of a conduction blockade. Supplemental oxygen is recommended if procedural sedation is planned for the block and a separate dedicated provider should act as a patient monitor. Emergency supplies for resuscitation should be immediately available when performing blocks. The ability to secure an airway or perform CPR necessitates the availability of endotracheal tubes, a laryngoscope, working suction, emergency drugs, an Ambu bag, and lipid emulsion designed for intravascular injection rescue.

D *Procedural Tools:* Assemble all equipment including ultrasound or nerve stimulator, appropriately sized needle, and properly labeled local anesthetic. Consideration should be made for administering subcutaneous local anesthetic injection at the skin site of needle entry with a 24 gauge or smaller needle. A wide variety of blunt tipped, insulated, and echogenic regional anesthesia needles/catheters are available and should be selected to best match the depth of the target nerve.

E *Sterile Preparation:* Observance of strict sterile technique is mandatory. The site of injection should be widely prepped with a microbicidal-based solution (e.g. chlorhexidine) and a barrier drape, including full body drape (and gown) for placement of a continuous perineural catheter. At a minimum, the anesthetist placing the block should wear a mask, hat, clean scrubs, and sterile gloves. Consideration should also be made for the administration of preprocedure antibiotics in the placement of perineural catheters.

F *Time Out:* Just before initiation of the procedure, a final time out should be conducted so as to verify the correct patient, procedure, and laterality. Site marking by both the anesthesia and surgical teams along with immediate reaffirmation of laterality prior to initiation of the procedure is an essential step to minimize the risk of a wrong-sided block.

G *Continued Monitoring and Confirmation:* The patient should be monitored continuously after placement for both local anesthetic toxicity and side effects from procedural sedation. Local anesthetic toxicity can occur up to 30 minutes following placement of a block and may manifest initially as neurologic symptoms (seizure or altered mental status) or with sudden cardiovascular symptoms as severe as total cardiovascular collapse. Therefore, patient monitoring during this period is essential. The assessment of block success should occur at an appropriate time frame following a block with consideration of the local anesthetic injected. In anticipation of a motor block, the patient should be prevented from ambulating and any affected limb appropriately padded; the patient should be warned of the potential for limb malposition injury.

Ⓗ *Transition of Care:* The patient should be prepared for the eventual dissipation of anesthesia. The patient and caregivers should be given clear guidelines about the anticipated time for the block to wear off, any expected side effects, and a contact number (if discharged to home) for questions or concerns. A clear plan for pain control should anticipate any pain medication requirements. Finally, to guide practice improvement and further care, follow-up should be performed recording the time of block resolution, the overall success of the block, patient satisfaction with regional anesthesia, and any problems.

SUGGESTED READING

ASA House of Delegates. (2015). ASA standards for basic anesthetic monitoring. [online] Available from *http://www.asahq. org.* [Accessed January, 2017].

Capdevila X, Bringuier S, Borgeat A. Infectious risk of continuous peripheral nerve blocks. Anesthesiology. 2009;110:182-8.

Edmonds CR, Liguori GA, Stanton MA. Two cases of a wrong-site peripheral nerve block and a process to prevent this complication. Reg Anesth Pain Med. 2005;30(1):99-103.

Hebl JR. The importance and implications of aseptic techniques during regional anesthesia. Reg Anesth Pain Med. 2006;31(4): 311-23.

Horlocker T, Wedel DJ, Rowlingson JC, et al. Regional anesthesia in the patient receiving antithrombotic or thrombolytic therapy: American Society of Regional Anesthesia and Pain Medicine Evidence-Based Guidelines (Third Edition). Reg Anesth Pain Med. 2010;35(1):64-101.

Phillips DP, Knizner TL, Williams BA. Economics and practice management issues associated with acute pain management. Anesth Clin. 2011;29(2):213-32.

The American Society of Regional Anesthesia and Pain Medicine. (2012). Checklist for treatment of local anesthetic systemic toxicity. [online] Available from *http://www.asra.com/checklist-for-local-anesthetic-toxicity-treatment-1-18-12.pdf.* [Accessed January, 2017].

CHAPTER 6

Evaluation and Preparation for Chronic Pain Procedure

Nagpal A, Fehl JE

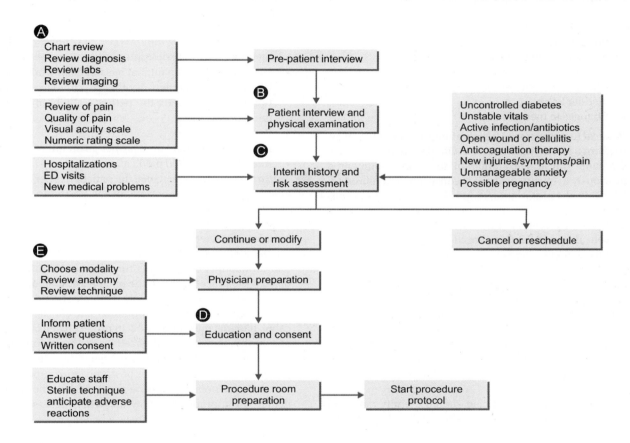

Outpatient interventional procedures and techniques can be very similar to those performed in the inpatient setting and have similar safety concerns. Chronic pain procedures are often performed in the ambulatory surgery or outpatient clinic setting. Since the patient will have less intensive postprocedural observation in the outpatient setting by comparison, the clinician should take special preparation and evaluation to ensure patient safety. Often, the patient's workup and evaluation was already completed at a previous clinic visit. Despite any previous workups, a thorough and focused examination must be performed at each patient visit to ensure the planned procedure is the best management for the patient. The patient should be well educated on pre- and postprocedure precautions to reduce the chance of periprocedural complications.

Ⓐ *Chart Review:* The physician performing the procedure should first perform a thorough chart review of the patient's diagnosis and previous procedures and ensure alternative treatment options have been ruled out. A simple chart review of previous visits can direct your history and examination, especially if a previous diagnosis has been given. The patient's allergies, previous imaging, and pertinent laboratory values should be reviewed. Any documented emergency room visits, hospital visits, or other pertinent clinic visits since the last evaluation should be analyzed. Special attention should be directed to use of anticoagulants or antiplatelet agents and diabetes.

Ⓑ *Patient Interview/History:* The patient interview is an essential source of information in pain management. Once in the patient's room, a focused history should be obtained. Verify the patient's subjective history of pain, function, location, radiation, and any changes since the last examination. A measure of pain in the treated area should be taken; the most commonly used are the visual analog scale and the numeric rating scale. These scales can aid in confirming a change in pain before and after the procedure. Most importantly, verification should be made that the planned procedure continues to be the most suitable option to improve the patient's pain.

Interim History: In planning for a procedure, recent changes in a patient's medical history may give reason to modify or cancel the planned procedure. Prior to discussing the procedure at hand, it is helpful to obtain a history from the patient including:

- Previous hospitalizations since last visit
- Recent accidents or injuries
- Changes in pain including location, duration, radiation, or intensity
- New pain-generating locations
- Recent infection and antibiotic use
- Changes in function, sensation, strength, or bowel/bladder habit
- Changes in mental status.

Physical Examination: After obtaining a thorough history, perform a focused examination. Often you can reproduce the same physical examination that was documented previously to ensure the pain is consistent and reproducible. This physical examination is beneficial to help confirm the planned procedure is appropriate ahead of time, and to have documentation to reference postprocedure as well. This examination should include a focused musculoskeletal examination, neurologic testing, and appropriate special tests to confirm or rule out the patient's diagnosis. A focused neurologic examination is particularly important if a diagnostic block is planned. To help alleviate patient concerns, communicate your findings with the patient throughout the examination. Discuss any new or different findings in the physical examination with the patient. These findings may require additional workup and a possible change in plan for the expected procedure.

C *Risk Assessment:* The clinician should identify risks and medical conditions that exclude the patient from having the planned procedure. For example, administering an intravenous (IV) steroid to an uncontrolled diabetic may place the patient at significant risk for diabetic ketoacidosis due to the expected increase in blood glucose level. A clinical protocol for preprocedure glucose monitoring is an essential preventative measure. A procedure may also have avoidable contraindications, such as using radiation during pregnancy. This risk may be avoided by performing the procedure with an alternative and safe modality such as ultrasound. Essential information should be gathered prior to setting up the procedure, and the clinician should have a low threshold for canceling or rescheduling. Significant time and effort can be saved when contraindications are identified promptly and before set-up for the procedure has begun. The duration of the visit should focus on patient education to address the patient's contraindication. Below is a nonexhaustive list of considerations for modifying, canceling, or rescheduling elective clinic procedures:

- Uncontrolled diabetes

- Unstable vitals including heart rate, blood pressure, respiratory rate, and temperature
- Active infection
- Current or recent antibiotic use
- Skin check reveals the injection site is compromised, such as an open wound or cellulitis
- Anticoagulation therapy incompatible with the procedure
- Uncorrected coagulopathy or bleeding disorders
- Recent accidents or injuries that have not been evaluated in the ED or by the primary care physician
- New unevaluated symptoms (i.e. new bowel/bladder incontinence, weakness, numbness, paresthesia, etc.)
- New uncontrolled pain that has not been worked up
- Unmanageable anxiety or other psychological condition that could affect the patient's ability to tolerate the procedure
- Possible pregnancy
- Patient unable to tolerate proper positioning
- Allergies to required medications

D *Education and Consent:* Once the patient has been evaluated and deemed appropriate for the procedure, proper consent must be obtained. During this process, it is also necessary to further educate the patient about the risks, benefits, expected outcomes, and possible alternatives. As many of procedures are performed in the outpatient and ambulatory setting, this time should be utilized to discuss the procedure with the patient and prepare them for postprocedure management. Patients should be educated on monitoring for the potential side effects. If applicable, patients must know how to protect insensate areas of skin that may be anesthetized by the procedure. They must also understand the use of analgesic adjuncts and provide proof of appropriate postprocedure supervision (i.e. a driver present). Ensure they will be able to participate in appropriate follow-up. When necessary, the patient must show that they have a reliable caregiver. The patient should verbalize their own understanding of the procedure, the risks and the benefits, and they should be given the opportunity to ask questions. Once the physician and the patient are satisfied with the communication, proper consent should be obtained. This usually includes a document that is signed by both the physician and patient documenting the previous discussion and the patient's acknowledgment of the risks and their willingness to go forward with the procedure.

E *Review of Anatomy and Procedure Technique:* Prior to each procedure the physician should go over all applicable anatomy, including the intended site of the injection, the anatomical landmarks, the sites that will be affected by invasive instrumentation, and possible areas to avoid including vessels and nerves. Medications to be used should be reviewed for any potential toxicity in the individual patient, based upon their medical history. The physician should ensure that he/she is comfortable with each aspect of the procedure and that your clinical staff is properly trained and prepared to assist you.

Choosing Interventional Modality: In the past, interventional procedures were often done "blind" or without the aid of imaging. Due to the escalation in technology and the increasing availability of ultrasound, CT, and other imaging, there are many modalities to consider when providing an interventional technique. The interventional imaging modality that will suit the procedure's need while ensuring reduction of the patient's overall risk is the best to use.

Sterile Technique: Sterile technique is paramount in protecting the patient from possible infection. The risk of infection is variable depending on the invasiveness of the procedure. As each procedure can carry its own risk of infection, the practitioner should ensure sterility of their field and sterility of the location of the equipment that is used for the procedure. Additionally, the use of a high-efficiency particulate absorber (HEPA) filter in the procedure room can decrease the incidence of infection. High-risk interventions, such as spinal cord stimulator placement or discography, may warrant preprocedural intravenous antibiotics.

Possible Adverse Reactions: Each procedure has its own potential risks. The physician performing the procedure must not only know the risks, but also be trained on the appropriate management of potential adverse reactions. Quick recognition and treatment of an adverse event is necessary in order to treat the adverse effect. Facilities that are involved with performing chronic pain procedures should be equipped to handle all potential catastrophes with fully functioning crash cart and advanced cardiac life support (ACLS)-trained personnel. Lipid emulsion rescue therapy should be available if nerve blocks are being performed. Possible acute conditions to consider include:

- Vasovagal syncope
- Local anesthetic toxicity
- Anaphylaxis
- High intrathecal block
- Spinal cord injury
- Intrathecal pump overdose
- Acute opioid withdrawal
- Acute baclofen withdrawal
- Pneumothorax
- Hypertension
- Anxiety or panic episode

SUGGESTED READING

Braxton K. Basic risk management for interventional procedures. In: Raj PP, Lou L, Erdine S, Staats PS (Eds). Interventional Pain Management, 2nd edition. Philadelphia, PA: Saunders; 2008.

Chahal HS, Urman RD. Emergencies in the pain clinic. In: Urman RD, Vadivelu N (Eds). Pocket Pain Medicine. Philadelphia, PA: Lippincott Williams & Wilkins; 2011.

Evans H, Nielson KC, Tucker MS, et al. Regional anesthesia for acute pain management in the outpatient setting. In: Sinatra RS, de Leon-Casosola OA, Ginsgerg B, Viscusi ER (Eds). Acute Pain Management. New York, NY: Cambridge University Press; 2009.

Fishman SM, Ballantyne JC, Rathmell JP. Bonica's Management of Pain, 4th edition. Philadelphia, PA: Lippincott Williams & Wilkins; 2010.

Psychological Evaluation

McGeary CA

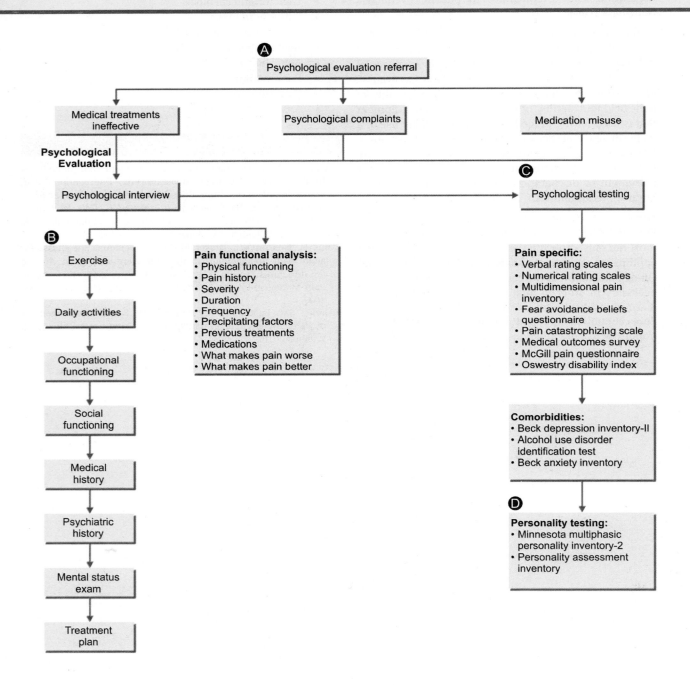

A Psychological evaluation referral

Medical treatments ineffective

Psychological complaints

Medication misuse

Psychological Evaluation

Psychological interview

C Psychological testing

B

Exercise

Daily activities

Occupational functioning

Social functioning

Medical history

Psychiatric history

Mental status exam

Treatment plan

Pain functional analysis:
• Physical functioning
• Pain history
• Severity
• Duration
• Frequency
• Precipitating factors
• Previous treatments
• Medications
• What makes pain worse
• What makes pain better

Pain specific:
• Verbal rating scales
• Numerical rating scales
• Multidimensional pain inventory
• Fear avoidance beliefs questionnaire
• Pain catastrophizing scale
• Medical outcomes survey
• McGill pain questionnaire
• Oswestry disability index

Comorbidities:
• Beck depression inventory-II
• Alcohol use disorder identification test
• Beck anxiety inventory

D **Personality testing:**
• Minnesota multiphasic personality inventory-2
• Personality assessment inventory

Because chronic pain encompasses biological, psychological, and social factors, it can be difficult to treat unless an interdisciplinary approach is adopted. The biopsychosocial model states that chronic pain is a combination of factors including biological (injury, medical problems), psychological (emotions and thoughts regarding pain experience) and social (family, friends, work). These factors interact to produce a patient's individual pain experience. A physician may consider referring a patient for a psychological evaluation if medical treatments alone are not producing optimal treatment results. A psychological evaluation can pinpoint both psychological and social dysfunction impacting pain. Most importantly, the use of psychological testing with pain patients can provide a medical provider insight into the patient's pain experience and help to identify viable treatment avenues.

A A physician may refer a chronic pain patient for a psychological evaluation when medical treatments are not effective, when psychological complaints are present or when there are concerns of medication misuse. There is high comorbidity between chronic pain and depression, anxiety, and substance abuse. However, a referral to a psychologist is recommended in any situation where a patient's psychological or social functioning is suspected to be significantly impacting (or is impacted by) their pain experience.

B When referring a patient for a psychological evaluation, it is important to find a clinician who is experienced working with pain patients. The clinician should be familiar with recent pain literature and pain psychometrics. The clinician should also have the appropriate training and knowledge to conduct a functional analysis of the patient's pain. A thorough functional analysis provides a synthesis of problems and variables that are associated with them. This information is useful to help develop an effective

treatment plan to address chronic pain. Many pain providers utilize numerical or visual rating scales to allow patients to rate the degree of pain they are experiencing. Many providers utilize this brief pain intensity rating as a diagnostic and outcome measure for pain treatment.

C Psychometric testing provides a wide array of information and is an important part of a thorough psychological evaluation for pain. The psychometric testing battery will include measures specific to pain but also measures of common pain comorbidities. Common measures will assess mood, pain intensity, quality of life, psychological coping, fear avoidance, disability, pain beliefs, and personality.

D Many researchers have tried to identify a "pain personality profile," but have been unsuccessful in their attempts. However, personality tests continue to be administered to individuals with chronic pain and can shed light on an individual's mental health functioning that may impact the chronic pain experience. Most frequently administered personality tests are the Minnesota Multiphasic Personality Inventory, 2nd edition (MMPI-2) and the Personality Assessment Inventory (PAI).

SUGGESTED READING

Engel GL. The biopsychosocial model and the education of health professionals. Ann NY Acad Sci. 1978;310(1):169-87.

Gatchel RJ. Comorbidity of chronic pain and mental health disorders: the biopsychosocial perspective. Am Psychol. 2004;59(8):795-805.

Karlin BE, Creech SK, Grimes JS, et al. The personality assessment inventory with chronic pain patients: psychometric properties and clinical utility. J Clin Psychol. 2005;61(12):1571-85.

McGeary DD, Gatchel RJ, McGeary CA, et al. Chronic pain assessment. In: Andrasik, F, Goodie J, Peterson AL (Eds). Biopsychosocial Assessment in Clinical Health Psychology: A Handbook. New York: The Guilford Press; 2015.

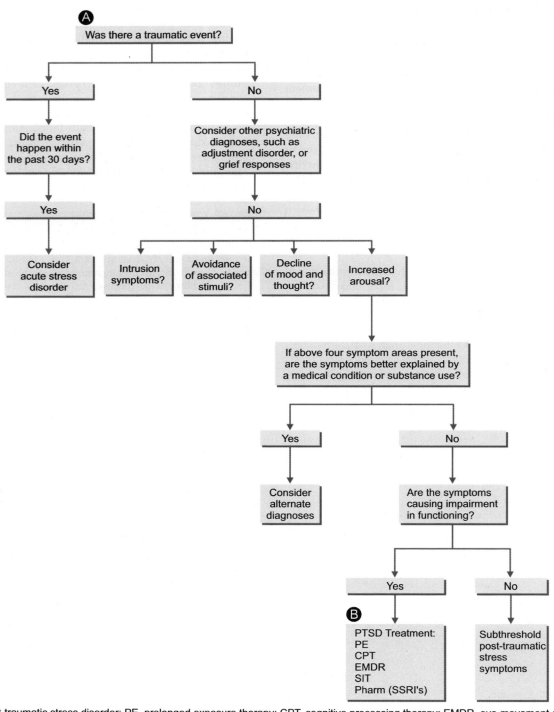

PTSD, post-traumatic stress disorder; PE, prolonged exposure therapy; CPT, cognitive processing therapy; EMDR, eye-movement desensitization and reprocessing; SIT, stress inoculation training; SSRI, selective serotonin reuptake inhibitors

Post-traumatic stress disorder (PTSD) is an anxiety disorder characterized by the development of chronic symptoms following exposure to one or more highly traumatic stressors. As many as 80% of persons meeting the criteria for PTSD also have comorbid diagnoses, most commonly depression, an anxiety disorder, or a substance abuse disorder. The lifetime prevalence of PTSD has been estimated to range from 1% to 14% and has been found to be twice as high in women (10.4%) as in men (5%). Increasing attention has been drawn to the co-occurrence of psychological trauma and physical symptoms. Recent studies have suggested a high prevalence of PTSD symptoms among chronic pain patients, though rates of co-occurrence vary based on the cause of the pain. Patients with accident-related pain demonstrate comorbid PTSD at a rate of 30–50%, whereas 80% of combat veterans reported both chronic pain and PTSD. Individuals with both physical symptoms and PTSD report higher levels of pain, lower quality of life, greater functional impairment, and more psychological distress than their counterparts with either pain or PTSD alone. PTSD symptoms often go undetected in patients presenting with pain complaints, yet such symptoms can complicate the clinical picture and adversely affect treatment outcome if not addressed. Consequently, increasing attention is being given to the importance of recognizing and treating PTSD in pain patients.

Ⓐ *Diagnosing PTSD:* The steps below provide an outline for diagnosing PTSD according to Diagnostic and Statistical Manual of Mental Disorders (DSM)-5 criteria.

- To qualify for a diagnosis of PTSD, a person first must have been exposed to a traumatic event in which he or she experienced, witnessed, or was confronted with an event or events that involved actual or threatened death or serious injury or a threat to the physical integrity of self or others. A similar response to a less severe stressor should be evaluated for grief or adjustment disorder.
- The event must have occurred more than 30 days ago. Within 30 days, symptoms of trauma-related distress are considered part of the normal recovery process. If, however, within 30 days the distress is impacting the individual's functioning, a diagnosis of acute stress disorder may be considered.
- The traumatic event is persistently re-experienced through intrusive, distressing recollections of the event, distressing dreams of the event, acting or feeling as if the event were recurring (e.g. flashbacks), intense psychological distress or physiological reactivity upon exposure to cues associated with the trauma.
- Persistent avoidance of external stimuli (e.g. people, places, conversations) and/or internal stimuli (e.g. thoughts, memories, feelings) associated with the trauma is present.
- Mood and thought conditions demonstrate decline, evidenced by at least two of the following: trouble remembering significant aspects of the trauma; negative beliefs about self, others, and/or the world; distorted thoughts about why the event happened resulting in inappropriate blame of self or others;

persistent negative emotions (e.g. fear, anger, or guilt); reduction of interest or participation in activities; withdrawal or distancing from others; and continual inability to experience positive emotion.

- Increased symptoms of arousal and reactivity beginning or worsening after the event must be present, manifested by at least two of the following: Difficulty falling or staying asleep, irritability or anger outbursts, reckless or self-destructive behavior, difficulty concentrating, hypervigilance, or an exaggerated startle response.
- Other causes must also be ruled out. Substance use and other medical conditions can sometimes present similarly. Rule out alternative diagnoses before proceeding.
- If all of the above criteria are met, intensity of symptoms is then considered. Either impairment in social, occupational or other important areas of functioning or significant emotional distress must be present.

Ⓑ *Treatment of Functionally Impairing PTSD:* Once a diagnosis of PTSD is established, treatment should be provided by a qualified clinician and should always include patient and family education. The patient should be involved in deciding which treatment to pursue. Treatment selection should take into account treatment efficacy for PTSD, the patient's treatment goals (e.g. symptom reduction versus fostering resilience or growth from the experience), possible difficulties or side effects, and patient motivation and willingness to engage in the proposed treatment as well as treatment length, cost, and the patient's availability of resources.

Cognitive and behavioral therapies have been the most widely studied and validated interventions for PTSD. They encompass a variety of techniques with those described in the list below having demonstrated replicated and high-quality empirical support. While these therapies have been shown to be effective in reducing symptoms of PTSD, not all patients benefit, and it is not yet clear what factors predict success with this treatment approach.

- *Prolonged Exposure (PE)*: This therapy involves progressive exposure to avoided memories through imagined and in-person exposure to the traumatic experience, reducing the conditioned fear response over time. It has been demonstrated to be effective with men and women as well as with a variety of traumas and lasts about 8–15 sessions.
- *Cognitive Processing Therapy (CPT)*: CPT incorporates imagined exposure through a trauma narrative with re-evaluation of thoughts and beliefs related to the event. The standard CPT protocol is 12 sessions and has been validated among veterans and female sexual assault survivors. An adapted version, CPT-C, that does not involve a trauma narrative has also proven efficacious.
- *Eye-Movement Desensitization and Reprocessing (EMDR)*: Similar to PE and CPT in efficacy, EMDR involves imagined exposure to memories and

sensations of the trauma concurrent with identifying distorted trauma-related thoughts alongside more adaptive alternatives. Typically, patients talk through their trauma memory while the clinician uses a side-to-side alternating stimulus, such as the clinician's finger moving left and right; however, research has suggested efficacy for treatment without the alternating stimulus component. Treatment length varies for EMDR.

- *Stress Inoculation Training (SIT)*: SIT trains patients to cope better with their anxiety-related trauma symptoms. Patients learn to practice skills in five areas: deep breathing, relaxation training, positive self-talk, assertiveness training, and thought stopping.

Pharmacotherapy is also used to treat PTSD. Selective serotonin reuptake inhibitors (SSRIs) are currently recommended as first-line pharmacotherapy for PTSD. In general, pharmacotherapy has been shown to reduce symptoms effectively, but it does not have a clear effect on the course of the disorder and, therefore, may be most effective as an adjunct to psychological and social treatments. It should be noted that benzodiazepines have been shown to not only be ineffective in treating PTSD, patients, but also to increase the patient's fear response; therefore, their use for PTSD is not recommended.

SUGGESTED READING

American Psychiatric Association. Diagnostic and Statistical Manual of Mental Disorders, 5th edition. Washington, DC: American Psychiatric Association; 2013.

Department of Veterans Affairs and Department of Defense. VA/DoD clinical practice guideline for management of post-traumatic stress; 2010.

Kessler RC, Sonnega A, Bromet E, et al. Post-traumatic stress disorder in the National Comorbidity Survey. Arch Gen Psychiatry. 1995;52:1048-60.

Otis D, Gregor K, Hardway C, et al. An examination of the comorbidity between chronic pain and post-traumatic stress disorder on US veterans. Psychological Services. 2010;7(3);126-35.

Otis D, Keane TM, Kerns RD. An examination of the relationship between chronic pain and post-traumatic stress disorder. J Rehabil Res Dev. 2003;40(5):397-406.

Resick PA, Monson CM, Chard KM. Cognitive processing therapy: Veteran/military version: Therapist and patient materials manual. Washington, DC: Department of Veterans Affairs, 2014.

Samson AY, Bensen S, Beck A, et al. Post-traumatic stress disorder in primary care. J Fam Pract. 1999;48:222-7.

CHAPTER 9

Assessment of Substance Abuse Potential

McGeary DD, Eckmann MS

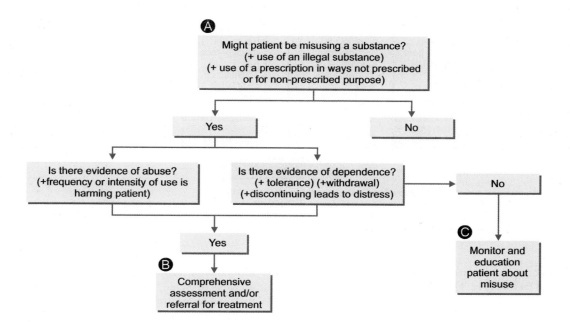

Substance abuse was recently redefined under the 5th revision of the Diagnostic and Statistical Manual of Mental Disorders (DSM-5) to include symptoms of both substance abuse and substance dependence under the same umbrella disorder (Substance Use Disorder; SUD). Furthermore, the DSM-5 allows for subcategories of SUD relative to specific substances (e.g. alcohol, alcohol use disorder; marijuana, cannabis use disorder; opioids, opioid use disorder). An SUD is diagnosed when abuse, dependence, or misuse of a substance is believed to cause significant and clinically-relevant functional impairment in one or more life domains (e.g. home life, work, school, etc.). Estimates of SUD among chronic pain samples are highly variable ranging from 3% to 48% point prevalence and 16% to 74% lifetime prevalence under older definitions of SUD. Although opioid medications have likely received the highest level of attention in chronic pain and SUD comorbidity research, other substance use disorders (e.g. alcohol use disorder) are also quite problematic in this population and should receive increasing attention in future research.

Ⓐ *Identifying Behaviors and Risks Associated with Misuse*: Mechanisms of comorbidity between chronic pain conditions and substance use disorder range widely, including iatrogenic effects of pain treatments (e.g. opioid medications), lack of knowledge about substance use disorder risks among pain treatment providers, poor response to other pain interventions, and emotional disruption caused/maintained by chronic pain, SUD, or both. Risk for SUD has been linked to genetic factors, and chronic pain-SUD comorbidity risk is likely higher among those with mental illness. Often, substance use is rewarded in chronic pain sufferers because use of the substance may lead to symptom improvement (e.g. pain becomes less noticeable, sleep seems easier). As tolerance develops for the substance, however, this reward is diminished and use of the substance can increase to the point where it leads to additional problems. Abuse of pain medications often is not self-reported to the treating physician due to stigma and fears of consequences, yet it manifests as aberrant behavior. These may include multiple reports of lost/stolen medications, unapproved increases in medication use, refusal to undergo any other rational treatment other than oral opioid-based medication, obtaining medications from multiple physicians. Evidence of prescription falsification, illicit drug use, drug tampering, and diverting medications, if found, is especially confirmative of medication abuse. Tools such as random urine drug tests (UDTs), combined with monitoring of prescription drug monitoring programs (PDMP, databases) and medical record review, can assist providers in detecting illicit behavior.

Ⓑ *Assessment and Treatment*: Because of the complexity of substance use in chronic pain, assessment can be difficult and should be guided by a comprehensive biopsychosocial

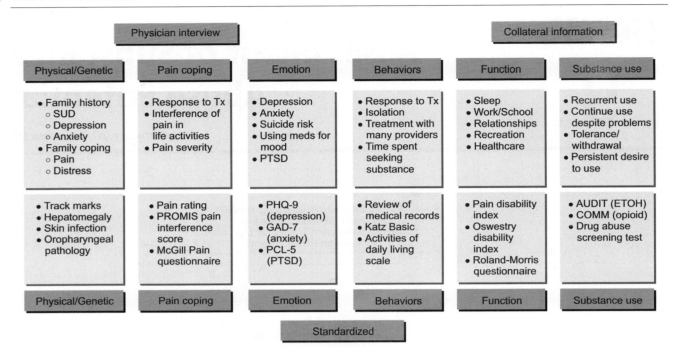

Fig. 1: Biopsychosocial assessment for substance use disorder in chronic pain
SUD, substance use disorder; PTSD, post-traumatic stress disorder; PROMIS, Patient-Reported Outcomes Measurement Information System; GAD, generalized anxiety disorder; PCL, Post-traumatic Stress Disorder Checklist; PHQ, The Patient Health Questionnaire; AUDIT, alcohol use disorders identification test; COMM, Current Opioid Misuse Measure

framework that captures physical, emotional, and behavioral factors **(Fig. 1)**. In 2012, the Substance Abuse and Mental Health Service Administration (SAMHSA) published a Treatment Improvement Protocol (TIP) in acknowledgment of the serious problems posed by chronic pain and SUD comorbidity. The SAMHSA TIP titled "Managing Chronic Pain in Adults with or in Recovery from Substance Use Disorders," offers detailed instructions for improving the quality of assessment and treatment in chronic pain patients with SUD. Specifically, pain providers interested in improving surveillance of substance use disorders in chronic pain patients should offer a refined assessment of:

- *Pain coping*—individuals coping poorly with pain are at increased risk of SUD
- *Emotional distress*—mental health history and emotional distress may be a cause or consequence of SUD
- *Behavior*—changes in behavior and social interaction may indicate a SUD
- *Collateral data*—review of medical records and discussions with patient's supportive others may clarify risk factors

C Patients on long-term therapy with controlled substances should be monitored for development of misuse, abuse, and addiction. Based on risk stratification, timing interval of UDT should be selected. Absence of expected medication and metabolites on testing may indicate binging, hoarding, or diversion. Presence of unprescribed medications or illicit substances can indicate abuse. Monitoring of the PDMP, if available, can detect "doctor shopping" in the absence of a confirmed medical rationale for having multiple treating (pain) providers. If abuse is detected, referral to addiction medicine and/or weaning of controlled substances may be warranted.

The SAMHSA TIP (which can be found at: *http://store.samhsa.gov/shin/content/SMA12-4671/TIP54.pdf*) offers numerous suggestions for assessment questions and standardized self-report measures to improve SUD assessment in chronic pain patients along with advice for treatment in this complex population.

SUGGESTED READING

American Psychiatric Association. Diagnostic and Statistical Manual of Mental Health Disorders: DSM-5 (5th edition). Washington, DC: American Psychiatric Publishing; 2013.

Atluri S, Akbik H, Sudarshan G. Prevention of opioid abuse in chronic non-cancer pain: an algorithmic, evidence-based approach. Pain Physician. 2012;15(3 Suppl):ES177-89.

Morasco BJ, Gritzner S, Lewis L, et al. Systematic review of prevalence, correlates, and treatment outcomes for chronic non-cancer pain in patients with comorbid substance use disorder. Pain. 2011;152(3):488-97.

Robinson RC, Gatchel RJ, Polatin P, et al. Screening for problematic prescription opioid use. Clin J Pain. 2001;17:220-8.

St. Marie B. Health care experiences when pain and substance use disorders co-exist: "Just because I'm an addict doesn't mean I don't have pain." Pain Med. 2014;15:2075-86.

Substance Abuse and Mental Health Services Administration (SAMHSA). Managing chronic pain in adults with or in recovery from substance use disorders. Treatment Improvement Protocol (TIP) Series 54. HHS Publication No. (SMA) 12-4671. Rockville, MD: Substance Abuse and Mental Health Services Administration; 2011.

CHAPTER 10

Substance Abuse and Chronic Pain

McGeary DD

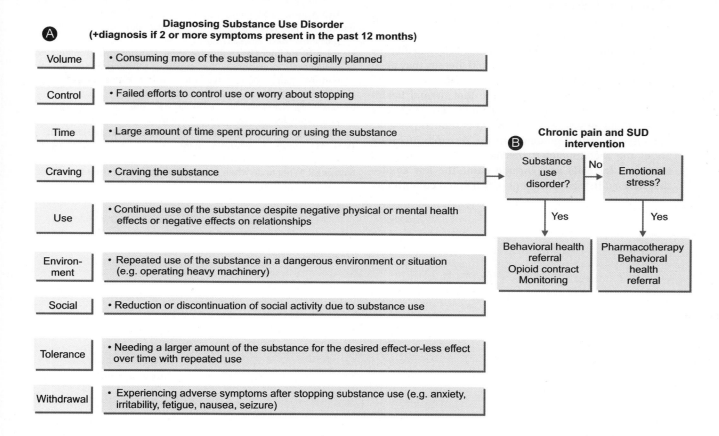

Diagnosing Substance Use Disorder
(+diagnosis if 2 or more symptoms present in the past 12 months)

Ⓐ

Volume	• Consuming more of the substance than originally planned
Control	• Failed efforts to control use or worry about stopping
Time	• Large amount of time spent procuring or using the substance
Craving	• Craving the substance
Use	• Continued use of the substance despite negative physical or mental health effects or negative effects on relationships
Environ-ment	• Repeated use of the substance in a dangerous environment or situation (e.g. operating heavy machinery)
Social	• Reduction or discontinuation of social activity due to substance use
Tolerance	• Needing a larger amount of the substance for the desired effect-or-less effect over time with repeated use
Withdrawal	• Experiencing adverse symptoms after stopping substance use (e.g. anxiety, irritability, fetigue, nausea, seizure)

Ⓑ **Chronic pain and SUD intervention**

Substance abuse (now referred to as "substance use disorder" as classified under the 5th revision of the Diagnostic and Statistical Manual of Mental Health Disorders; DSM-5) is a significant problem among people with chronic pain. Individuals with substance use disorder (SUD) are at a higher risk of comorbid chronic pain than those without SUD and are more likely to be diagnosed with a comorbid mental health problem. Unfortunately, chronic pain patients with SUD are likely to respond poorly to treatment and both problems are likely to exacerbate one another, leading to increased symptom severity. Comorbid mental health conditions may further worsen symptoms and erode response to treatment for either condition.

Opioid medications have generated the greatest amount of attention in research on chronic pain and substance use disorder comorbidity. Not only does SUD in chronic pain cause concern for patients entering treatment with opioids, but opioid medications can introduce risk for SUD in and of themselves (so much so that the DSM-5 now allows for a SUD subcategory specific to opioid medications; "Opioid Use Disorder"). It is important to note, however, that rates of substance use disorder related to alcohol and other illicit substances are also quite high among chronic pain sufferers and should be monitored closely when risk is identified.

Ⓐ *Diagnosis*: Substance use disorders (based on the DSM-5 definition) include characteristics of both abuse and dependence. A positive diagnosis of SUD must include a significant, clinical impact of substance use on functioning and quality of life, as well as other characteristics of abuse, dependence or misuse such as impaired control of substance use, craving the substance, persistent use despite negative health and social effects, persistent use despite efforts to discontinue or decrease use, increasing time spent procuring the substance, craving the substance, repeated use of the substance in dangerous situations (e.g. operating a motor vehicle), tolerance, and withdrawal.

B *Management of SUD*: Factors underlying substance use disorder and chronic pain comorbidity are complex, so assessment and intervention should tap multiple dimensions including physical, emotional, functional, behavioral, and environmental factors. Chronic pain patients should be regularly screened for SUD, especially when treated with opioid medications. Some have encouraged the use of "opioid consents" or "opioid agreements" to explicitly outline how SUD risk will be monitored and addressed in the context of opioid therapy for chronic pain. In some cases, opioid therapy may need to be discontinued if other substance use disorders arise/worsen during its use. Most agree that mental health conditions (which are common in both SUD and chronic pain) should be assessed and treated as soon as possible, but there is limited guidance in the research literature about the recommended mechanism(s) and order of treatment for SUD and chronic pain. The few studies that have addressed treatment of SUD-pain comorbidity generally recommend an integrated behavioral health intervention approach (e.g. combining elements of motivational interviewing and cognitive-behavioral therapies that can reasonably address chronic pain, SUD, and emotional distress symptoms concurrently).

SUGGESTED READING

American Psychiatric Association. Diagnostic and Statistical Manual of Mental Health Disorders: DSM-5 (5th edition). Washington, DC: American Psychiatric Publishing; 2013.

Ballantyne JC. Treating pain in patients with drug-dependence problems. BMJ. 2013;347:f3213.

Haibach JP, Beehler GP, Dollar KM, et al. Moving toward integrated behavioral intervention for treating multimorbidity among chronic pain, depression, and substance-use disorders in primary care. Med Care. 2014;52:322-7.

Morasco BJ, Duckart JP, Dobscha SK. Adherence to clinical guidelines for opioid therapy for chronic pain in patients with substance use disorder. J Gen Intern Med. 2011;26(9):965-71.

Pohl M, Smith L. Chronic pain and addiction: Challenging co-occurring disorders. J Psychoactive Drugs. 2012;44(2):119-24.

Savage SR. What to do when pain and addiction coexist. J Fam Pract. 2013;62(6):S10-6.

Sleep Disturbances and Chronic Pain

Keizer BM, Lai TT

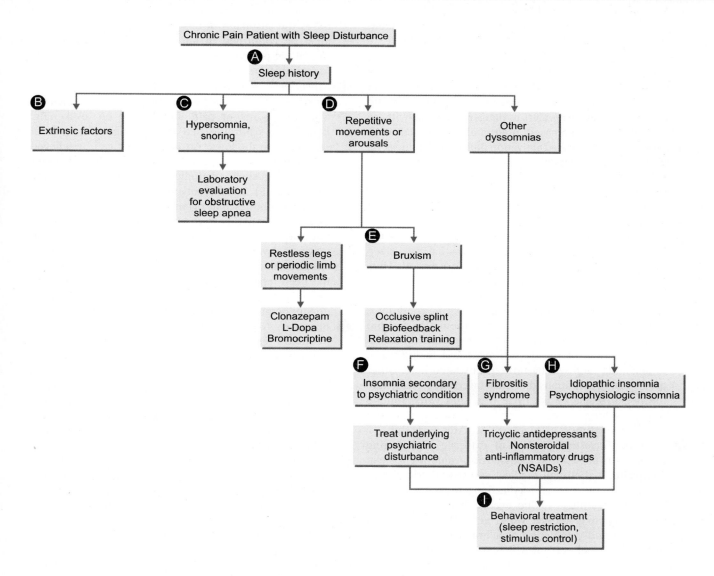

Sleep disturbances are common among chronic pain patients; complaints of poor sleep occur in up to 70% in some reported series. According to the most recent National Sleep Foundation 2015 poll, 63% of chronic pain sufferers reported that poor sleep significantly impacted both their pain experience and their daily function. Indeed, people with chronic pain averaged 42 minutes less sleep when compared with people without chronic pain. Due to the brain region and neural network overlap between sleep regulation and nociception, sleep and pain exhibit a bidirectional relationship. That is, inadequate sleep exacerbates pain which, in turn, causes microarousals that disturb sleep continuity and quality. Another factor that complicates the treatment of chronic pain patients is the negative reciprocal relationship between pain medications and sleep disruption. Increased pain medications diminish sleep quality that intensifies the patient's pain experience.

Research using electroencephalogram (EEG) indicates that every class of drug used to treat chronic pain (i.e. opioids, benzodiazepines, tricyclic antidepressants [TCAs], membrane stabilizers, and serotonin-norepinephrine reuptake inhibitors [SNRIs]) exhibit some types of negative impact on the overall sleep architecture. Opioids are especially disruptive in that they suppress both slow wave and rapid eye movement (REM) while simultaneously disrupting important *gamma-aminobutyric acid* (GABA) transmission that would normally promote sleep. Several studies have also linked chronic opioid use with ataxic breathing and central sleep apneas. With opioid prescriptions for chronic pain nearly doubling between 2000 and 2010, providers must take into account the negative sleep effects of prescribing this potent analgesic drug.

The main individual predisposing condition that contributes to sleep difficulty is a tendency towards cognitive hyperarousal. Hyperaroused people exhibit difficulty in concentrating and are easily startled, irritable, prone to anger, agitated, and hyperalert to danger. Specifically, these individuals exhibit increased prefrontal cortex activation during sleep and decreased activation during wakefulness. As an extreme example, patients who suffer from untreated post-traumatic stress disorder may perseverate in hyperarousal especially at night time, leading to severe sleep disturbance or inability to initiate and maintain sleep as well as frequent nightmares.

Ⓐ *Evaluation*: According to the World Health Organization ICD-10, a patient would be classified as having a sleep disturbance (insomnia) if they report one of the following: difficulty in initiating sleep, difficulty in maintaining sleep, or nonrestorative sleep despite adequate opportunity. The 3-P model of insomnia (i.e. predisposing conditions, precipitating circumstances, and perpetuating factors) is largely viewed as the most comprehensive model for accounting for the development and maintenance of insomnia and will be further illustrated here. Other predisposing conditions that must be considered include the person's sleep-wake cycle (e.g. shift work, routine travel resulting in jet lag, etc.), age, and their innate circadian rhythms (i.e. "night owl" working early shifts).

Ⓑ *Extrinsic Factors*: A variety of extrinsic precipitating factors also need to be assessed in evaluating a sleep complaint. A thorough medical and psychiatric history along with the use of medications must be elicited. Increasing numbers of life events that are viewed as threatening (e.g. family, work, school), coupled with the worry and rumination over impaired sleep, results in the release of cortisol which subsequently adversely affects sleep architecture. The release of cortisol has been shown to exhibit earlier time to arise, delayed time to sleep initiation, less REM sleep, and increased nocturnal awakenings. A sleep log documenting hours spent in bed, time asleep, and daytime naps, may yield useful data for the initial assessment. A collateral history from the bed partner, including information about the frequency and types of movements, arousals, and any respiratory abnormalities, is often critical in arriving at a tentative diagnosis. The perpetuating factors of insomnia include poor sleep hygiene (e.g. excessive napping, watching television in bed, caffeine prior to bed), noisy sleep environment, and the inappropriate use of alcohol, stimulants, or sedative hypnotic medications. In addition, dysfunctional cognitions about the consequences of poor sleep and fear of night time awakening due to pain, combined with worry about routine daily stressors, add to the challenge of managing this condition.

Ⓒ *Hypersomnia*: Disorders of excessive daytime sleepiness are sometimes termed hypersomnias. A complaint of hypersomnia accompanied by loud, irregular snoring raises the suspicion of obstructive sleep apnea, which must be confirmed in an overnight laboratory study (nocturnal polysomnography). Associated features may include hypertension, obesity, and morning headaches.

Ⓓ *Repetitive Movements*: Disorders associated with repetitive movements during sleep may be associated with complaints of pain and fatigue on awakening. Restless legs syndrome (RLS) consists of creeping, painful sensations in the lower extremities that can be relieved only by movement and may be associated with difficulties in initiating sleep. Periodic limb movements during sleep (PLMS) are stereotyped, repetitive movements of the extremities that occur during sleep. Virtually all patients with RLS have PLMS, although the converse is not true. The incidence of PLMS increases with age and may occur without an associated complaint of disturbed sleep. Clonazepam, 0.5–2.0 mg, or temazepam, 30 mg, has been reported to be effective. Reports of successful treatment with bromocriptine and L-Dopa may implicate dopaminergic mechanisms in the etiology of the disorder.

Ⓔ *Bruxism*: Nocturnal bruxism (tooth grinding) is frequently associated with complaints of facial pain and may involve destruction of dental and joint tissue. The cause is unknown, although psychosocial stressors are frequently implicated as trigger factors. Treatment generally consists of an occlusive splint or night guard. Biofeedback or relaxation training may be helpful in some cases; although the clinical efficacy for bruxism remains to be established.

Ⓕ *Insomnia Secondary to Psychiatric Condition*: Psychiatric conditions, particularly anxiety and depression, are often associated with disturbed sleep, although the presence of psychiatric symptoms should not preclude investigation of other possible etiologies.

Ⓖ *Pain*: Chronic musculoskeletal pain, in the absence of specific laboratory findings or evidence of connective tissue or metabolic disease, has been labeled fibrositis, fibromyalgia, or myofascial pain. The disorder is frequently associated with complaints of nonrestorative sleep. Nocturnal polysomnography in such patients often demonstrates alpha-frequency (8–11.5 Hz) intrusions in the EEG, or non-rapid eye movement sleep. The alpha EEG finding is also observed during febrile illness and postviral syndromes, but is generally absent in insomnia or depressive disorders. Treatment generally consists of a sedating tricyclic (e.g. amitriptyline) in conjunction with nonsteroidal anti-inflammatory analgesics. The use of short half-life benzodiazepines such as triazolam is generally discouraged, although benzodiazepines with intermediate range half-lives (e.g. nitrazepam) have proved useful in some cases. Behavioral approaches to treatment may often be helpful.

H *Idiopathic or Psychophysiologic Insomnia*: Idiopathic insomnia is a childhood onset disorder of initiating or maintaining sleep that cannot be attributed to other psychiatric or medical factors. Psychophysiologic, or "learned" insomnia, usually has an adult onset and is associated with agitation and somaticized tension. Patients in both groups are frequently prescribed benzodiazepines; however, the chronic nature of the complaint may lead to problems with tolerance or dependence. Ultimate resolution of the disturbance often requires some form of behavioral intervention.

I *Behavioral Treatment:* Chronic pain patients typically report spending much time in bed or at rest, although they also describe their sleep as disturbed and frequently nonrestorative. Cognitive behavioral approaches to insomnia have proven effective and include such therapies as cognitive behavioral therapy for insomnia (CBT-I), stimulus control therapy (SCT), sleep restriction therapy (SRT), and sleep hygiene and education (SHE). Cognitive and behavioral approaches to sleep disturbances focus on modifying maladaptive sleep behaviors and cognitions. SCT focuses on altering cues in the sleep environment that may be associated with arousal rather than sleep. SRT titrates the amount of time spent in bed to the patient's sleep efficiency—a ratio of sleep time to the amount of time spent in bed. SHE focuses on educating the patient about sleep processes, circadian rhythms, and individual sleep behaviors. The aforementioned approaches, and combinations thereof, may help consolidate the sleep phase and improve the subjective quality of sleep.

SUGGESTED READING

Bootzin RR, Epstein DR. Understanding and treating insomnia. Annu Rev Clin Psychol. 2011;7:435-58.

Daubresse M, Chang HY, Yu Y, et al. Ambulatory diagnosis and treatment of nonmalignant pain in the United States, 2000-2010. Med Care. 2013;51(10):870-8.

Drewes AM, Nielsen KD, Arendt-Nielsen L, et al. The effect of cutaneous and deep pain on the electroencephalogram during sleep--an experimental study. Sleep. 1997;20(8):632-40.

Institute of Medicine (US) Committee on Advancing Pain Research, Care, and Education. Relieving Pain in America: a Blueprint for Transforming Prevention, Care, Education, and Research. Washington (DC): National Academies Press (US); 2011.

Lydic R, Baghdoyan HA. Neurochemical mechanisms mediating opioid-induced REM sleep disruption. In: Lavigne G, Sessle BJ, Choinière M, Soja PJ (Eds). Sleep and Pain. Seattle: International Association for the Study of Pain (IASP). Press; 2007. pp. 99-122.

Mogri M, Khan MI, Grant BJ, et al. Central sleep apnea induced by acute ingestion of opioids. Chest. 2008;133(6):1484-8.

Morin CM. Insomnia, Psychological Assessment and Management. New York: Guilford Press; 1993.

Prinz PN, Bailey SL, Woods DL. Sleep impairments in healthy seniors: roles of stress, cortisol, and interleukin-1 beta. Chronobiol Int. 2000;17(3):391-404.

Rodenbeck A, Huether G, Rüther E, et al. Interactions between evening and nocturnal cortisol secretion and sleep parameters in patients with severe chronic primary insomnia. Neurosci Lett. 2002;324(2):159-63.

Steriade M, McCarley RW. Brain Control of Wakefulness and Sleep, 2nd edition. New York: Plenum Press; 2005.

Sternberg M, Baghdoyan HA, Lydic R. A circular conundrum for pain medicine: sleep disruption worsens pain and pain medications disrupt sleep. In: Brummett CM, Cohen SP (Eds). Managing Pain: Essentials of Diagnosis and Treatment. New York: Oxford University Press; 2013. pp. 164-82.

World Health Organization. The ICD-10 classification of mental and behavioural disorders: clinical descriptions and diagnostic guidelines. Geneva: World Health Organization; 1992.

Mood Disorders and Chronic Pain

McGeary DD

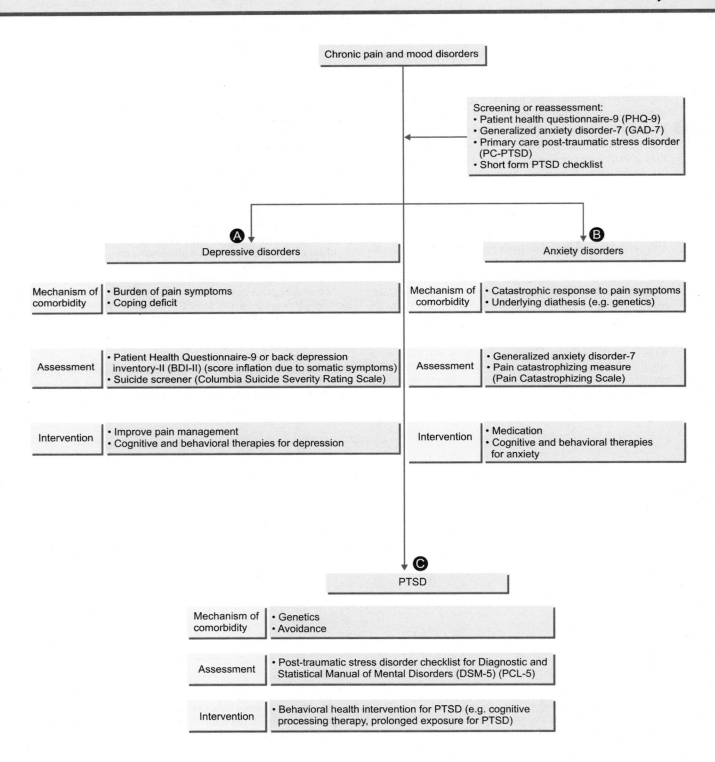

For the purpose of this chapter, "mood disorder" is interpreted as the "depressive disorders" and "anxiety disorders" chapters of the Diagnostic and Statistical Manual of Mental Disorders (DSM-5). This chapter will also include a review of "trauma and stressor-related disorders" from the DSM-5 (e.g. post-traumatic stress disorder [PTSD]). Mood disorders have long been linked to chronic pain. Prevalence of mood disorders among chronic pain populations range from 11% to 56% with depressive disorders representing the most common mood comorbidity. Past examinations of mechanisms underlying the high rate of mood disorders in chronic pain center around a diathesis-stress model in which individuals with chronic pain are hypothesized to have characteristics putting them at risk for mood disorders that are exacerbated or triggered after pain onset. Considering the potential of such disorders to complicate adherence to care plans including pain pharmacotherapy with controlled substances, screening and periodic reassessment of the chronic pain patient for mood disorders is warranted.

A *Depressive Disorders*: Depressive disorders (e.g. major depressive disorder) are a very common part of chronic pain experience. Although mechanistic studies of depression in chronic pain are ongoing, many agree that pain-related discomfort, disability and symptom burden contribute significantly to depression, and depression symptoms increase in intensity as pain-related somatic symptoms increase in number. Identifying effective methods of depression management in chronic pain are vital due to the deleterious effects of depression on quality of life and function as well as the increase in risk of suicide due to depression comorbidity. Depression has also been linked to increased risk of opioid medication misuse. Clinicians can assess for depression with commonly available screening tools (like the Patient Health Questionnaire-9), though many depression screeners are likely to result in artificially inflated depression scores due to somatic items assessed for depression (e.g. low energy, poor sleep). Interestingly, recommendations for intervention generally describe effective pain management (versus targeted depression interventions), which fits the hypothesized model that depression is a function of pain-related symptom burden.

B *Anxiety Disorders*: Anxiety disorders (e.g. panic disorder, generalized anxiety disorder) are less common in chronic pain, but still present in a large number of pain sufferers. Recent psychological conceptualizations of chronic pain have emphasized "catastrophic" thoughts about pain that drive anxiety and poor pain coping behaviors. Chronic pain patients with comorbid anxiety disorders are more disabled than those without anxiety, and more severe anxiety symptoms have been linked to increased severity of disability. Anxiety symptoms can be screened using brief measures like the generalized anxiety disorder-7 (GAD-7) item scale. Whereas depression symptoms appear to be best addressed with improved pain management, much of the research on comorbid anxiety intervention supports targeting the anxiety symptoms directly through medication and/or psychotherapeutic intervention.

C *Post-traumatic Stress Disorder:* A recent shift in focus to pain comorbidities in military populations has highlighted the unique problem of comorbid chronic pain and PTSD. PTSD is a psychiatric condition characterized by symptoms of avoidance (e.g. avoiding stimuli or situations that remind a person of trauma), negative alterations in cognition and mood, alterations in arousal and reactivity (e.g. jumpiness in response to loud noises), and symptom intrusion (i.e. flashbacks). Multiple mechanisms are likely to underlie pain and PTSD comorbidity including pre-existing (e.g. genetic) factors, components of both diagnoses that mutually maintain them (e.g. pain sufferers and PTSD sufferers may both avoid social activity), and other polymorbid diagnoses like depression. Several screening tools are available, such as the primary care PTSD (PC-PTSD) screen and the short form of the PTSD checklist. There is little available evidence guiding treatment of comorbid pain and PTSD, but targeted behavioral intervention for PTSD is recommended.

SUGGESTED READING

American Psychiatric Association. Diagnostic and Statistical Manual of Mental Health Disorders: DSM-5, 5th edition. Washington DC: American Psychiatric Publishing; 2013.

De Heer EW, Gerrits MM, Beekman AT, et al. The association of depression and anxiety with pain: a study from NESDA. PLoS One. 2014;9(10):e106907.

Dersh J, Gatchel RJ, Mayer T, et al. Prevalence of psychiatric disorders in patients with chronic disabling occupational spinal disorders. Spine (Phila Pa 1976). 2006;31(10):1156-62.

Dersh J, Polatin PB, Gatchel RJ. Chronic pain and psychopathology: research findings and theoretical considerations. Psychosom Med. 2002;64(5):773-86.

Katzman MA, Pawluk EJ, Tsirgielis D, et al. Beyond chronic pain: how best to treat psychological comorbidities. J Fam Pract. 2014; 63(5):260-4.

McGeary D, Moore M, Vriend CA, et al. The evaluation and treatment of comorbid pain and PTSD in a military setting: an overview. J Clin Psychol Med Settings. 2011;18(2):155-63.

Wasan AD, Butler SF, Budman SH, et al. Psychiatric history and psychologic adjustment as risk factors for aberrant drug-related behavior among patients with chronic pain. Clin J Pain. 2007; 23(4):307-15.

CHAPTER
13

Obesity and Chronic Pain

Fehl JE, Nouri G

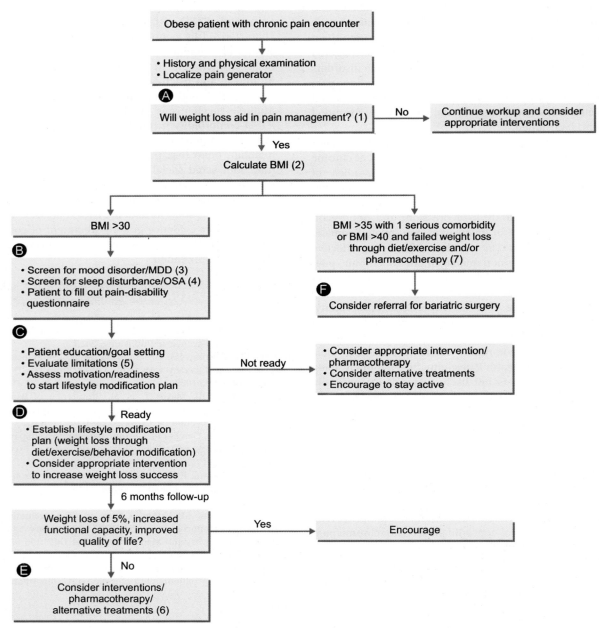

1. Weight loss has been shown to improve chronic pain caused by generalized or widespread pain, chronic headaches, fibromyalgia, pain from osteoarthritis, as well as musculoskeletal, joint and back pain; 2. BMI, body mass index. Calculated by dividing weight in kilograms by height in meters squared; 3. MDD, major depressive disorder; 4. OSA, obstructive sleep apnea; 5. Pain, range of motion limitations, finances, support, comorbidities; 6. Acupuncture for pain relief and weight loss. Osteopathic manipulative medicine combined with specific exercises; 7. Medications that are US Food and Drug Administration (FDA)-approved for short-term use (less than 3 months) are: benzphetamine, diethylpropion, phendimetrazine, phentermine, and phentermine/topiramate combination. Medications that are FDA-approved for long-term use (more than 6 months) are: orlistat, lorcaserin, naltrexone/bupropion combination

Obesity is defined as an excess of body fat sufficient to adversely affect health. The body mass index (BMI) is commonly used to define obesity and has been classified per the World Health Organization (WHO). Obesity Class I is BMI of 30–34.9 kg/m^2, Class II is BMI of 35–39.9 kg/m^2, and class III is BMI of greater than or equal to 40 kg/m^2, based on estimates by the WHO, 13% of adults worldwide were obese in 2014. In the United States, these estimates far exceed world averages, with 35% of adults being obese. The prevalence of chronic pain is comparable to prevalence of obesity worldwide. Studies have shown that approximately 40% of obese people suffer from chronic pain, and obese adults have 2–4 times greater likelihood of experiencing chronic pain compared to nonobese individuals. Comorbidity of obesity and chronic pain significantly reduces health-related quality of life and decreases functional capacity.

Accumulating evidence suggests that pain and obesity are significantly associated with each other. The potential mechanisms of this association are unclear but are likely complex, bidirectional, and mediated by various factors. Such factors include biomechanical or structural changes associated with obesity, inflammatory mediators, mood disturbances, poor sleep, and lifestyle issues. Obesity has been related to several chronic pain conditions, such as fibromyalgia, knee and back pain caused by degenerative joint disease, and neck pain. Obesity is a risk factor for developing pelvic pain, abdominal pain, neuropathic pain, chronic headaches, first time sciatica, tendinopathy and fractures. Nevertheless, weight gain can occur as a result of chronic pain through the vicious cycle of chronic pain → inactivity → obesity. Some of the behaviors involved in this vicious cycle are eating analgesia due to frustration associated with functional limitation, pain catastrophizing, and kinesiophobia.

A First, it should be determined if weight loss will be beneficial in relieving patient's chronic pain. Weight loss has been shown to improve chronic pain caused by generalized or widespread pain, chronic headaches, fibromyalgia, pain from osteoarthritis, as well as musculoskeletal, joint and back pain. If a patient's chronic pain is not attributed to their obesity, then further workup and treatment modalities should be used.

B Screening and treating for depression and sleep disturbances are essential in managing obesity-related pain. Depression facilitates and maintains the chronic pain-obesity vicious cycle through behaviors such as low self-efficacy, loss of motivation, and emotional eating. Sleep disturbances such as obstructive sleep apnea (OSA) cause weight gain and the majority of people with OSA are obese.

C Education about the importance of a lifestyle modification program, which includes weight loss and behavioral modifications, should be provided for improving pain, quality of life, and functional capacity. Patient motivation and readiness should be assessed, as they are affected by many factors. If the patient is not ready for a lifestyle modification program, he or she should be encouraged to become or stay active, as any physical activity is advantageous over sedentary behavior for relieving chronic pain.

D Before considering weight loss in a medically complicated patient, patient's primary care physician and other relevant specialists should be consulted regarding safety of weight loss. If weight loss is deemed safe, patient should be referred to a supervised weight loss program, under the direction of nutritionists, trainers, therapists and counselors. Some patients may require interventions and pharmacological pain management before starting their exercise program to increase weight loss success. Prior to initializing an aerobic exercise program patient should start with a resistance exercise program in order to develop joint stability and muscle strength. An exercise program should include a multimodal program, with a combination of aerobic exercise (3 times per week) and resistance exercise programs (2 times per week). To improve adherence, patients may need to start with walking on an incline at a slower speed, or perform non-impact exercises such as pool exercises, cycling, and elliptical machines. Patients should follow a diet compromising of lower caloric intake (at least 810 kcal/day) of high quality, nutrient dense foods.

E For patients with class I obesity and above who have failed to lose weight with weight loss and exercise alone, pharmacotherapy for weight loss can be utilized. Medications that are US Food and Drug Administration (FDA)-approved are expensive, have shown to facilitate modest weight loss, and there are concerns about their long-term use safety. There are also limited published studies on their effect on chronic pain.

F Bariatric surgery can be considered for class III obesity without comorbidities, class II obesity with at least one serious comorbidity, or class I with uncontrolled diabetes and/or metabolic syndrome. A lifestyle modification program and pharmacotherapy for weight loss are usually attempted before considering bariatric surgery. Bariatric surgery usually results in a larger degree of weight loss than lifestyle and/or pharmacotherapy therapy alone. Serious postoperative complications include changes in absorption, which cause nutritional deficiencies, and the need for reoperation, as well as surgical wound infections.

SUGGESTED READING

Ambrose, KR, Golightly YM. Physical exercise as non-pharmacological treatment of chronic pain: Why and when. Best Pract Res Clin Rheumatol. 2015;29(1):120-30.

McVinnie DS. Obesity and pain. Br J Pain. 2013;7(4):163-70.

Narouze S, Souzdalnitski D. Obesity and chronic pain: systematic review of prevalence and implications for pain practice. Reg Anesth Pain Med. 2015;40(2):91-111.

Okifuji A, Hare BD. The association between chronic pain and obesity. J Pain Res. 2015;8:399-408.

Vincent HK, Adams MC, Vincent KR, et al. Musculoskeletal pain, fear avoidance behaviors, and functional decline in obesity: potential interventions to manage pain and maintain function. Reg Anesth Pain Med. 2013;38(6):481-91.

Zdziarski LA, Wasser JG, Vincent HK. Chronic pain management in the obese patient: a focused review of key challenges and potential exercise solutions. J Pain Res. 2015;8:63-77.

CHAPTER 14

Disability and Dysfunction

McGeary DD, Eckmann MS

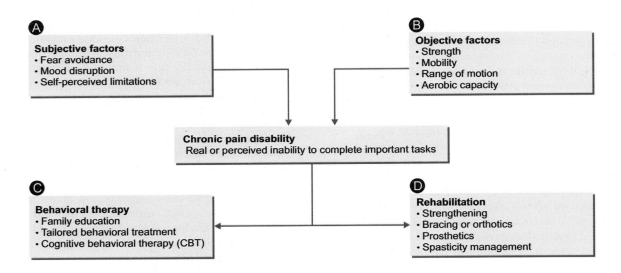

Over the past two decades, disability and dysfunction have emerged as major concepts in chronic pain experience and assessment. Although definitions widely vary, most define "disability" in terms of functional capacity for completing activities of daily living, work-related activities, home activities, and other activities of mastery and enjoyment. Since 2010, both the National Institutes of Health (NIH) and the Department of Defense have strongly emphasized disability and dysfunction as part of their respective definitions of chronic pain. The NIH Pain Consortium established a Task Force of standards of pain measurement in which they emphasized classification of chronic low back pain by the "impact" of pain on function and "normal" activity. This impact definition was strongly integrated into the standardized NIH Patient-Reported Outcomes Measurement Information System (PROMIS) assessment representing almost one-third of all items in the PROMIS short form measure. The Department of Defense Pain Management Task Force published its final report in 2010 in which they highly emphasized the contribution of "level of function" and "quality of life" to chronic pain conceptualization and assessment. Measures of functional disability have been incorporated into the Department of Defense Pain Assessment Screening Tool and Outcomes Registry (PASTOR), which also includes elements of the NIH PROMIS assessment.

Pain-related disability has widespread impact on adjustment to chronic pain vis-a-vis mood dysregulation, cognitions of burdensomeness, socioeconomic stress related to decreased work attendance and potential job loss, and inability to access external coping resources for pain management (i.e. inability to socialize and attend medical appointments for pain). Numerous models have been developed to explain the relationship between disability and chronic pain, though most recent models describe a "fear avoidance" mechanism in which concerns about pain exacerbation with activity result in functional deactivation and physical deconditioning.

A *Subjective Measures*: Pain-related disability is assessed in one of two ways. There are excellent "subjective" self-report measures of disability in which the pain sufferer is asked to rate the extent to which chronic pain affects their ability to complete daily tasks. These measures are easy to use, often require 5–10 minutes to complete, and their results highly correlate with other measures of pain and emotional adjustment.

B *Objective Measures*: Disability can also be assessed through "objective" measures of lifting capacity, aerobic capacity, gait, and range of motion. A skilled assessor (often a physical or occupational therapist) can assess function, self-limiting, motivation, and effort to give a comprehensive description of function in multiple domains. These objective measures are not as highly correlated with other domains of pain coping as subjective disability measures, but objective disability measures do offer excellent work-related disability assessment to the extent that functional capacity tests mimic work requirements. However, because objective tests require more specialized and costly assessment, disability assessment should begin with subjective measures (like the Oswestry Disability Index, a free-to-use measure that represents the gold standard in subjective disability assessment).

C *Behavioral Intervention:* Once disability is determined, the comorbid behavioral challenges versus biomechanical and neurologic challenges should be addressed concurrently. Available evidence suggests that "tailored behavioral treatment" targeting specific "fear avoidance" and other maladaptive behavior patterns is beneficial over exercise alone. Cognitive behavioral therapy (CBT) for the patient may need supplementation in the form of family education to ensure that pain-disability promoting behaviors are not inadvertently rewarded in the home setting. Prior to initiation of formal psychotherapy, providers can incorporate motivational interviewing and prescribe a graded home exercise regimen within the patient's individual safe physical limits.

D Biomechanical or neurologic deficits, especially which result in limb or trunk weakness, spasticity, or deformity, may require specific treatment and adaptation. Physical therapy, orthotics, external bracing, prosthetics, or even intrathecal therapy may be needed to improve functional outcome. Depending on the complexity or level of injury (e.g. spinal cord injury, traumatic brain injury, or amputation), a referral to a physical medicine specialist may be warranted to coordinate long-term clinical objectives.

SUGGESTED READING

Deyo RA, Dworkin SF, Amtmann D, et al. Report of the NIH Task Force on research standards for chronic low back pain. J Pain. 2014;15(6):569-85.

Gatchel RJ, McGeary DD, McGeary CA, et al. Interdisciplinary chronic pain management: past, present, and future. Am Psychol. 2014;69(2):119-30.

Office of the Army Surgeon General. (2010). Pain Management Task Force. Final Report. Providing a Standardized DoD and VHA Vision and Approach to Pain Management to Optimize the Care for Warriors and their Families. [online] Available from *www.regenesisbio.com/pdfs/journal/pain_management_task_force_report.pdf*. [Accessed January, 2017].

Ratzon NZ, Amit Y, Friedman S, et al. Functional capacity evaluation: does it change the determination of the degree of work disability? Disabil Health J. 2015;8(1):80-5.

Senlöf P, Denison E, Lindberg P. Long-term follow-up of tailored behavioural treatment and exercise based physical therapy in persistent musculoskeletal pain: A randomized controlled trial in primary care. Eur J Pain. 2009;13(10):1080-8.

Van der Meer S, Reneman MF, Verhoeven J, et al. Relationship between self-reported disability and functional capacity in patients with whiplash associated disorder. J Occup Rehabil. 2014;24(3):419-24.

World Health Organization. (1976). International Classification of Impairments, Disabilities, and Handicaps. [online] Available from *apps.who.int/iris/bitstream/10665/41003/1/9241541261_eng.pdf*. [Accessed January, 2017].

Zale EL, Lange KL, Fields SA, et al. The relation between pain-related fear and disability: a meta-analysis. J Pain. 2013;14(10): 1019-30.

CHAPTER 15

Pain Measurement

McGeary CA

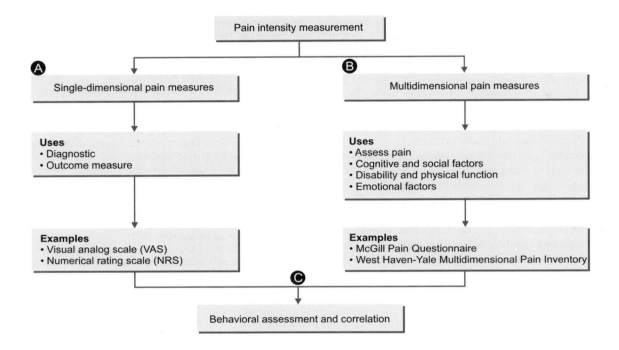

Pain is a subjective experience which can make its assessment difficult. Individual pain experience is not predicated on sensory experience alone, but is influenced by multiple factors, which include emotional state, psychological well-being, physical state, and comorbid conditions. Pain measurement may need to be adapted to individuals based on the confluent factors that impact pain. Pain measurement consists of both single dimensional and multidimensional assessment tools.

Ⓐ Pain is often initially assessed by physicians using a single dimensional pain intensity rating scale particularly since the Joint Commission identified pain as the "fifth vital sign." The most common of these assessments include the visual analogue scale and the numerical rating scale. These assessments are similar as they often assess pain on a rating scale (e.g. on a scale from 0 to 10). These scales can be helpful as a diagnostic tool or for tracking severity of pain across appointments or procedures, but to understand a patient's subjective pain experience, multidimensional pain assessments are more appropriate.

Ⓑ Self-report multidimensional tools not only assess pain, but social and cognitive factors, disability and physical function, and emotional factors that can contribute to pain. Information gathered from multidimensional assessments (along with a diagnostic interview and physical examination) can be used to treat chronic pain holistically. Common multidimensional assessments for pain are the McGill Pain Questionnaire (MPQ) and the West Haven-Yale Multidimensional Pain Inventory (WHYMPI). The MPQ is divided into three sections that measure pain intensity, how pain changes over time, and how pain is experienced. The MPI is divided into 12 subscales that measure daily activities, quality of social support, and pain impact.

Ⓒ In addition to using single-dimensional or multidimensional assessments alone or in combination, behavioral assessment methods should be employed. Behavioral assessments include clinician observations of pain behaviors during appointments such as a patient's gait, posture, bracing, rubbing, and grimacing, use of a pain diary to determine time of day or activities that exacerbate pain, and use of a pain drawing to determine location of pain.

SUGGESTED READING

Kerns RD, Turk DC, Rudy TE. The West Haven-Yale Multidimensional Pain Inventory (WHYMPI). Pain. 1985;23(4):345-56.

Lorenz KA, Sherbourne CD, Shugarman LR, et al. How reliable is pain as the fifth vital sign? J Am Board Fam Med. 2009;22(3):291-8.

Melzack R, Torgerson WS. On the language of pain. Anesthesiology. 1971;34(1):50-9.

Ramamurthy S, Alanmanou E, Rogers J. Decision Making in Pain Management, 2nd edition. Philadelphia: Elsevier; 2006.

Scott J, Huskisson EC. Graphic representation of pain. Pain. 1976; 2(2):175-84.

Stahmer SA, Shofer FS, Marino A, et al. Do quantitative changes in pain intensity correlate with pain relief and satisfaction? Acad Emerg Med. 1998;5(9):851-7.

CHAPTER
16

Provocation Discography

Feldman AT, Goff BJ

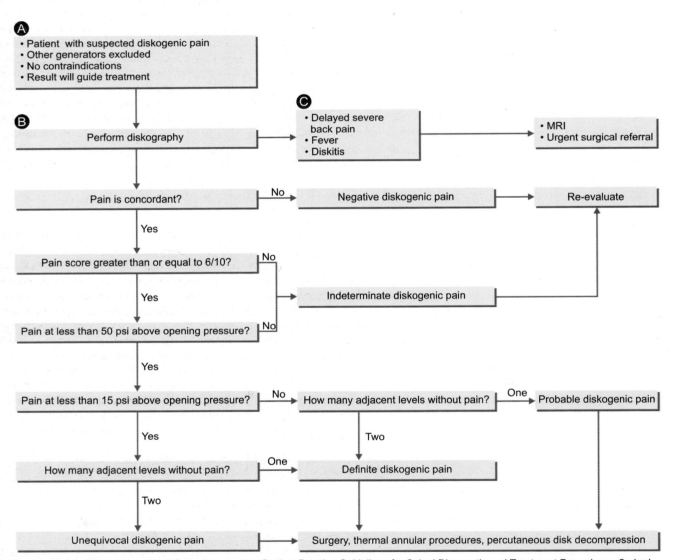

A
- Patient with suspected diskogenic pain
- Other generators excluded
- No contraindications
- Result will guide treatment

B Perform diskography

C
- Delayed severe back pain
- Fever
- Diskitis

- MRI
- Urgent surgical referral

Pain is concordant? — No → Negative diskogenic pain → Re-evaluate

Yes ↓

Pain score greater than or equal to 6/10? — No → Indeterminate diskogenic pain → Re-evaluate

Yes ↓

Pain at less than 50 psi above opening pressure? — No → Indeterminate diskogenic pain

Yes ↓

Pain at less than 15 psi above opening pressure? — No → How many adjacent levels without pain? — One → Probable diskogenic pain

Two ↓ Definite diskogenic pain

Yes ↓

How many adjacent levels without pain? — One → Definite diskogenic pain

Two ↓

Unequivocal diskogenic pain → Surgery, thermal annular procedures, percutaneous disk decompression

Probable diskogenic pain → Surgery, thermal annular procedures, percutaneous disk decompression

Source: Adapted from International Spine Intervention Society Practice Guidelines for Spinal Diagnostic and Treatment Procedures, 2nd ed.
Acknowledgments: The view(s) expressed herein are those of the author(s) and do not reflect the official policy or position of Brooke Army Medical Center, the U.S. Army Medical Department, the U.S. Army Office of the Surgeon General, the Department of the Army and Department of Defense or the U.S. Government.

Discogenic pain secondary to internal disc disruption is a significant etiology of lower back pain, a condition that costs the United States health system up to 100 billion dollars yearly. In 1994, Schwarzer et al. reported an oft-cited 39% prevalence of discogenic pain while more recently, Verrills et al. suggest a lower prevalence of 21.8% by investigating a larger population and incorporating updated procedural recommendations. While magnetic resonance imaging (MRI) is relatively sensitive in identifying pathological discs, provocative discography remains a useful tool for evaluating discogenic pain as there is a significant prevalence of asymptomatic patients with MRI changes.

As the intervertebral disc ages, degeneration can lead to height loss and fissuring of the annulus fibrosis. Height loss does not necessarily directly cause pain, however, the annular tears allow for nociceptive nerve ingrowth that responds to inflammatory cytokines. This is a suggested etiology of discogenic pain. While routine imaging (radiography, computed tomography [CT], magnetic resonance [MR]) can indicate the shape of each disc, provocation discography is the only modality, which can assist in determining whether a disc is intrinsically painful. The goal is to stimulate the disc by increasing the intervertebral disc pressure and reproducing the patient's pain. It can be done in the cervical, thoracic, or lumbar discs, with the latter being the most common.

A *Candidates for Discography:* Lumbar discogenic pain is typically a deep, dull midline aching in the low back that might radiate to the gluteal areas but rarely more distal. It usually worsens with axial loading, increased intra-abdominal pressure and after sudden bending or twisting. Provocation discography is indicated in patients who have failed conservative therapy for pain that has been present for over 4 months and is consistent with the description above. Other common pain generators such as the zygapophyseal and sacroiliac joints should have also been ruled out and the patient should have such significant pain that they are considering either surgery or more invasive interventional pain procedures. Disc stimulation should not be performed on patients who are not candidates for definitive management of discogenic pain (surgery, thermal annular procedures or percutaneous disc decompression). Other contraindications include the existence of sensory or motor loss, discitis, disc herniation with acute radiculopathy, local skin infection, coagulopathies, allergy to contrast material, and pregnancy. Contrast allergy may be pretreated with antihistamines and corticosteroids. The patient's mental status is crucial for effective discography since they must be able to effectively communicate their pain during the procedure to meet criteria. Additionally, the presence of somatization and significant psychological distress may confound the results of discography.

B *Disc Provocation:* Techniques for obtaining intradiscal access are thoroughly explained in the Practice Guidelines for Spinal Diagnostic and Treatment Procedures published by the Spine Intervention Society. Regardless of method, good practice includes infection prevention with preprocedural antibiotics, strict attention to sterile technique and incorporation of a two-needle technique to prevent the needle that accesses the disc from traversing the skin. During injection of contrast, the following data points need to be recorded at each disc: the opening pressure when contrast appears in the disc, the pressure at which the patient feels pain, the numerical rating for the pain and whether it is the same as their baseline pain. The International Association for the Study of Pain and the Spine Intervention Society have four criteria for diagnosing discogenic pain: (1) stimulation causes concordant pain, (2) the pain is rated at least 6 out of 10 on a numerical scale, (3) the pain is at a pressure less than

50 psi or less than 15 psi above opening pressure, and (4) stimulation of adjacent discs are either not painful or produce pain that is discordant at a pressure greater than 15 psi above opening pressure. Whether a test is positive or negative can be determined by categorizing it using the above criteria as outlined in the algorithm.

C *Complications:* Complications of discography include discitis, nerve root injury, accelerated disc degeneration, intravascular injection, bleeding, infection, reaction to medications used, and dural puncture among other risks. Pneumothorax and spinal cord injury are possible with cervical and thoracic procedures. Discitis is of specific concern with these procedures due to the inherent treatment limitations as well as morbidity. Patients usually present 2–4 weeks after the procedure complaining of severe back pain. Treatment is limited due to the lack of vascularity in the intervertebral disc which would provide access for the immune system or antibiotics. Besides complete history and physical, laboratory evaluations such as complete blood count, erythrocyte sedimentation rate, and MRI are indicated. In addition to discitis, any of the above complications warrant timely evaluation to facilitate early treatment.

A recent systematic review of the evidence by Manchikanti et al. described the evidence supporting the accuracy of provocation discography as fair, though it is still debatable based on the lack of outcome data in those who undergo surgical procedures. There is currently limited data supporting the use of discography prior to surgery, however, the argument can be made that properly performed discography may be able to limit unnecessary spinal fusions. Provocation discography may also accelerate disc degeneration and should be performed only when the need for information is weighed carefully. When performed according to the International Association for the Study of Pain (IASP)/Spine Intervention Society (SIS) guidelines, the false positive rate is only 9.3% (6.0% per disc evaluated). Ultimately, provocation discography is a useful tool in determining whether the source of a patient's pain is the intervertebral disc.

SUGGESTED READING

Bogduk N (Ed). International Spine Intervention Society Practice Guidelines for Spinal Diagnostic and Treatment Procedures, 2nd edition. San Francisco, CA: International Spine Intervention Society; 2013.

Carragee EJ, Don AS, Hurwitz EL, et al. 2009 ISSLS Prize Winner: Does discography cause accelerated progression of degeneration changes in the lumbar disc: a ten-year matched cohort study. Spine (Phila Pa 1976). 2009;34(21):2338-45.

Lu Y, Guzman JZ, Purmessur D, et al. Nonoperative management for discogenic back pain: a systematic review. Spine. 2014;39(16):1314-24.

Manchikanti L, Benyamin RM, Singh V, et al. An update of the systematic appraisal of the accuracy and utility of lumbar discography in chronic low back pain. Pain Physician. 2013;16: SE55-95.

Verrills P, Nowesenitz G, Barnard A. Prevalence and characteristics of discogenic pain in tertiary practice: 223 consecutive cases utilizing lumbar discography. Pain Med. 2015;16:1490-9.

CHAPTER 17

Imaging Studies

Huynh L, Levin JE, Kennedy DJ

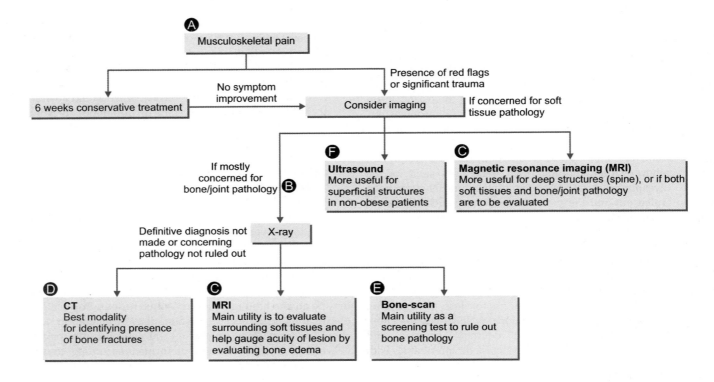

Practice guidelines recommend against the routine use of imaging in patients presenting with musculoskeletal pain. For most musculoskeletal conditions, the majority of pain resolves without any intervention. While the use of imaging may seem relatively benign, the risk is actually quite substantial. Risks associated with routine imaging include unnecessary radiation exposure, labeling patients with anatomic diagnoses that are not the true cause of their symptoms, and increased rates of surgery without improved outcomes. Some rationalize that obtaining imaging may provide reassurance to both patients and practitioners. However, this goal must be balanced by the fact that studies have demonstrated a lesser sense of well-being and higher rates of pain with lower overall health status in those who obtain imaging studies.

Ⓐ *Workup of Musculoskeletal Pain*: The purpose of imaging studies should be to provide accurate anatomic information that can be correlated to a patient's symptoms. Ideally, these findings should affect the therapeutic decision-making process. Immediate imaging may be appropriate for patients who exhibit red flags, such as those with neurologic symptoms from the spine due to progressive weakness, saddle anesthesia, bowel or bladder changes.

Other reasons to consider imaging include unexplained weight loss, fevers, or in those with a suspected fracture or significant trauma. Some at risk patient populations may also warrant earlier imaging including patients that are susceptible to infections such as intravenous (IV) drug users, those with a suspected systemic disease, or even those with a history of cancer. Early imaging may also be obtained in cases where specific treatment options may require advanced imaging, such as those receiving an epidural injection for acute radicular pain from a suspected disc herniation. Otherwise, imaging should typically be reserved for patients with persistent symptoms despite an adequate trial of conservative treatment or those with sufficient duration of symptoms to account for natural history.

The following are the various imaging studies commonly obtained for diagnostic purposes:

Ⓑ *X-ray*: X-rays have the advantage of being relatively easy and inexpensive to obtain. They provide details of bony anatomy and alignment, which can be helpful in evaluating for fractures, osteoarthritis of joints, or spinal instability (such as from spondylolisthesis). They can also show advanced signs of malignancy or osteomyelitis if the disease has significantly progressed. It is no longer recommended to obtain oblique views of the lumbar spine to evaluate for spondylolysis (pars defects), as these views expose patients to a substantial dose of radiation without providing significant diagnostic information that alters management. X-rays also have the advantage of being able to take multiple views (anterior-posterior, lateral, oblique, etc.) to show specific anatomic structures. They can also be taken with the patient in different positions to show the dynamic nature of a structure, such as flexion and extension views of the lumbar spine, which may be helpful in some conditions such as spondylolisthesis.

(C) *Magnetic Resonance Imaging (MRI):* MRI uses interaction between magnetic forces and radio waves to create detailed images of the body. The advantages of MRI include excellent visualization of soft tissue and neurologic structures with no exposure to ionizing radiation. Additionally, MRIs are oftentimes useful in the evaluation of edema in order to establish the acuity of conditions such as tendinopathies, muscle tears, and vertebral body compression fractures; MRIs increase sensitivity for fractures when compared to X-rays. The disadvantages of MRI are the high cost and the requirement for patients to remain still in a small, enclosed space. Open MRIs were developed to accommodate claustrophobic patients; however, the image quality is not currently on par with closed MRIs. Lastly, as with all imaging tests, anatomic abnormalities are ubiquitous in asymptomatic individuals. MRIs may carry the highest risk of demonstrating asymptomatic findings that may lead to inappropriate treatment or a diminished sense of well-being.

(D) *Computed Tomography (CT):* CT scans use multiple X-rays to produce cross-sectional layers to provide detailed views of the body. CT scans provide high quality images of the bony structures. CT scans are typically more readily available than MRI, and the cost is substantially less. They may have increased sensitivity for bony pathology and fractures, even when compared to an MRI. They also may be used to evaluate patients who are unable to obtain an adequate MRI due to claustrophobia, body habitus, or obscured images from metallic artifact. Other MRI contraindications such as pacemakers or spinal cord stimulators, may make CT scans the imaging modality of choice when cross sectional evaluation is indicated. Disadvantages of CT scans include exposure to ionizing radiation and poor visualization of soft tissue. The average effective radiation dose of a CT spine is 6 mSv as compared to 1.5 mSv for a lumbar spine X-ray, and 6.3 mSv for bone scan.

(E) *Bone Scan:* Bone scan is a nuclear imaging test that can detect abnormalities in bone turnover. Prior to scanning, the patient is injected with a small amount of radioactive material, such as technetium-99m-MDP. Then, the patient is scanned with a gamma camera. There are variants of scanning including limited scan, whole-body scan, three-phase scan, and single-photon emission computed tomography (SPECT) imaging. Bone scans are useful in detecting occult fractures, inflammatory processes such as osteomyelitis and metastatic disease. Bone scans can detect even as small as a 5% change in bone turnover, whereas radiographs and CT detect lucency after 40–50% of the bone minerals have already been lost. The disadvantage to bone scan is the increased radiation exposure compared to MRI and X-ray. Additionally, while bone scans are very sensitive for bony turnover, they may stay positive for 6–9 months after clinical resolution of the disorder. Thus, they may be more useful as a screening test to rule out a condition, rather than as a definitive diagnostic test.

(F) *Ultrasound (US):* US imaging is based on the interaction of high frequency sound waves with tissues it encounters. The US transducer emits sound waves that are then reflected back to the transducer to produce an image. The advantage of US is the lack of radiation exposure and the lower cost than CT/MRI. US is especially useful for dynamic scanning of joints, such as when evaluating for shoulder impingement. Disadvantages of US include greater variance in image quality, limited ability to visualize deeper structures, especially in obese patients, and variability in quality which is dependent upon the skill of the operator.

SUGGESTED READING

Brenner AI, Koshy J, Morey J. The bone scan. Semin Nucl Med. 2012;43(1):11-26.

Kendrick D, Fielding K, Bentley E, et al. Radiography of the lumbar spine in primary care patients with low back pain: randomized controlled trial. BMJ. 2001;322(7283):400-5.

Mettler FA, Huda W, Yoshizumi TT, et al. Effective doses in radiology and diagnostic nuclear medicine: a catalog. Radiology. 2008;248(1):254-63.

Modic MT, Obuchowski NA, Ross JS, et al. Acute low back pain and radiculopathy: MR imaging findings and their prognostic role and effect on outcome. Radiology. 2005;237(2):597-604.

Rhea JT, DeLuca SA, Llewellyn HJ, et al. The oblique view: An unnecessary component of the initial adult lumbar spine examination. Radiology. 1980;134(1):45-7.

Srinivas SV, Deyo RA, Berger ZD. Application of "less is more" to low back pain. Arch Intern Med. 2012;172(13):1016-20.

Electromyography and Nerve Conduction Studies (Upper/Lower)

Nagpal A, Benfield JA

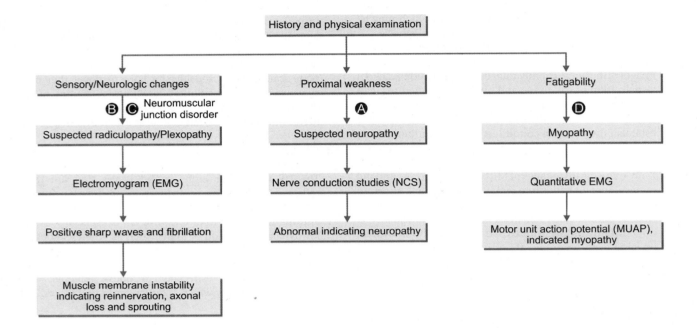

An electromyogram (EMG) is an extension of the history and physical examination. It uses sensory and motor nerve conduction studies (NCS) and qualitative or quantitative needle EMG to diagnose a variety of nervous system disorders along the motor unit, including damage to anterior horn cells, peripheral nerves, the neuromuscular junction, and muscle fibers. These conditions range from anterior lateral sclerosis, myopathies, myasthenia gravis, Guillain-Barré syndrome, plexopathies, motor radiculopathies, Carpal tunnel syndrome and peripheral neuropathies. Sensory and motor NCS provide information on large myelinated nerves by stimulating the nerve and recording its associated action potential with electrodes placed on a patient's skin. Qualitative and quantitative needle EMG investigate a variety of pathologies by assessing rest and insertional activity, motor unit action potential and the ability to recruit muscle fibers in normal, myogenic, or neurogenic patterns. There are some limitations, as temperature of the extremity will significantly alter the NCS. Electrical interference is ubiquitous, and proper techniques should be employed to minimize this. Time duration after a significant injury requires 7–21 days for demyelination to be seen with EMG. Edema in the extremities limits the ability of surface electrodes, in NCS, to record action potentials and increases the risk for soft tissue injury during needle examination. Additionally, patients on chemical anticoagulation may have a limited ability for needle examination. In conclusion, EMG evaluations can be helpful in locating nerve lesions but rarely delineates the etiology. It does however, differentiate axonal from demyelinating lesions and establish localization (unilateral, symmetric, asymmetric, sensory and/or motor involvement), but responsibility for the final diagnosis lies with the clinician.

Ⓐ *Focal Entrapment and Peripheral Neuropathies*: A variety of peripheral nerves can be studied. However, the median, ulnar, radial, common fibular, tibial, and sural nerves are the most commonly studied. NCS distinguish location, sensory and/or motor fiber or nerve involvement, presence of demyelination, axonal injury and/or conduction block. Qualitative EMG is used to for evaluation of muscle denervation and nerve localization. Unilateral lesions can involve comparing NCS and qualitative EMG to the asymptomatic contralateral limb. This allows for improved evaluation and accuracy in identifying a nerve lesion. For example, it is recommended to evaluate the asymptomatic limb in a fibular nerve lesion in cases of foot drop. In peripheral neuropathies of the upper or lower extremities, three limbs are tested for evaluation for a generalized peripheral neuropathy versus one affecting only upper or lower extremities.

B *Radiculopathies:* NCS and EMG are mandatory for an appropriate radiculopathy evaluation. Evaluation involves examination of 5–7 muscles per limb, including paraspinal muscles, for rest and insertional activity, presence of denervation potentials, and neurogenic recruitment. A radiculopathy is defined by finding two or more muscles in the same myotome with different peripheral nerve innervation with membrane instability illustrated through denervation potentials (i.e. positive sharp waves and fibrillation potentials) and/or a neurogenic recruitment pattern. In mild or moderate cases, NCS are normal. However, severe cases involving more than 80% axonal damage abnormal motor NCS can be seen. Needle EMG is imperative for acuity, localization and grading of the radiculopathy.

C *Plexopathies:* Brachial, lumbar, and sacral plexopathies can be evaluated using NCS and qualitative EMG. Appropriate sensory and motor NCS need to be performed as well. NCS aid in localizing plexopathies into pre- or postdorsal ganglion lesions. Motor NCS need to be completed including a close analysis for any decrease in amplitude allowing for an approximation axonal loss. Unilateral plexopathies involve comparison to the asymptomatic side. Sensory and motor NCS changes appear between 5–10 days and 2–7 days, respectively.

Qualitative EMG needle examination will show increased activity, denervation potentials, and decreased recruitment between 7 days and 30 days. When referring or evaluating a patient for a plexopathy, 14–21 days postinjury should be allowed prior to examination unless a baseline examination is wanted.

D *Myopathies and Neuromuscular Junction (NMJ) Disorders:* Myopathies are rare, diverse and complex and require quantitative EMG. Assessment of motor unit size, recruitment, and quantity of motor units recruited in addition to insertional and rest activity for a myopathic recruitment pattern is necessary. NCS are usually normal with exception of a possible decrement in motor NCS amplitude. Neuromuscular junction disorders like myasthenia gravis can be evaluated using a special NCS technique known as repetitive stimulation. Myopathy and NMJ testing require an experienced electromyographer. Coinciding laboratory studies should be ordered along with the quantitative EMG testing in myopathies.

SUGGESTED READING

Dumitru D, Amato AA, Zwaats MJ, et al. Electrodiagnostic Medicine, 2nd edition. Philadelphia: Hanley and Belfus; 2002.

CHAPTER
19

Small Fiber Neuropathy

Bhavaraju-Sanka R

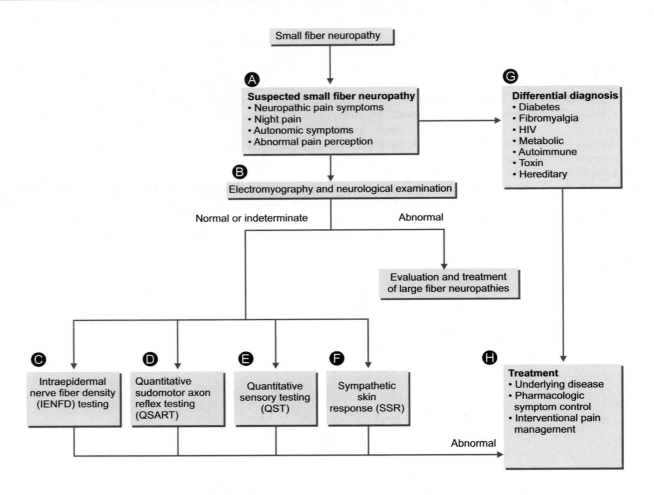

INTRODUCTION

Small fiber neuropathy is defined as a disorder of sensory nerves caused by abnormalities in thinly myelinated A delta fiber (Aδ) and unmyelinated C nerve fibers **(Fig. 1)**. It causes a painful neuropathy that can be difficult to diagnose. Recent electrophysiological and histological methods have been developed to help improve the diagnosis.

These nerve fibers are the smallest diameter fibers and are responsible for generation of sense of pain in response to noxious mechanical, thermal, and chemical stimulation. The Aδ fibers also perform preganglionic sympathetic and parasympathetic functions while C fibers play a role in postganglionic functions of the sympathetic and parasympathetic nervous systems. The myelinated Aδ

fibers respond to cold perception and pain. These fibers are abundant in the peripheral nerves.

DIAGNOSTIC CRITERIA

Stewart et al. defined small fiber neuropathy as a sensory neuropathy manifested by paresthesias that are typically painful, along with abnormal findings of small-fiber function on at least one of the following: (1) neurological examination; (2) specialized electrodiagnostic testing; (3) or pathological studies. Though, small fiber neuropathy can coexist with large fiber neuropathy, presence of predominant large fiber dysfunction like reduced proprioception at toes, absent or reduced vibration at ankles, distal weakness or atrophy, generalized areflexia, or abnormal routine nerve conduction

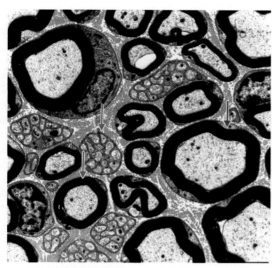

Fig. 1: Electron micrograph of the sural nerve. The blue arrow shows a large diameter myelinated fiber, the purple arrow marks a small diameter myelinated fiber and the red arrow marks a Remak bundle in which one non-myelinating Schwann cell associates with multiple unmyelinated C-fibers which are ensheathed in Schwann cell pockets
Source: Themistocleous AC, et al. (2014).

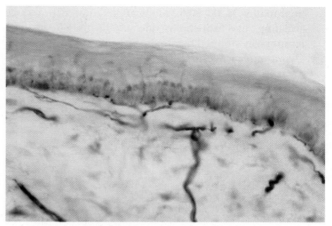

Fig. 2: Normal intraepidermal nerve fiber density (IENFD)

studies of electromyography are considered exclusion for diagnosis of small fiber neuropathy.

INCIDENCE

The exact incidence and prevalence of small fiber neuropathy is unknown. Studies to assess the epidemiology were limited due to absence of widely accepted diagnostic criteria and testing. A study in Netherlands published in 2013 estimated the minimal incidence to be 11.73 (95% confidence interval 7.12–18.22) cases/100,000 inhabitants with a minimum prevalence of 52.95 (95% confidence interval 42.47–65.23) cases/100,000. These values are expected to be higher as awareness of this condition increases and the diagnostic testing becomes more widely available.

A *Clinical Presentation:* Symptoms include burning, tingling, itching, prickly pain, shooting pain, electrical shock like pain, achy pain and sensitivity to normal or noxious stimulation, and tight or cold feeling in extremities. All the symptoms tend to be worse at night and disturb sleep. Symptoms are often length dependent (worse distally then proximally) but certain small fiber neuropathies can cause patchy or non-length-dependent symptoms affecting face/trunk, etc.

Symptoms of abnormal autonomic function may be present. These include reduced or increased sweating, skin discoloration, dry eyes, dry mouth, loss of hair growth in arms and legs, abnormal light sensitivity due to accommodation changes, orthostatic intolerance/hypotension, early satiety, fullness, bloating, constipation and/or diarrhea, urinary urgency, hesitancy, incomplete emptying, incontinence, erectile dysfunction, etc.

Examination typically shows abnormalities in temperature and pain perception with relatively preserved vibration and proprioception. In many patients, the neurological examination may be completely normal. There is no weakness, muscle atrophy, or abnormal reflex.

B *Diagnostic Workup:* Routine nerve conduction studies evaluate the large nerve fibers are normal. But, due to coexistence of mild large fiber neuropathy in some of these patients, mild abnormalities in sensory nerve conduction studies (like abnormal sural sensory response) may be seen. Various other methods are available for evaluation of small nerve fiber function.

C *Intraepidermal Nerve Fiber Density (IENFD) Testing:* Skin punch biopsy for evaluation of IENFD testing is a well-validated and reproducible testing method for evaluation of small fiber neuropathy. It can be performed at bedside but needs a specialized pathology laboratory with trained neuropathologist for interpretation. It has 92% sensitivity for diagnosis of small fiber neuropathy. A 3 mm punch biopsy at the distal leg (10 cm above the lateral malleolus) is the suggested site to confirm the diagnosis. Other common sites of testing include foot, distal thigh, proximal thigh, or other sites based on symptoms. A proximal site may help differentiate a length-dependent from a non-length-dependent neuropathy. Normal density varies with age, gender and body site. Rabbit polyclonal anti-PGP 9.5 antibodies are used to stain the nerve fibers **(Figs 2 and 3)**. The density is calculated in at least three sections as the number of IENF per length of the section (IENF/mm).

D *Quantitative Sudomotor Axon Reflex Testing (QSART):* This test measures stimulated sweat output using axon reflex. Acetylcholine is iontophoresed to cause sweating by axon reflex using specialized sweat capsule. Relative change in humidity of nitrogen gas is measured and plotted as a graph **(Fig. 4)**. The area under the curve is measured to quantitatively evaluate sweating. Normal values are available for foot, distal leg, proximal leg and forearm. It needs special equipment and thus not widely available. The sensitivity of QSART in small fiber neuropathy is 60–80%. Medications that can reduce sweating like anticholinergic medications must be temporarily stopped before the test.

E *Quantitative Sensory Testing (QST):* QST utilizes measuring temperature and vibratory thresholds to assess small and large nerve fibers respectively. Special equipment is available for clinical and research use.

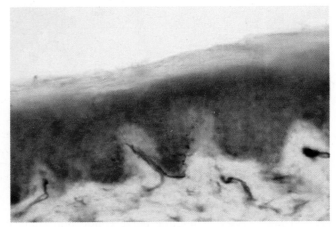

Fig. 3: Reduced intraepidermal nerve fiber density (IENFD)

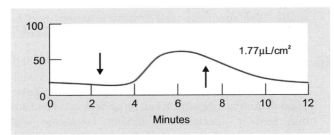

Fig. 4: QSART graph showing relative change in humidity of nitrogen gas

QST can be abnormal in disorders of the central nervous system and peripheral nervous system. The sensitivity ranges from 60% to 85%.

F *Sympathetic Skin Response (SSR):* SSR is an older widely available and inexpensive method to assess the small nerve fibers. It utilizes the reflex change in sweat-related skin electrical potential that can be elicited by unexpected stimuli like electrical shock to a nerve. It can be measured using routine electromyographic equipment. The sensitivity and specificity of this test in detecting small fiber neuropathy is low. The response amplitude declines with habituation. One study (Evans et al.) showed that it was abnormal in only 10% of patients with suspected small fiber neuropathy.

G *Etiology:* Small fiber neuropathy can be seen secondary to many common and uncommon disorders. A systematic assessment for the cause is recommended unless the patient has a known pre-existing condition like diabetes or human immunodeficiency virus (HIV) infection. The most common etiology is diabetes mellitus and small fiber neuropathy has been reported in patients with impaired glucose tolerance or abnormal fasting glucose levels. Other causes are included in the table below **(Table 1)**. Autoimmune disorders especially Sjögren's syndrome can cause small fiber neuropathy. Diagnosis may be difficult as neuropathy can be the presenting manifestation even before the onset of Sicca symptoms. Various toxins like alcohol can also cause small fiber dysfunction. HIV infection typically causes a predominant small fiber dysfunction. Idiopathic small fiber neuropathy is also very common and is the cause in most of the elderly patients above the age of 60 years. Some of these patients may have an inflammatory or autoimmune basis to them and some studies have shown improvement with immunomodulatory treatments. Some recent articles also showed that 40–60% of patients diagnosed of fibromyalgia had reduced IENFD suggesting some of them may have unrecognized small fiber neuropathy.

Table 1: Etiology of small fiber neuropathy	
Condition	*Recommended testing*
Diabetes or impaired glucose tolerance	HbA1C or oral glucose tolerance
B12 deficiency	B12, methylmalonic acid
Metabolic	Thyroid function tests, lipid panel
Sjögren's syndrome	SSA, SSB, Schirmer test, Rose Bengal corneal staining, minor salivary gland biopsy
Other connective tissue disorders	ANA, DS-DNA
Autoimmune	Voltage-gated potassium channel antibody, nicotinic acetylcholine receptor antibody
Sarcoidosis	Angiotensin converting enzyme level, chest X-ray
Celiac disease	Gliadin antibody, tissue transglutaminase antibody
Amyloidosis/Paraproteinemia	Immunofixation, quantitative immunoglobulins, light chains
Toxic (Chemo/alcohol/drugs)	History
Hereditary	Genetic testing for HSAN I, HSAN II, SCN9A, SCN 10A, Fabry's disease, Tangier's disease

ANA, antinuclear antibodies; DS-DNA, double stranded DNA, SSA, Sjögren's syndrome A; SSB, Sjögren's syndrome B

Box 1: Medications to treat small fiber neuropathy

Anticonvulsants
Gabapentin
Pregabalin
Topiramate
Lamotrigine
Tricyclics
Amitriptyline
Nortriptyline
SNRI (Serotonin–norepinephrine reuptake inhibitor)
Venlafaxine
Duloxetine
Milnacipran
Sodium channel blockers
Carbamazepine
Oxcarbazepine
Mexiletine
Lidocaine patch
Lidocaine infusion
Others
Topical capsaicin
Alpha lipoic acid
Opioid analgesics

H *Treatment:* Treatment of small fiber neuropathy is symptomatic unless an underlying cause is found. Medications currently available can reduced the pain between 20–40%. Patient should be made aware of this, so realistic goals and expectations can be set. Medications include anticonvulsants, tricyclic antidepressants, serotonin norepinephrine reuptake inhibitors, sodium channel blockers, opioids and others **(Box 1)**. Medications can be used as monotherapy or in combination. Other agents that have been reported to help in literature are tramadol, alpha lipoic acid. Other modalities that have been reported to be helpful include spinal cord stimulators and intrathecal morphine pumps. Larger long term, randomized studies are needed to prove their benefit. Nonpharmacological methods that have been tried include warm water or cold-water soaks, aspirin soaks, massage and elevation.

Treating the underlying condition is recommended where a cause has been identified. Studies have shown that diet control and exercise can show improvement in IENFD in patients with diabetes. In suspected autoimmune small fiber neuropathies, small case studies have shown improvement with intravenous immunoglobulin. It has been reported to help neuropathies associated with sarcoidosis, celiac disease and Sjogren's syndrome.

SUGGESTED READING

Devigili G, Tugnoli V, Penza P, et al. The diagnostic criteria for small fiber neuropathy: from symptoms to neuropathology. Brain. 2008;131:1912-25.

Kluding PM, Pasnoor M, Singh R, et al. The effects of exercise on neuropathic symptoms, nerve function and cutaneous innervation in people with diabetic peripheral neuropathy. J Diabetes Complications. 2012;26(5):424-9.

Lacomis D. Small fiber neuropathy. Muscle Nerve. 2002;26:173-88.

Lauria g, Hsieh ST, Johansson O, et al. European federation of Neurological Societies/Peripheral Nerve Society Guidelines on the use of skin biopsy in the diagnosis of small fiber neuropathy. Report of a joint task force of the European Federation of Neurological Societies and Peripheral Nerve Society. Eur J Neurol. 2010;17:903-12.

McIlduff CE, Rutkove SB. Critical appraisal of use of ahlph lipoic avid (thioctic acid) in the treatment of symptomatic diabetic polyneuropathy. Ther Clin Risk Manag. 2011;7:377-85.

Peters MJ, Bakkers M, Merkies IS, et al. Incidence and prevalence of small fiber neuropathy. A survey in the Netherlands. Neurology. 2013;81(15):1356-60.

Themistocleous AC, Ramirez JD, Sierra J, et al. The clinical approach to small fibre neuropathy and painful channelopathy. Pract Neurol. 2014;14:368-79.

CHAPTER 20

Differential Epidural/ Spinal Blockade

Boies BT

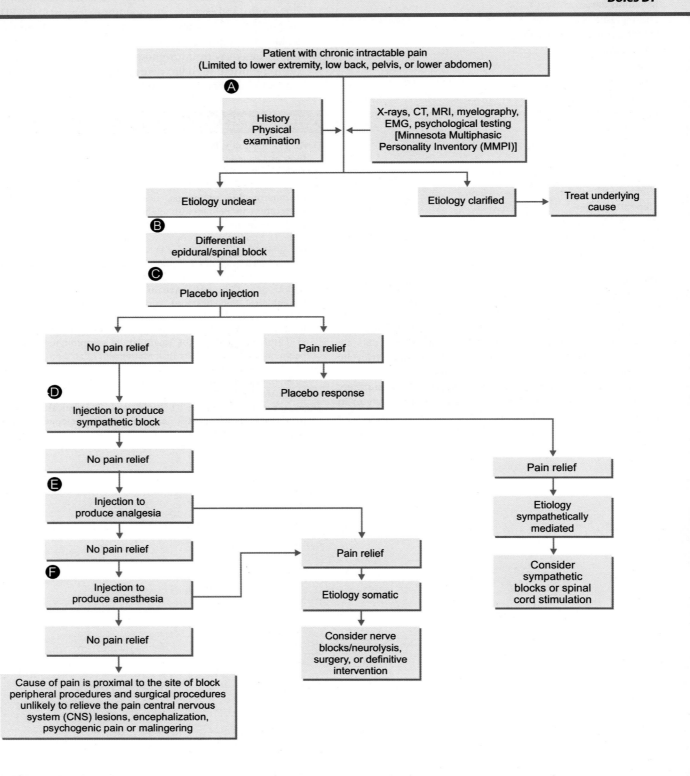

Patient with chronic intractable pain
(Limited to lower extremity, low back, pelvis, or lower abdomen)

A History Physical examination

X-rays, CT, MRI, myelography, EMG, psychological testing [Minnesota Multiphasic Personality Inventory (MMPI)]

Etiology unclear

Etiology clarified → Treat underlying cause

B Differential epidural/spinal block

C Placebo injection

No pain relief

Pain relief

Placebo response

D Injection to produce sympathetic block

No pain relief

Pain relief

Etiology sympathetically mediated

Consider sympathetic blocks or spinal cord stimulation

E Injection to produce analgesia

No pain relief

Pain relief

Etiology somatic

Consider nerve blocks/neurolysis, surgery, or definitive intervention

F Injection to produce anesthesia

No pain relief

Cause of pain is proximal to the site of block peripheral procedures and surgical procedures unlikely to relieve the pain central nervous system (CNS) lesions, encephalization, psychogenic pain or malingering

Many patients are referred to the pain clinic with chronic pain problems of unknown etiology despite extensive evaluation. Theoretically, specifically blocking different nerve fiber types could determine the mechanism of pain (sympathetically-mediated/visceral, somatic, or central in origin). The differential epidural/spinal block was developed to do this by taking advantage of differential sensitivity of nerve fibers to local anesthetic agents **(Table 1)**.

The differential spinal block was first described by Sarnoff and Arrowood (1946) and later modified by Raj and Ramamurthy (1988) to include differential epidural blocks. A modified retrograde spinal block has also been described. While this procedure is the most useful for patients with pain in the lower extremities, lower abdomen, pelvis, or low back given its neuraxial nature, the epidural form can also be safely used for thoracic pain.

However, more recent analysis of this procedure has called its validity into question. First, it is unlikely that one could reliably block just one type of fiber without causing partial blockade of others, as the local anesthetic concentration required to block each fiber type likely is described by overlapping Gaussian distributions. Furthermore, intrathecal blockade of roots only below L2 will leave sympathetic fibers unaffected, as all white rami communicantes, and thus the sympathetic outflow from the spinal cord exits the cord between T1 and L2. Additionally, the premise behind the procedure is that only afferent fibers are affected, with no mention of the pain-modulating descending inhibitory fibers that may be blocked at various concentrations of local anesthetic as well. Finally, prolonged pain relief that extends beyond the expected duration of action of a local anesthetic is a well-known phenomenon to practicing pain physicians and may relate to changes in central processing. Return of pain, therefore, may be delayed past the return of normal function of a specific fiber type, reducing the specificity of the procedure. These represent just some of the considerations that may limit the usefulness of this procedure from a diagnostic perspective.

Nonetheless, with these caveats being presented, both the traditional and modified retrograde techniques for performing this procedure are described below:

A A thorough history and physical examination is required in the initial evaluation of all patients with pain. Additional studies such as imaging and electromyography (EMG)/nerve conduction are performed as indicated. Psychological testing completes the initial evaluation. At this point, a diagnosis can usually be ascertained and treatment may begin. If the etiology is still unclear, a differential block can be considered.

B The differential block can be performed as a progressive spinal or retrograde (modified) spinal, continuous spinal, or continuous epidural block. An advantage of the continuous technique is that patients do not have to lie on their side with a needle in place for the duration of the entire procedure. Disadvantages of the epidural technique are slower onset and less clear endpoints. Since these patients are receiving a central neuraxial block, the usual monitoring, IV access, and airway resuscitation equipment should be immediately available.

C Perform the spinal or epidural block in the usual manner. For the spinal technique (noncontinuous), patients must remain on their side with the needle in the subarachnoid space during the entire procedure. In order to provide proper patient blinding for this diagnostic injection, all injections should be made with syringes that have the same volume and appearance. The sensation in the affected area is tested with pinprick (to evaluate Aδ and C fiber pathways) and sympathetic function (to evaluate B fiber pathways) with the cutaneous temperature probe or sympathogalvanic response immediately before and also 5 minutes after each injection. Whether an epidural or spinal technique is chosen, the initial injection should be with 0.9% saline as a placebo. Pain relief following this injection is considered a placebo response; however, a placebo response does not rule out organic etiology because 30–35% of patients whose pain is of an organic etiology can obtain significant pain relief with a placebo.

Table 1: Classification of nerve fibers on the basis of fiber size (relating fiber size to fiber function and sensitivity to local anesthetics)

Group	Fiber	Conduction	Modality	Sensitivity to local anesthetics (Subarachnoid procaine)
A (Myelinated) Alpha	20 µm	100 mps	Large motor, proprioception (reflex activity)	1%
Beta	20 µm	100 mps	Small motor, touch, and pressure	1%
Gamma	20 µm	100 mps	Muscle spindle fibers (muscle tone)	1%
Delta	4 µm	5 mps	Temperature and sharp pain Possibly touch	0.5%
B (myelinated)	3 µm	3–14 mps	Preganglionic autonomic fibers	0.25%
C (unmyelinated)	0.5–1 µm	1.2 mps	Dull pain, temperature, touch (like delta, but slower)	0.5%

MPS, meters per second

Source: With permission from Ramamurthy S, Winnie AP: Regional anesthetic techniques for pain relief. Semin Anesth. 1985;4:237-46.

D If the patient receives no pain relief with the placebo, inject a low concentration of local anesthetic (0.25% procaine for spinal or 0.25–0.5% lidocaine for epidural) to produce a sympathetic block. If the pain is relieved with a confirmed sympathetic block and with intact sensation, the pain could be sympathetically mediated. This patient's pain may respond to a series of sympathetic blocks or spinal cord stimulation. Misdiagnosis can occur if presence of sympathetic block and absence of sensory block is not verified.

E If the patient continues to have pain, inject a higher concentration of local anesthetic (0.5% procaine for spinal, 0.5–1% lidocaine for epidural). If pain is relieved after loss of sensation to pinprick, a somatic etiology is possible, and the patient may be a candidate for further peripheral nerve blocks or surgery.

F If the pain is not relieved with a sensory nerve block, inject a concentration of local anesthetic (1% or higher concentration of procaine for spinal, 1–2% lidocaine for epidural) to more completely block sensory (Aβ) and motor (Aα) fibers. If the pain is relieved, a somatic etiology is possible and peripheral nerve blocks or surgery may be helpful. If the patient obtains no pain relief with complete somatic nerve block, the etiology of the pain may be proximal to the site of the block, and possibly neither peripheral blocks nor surgical procedures will be of benefit. No pain relief with this procedure can occur in the case of central nervous system (CNS) lesions, encephalization, malingering, or psychogenic pain.

The differential sensory block is independent of the local anesthetic injected in the epidural space, so one could potentially use an alternative to lidocaine, though lidocaine was mentioned here given its speed of onset and short duration of action.

Complications of the differential epidural/spinal block procedure are the same as those associated with other spinal or epidural procedures. These include hypotension secondary to sympathetic block, postdural puncture headache, nerve or spinal cord injury, backache, infection, bleeding, and hematoma.

DIFFERENTIAL BLOCK—MODIFIED TECHNIQUE

With this technique, the indications and the patient preparation are similar to that of the standard differential epidural and spinal technique. After injection of the placebo, if the pain persists, a high concentration of local anesthetic such as 5% procaine for spinal or 2% lidocaine for epidural is injected to ensure good sympathetic, sensory, and motor block. The spinal needle is removed and the patient is turned to the supine position. If the patient has no pain relief despite having a significant sympathetic, sensory, and motor block in the painful area, then the etiology may be proximal to the site of block. This patient may not benefit from procedures such as injections or surgery. Proximal etiology such as CNS lesions, encephalization, malingering, or psychogenic pain is to be considered.

If the patient has pain relief, then the etiology could potentially be either sympathetic or somatic. The patient is observed for return of pain while the sensory and sympathetic blocks are simultaneously monitored. If the pain relief is present only for the duration of sensory block, then a somatic etiology is possible. If the pain relief persists even after recovery from the sensory block, then this patient has a pain condition in which long-term pain relief follows temporary interruption of sympathetic and somatic pathways. This patient could have sympathetically mediated pain or a condition that may be relieved by repeated local anesthetic blocks.

This technique has several advantages. Patients do not have to lie on their side after injection of the local anesthetic. This is comfortable for the patient and also facilitates examination of the patient to evaluate the effectiveness of the local anesthetic block while attempting to reproduce the painful maneuvers. The time required to perform this technique is much shorter than that for the classical technique, especially when the pain is not likely to be relieved despite significant sensitive motor block. Endpoints are also much better defined than in the classical technique.

SUGGESTED READING

Fink BR. Mechanisms of differential axial blockade in epidural and subarachnoid anesthesia. Anesthesiology. 1989;70(5):851-8.

Hogan QH, Abram SE. Neural blockade for diagnosis and prognosis. A review. Anesthesiology. 1997;86(1):216-41.

Raj PP, Ramamurthy S. Differential nerve block studies. In: Raj P (Ed). Practical Management of Pain. Chicago: Year Book; 1988. p. 173.

Sarnoff SJ, Arrowood JG. Differential spinal block; a preliminary report. Surgery. 1946;20:150-9.

White JL, Stevens RA, Beardsley D, et al. Differential epidural block. Does the choice of local anesthetic matter? Reg Anesth. 1994;19(5):335-8.

Diagnostic Neural Blocks

Patel S, Roe TC

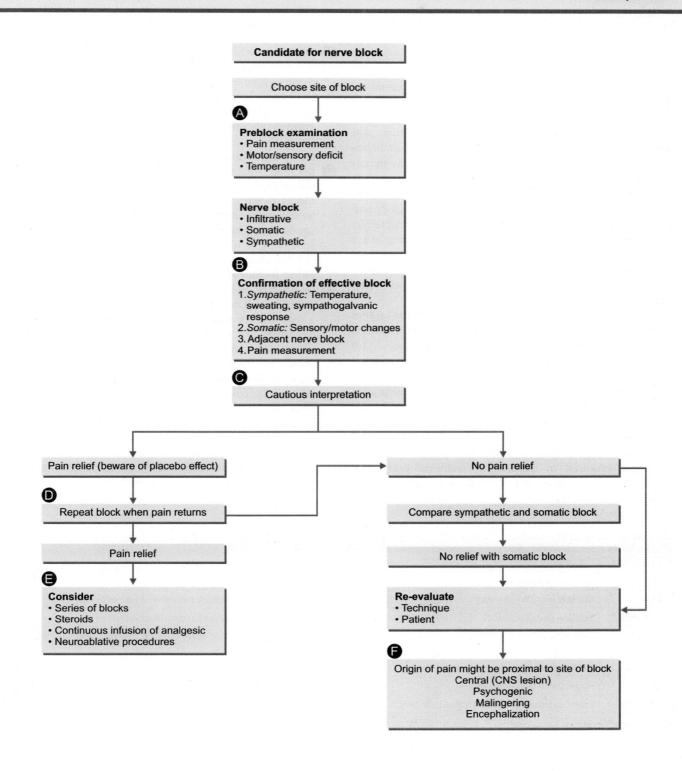

Diagnostic nerve blocks are frequently called upon to assist the physician faced with the complexity of chronic pain. In patients with acute pain, the stimulus creates impulses in nociceptors and the conduction of these signals can be blocked by local anesthetics before they are perceived in the central nervous system (CNS). With chronic pain, the site of generation and the mechanism of maintenance of nociceptor activity are not always clear. There is a complex interplay of peripheral and central mechanisms involving nociceptor activity, sympathetic contribution, spinal processing, plasticity, and convergent input. The issues that compound the complexity of a patient's pain include psychosocial, financial, and sometimes legal factors.

Local anesthetics do not block sensory and motor modalities equally. There is progressive interruption of nerve conductance that is dependent on local anesthetic concentration, local anesthetic's inherent properties, and nerve fiber characteristics. Nerve blocks with local anesthetics in high concentration interrupt both afferent and efferent neural conduction; in contrast, with low concentrations of local anesthetics this interruption might become selective. Thus, neural conduction in small fibers (A-δ) and nonmyelinated nerve fibers (C fibers) may be interrupted by low-dose anesthetics, whereas there is only a modest effect on large myelinated fibers, which are predominantly motor or proprioceptive agents. Commonly, disappearance of pain perception is first, followed by cold, warmth, touch, deep pressure, and loss of motor function.

The limitations of a diagnostic nerve block should be kept in mind because these blocks are simply useful additions to the available diagnostic and prognostic tools. Full evaluation of the patient and the pain problem is warranted for determining if a nerve block is appropriate. A review of the available investigations is performed, and new studies are ordered if necessary. A psychological or psychiatric evaluation can provide additional insight.

The decision to block a specific site depends on the painful body part **(Table 1)**. Performance of the regional anesthesia technique requires, in addition to technical excellence, knowledge of anatomic and physiologic foundations and limitations of the procedure. Physicians should be prepared to deal with potential side effects and complications. Diagnostic nerve blocks performed in the appropriate settings, combined with a patient's complete clinical picture, can provide valuable additional information in determining the cause of persistent pain.

(A) Before the block is performed, a pain measurement (e.g. the visual analog scale) is applied, any motor or sensory deficit is determined, and the temperature over the affected area is recorded. These indicators are then compared to those on the contralateral site and documented.

(B) Once a nerve block is performed, it is essential to confirm that the targeted nerve has been reached. It is also useful to know if an undesired blockade has occurred, such as blockage of an adjacent nerve. The postblock examination includes assessment of temperature, sweating, and the sympathogalvanic response to evaluate the sympathetic response. Any sensory and motor change should be documented and a new pain measurement undertaken.

(C) Because treatment often depends on an accurate diagnosis, cautious interpretation of diagnostic nerve blocks is warranted. The sensitivity of such blocks can be enhanced during their performance by fluoroscopic, sonographic, or computed tomographic guidance. The specificity of blocks is more difficult to control. Some of the factors that decrease the specificity of diagnostic blocks include placebo effects and expectation bias.

(D) In practice, pain relief of more than 50% and/or 50% improvement in function after a confirmed block warrants a repeat block when the pain returns for confirmation. Otherwise, the likelihood of pain generation from that nerve innervation is very unlikely and other sources should be considered. If a confirmed sympathetic block does not result in pain relief (for example an extremity affected by complex regional pain syndrome [CRPS]), then consider a somatic block of the same structure.

(E) If the relief can be consistently reproduced, consider a block at regular intervals, continuous infusion of analgesic, injection of steroids, or a neuroablative procedure. Use these analgesic techniques to augment participation in physical therapy and a home exercise regimen. Keep in mind that relief obtained with a nerve block may help

Table 1: Site of block		
Site of pain	*Sympathetic*	*Somatic*
Head	Stellate ganglion block	C2 block; trigeminal block (or branches)
Neck	Stellate ganglion block	Cervical plexus block (or individual nerve)
Upper Ext	Stellate ganglion block	Brachial plexus block (or individual nerve)
Thorax	*Low dose*: Thoracic epidural; paravertebral block; intercostal block	Thoracic epidural; paravertebral block; intercostal block
Abdomen	Celiac plexus block; splanchnic block	Paravertebral block; intercostal block
Pelvis	Superior hypogastric block	Caudal, epidural, saddle, sacral root block
Lower Ext	Lumbar paravertebral sympathetic block	Lumbar plexus somatic block or Sciatic/Femoral block

Source: Modified from Ramamurthy S, Winnie AP (1985).

predict the response to neural decompression, but its value for predicting the response to neuroablation is controversial. Moreover, the available studies raise doubt as to whether analgesia after sympathetic blockade necessarily indicates a sympathetic contribution to pain.

F If there is no pain relief after a confirmed block, consider that the origin of pain might be proximal to the site of the block. The etiologies might include a CNS lesion, a psychogenic process, malingering, or encephalization.

SUGGESTED READING

Buckley FP. Regional anesthesia with local anesthetic. In: Loeser JD (Ed). Bonica's Management of Pain, 3rd edition. Philadelphia: Lippincott Williams & Wilkins; 2001.

Curatolo M. Regional anesthesia in pain management. Curr Opin Anaesthesiol. 2016;29:614-9.

Hayek SM, Shah A. Nerve blocks for chronic pain. Neurosurg Clin N Am. 2014;25:809-17.

Hogan QH, Abram SE. Neural blockade for diagnosis and prognosis: a review. Anesthesiology. 1997;86:216-41.

Lin Y, Liu S. Local anesthetics. Clinical Anesthesia, 7th edition. Philadelphia: Lippincott Williams & Wilkins; 2013.

Raja SN. Nerve blocks in the evaluation of chronic pain: a plea for caution in their use and interpretation. Anesthesiology. 1997;86:4-6.

Ramamurthy S, Winnie AP. Regional anesthetic techniques for pain relief. Semin Anesth. 1985;4:237-46.

Smith H, Youn Y, Guay RC, et al. The role of invasive pain management modalities in the treatment of chronic pain. Med Clin North Am. 2016;100:103-15.

SECTION 2

Acute Pain

Maxim S Eckmann

Patient-Controlled Analgesia

Hilliard PE, Chen J

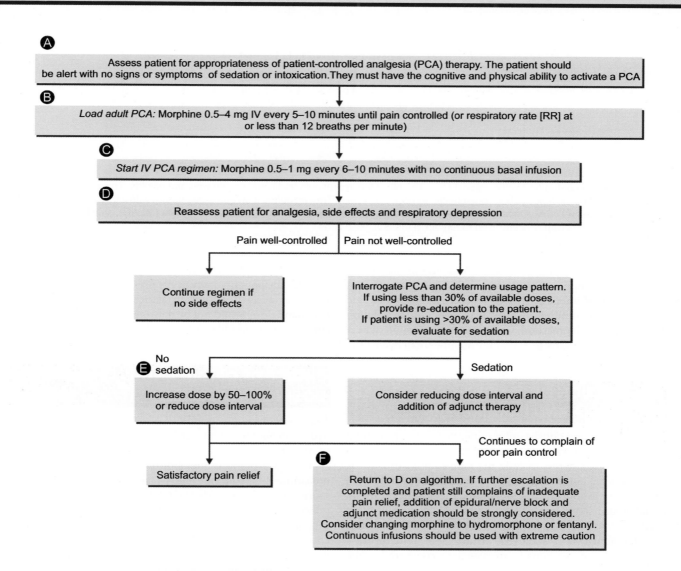

A — Assess patient for appropriateness of patient-controlled analgesia (PCA) therapy. The patient should be alert with no signs or symptoms of sedation or intoxication. They must have the cognitive and physical ability to activate a PCA

B — *Load adult PCA:* Morphine 0.5–4 mg IV every 5–10 minutes until pain controlled (or respiratory rate [RR] at or less than 12 breaths per minute)

C — *Start IV PCA regimen:* Morphine 0.5–1 mg every 6–10 minutes with no continuous basal infusion

D — Reassess patient for analgesia, side effects and respiratory depression

Pain well-controlled | Pain not well-controlled

Continue regimen if no side effects

Interrogate PCA and determine usage pattern. If using less than 30% of available doses, provide re-education to the patient. If patient is using >30% of available doses, evaluate for sedation

E — No sedation | Sedation

Increase dose by 50–100% or reduce dose interval

Consider reducing dose interval and addition of adjunct therapy

Satisfactory pain relief

Continues to complain of poor pain control

F — Return to D on algorithm. If further escalation is completed and patient still complains of inadequate pain relief, addition of epidural/nerve block and adjunct medication should be strongly considered. Consider changing morphine to hydromorphone or fentanyl. Continuous infusions should be used with extreme caution

ROLE OF PATIENT-CONTROLLED ANALGESIA IN THE ACUTE PAIN MANAGEMENT CONTINUUM

Patient-controlled analgesia (PCA) is a mainstay in the spectrum of pain management for acute postsurgical pain. Optimal perioperative analgesia is best achieved with a multimodal approach that includes oral medications (nonsteroidal anti-inflammatory drugs [NSAIDs], acetam-inophen, adjuncts), intravenous (IV) PCA and regional anesthesia. When used properly, it is theorized that IV PCA provides effective analgesia due to maintenance of the serum minimum effective analgesic concentration (MEAC). Small, frequent IV dosing of opioid medication allows the serum concentration of opioid to remain within the MEAC, thereby providing the patient with a consistent level of analgesia **(Fig. 1)**. The advantages of IV PCA use include better pain control compared to non-PCA and increased patient satisfaction due to less administrative delays compared to

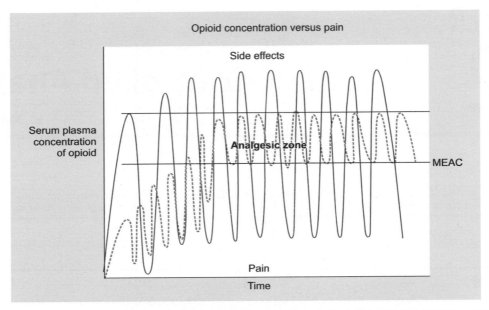

Fig. 1: Opioid concentration plotted against time. The black line represents traditional dosing with oral opioids. The variability in serum concentration of opioid leads to both side effects and persistent pain. The red dotted line represents dosing with intravenous (IV) patient-controlled analgesia (PCA). Once IV boluses are above the minimum effective analgesic concentration (MEAC), small frequent doses of opioid allow the serum concentration to remain in the analgesic zone

intramuscular (IM) or IV administration. The limitations of IV PCA use include technical pump errors (programing PCA dosing), risk of infection due to IV access and opioid side effects (nausea, vomiting, pruritus, urinary retention, sedation and respiratory depression). Unauthorized activation of PCA therapy by a third party (e.g. a family member) can bypass the safety advantage of PCA.

DESCRIPTION OF PATIENT-CONTROLLED ANALGESIA AND PARAMETERS

An IV PCA system consists of a computerized pump and a syringe of IV medication connected to the patient's IV line. PCA pump parameters include the following: loading dose, demand dose, continuous infusion rate, and depending on PCA, 1-hour, 4-hour and 24-hour limits. The loading dose is an initial bolus used to increase the serum opioid concentration until the patient experiences effective analgesia. Once effective analgesia is achieved, an available demand dose with temporal constraints (a smaller dose compared to the initial bolus) maintains the MEAC and is delivered when the patient activates the PCA delivery by pressing the demand button. The continuous infusion option provides a steady infusion of IV medication, regardless of demand dosing.

Built-in safeguards to IV PCA include the 1-hour limit, 4-hour limit and patient-initiated delivery. More recent developments include end-tidal CO_2 monitoring of respiratory rate with an automatic lock out below a predetermined threshold. The 1- and 4-hour limits prevent the patient from exceeding a prespecified accumulated

dosage of opioid medication. The patient-initiated delivery requires the patient to physically press the demand button to receive a dosage. Theoretically, if the patient was too sedated, a demand dose would not be delivered and the serum opioid concentration should continue to decline, thereby preventing progression to respiratory arrest.

CHOICE OF OPIOID AND DOSING PARADIGMS

The most commonly used IV PCA opioids include morphine, hydromorphone and fentanyl. Morphine is the most studied, most commonly used and the "gold standard" opioid for IV PCA. Morphine is metabolized by the liver to inactive morphine-3-glucuronide (M3G) and an active metabolite, morphine-6-glucuronide (M6G). M6G provides an analgesia effect, but also contributes to the opioid side effects. Since M6G is cleared by the kidney, delayed side effects of sedation, confusion and respiratory depression can occur hours after the last PCA dose with patients who have renal insufficiency, secondary to accumulation of M6G.

Hydromorphone is a commonly used alternative to morphine for patients with renal failure. Hydromorphone is approximately five times as potent as morphine and is metabolized by the liver to an inactive glucuronide metabolite. Fentanyl is a lipophilic opioid and does not have any active metabolites, making it a good option for patients with renal insufficiency. Due to the rapid effect site equilibration time and short duration of analgesia, it is often administered with a continuous infusion.

Table 1: Initiation of adult patient-controlled analgesia (PCA) should take into consideration patient's recent exposure to opioid-based medication. Categories of opioid usage based upon University of Michigan Opioid Guidelines

Opioid	Adult opioid naïve* initial bolus dose and time interval	Adult opioid tolerant[†] bolus dose and time interval	Adult opioid highly tolerant[‡] basal infusion, bolus dose and time interval
Morphine	0.5–1 mg[§] q 6–10 minutes	2–3 mg[§] q 6–10 minutes	2–3 mg[§] q 6–10 minutes and basal infusion in mg/hr equal to bolus dose
Hydromorphone	0.1 mg[§] q 6–10 minutes	0.3–0.04 mg[§] q 6–10 minutes	0.3–0.4 mg[§] q 6–10 minutes and basal infusion in mg/hr equal to bolus dose

* *Opioid naïve*: Patient taking less than 80 mg by mouth morphine equivalents (PO MEQ) per day prior to initiation of PCA.
[†] *Opioid tolerant*: Patient taking between 80 and 120 mg PO MEQ per day.
[‡] *Opioid highly tolerant*: Patient taking buprenorphine greater than 8 mg per day or greater than 120 mg PO MEQ per day.
[§] May bump up bolus dose by 50–100% if pain not well-controlled after 2 hours of therapy.

FUTURE DEVELOPMENTS

From a macroscopic conceptual level, PCA is not restricted to one type of medication or one route of administration. Although PCA frequently refers to IV administration of opioid medications, recent PCA iterations have included opioid medications administered through the transdermal, intranasal, and sublingual routes. While the mode of administration of medication is variable, the central tenet of patient controlled on-demand dosing remains unchanged. Some of the newer developments in PCA technology include transdermal or intranasal fentanyl and sublingual sufentanil.

A Assess the patient prior to initiation of PCA therapy. The patient should demonstrate understanding of the concept and be physically and cognitively able to activate a PCA button. PCA therapy should be avoided in patients who are sedated or show signs and/or symptoms of intoxication. Therapy should be initiated with caution in patients with obstructive or central sleep apnea or in patients with morbid obesity.

B Choose medication appropriate for the patient, taking into account medical comorbidities and allergy status. Initial loading of medication may be necessary to achieve serum plasma concentrations in the analgesic zone. This may require frequent bolus dosing. Care should be taken to avoid narcotization and respiratory depression.

C Once pain is reasonably controlled or patient is satisfied, the patient will assume responsibility of self-administered dosing. The initial PCA settings should be determined by patient age, degree of pain, history of previous or active opioid tolerance and medical comorbidities. **Table 1** offers some guidance on initiation of therapy.

D The patient should be reassessed after initiation of therapy with particular attention to side effects and respiratory depression. If pain is adequately controlled and the patient is tolerating the regimen with no untoward side effects, continue therapy. If pain is not well-controlled,

interrogate the PCA to determine usage by the patient. If the patient is utilizing less than 30% of available doses, re-educate the patient on use of the PCA and encourage its use. If the patient is utilizing greater than 30% of available doses, assess for sedation and respiratory depression.

E If the patient is sedated, consider reducing dose or bolus interval and the addition of adjuncts that will not contribute to further sedation (acetaminophen, NSAIDs, epidural, regional block, etc.) If the patient is not sedated, increase the bolus dose by 50–100% or decrease the time interval if it is greater than every 6 minutes.

F Reassess the patient. If pain is well-controlled, no changes are indicated. If pain is poorly controlled and patient is not sedated, repeat the algorithm starting at letter B. Strong consideration should be given to addition of adjuncts and/or nerve blocks/epidural therapy. If after working through the algorithm a second time, the pain is still not well-controlled, consider changing to a different opioid-based medication. Use of continuous infusion is generally discouraged as it has been shown to be a risk factor for respiratory depression.

SUGGESTED READING

Grass JA. Patient-controlled analgesia. Anesth Analg. 2005;101 (5 Suppl):S44-61.

McNicol ED, Ferguson MC, Hudcova J. Patient controlled opioid analgesia versus non-patient controlled opioid analgesia for postoperative pain. Cochrane Database Syst Rev. 2015;(6): CD003348.

Osborne R, Joel S, Slevin M. Morphine intoxication in renal failure: the role of morphine-6-glucuronide. Br Med J (Clin Res Ed). 1986;293(6554):1101.

Palmer PP, Miller RD. Current and developing methods of patient-controlled analgesia. Anesthesiol Clin. 2010;28(4): 587-99.

Rathmell JC, Wu CL, Sinatra RS, et al. Acute post-surgical pain management: a critical appraisal of current practice, December 2-4, 2005. Reg Anesth Pain Med. 2006;31(4 Suppl 1):1-42.

Epidural Analgesia

Rana MV, Kusper TM

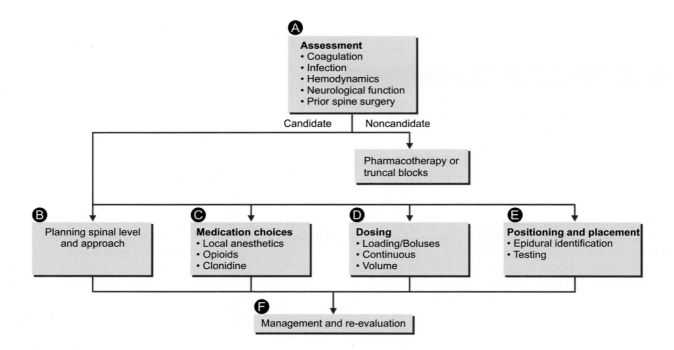

The epidural space is a central axis target point for the administration of agents for analgesic purposes. The term describes the potential space located dorsal to the vertebral body. It is an oval conduit composed of various tissues: blood vessels, lymphatic structures, and fat. The epidural space spans cranially from the foramen magnum to the sacral hiatus distally. The boundaries of the posterior epidural space, which is most practical for interventional access, are the dura mater ventrally and just past the laminar shelf of the vertebra and the ligamentum flavum dorsally. Uptake of agents occurs via fat and vascular uptake, with some agent diffusing through the dura and nerve roots, accounting for a dual systemic and local mechanism of analgesia. Evaluation and management steps are outlined in **Figure 1**.

Ⓐ *Assessment:* Epidural medication serves to alter pain signals throughout the entire spine. Assessment for placement of an epidural begins with a careful review of the medical history ensuring that no contraindications exist for therapy including neurological dysfunction, coagulation abnormality, and the presence of infection. Anesthesiologists should be aware of prior surgical access in the area of proposed epidural placement as access via the loss-of-resistance technique may not be valid with

altered tissue integrity. Assessment of hemodynamic status is important as hypotension may result from administration of local anesthetic agents. Pretreatment with fluids may mitigate the hypotensive response, while choosing an opioid-only regimen may decrease the sympathectomy-induced hypotension. Patients who cannot receive epidural analgesia may still be candidates for truncal compartment blocks or systemic pharmacotherapy based on risk profile.

Ⓑ *Anatomic Target:* Epidural placement mandates knowledge of surgical incisional area to ensure appropriate anatomical coverage. An epidural should be placed in the thoracic region for xiphoid to pubis incisions, thoracic procedures, and abdominal incisions. The lumbar epidural space should be the target for surgeries in the lower abdominopelvic region and the lower extremities. Access to the epidural space with regards to needle angulation also varies depending on the targeted location. For example, a paramedian approach to the epidural space is undertaken to obtain loss of resistance to avoid the overhanging thoracic vertebral body spinous process. A midline approach is routinely performed for lumbar epidural considerations. There is no consensus

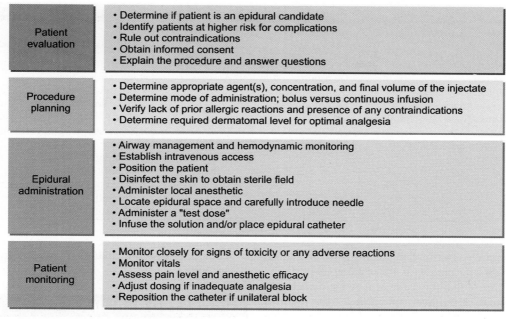

Fig. 1: Approach to epidural anesthesia

in the literature on the optimal insertion distance of the epidural catheter. D'Angelo et al. examined various insertion lengths and, although they did not find an optimal length, concluded that 6 cm might be preferred over 4 cm since it requires less frequent replacement. Other investigators, such as Beilin et al., reported that 5 cm provides satisfactory analgesia.

C *Medication Choice:* The choice of epidural drug should be tailored for the analgesic indication. Agents may be delivered intermittently via a bolus approach or by a continuous infusion. Drugs utilized include preservative-free local anesthetics, opioids, clonidine and other agents to counteract the nociceptive signal. Surgery requiring anesthetic depth along with motor block would be best served by a local anesthetic. The benefit of this blockade is counterbalanced by a risk of sympathectomy-induced hypotension. On the contrary, if motor block is not required but analgesia is, an opioid such as fentanyl may be better suited for the epidural; however, the benefits of these agents are counterbalanced by the risk of sedation, respiratory depression, nausea/vomiting, itching, and urinary retention. Opioids and local anesthetics have been combined to produce synergistic effects with fewer side effects of the individual component drugs.

D *Dosing:* Once a particular drug has been chosen for epidural administration, the anesthesiologist must consider certain factors when determining dose volume drug delivery. The dose and volume of the drug is a function of drug properties, spine level of epidural drug administration, target location of drug, patient considerations. If the epidural is placed in the thoracic region and has a corresponding target in the thoracic region, a smaller dose of agent is required to target nerves,

versus a lumbar epidural for the same thoracic target. This applies both to local anesthetics and opioid drugs.

E *Positioning and Placement:* After obtaining informed consent, the patient is placed in the sitting position, slouching to open up the target epidural space as extension of the spine limits the translaminar space. Alternatively, the patient may be placed in the lateral decubitus position but should flex the cervical spine and bend the knees to round the back. Intravenous access, nasal cannula, and standard American Society of Anesthesiologists (ASA) monitors are required prior to proceeding. The skin is prepped with chlorhexidine and draped. Mild conscious sedation is not mandatory but may be instituted if desired. Local anesthesia is delivered for the skin and subcutaneous tissues, followed by the placement of the Tuohy needle to access the epidural space. On average the ligamentum flavum is encountered at 4.5 cm depth but significant variability is possible depending on the angle of approach and patient body habitus. A tactile spongy sensation is felt when this occurs, and this tightens near the end of traversing the ligament. For the loss-of-resistance technique, the needle hub is connected to a syringe filled with air or saline (the syringe may be glass or siliconized plastic). A loss of resistance is sought with advancement of the needle intermittently while assessing with the attached syringe plunger, or continuous advancement with the needle and continued pressure on the syringe. Next, a catheter is inserted, ensuring that the catheter is no more than 5 cm in the epidural space to decrease the risk of epidural vein cannulation and/or lateral placement if undesired. This is secured in position. Aspiration is performed to ensure that the needle/catheter is not intravascular or

Table 1: Adverse effects of epidural anesthesia

Effects related to the needle and catheter placement	*Effects related to the presence of an catheter in the epidural space*	*Effects related to epidural medication*
• Postdural puncture headache • Subdural hematoma • Intravascular injection • Air embolism (pneumocephalus) • *Mechanical trauma*: Back pain, hematoma • Nerve injury • Transient/persistent neuropathy • Pneumothorax • Hemothorax	• Spinal hematoma • *Neuraxial infection*: Abscess, meningitis • Catheter migration	• Drug errors • Allergic reaction • Chemical irritation • Local anesthetic systemic toxicity (LAST) • Respiratory depression or apnea • Hypotension • Nausea/vomiting • Urinary retention • Motor paralysis, including muscles of respiration • High spinal anesthesia

accessing cerebrospinal fluid and blood. Next, a test dose of 3 mL of 2% lidocaine with 1:200,000 epinephrine is injected to ensure that the catheter is not subarachnoid or intravascular. A positive aspirate/test dose requires adjustment/replacement of the catheter. A positive meniscus drop test is fairly specific against vascular or intrathecal insertion in the event of negative aspiration. Vital signs are regularly assessed thereafter in the patient.

F *Management:* During long-term management of the catheter on rounds for the patient, the anesthesiologist should perform investigation particularly if analgesia is considered insufficient or there are reported side effects. In this case, the location of the catheter to ensure that the catheter has not migrated from initial placement. Presence and distribution of sensory and motor block should be evaluated. Also, inquiring about side effects including weakness, itching, nausea/vomiting, constipation, and urinary retention should be performed. Assessment of respiratory function and mental status are crucial to avoid respiratory sedation and depression. The anesthesiologist must also be vigilant to infections in a catheter used in situ greater for extended periods (>3 days) but should do daily inspection. Vigilance against neurologic complications should also be present. Adverse effects or complications from epidural anesthesia are summarized in **Table 1**.

SUGGESTED READING

Beilin Y, Bernstein HH, Zucker-Pinchoff B. The optimal distance that a multiorifice epidural catheter should be threaded into the epidural space. Anesth Analg. 1995;81(2):301-4.

Bromage PR. Epidural Analgesia. Philadelphia: WB Saunders; 1978. p. 8.

Cousins MJ, Mather LE. Intrathecal and epidural administration of opioids. Anesthesiology. 1984;61:276-310.

Eisenach JC. Pain relief in obstetrics. In: Raj PP (Ed). Practical Management of Pain. St. Louis: Mosby Year Book; 1992. p. 391.

Elliott RD. Continuous infusion epidural analgesia for obstetrics: bupivacaine versus bupivacaine-fentanyl mixture. Can J Anaesth. 1991;38:303-10.

Hoefnagel A, Yu A, Kaminski A. Anesthetic complications in pregnancy. Crit Care Clin. 2016;32(1):1-28.

Loeser JD, Cousins MJ. Contemporary pain management. Med J Aust. 1990;153:208-12.

Mulroy MF. Regional Anesthesia. Boston: Little Brown; 1989. p. 93.

Raj PP, Pai U. Techniques of nerve blocking. In: Raj PP (Ed). Handbook of Regional Anesthesia. New York: Churchill Livingstone; 1985. p. 237.

Wheatley RG, Schug SA, Watson D. Safety and efficacy of post-operative epidural analgesia. Br J Anaesth. 2001;87(1):47-61.

Acute Herpes Zoster

Guthmiller KB, Thorsted RS

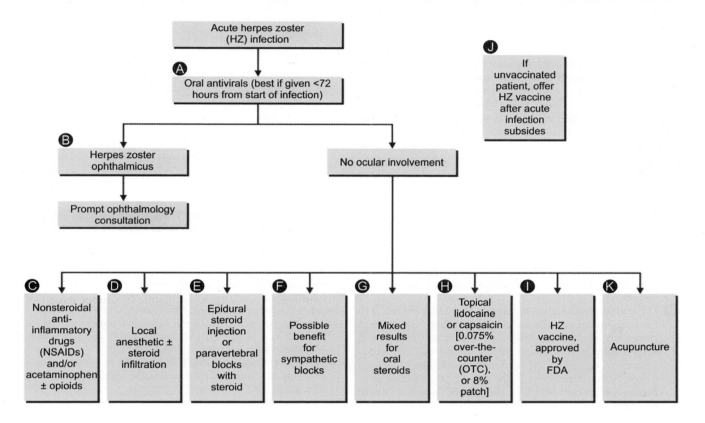

Acute herpes zoster (HZ), also known as shingles, is an infectious disease involving reactivation of the varicella-zoster virus (VZV), which resides primarily within the dorsal root ganglia. The estimated lifetime risk of developing HZ is up to 30% with a dramatic increased risk after age 50. In North America, the incidence rate of HZ ranges between 3/1,000 and 5/1,000 person-years. The recurrence rate is about 5%. Elderly and immunocompromised individuals are most often affected. Within 2–3 days of the start of viral replication, patients first develop a paresthesia, which is followed a short time later by a unilateral dermatomal vesicular rash and acute neuritis; the rash crusts over in 3–4 weeks. Occasionally, a pain prodrome may be experienced in the affected dermatome prior to onset of the rash. Pain with HZ is a combination of normal and neuropathic pain that reflects acute tissue and neural injury. Acute herpetic neuralgia may be defined as pain lasting 30 days after the onset of the rash, while subacute herpetic neuralgia is defined as pain lasting from 30 days to 120 days after the onset of the rash. Postherpetic neuralgia (PHN) is defined as pain lasting more than 120 days after the onset of the rash. The thoracic and trigeminal dermatomes are the most frequent sites of rash, although any dermatome

could be involved, and in immunocompromised individuals dissemination of the rash may occur. A thorough history and physical examination are important for delineating the dermatomal distribution involved, and the time since the onset of symptoms. Most cases of HZ can be diagnosed clinically, although atypical rashes may require a direct immunofluorescence assay for VZV antigen or a polymerase chain reaction assay for VZV DNA in cells from the base of lesions after they are unroofed. The goals of therapy are pain relief, decreasing viral replication, and prevention of PHN.

A Oral antiviral agents have been shown in numerous studies to be effective in decreasing viral replication but only if administered within 72 hours of the onset of the rash, regardless of age or degree of pain. Oral antiviral drug dosages are as follows: either acyclovir 800 mg five times daily for 7 days, valacyclovir 1,000 mg three times daily for 7 days, or famciclovir 500 mg three times daily for 7 days. Valacyclovir or famciclovir is preferable to acyclovir because of ease of dosing and higher levels of antiviral drug activity. Unfortunately, antiviral agents have not been shown to decrease the incidence of PHN.

B Herpes zoster ophthalmicus is caused by VZV reactivation within the trigeminal ganglion, which may lead to permanent blindness and should be treated promptly by an ophthalmologist. Oral antiviral agents should be prescribed immediately if symptoms have been present for less than 72 hours.

C Analgesia is of utmost concern to the patient as this syndrome may be extremely painful. The course of the acute eruption is brief, so oral opioids may be administered in the short term, especially when combined with nonsteroidal anti-inflammatory drugs (NSAIDs). If the pain is not as severe, NSAIDs or acetaminophen may be all that is needed.

D If the painful area is small, locally infiltrated anesthetics mixed with glucocorticoids have been advocated as a way to avoid other more invasive treatments.

E Epidural injections and paravertebral blocks with local anesthetics, combined with steroids given soon after onset of HZ, might lead to a long-term decrease in pain and allodynia; however, studies vary in the number, frequency, and duration of the blocks and an optimal number and interval is difficult to determine. One prospective study evaluated 485 patients at 12 months and revealed an incidence of 22% of PHN in the group that received intravenous acyclovir and prednisolone versus 1.6% in the group that received epidural bupivacaine and methylprednisolone. The patients in the interventional group received their epidural injections every 3–4 days for three weeks, a practice that is not without substantial risk of suppression of the adrenal axis. Other neuraxial interventional studies have not demonstrated such robust results.

F Unfortunately, there is limited or low-quality evidence to recommend for or against several procedural modalities to treat PHN, including spinal cord stimulation, intrathecal drug delivery, intrathecal steroids, and pulsed radiofrequency treatment. Sympathetic nerve blocks should generally be avoided in PHN due to inconsistent low-quality evidence indicating no benefit, however might be effective in reducing the pain associated with HZ. For further information, see Chapter on Postherpetic Neuralgia.

G Oral steroids have been used to treat HZ with mixed results. Pain and inflammation appear to be reduced; however, no decrease in the incidence of PHN has been demonstrated. There is some concern of systemic HZ dissemination associated with the use of steroids in immunocompromised patients, such as those with acquired immunodeficiency syndrome.

H Commonly used topical treatments include lidocaine and capsaicin. 0.075% capsaicin was found to be useful compared to placebo when applied three to four times daily, and an 8% patch was noted to provide statistically significant improvement in pain scores compared to placebo (0.04% capsaicin). A randomized controlled trial (RCT) and two-open label studies suggested benefit for the 5% lidocaine patch.

I The HZ vaccine has been shown to be moderately effective in reducing the incidence of HZ and is recommended for persons 60 years of age or older, although it was recently approved by the US Food and Drug Administration (FDA) for persons as young as 50 years of age. It appears to be moderately effective in preventing the development of PHN. The Centers for Disease Control and Prevention (CDC) states and other literature suggests that individuals with a history of zoster can be vaccinated, on the basis that experiencing a zoster infection does not prevent a subsequent episode. When to administer the vaccine in these cases is uncertain; however, it can probably be delayed for some time as the risk for reinfection for a couple of years is low. Zoster vaccination is not recommended in individuals who have received the varicella vaccine, or in pregnant women.

J Additional therapeutic options that have been useful in treating severe unresponsive pain include use of gabapentinoids and tricyclic antidepressants. Despite the administration of complex drug combinations, pain control is often unsatisfactory.

K Acupuncture may offer an addition mode of pain relief. In an RCT comparing acupuncture and standard analgesic therapy, acupuncture showed a significant and similar degree of pain relief for acute herpetic pain. The study was limited due to small sample size and no control arm for mock acupuncture.

SUGGESTED READING

Chen N, Li Q, Zhou M, et al. Antiviral treatment for preventing postherpetic neuralgia. Cochrane Database of Syst Rev. 2014; 2:CD006866.

Cohen JI. Clinical practice: herpes zoster. N Engl J Med. 2013;369: 255-63.

Cohen JI. Herpes zoster. N Engl J Med. 2013;369:1766-7.

Dworkin RH, Gnann JW, Oaklander AL, et al. Diagnosis and assessment of pain associated with herpes zoster and postherpetic neuralgia. J Pain. 2008;9(1):S37-44.

Dworkin RH, O'Connor AB, Kent J, et al. Interventional management of neuropathic pain: NeuPSIG recommendations. Pain. 2013;154: 2249-61.

Gan EY, Tian EA, Tey HL. Management of herpes zoster and postherpetic neuralgia. Am J Clin Dermatol. 2013;14:77-85.

Han Y, Zhang J, Chen N, et al. Corticosteroids for preventing postherpetic neuralgia. Cochrane Database Syst Rev. 2013;3: CD005582.

Harpaz R, Ortega-Sanchez IR, Seward JF. (2008). Prevention of herpes zoster: recommendations of the Advisory Committee on Immunization Practices (ACIP). MMWR Recomm Rep. 2008; 57:1-30.

Kawai K, Gebremeskel BG, Acosta CJ. Systematic review of incidence and complications of herpes zoster: towards a global perspective. BMJ Open. 2014;4:e004833.

Oaklander AL. Mechanisms of pain and itch caused by herpes zoster (shingles). J Pain. 2008;9:S10-8.

Schmader KE, Dworkin RH. Natural history and treatment of herpes zoster. J Pain. 2008;9(1):S3-9.

Ursini T, Tontodonati M, Manzoli L, et al. Acupuncture for treatment of severe acute pain in herpes zoster: results of a nested, open-label, randomized trial in the VZV Pain Study. BMC Complement Altern Med. 2011;11:46.

Van Wijck AJ, Wallace M, Mekhail N, et al. Herpes zoster and postherpetic neuralgia. Pain Practice. 2011;11(1):88-97.

Acute Upper Extremity Pain

Patel S, Soliman S

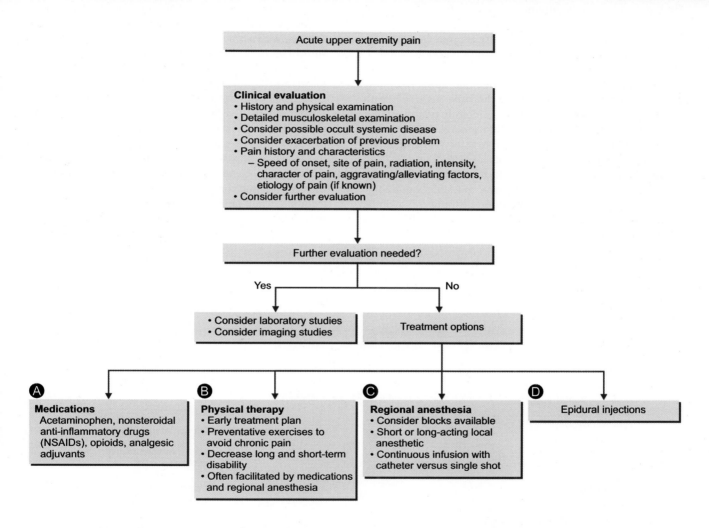

The upper extremities are common sites for acute pain or chronic pain with acute exacerbations. The most common etiologies of upper extremity pain include trauma, tumor, infection, and neuropathic pain (including radicular pain). Successful treatment of acute upper extremity pain usually involves a multifaceted approach utilizing medications, physical therapy (PT), and regional anesthesia depending on the etiology. If the cause of acute pain is not obvious, one needs to be sure to be aware of underlying pathology including stroke, ischemia, and venous thrombosis.

A Treatment of acute upper extremity pain is usually aided by the use of analgesic medications such as nonsteroidal anti-inflammatory drugs (NSAIDs), acetaminophen,

and opioids. Antispasmodic (muscle relaxants) medications may be considered if severe muscle spasms are a significant component of the pain. Optimal pharmacologic therapy often includes a combination of several medications. NSAIDs should always be considered in acute pain with a musculoskeletal etiology. The side effects should also be considered, which range from an antiplatelet to gastrointestinal (GI) to kidney effect. Regarding the GI system, it is important to keep in mind the top three risk factors: (1) a prior history of GI ulcers, (2) age, and (3) concomitant aspirin use. Besides oral NSAIDs, topical NSAIDs should always be considered, especially if the pain is localized and the avoidance of systemic side effects is desired. From a large, recent study, it was determined that the number needed to treat (NNT) with topical NSAIDs is below 4. Treatment in this study was determined to be 50% pain relief with a 6- to 14-day period. Additionally, it was found not all formulations of topical anesthetic had the same results. For example, regarding diclofenac, Emulgel® had the lowest NNT of 1.8 whereas diclofenac plasters had a NNT of 3.2. Ibuprofen had a NNT of 3.9 and ketoprofen had a NNT of 2.5.

B Physical therapy is extremely important for the successful treatment of acute pain and the prevention of chronic pain and permanent disability. PT is often facilitated by medications and regional anesthetic techniques.

C There are many effective regional anesthetic techniques available for relief and control of acute upper extremity pain. Regional anesthesia has become very safe with the advent of ultrasonography to identify neurovascular structures and guide needle placement; however, the practitioner should be prepared to intervene if there are complications. Regional anesthesia can reduce pain from neuralgias or provide analgesia to augment PT. Neural innervation of the painful area, possible neurologic focus for pain, and any contraindications to regional anesthesia should be considered. It may be difficult to determine which nerves are involved with the production

of pain in an injured or painful extremity. The cutaneous innervation of an extremity is highly variable, with much overlap of adjacent nerves **(Fig. 1)**. In addition, the innervation of the underlying muscles (myotomes) and bones (sclerotomes) is often not the same as that of the overlying skin. Always consider the differential innervation of the involved structures to avoid developing an unsatisfactory regional anesthesia plan **(Table 1)**.

Nerve injections can be extremely valuable in acute upper extremity pain. These are often used in cases such as complex regional pain syndrome (CRPS), postsurgical, or those with a brachial plexus tension sign. It is useful to categorize nerve blocks of the upper extremity into two groups: (1) blocks performed at the level of the brachial plexus and (2) those performed at the level of the terminal nerve. Blocks at the level of the brachial plexus can be further subdivided by the specific approach utilized to perform the block (i.e. supraclavicular, infraclavicular, axillary). There are many supraclavicular approaches to the brachial plexus including interscalene, subclavian perivascular, classic supraclavicular, and parascalene blocks. Potential complications should be considered; for example, when performing an interscalene nerve block, there is an almost 100% incidence of transient ipsilateral diaphragmatic paresis. Of greater concern, however, is the

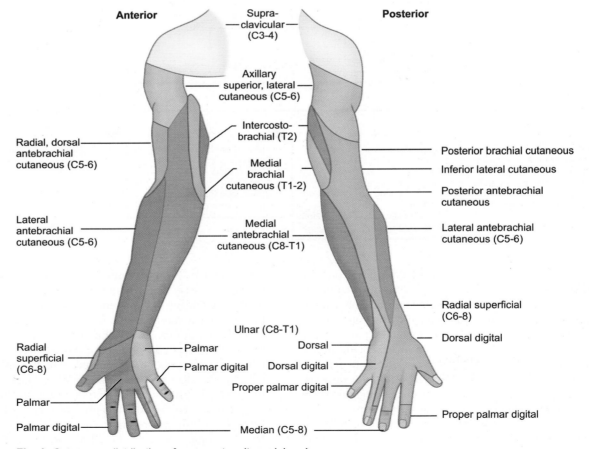

Fig. 1: Cutaneous distribution of upper extremity peripheral nerves

Table 1: Blocks for nerves of upper extremities	
Nerves of the upper extremities	*Methods of blocking (cervical epidural)*
Cervical plexus	
Supraclavicular nerves (C3, C4)	Interscalene brachial plexus block (dependent on proximal spread to cervical plexus) Deep or superficial cervical plexus block Necessary to block for most shoulder procedures
Brachial plexus	
Musculocutaneous (C5-7)	Supra/infraclavicular approaches to brachial plexus block (most reliably blocked with supraclavicular approaches) Isolated musculocutaneous nerve block in coracobrachialis muscle
Lateral cutaneous nerve of forearm	Any type of musculocutaneous nerve block Proximal or midhumeral block Isolated lateral cutaneous nerve of the forearm block in antecubital fossa
Axillary (C5, C6)	Supra/infraclavicular approaches to brachial plexus block Variable success with axillary approaches
Radial (C5-8)	Supra/infraclavicular approaches to brachial plexus block Axillary approach to brachial plexus Proximal or midhumeral block (not reliable for procedures above the elbow) Elbow/wrist block
Posterior cutaneous nerve of arm	Supra/infraclavicular approaches to brachial plexus block Axillary approach to brachial plexus
Lower lateral cutaneous nerve of arm	Supra/infraclavicular approaches to brachial plexus block Axillary approach to brachial plexus Proximal humerus block
Posterior cutaneous nerve of forearm	Supra/infraclavicular approaches to brachial plexus block Axillary approach to brachial plexus Proximal or midhumeral block
Median (C6-8, T1)	Supra/infraclavicular approaches to brachial plexus block Axillary approach to brachial plexus Proximal or midhumeral block Elbow/wrist block
Ulnar (C8, T1)	Supra/infraclavicular approaches to brachial plexus block (not reliably blocked with interscalene block) Axillary approach to brachial plexus Proximal or midhumeral block Elbow/wrist block
Median cutaneous nerve of forearm (C8, T1)	Supra/infraclavicular approaches to brachial plexus block (not reliably blocked with interscalene block) Axillary approach to brachial plexus Proximal or midhumeral block Elbow block
Median cutaneous nerve of arm (T1)	Not reliably blocked by many approaches to the brachial plexus Field block of very proximal humerus in axilla
Intercostobrachial (T2)	Not blocked by any approach to brachial plexus Field block of very proximal humerus in axilla

Source: Copyright © Beyer JA and Anderson DM (January 2002).

possibility of developing permanent diaphragm paralysis, which is a potential complication.

The intercostobrachial nerve (T2) and the medial cutaneous nerve of the arm (T1) innervate the medial aspect of the arm proximal to the elbow. These nerves are poorly anesthetized with many approaches to the brachial plexus, so a supplemental field block may be required to achieve analgesia or anesthesia (e.g. tourniquet pain).

Supraclavicular approaches to the brachial plexus are highly effective for pain originating in the shoulder and arm. If the pain is originating in the shoulder and an interscalene approach is not used, it may be necessary to block the cervical plexus for skin analgesia. Pneumothorax is a relevant risk for the supraclavicular block but incidence is low with the modern use of ultrasound needle guidance.

Infraclavicular and axillary approaches to the brachial plexus are highly effective for relieving pain mediating from the hand, forearm, and arm. The literature describes many types of infraclavicular and axillary blocks. These approaches have enjoyed popularity owing to their favorable side effect and safety profiles.

Blocks performed at the elbow, wrist, and digits can be highly effective for relieving localized pain or "rescuing" an incomplete block. Many operations can be performed with a limited distal block, but prolonged tourniquet use (>20 minutes) may not be tolerated by the patient.

D Both interlaminar and transforaminal epidural steroid injections may be performed for radicular pain that leads to the arms. For acute radicular pain, the cause is often times a bulging disc in the cervical region. If this is the case, it is best to perform the interlaminar injection early for optimal results. Regarding cervical transforaminal injections, these should only be done with care but can have excellent results. From a recent, smaller-sized study of those with cervical radiculopathy that were potential candidates for spine surgery, a transforaminal injection prevented 70% of those from proceeding to surgery and dropped their visual analog score by 4.4 units. A large study examining 4,265 epidural steroid injections, including 161 cervical interlaminar epidural steroid injections had relatively few complication rates. The most common complaint among all epidural steroid injections was increased pain, being present at 1.1% of the time. Overall complication rate was 2.4% with no major complications being noted.

SUGGESTED READING

Amr Y, Yousef A. Evaluation of efficacy of the perioperative administration of venlafaxine or gabapentin on acute and chronic postmastectomy pain. Clin J Pain. 2010;26(5):381-5.

Bonica JJ, Cailliet R, Loeser JD. General considerations of pain in the neck and upper limb. In: Loeser JD (Ed). Bonica's Management of Pain, 3rd edition. Philadelphia: Lippincott Williams & Wilkins; 2001. pp. 969-1002.

Brown DL, Bridenbaugh LD. The upper extremity: somatic block. In: Cousins MJ, Bridenbaugh PO (Eds). Neural Blockade in Clinical Anesthesia and Management of Pain, 3rd edition. Philadelphia: Lippincott-Raven; 1998. pp. 345-71.

Brown DL. Atlas of Regional Anesthesia, 2nd edition. Philadelphia: WB Saunders; 1999.

DeLaunay L, Chelly JE. Indications for upper extremity blocks. In: Chelly JE (Ed). Peripheral Nerve Blocks: A Color Atlas. Philadelphia: Lippincott Williams & Wilkins; 1999. pp. 17-27.

Derry S, Moore R, Gaskell H, et al. Topical NSAIDs for acute musculoskeletal pain in adults. Cochrane Database Syst Rev. 2015;6:CD007402.

Kaufman M, Elkwood A, Rose M, et al. Surgical treatment of permanent diaphragm paralysis after interscalene nerve block for shoulder surgery. Anesthesiology. 2013;119(2):484-7.

McGrath J, Schaefer M, Malkamaki D. Incident and characteristics of complications from epidural steroid injections. Pain Med. 2011;12(5):726-31.

Sostres C, Gargalla C, Arroyo M, et al. Adverse effects of non-steroidal anti-inflammatory drugs (NSAIDs, aspirin and coxibs) on upper gastrointestinal tract. Best Pract Res Clin Gastroenterol. 2010;24(2):121-32.

Vester-Andersen T, Christiansen C, Hansen A, et al. Interscalene brachial plexus block: area of analgesia, complications and blood concentrations of local anesthetics. Acta Anaesthesiol Scand. 1981;25:81-4.

Acute Lower Extremity Pain

Mitchell B, William JG

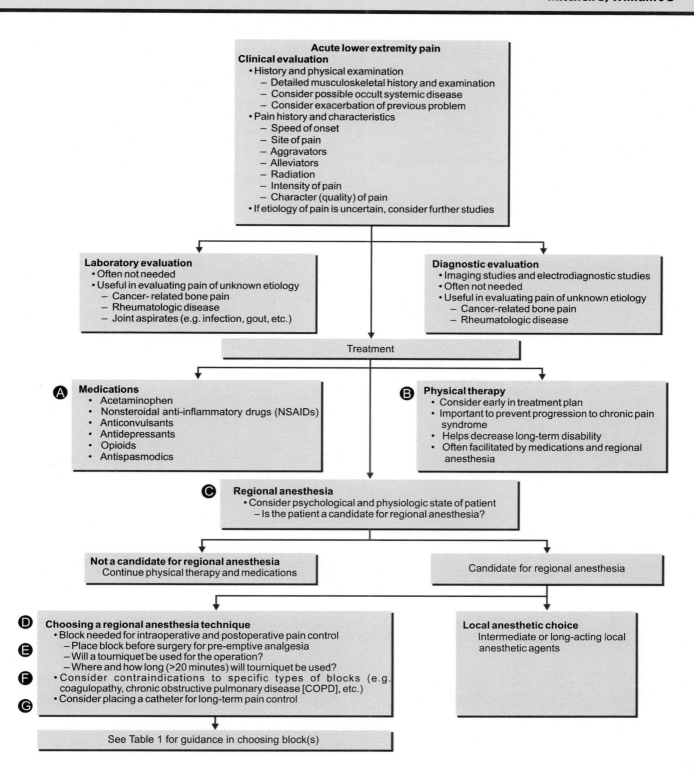

Acute lower extremity pain
Clinical evaluation
- History and physical examination
  - Detailed musculoskeletal history and examination
  - Consider possible occult systemic disease
  - Consider exacerbation of previous problem
- Pain history and characteristics
  - Speed of onset
  - Site of pain
  - Aggravators
  - Alleviators
  - Radiation
  - Intensity of pain
  - Character (quality) of pain
- If etiology of pain is uncertain, consider further studies

Laboratory evaluation
- Often not needed
- Useful in evaluating pain of unknown etiology
  - Cancer- related bone pain
  - Rheumatologic disease
  - Joint aspirates (e.g. infection, gout, etc.)

Diagnostic evaluation
- Imaging studies and electrodiagnostic studies
- Often not needed
- Useful in evaluating pain of unknown etiology
  - Cancer-related bone pain
  - Rheumatologic disease

Treatment

Ⓐ Medications
- Acetaminophen
- Nonsteroidal anti-inflammatory drugs (NSAIDs)
- Anticonvulsants
- Antidepressants
- Opioids
- Antispasmodics

Ⓑ Physical therapy
- Consider early in treatment plan
- Important to prevent progression to chronic pain syndrome
- Helps decrease long-term disability
- Often facilitated by medications and regional anesthesia

Ⓒ Regional anesthesia
- Consider psychological and physiologic state of patient
  - Is the patient a candidate for regional anesthesia?

Not a candidate for regional anesthesia
Continue physical therapy and medications

Candidate for regional anesthesia

Ⓓ Choosing a regional anesthesia technique
Ⓔ
Ⓕ
Ⓖ
- Block needed for intraoperative and postoperative pain control
  - Place block before surgery for pre-emptive analgesia
  - Will a tourniquet be used for the operation?
  - Where and how long (>20 minutes) will tourniquet be used?
- Consider contraindications to specific types of blocks (e.g. coagulopathy, chronic obstructive pulmonary disease [COPD], etc.)
- Consider placing a catheter for long-term pain control

Local anesthetic choice
Intermediate or long-acting local anesthetic agents

See Table 1 for guidance in choosing block(s)

The lower extremity is a common site for acute pain or chronic pain with acute exacerbations. The common etiologies include traumatic, degenerative, oncologic, infectious, ischemic, and neuropathic (including radicular pain). Lower extremity pain may also be referred from intervertebral discs, facet joints, and sacroiliac joints. Successful treatment of acute lower extremity pain can be optimized utilizing a multimodal approach with medications, physical therapy (including modalities such as ice or heat), graded exercise, and interventional procedures such as regional anesthesia **(Table 1)**. In a nonsurgical patient, regional anesthesia may also be useful for helping to break the pain cycle.

Ⓐ Pharmacologic treatment of acute lower extremity pain typically includes analgesic medications such as nonsteroidal anti-inflammatory drugs (NSAIDs), acetaminophen, anticonvulsants (e.g. gabapentin or pregabalin), antidepressants, and opioids. Antispasmodic (muscle relaxants) medications may be considered when severe muscle spasms are a significant component of the pain.

Ⓑ Physical therapy can play an important role in the successful treatment of acute pain as well as the prevention of chronic pain and permanent disability. Physical therapy may be the primary focus of the treatment plan, but it is often facilitated by the addition of medications and regional anesthesia techniques.

Ⓒ Regional anesthesia can be a valuable tool for the relief and control of acute lower extremity pain. Prior to choosing a technique, the patient's specific needs must be determined by answering the following questions:

- Is the patient a suitable candidate?
- Which nerves are involved in the production of pain?
- Will a tourniquet be used?
- Is anesthesia or analgesia required?
- What are the potential complications associated with each regional technique?
- Would the patient benefit from a long-term technique such as a continuous epidural or peripheral nerve catheter?
- What is your experience and expertise?

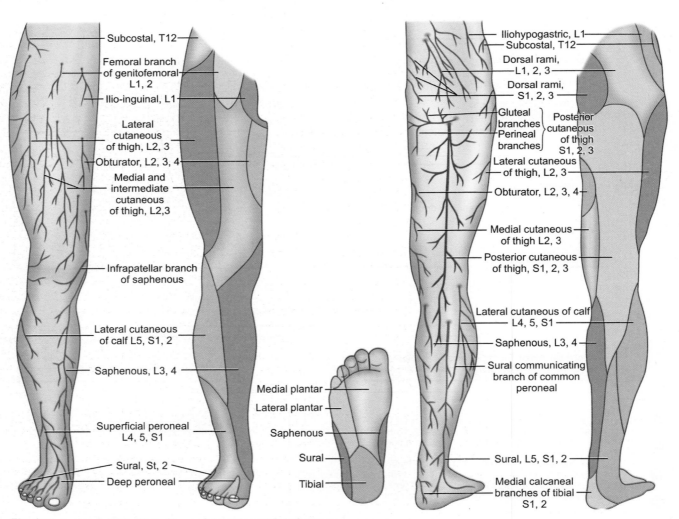

Fig. 1: Cutaneous distribution of lower extremity peripheral nerves

Table 1: Methods for blocking nerves of the lower extremities	
Nerves of the lower extremities	*Blocking methods (intrathecal or epidural)*
Lumbar plexus	
Lateral femoral cutaneous (L2, 3)	Isolated lateral femoral cutaneous nerve block 3-in-1 block Fascia iliaca block Psoas compartment block (posterior approach to lumbar plexus)
Femoral (L2-4)	Isolated femoral nerve block 3-in-1 block Fascia iliaca block Psoas compartment block (posterior approach to lumbar plexus)

Saphenous	Any type of femoral nerve block
	Isolated saphenous nerve block
	    Subsartorial (trans-sartorial) block
	    Femoral paracondylar block
	    Below-knee field block

Obturator (L2-4)	Isolated obturator nerve block Mansour's parasacral sciatic block (nerve in same fascial plane) Psoas compartment block (posterior approach to lumbar plexus) 3-in-1 block (not reliable)
Sacral plexus	Mansour's parasacral sciatic block
Sciatic (L4-S3)	Multiple approaches to posterior sciatic nerve block Anterior approach to sciatic nerve block Lateral approach to sciatic nerve block Popliteal fossa block (performed knee joint line)
Common peroneal	Any type of sciatic nerve block Isolated common peroneal nerve block at fibular head
Lateral sural cutaneous	Sciatic or common peroneal nerve block
Superficial peroneal	Sciatic or common peroneal nerve block Part of classic ankle block
Deep peroneal	Sciatic or common peroneal nerve block Isolated deep peroneal nerve block at ankle Part of classic ankle block
Tibial	Sciatic nerve block
Plantar nerves of the foot	
Medial calcaneal branches	Sciatic nerve block
Sural (contribution from calcaneal peroneal)	Part of classic ankle block
Lateral calcaneal branches	
Posterior cutaneous nerve of thigh (S1-3)	
	Isolated posterior cutaneous nerve of the thigh block Not a branch of the sciatic nerve More likely to block with higher approaches to sciatic nerve Most reliably blocked by Mansour's parasacral sciatic block

Source: Copyright © Beyer JA and Anderson DM (January 2002).

The cutaneous innervation of an extremity is highly variable, with much overlap of adjacent nerves **(Fig. 1).** In addition, the innervation of the underlying nerves (dermatomes), muscles (myotomes), and bones (sclerotomes) is often not the same as that of the overlying skin. One must always consider the differential innervation of the involved structures to avoid developing an unsatisfactory regional anesthetic plan.

D A subarachnoid or epidural block with local anesthetics and/or opioids are effective methods for treating acute lower extremity pain, especially when both lower extremities are involved. A continuous lumbar epidural can provide prolonged analgesia for hospitalized patients. A notable challenge is the relative inability to provide only unilateral anesthesia or analgesia with neuraxial anesthetic techniques. Respiratory depression, hemodynamic instability, urinary retention, sedation, postdural puncture headache, local anesthetic toxicity, epidural hematoma/abscess, and pruritus are all potential complications or side effects associated with neuraxial anesthesia.

E A combined lumbar plexus and sciatic nerve block may be effective in managing acute pain involving the entire lower extremity. This method provides better postoperative pain relief than general anesthesia and offers more hemodynamic stability than spinal or epidural anesthesia. There are several reliable approaches to the lumbar plexus and sciatic nerve block. The posterior approach to the lumbar plexus (psoas compartment block) offers many advantages, as it reliably blocks all three nerves of the lumbar plexus (i.e. femoral, lateral femoral cutaneous, and obturator). This approach is preferred in patients who have had a prior operation near the femoral vasculature. The parasacral approach is advantageous to more distal sciatic blocks as it reliably blocks both the obturator nerve and the posterior cutaneous nerve of the thigh. Blockade of the obturator nerve can be helpful when treating hip or knee pain. Both the parasacral approach to the sciatic nerve and the posterior approach to the lumbar plexus allow for placement of a catheter for continuous infusions of local anesthetic solutions.

F A more specific block or combination of blocks may also be advantageous for acute pain management of the lower extremity when a specific region is involved. A saphenous nerve block is highly effective for treating pain localized in the medial aspect of the leg. Several approaches for blocking the saphenous nerve have been described, but the subsartorial approach immediately above the knee is the least technically demanding. A common peroneal nerve block is extremely effective for managing pain localized in the lateral aspect of the leg. A lateral femoral cutaneous nerve block is effective for treating pain localized in the lateral thigh. An isolated femoral nerve block effectively controls pain originating in the knee, femur, or hip. Preoperative femoral nerve block in patients with a fractured femur or hip can facilitate movement and positioning in the operating room. The addition of a lateral femoral cutaneous nerve block can manage the pain associated with the skin incision with orthopedic intervention of hip and femoral fractures.

G Ultrasound has been shown to reduce procedure times compared to nerve stimulation alone as well as improve patient satisfaction scores. Sonographic ability to identify key structures (e.g. arteries/veins) probably improves injection safety. This imaging modality has been widely utilized to perform a variety of regional anesthesia procedures in the lower extremity and has become one of the most common tools used for nerve localization.

SUGGESTED READING

Aksoy M, Dostbil A, Ince I, et al. Continuous spinal anaesthesia versus ultrasound-guided combined psoas compartment-sciatic nerve block for hip replacement surgery in elderly high-risk patients: a prospective randomized study. BMC Anesthesiol. 2014;14:99.

Chou R, Huffman LH. Nonpharmacologic therapies for acute and chronic low back pain: a review of the evidence for an American Pain Society/American College of Physicians Clinical Practice guideline. Ann Intern Med. 2007;147(7):492-504.

Fritz JM, Magel JS, McFadden M, et al. Early physical therapy versus usual care in patients with recent-onset low back pain: a randomized clinical trial. JAMA. 2015;314(14):1459-67.

Frontera W. DeLisa's Physical Medicine and Rehabilitation: Principles and Practice, 5th edition. Philadelphia, PA: Lippincott Williams & Wilkins; 2010.

Koc Z, Ozcakir S, Sivrioglu K, et al. Effectiveness of physical therapy and epidural steroid injections in lumbar spinal stenosis. Spine (Phila Pa 1976). 2009;34(10):985-9.

Lamb SE, Lall R, Hansen Z, et al. A multicentred randomised controlled trial of a primary care-based cognitive behavioural programme for low back pain. The Back Skills Training (BeST) trial. Health Technol Assess. 2010;14(41):1-253, iii-iv.

Laplante BL, Ketchum JM, Saullo TR, et al. Multivariable analysis of the relationship between pain referral patterns and the source of chronic low back pain. Pain Physician. 2012;15(2):171-8.

Neal JM, Brull R, Horn JL, et al. The second American Society of Regional Anesthesia and Pain Medicine evidence-based medicine assessment of ultrasound-guided regional anesthesia: executive summary. Reg Anesth Pain Med. 2016;41(2):181-94.

Stanos S, Tyburski M, Harden N. Chronic pain. In: Cifu D (Ed). Braddom's Physical Medicine and Rehabilitation, 5th edition. Philadelphia, PA: Elsevier; 2016. pp. 809-33.

Waldman S. Atlas of Interventional Pain Management, 4th edition. Philadelphia, PA: Elsevier Saunders; 2015. pp. 500-13.

Acute Thoracic Pain

Walker TV, Day M

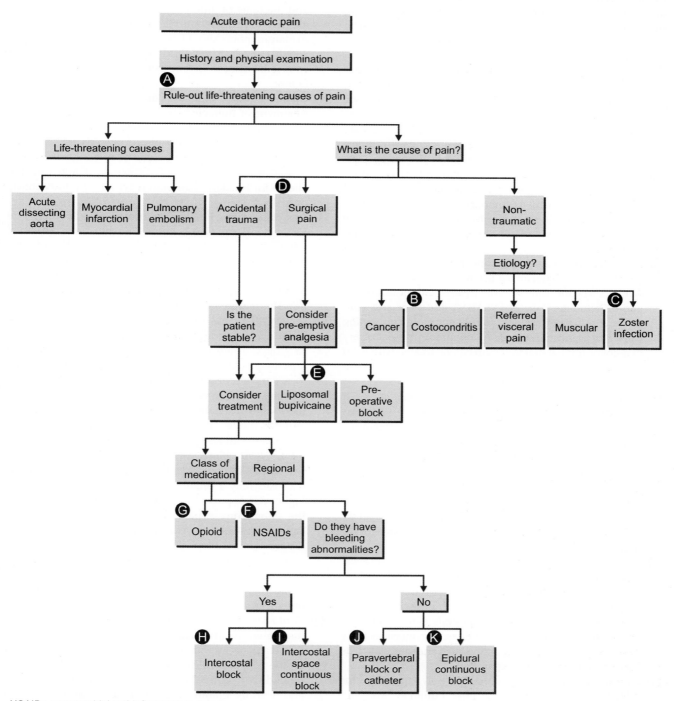

NSAIDs, nonsteroidal anti-inflammatory drugs

The thorax consists of a skeletal structure including ribs, thoracic vertebrae (T1-T12), clavicle, and sternum. Its viscera include the heart, aorta, aortic arch, vena cava, lungs, pleura, and esophagus. The thoracic innervation originates from the spine. The mixed nerve exits the spine via the neuroforamen and divides into the ventral and dorsal branches. The ventral branch continues as the intercostal nerve and traverses around the thorax, safely adhering to the caudal side of each of the ribs. The autonomic component, the white ramus communicans, also branches off of the nerve root and joins the sympathetic chain that runs vertically along the thoracic vertebrae. Visceral afferents from the thoracic pleural structures enter the spinal cord via the gray rami communicantes of the same nerve roots at T2-T6.

A *Evaluation*: Pain in the thorax does not always originate from the thorax but can be referred. Pain from the gallbladder and/or liver can present as shoulder or right lower thoracic pain; splenic pain as the left lower thoracic pain; or the stomach as mid back pain. Likewise, other visceral pain such as acute chest pain radiates as dull tightness to the arms or neck; the sharp pain caused by pleurisy, may feel like the ripping sensation of an aneurysm. It is necessary to rule out myocardial infarction, aneurism, pulmonary embolism and other life-threatening diseases by obtaining thorough history and physical examination prior to fully masking the pain symptoms.

B Costochondritis can be very concerning to patients and its pain can be mistaken for acute coronary syndrome (ACS). While costochondritis is easily treated with nonsteroidal anti-inflammatory drugs (NSAIDs) and heat and cold packs, it remains necessary to rule out more concerning causes of acute chest pain by obtaining the necessary diagnostic tests. Refractory pain can be treated with local anesthetic/steroid injections into the costochondral, and sometimes the costosternal, junction.

C Herpes zoster is difficult to identify in its early stages. It should be suspected if the patient has a history of varicella-zoster infection and the pain follows a dermatome. Diagnosis can be easily made after the pustules are present over an erythematous base. The diagnoses can be made clinically. Treatment is limited to antivirals and adequate pain control. Refractory cases can be treated with interventional therapy consisting of subcutaneous local anesthetic/steroid injections of the active pustules, thoracic sympathetic blocks, epidural steroid injections, or intercostal nerve blocks.

D Surgery or trauma are other common causes of thoracic pain, which may include open-heart surgery, video-assisted thoracoscopy, thoracotomy, or fractured ribs. Surgical and traumatic pain have historically been treated with NSAIDs, opioids, epidurals, single-shot local anesthetic and short-term catheters, but more recently have also used with longer acting local anesthetic such as liposomal bupivacaine (Exparel^{TM}).

E Liposomal bupivacaine, although only approved for infiltration of the soft tissue after bunionectomy and hemorrhoidectomy, is gaining acceptance as an adjunct for pain relief in surgical incisions, especially abdominal reconstruction and joint arthroplasty. It provides pain relief for up to 3 days after the injection. It should not be mixed with lidocaine in the same syringe or injected into the same area as lidocaine within 20 minutes of injection. Doing so can cause immediate release of the bupivacaine from its liposomes and may cause local anesthetic toxicity.

F *Multimodal Pharmacotherapy*: NSAIDs and acetaminophen have been used as part of multimodal pain relief, and the relief of thoracic pain is not any different. They are used in conjunction with thoracic-specific pain relief. Acetaminophen should be used with caution in those with liver disease, and NSAIDs used with caution in those with renal disease as they can hasten the progression to failure.

G *Opioid Therapy*: Opioids, commonly used as effective treatment of thoracic pain, carry with them some side effects such as nausea, vomiting, respiratory depression, or constipation. Despite these effects, opioids are beneficial because they can be used alone or in conjunction with other forms of pain relief. Opioids are a reasonable choice for breakthrough pain relief either intravenously or orally.

H *Intercostal Block*: Single-shot local anesthetic intercostal nerve blocks can give 3–4 hours of relief, possibly longer, depending on the choice of local anesthetic. There is also more rapid uptake in the thorax as compared to other parts of the body and consequently local anesthetic toxicity is a higher risk especially if multiple injections are done or they are repeated.

I *Intercostal Space Continuous Block*: Short-term local anesthetic infusion catheters can be left in place for up to 7 days. When placed over the intercostal space, the anesthetic follows the fascial planes and can act similarly to a paravertebral block. Unlike epidurals, the patient, primary care physician, or other provider can remove them after discharge. This offers the benefit of having another mode of pain control for a longer duration combined with rescue oral pain medication.

J *Paravertebral Block*: A paravertebral blockade has fewer side effects as compared to a thoracic epidural block as it causes only a unilateral sympathectomy. It carries a higher risk of pneumothorax, but a lower risk of injuring the spinal cord. A patient may be discharged with the catheter that can be removed at home or in the office. A paravertebral block poses less of a risk with those on anticoagulation as compared to that of an epidural as it does not reside in the spinal canal. Continuous paravertebral catheters provide comparably positive outcomes in chest wall injury to epidural catheters.

K *Continuous Epidural Block*: In spite of previously mentioned methods, an epidural is still considered the gold standard for thoracic pain relief. Side effects depend on the type of medication used and include, but are not limited to, hypotension, bradycardia, urinary retention, and pruritus. Epidurals should be used with caution in those with bleeding abnormalities, or those who are on anticoagulation therapies as bleeding within a closed space (the spinal canal) could lead to permanent or long-lasting neurological deficits.

SUGGESTED READING

Barrington JW. Efficacy of periarticular injection with a long-acting local analgesic in joint arthroplasty. Am J Orthop (Belle Mead NJ). 2015;44(10 Suppl):S13-6.

Fayezizadeh M, Petro CC, Rosen MJ, et al. Enhanced recovery after surgery pathway for abdominal wall reconstruction: pilot study and preliminary outcomes. Plast Reconstr Surg. 2014;134 (4 Suppl 2):151S-9S.

Hutchins J, Sikka R, Prielipp RC. Extrapleural catheters: an effective alternative for treating postoperative pain for thoracic surgical patients. Semin Thorac Cardiovasc Surg. 2012;24(1):15-8.

Pacira Pharmaceuticals, Inc. (2016). Highlights of prescribing information (for Exparel). [online] Available from *http://www. exparel.com/hcp/pdf/EXPAREL_Prescribing_Information.pdf.* [Accessed January, 2017].

Richard BM, Rickert DE, Doolittle D, et al. Pharmacokinetic Compatibility Study of lidocaine with EXPAREL in Yucatan miniature pigs. ISRN Pharm. 2011;2011:582351.

CHAPTER 28

Acute Vertebral Pain

Moore CC, Anitescu M

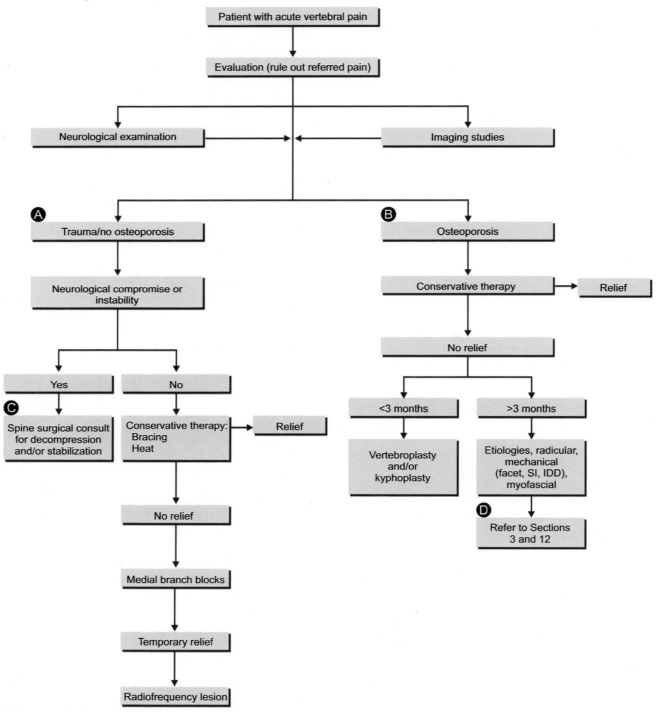

IDD, internal disc disruption; SI, sacroiliac

Severe acute pain overlying the spine has numerous causes. A thorough history, physical examination (especially neurologic examination), laboratory tests, and imaging studies are necessary to rule out referred pain from the abdominal and thoracic viscera (e.g. esophagus, heart, aorta, gallbladder, pancreas, etc.). Identifying the generator of acute axial pain is essential in delineating subsequent treatment plan to improve the acute condition.

A *Trauma*: Patients with acute vertebral pain after trauma expeditiously undergo neurologic examination and imaging studies. Patients with acute and significant neurologic compromise or instability revealed on the magnetic resonance imaging (MRI) are emergently evaluated by a neurosurgeon for possible decompression and stabilization. Vertebral fractures (particularly those involving the neural arch) that have compressed the spinal cord owing to a displaced fragment or a burst vertebrae, are considered for surgical intervention. Depending on the degree of neural canal compromise and the presence or absence of cauda equina symptoms—back pain with pain, numbness or weakness in one or both legs, saddle anesthesia, bowel or bladder dysfunction— conservative measures and braces may be of benefit. An acute traumatic vertebral compression fracture can heal in 6–8 weeks. If fractures are nondisplaced and stable without neurologic compromise, treatment is with bracing, heat, and analgesics. If the pain continues, epidural steroid injections are tried. As a next step, medial branch blocks with local anesthetics may be beneficial. Radiofrequency lesion of the medial branches may prolong pain relief for 6–9 months. In the very rare case of a fractured vertebral body that heals poorly with persistent edema confirmed by MRI images as well as persistent pain despite extensive conservative regimen with muscle relaxants, neuraxial interventions, anti-inflammatories and physical therapy, vertebral augmentation techniques (e.g. vertebroplasty or balloon kyphoplasty) are considered to stabilize the vertebrae **(Figs 1A and B)**.

B *Osteoporosis*: Elderly individuals, especially women with osteoporosis or patients who have been treated with steroids for asthma and rheumatoid arthritis, may suffer acute pain from a vertebral compression fracture. These patients receive conservative therapy with bracing, heat, and nonopioid and opioid analgesics. Physical therapy with early mobilization and stretching exercises decreases muscle spasm. However, in severe osteoporosis, a fracture may progress with height loss during aggressive mobilization. Often, older patients with osteoporotic vertebral body fractures may be incapacitated because of severe pain. In these cases, early intervention may be needed with spine augmentation to preserve as much functional capacity as possible. These interventions also are considered for patients with severe persistent pain lasting longer than 6 weeks despite conservative therapy or for patients with progressive neurologic deficit **(Figs 2A and B)**.

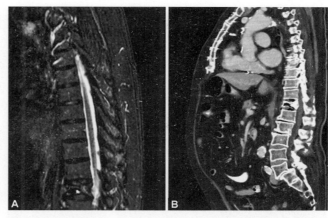

Figs 1A and B: Avascular necrosis of vertebral body (Kummel sign) in a patient with a 6-month-old compression fracture; visible edema and fluid accumulation seen in the T12 vertebral body on (A) magnetic resonance imaging (MRI) and (B) computed tomography (CT); patient underwent kyphoplasty for persistent debilitating pain

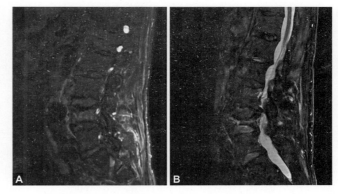

Figs 2A and B: Progression of osteoporotic fracture in a 94-year-old patient. Vertebral height significantly decreased in 4 months

C *Infection and Hematoma:* An epidural or intervertebral abscess may form after a procedure, epidural injection or in patients with endocarditis can develop epidural or intravertebral abscess. Symptoms include back pain, progressive neurological deficit, and fever. Diagnosis is established by computed tomography (CT) scans or MRI, preferably with contrast. Patients are evaluated by spine surgery consultants for emergent decompressive surgery along with antimicrobial treatment.

Epidural hematoma may form after needle placement in patients with bleeding and clotting disorders who are taking anticoagulants. After diagnosis and neurologic evaluation and imaging studies, neurosurgical consultants evaluate the patient for early (<24 hours) decompression to prevent long-term neurologic deficits.

An epidural abscess or hematoma is often considered a surgical emergency. Rapid accumulation of blood can progress quickly from back pain to paralysis within 6–8 hours; therefore, prompt recognition and intervention are warranted **(Fig. 3)**.

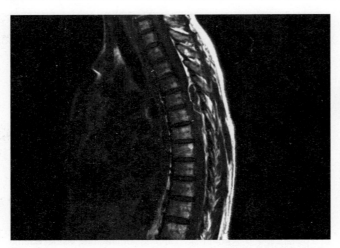

Fig. 3: Acute onset epidural hematoma after epidural catheter placement; notice significant compression on the spine and signal cord changes in the thoracic area

D *Discogenic and Mechanical Pain:* After the workup and diagnosis, patients with acute pain secondary to radicular, facet joint, discogenic, and myofascial causes should be treated as outlined in Sections 3 and 12.

SUGGESTED READING

Diamond TH, Champion B, Clark WA. Management of acute osteoporotic vertebral fractures: a nonrandomized trial comparing percutaneous vertebroplasty with conservative therapy. Am J Med. 2003;114:257-65.

Epstein NE. Timing and prognosis of surgery for spinal epidural abscess: a review. Surg Neurol Int. 2015;6(Suppl 19):S475-86.

Kendler DL, Bauer DC, Davison KS, et al. Vertebral fractures: clinical importance and management. Am J Med. 2016;129(2):221.e1-10.

Loeser JD. Bonica's Management of Pain, 3rd edition. Philadelphia: Lippincott Williams & Wilkins; 2001.

CHAPTER
29

Acute Abdominal Pain

Prust SM, Wallisch BJ

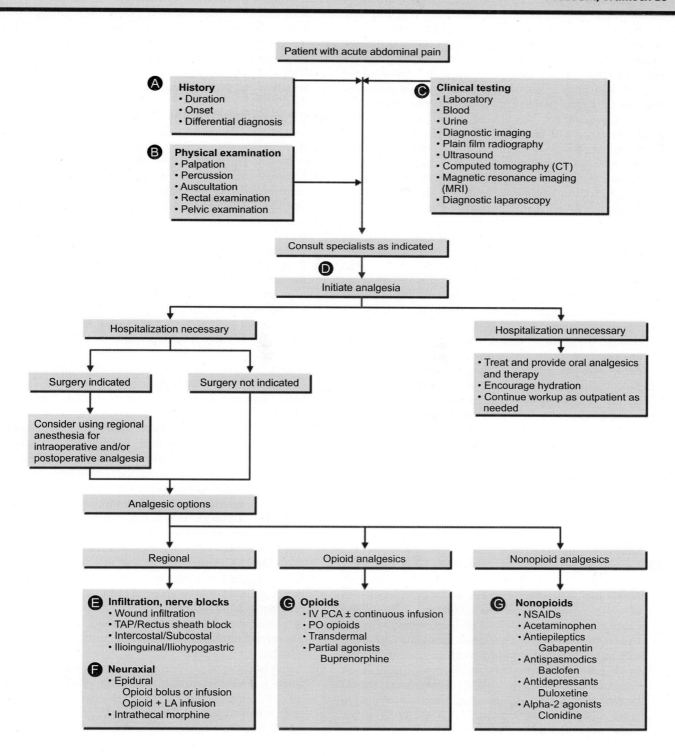

Patient with acute abdominal pain

A History
- Duration
- Onset
- Differential diagnosis

B Physical examination
- Palpation
- Percussion
- Auscultation
- Rectal examination
- Pelvic examination

C Clinical testing
- Laboratory
- Blood
- Urine
- Diagnostic imaging
- Plain film radiography
- Ultrasound
- Computed tomography (CT)
- Magnetic resonance imaging (MRI)
- Diagnostic laparoscopy

Consult specialists as indicated

D Initiate analgesia

Hospitalization necessary

Hospitalization unnecessary
- Treat and provide oral analgesics and therapy
- Encourage hydration
- Continue workup as outpatient as needed

Surgery indicated

Surgery not indicated

Consider using regional anesthesia for intraoperative and/or postoperative analgesia

Analgesic options

Regional

Opioid analgesics

Nonopioid analgesics

E Infiltration, nerve blocks
- Wound infiltration
- TAP/Rectus sheath block
- Intercostal/Subcostal
- Ilioinguinal/Iliohypogastric

F Neuraxial
- Epidural
  Opioid bolus or infusion
  Opioid + LA infusion
- Intrathecal morphine

G Opioids
- IV PCA ± continuous infusion
- PO opioids
- Transdermal
- Partial agonists
  Buprenorphine

G Nonopioids
- NSAIDs
- Acetaminophen
- Antiepileptics
  Gabapentin
- Antispasmodics
  Baclofen
- Antidepressants
  Duloxetine
- Alpha-2 agonists
  Clonidine

Abdominal discomfort is a common complaint stemming from a wide variety of causes. Although usually arising from the viscera or the parietal peritoneum, it may also result from referred pain or an intrathoracic disease process. This makes the differential diagnosis difficult and extensive. Referred pain may be experienced in the skin and body wall. A common example is inguinal and testicular pain from ureteral stones. Visceral pain is typically dull, and aching in nature, vague, diffuse, midline or difficult to pinpoint, and may be due to spasm of smooth muscle, stretch of organ capsule, inflammation or ischemia, chemical or mechanical irritation, mesenteric ischemia, and tissue acidosis. Parietal pain conversely is sharp or stabbing, and localized or referred. Both sources are accompanied by reflex guarding, tenderness, hyperalgesia, and (when severe) nausea or vomiting. Sympathetic stimulation including sweating or vagal stimulation with bradycardia is also possible.

A A complete history is important to rule out both systemic and extra-abdominal diseases such as diabetes mellitus, uremia, porphyria, sickle cell crisis, black widow spider bite, lead poisoning, trauma, acute myocardial infarction, pulmonary embolism, pneumothorax, spinal cord compression, herpetic problems, and psychological disorders. Severe pain lasting longer than 6 hours in a previously healthy patient is an "acute abdomen" and requires immediate evaluation and may require surgical intervention. Onset should be classified as sudden (rupture, perforation, embolism), rapid (acute inflammation, colic, torsion, obstruction, toxic or metabolic disease), or gradual (chronic inflammation, ectopic pregnancy, tumor, infarct). The quality is described as sharp (cutaneous or somatic, including nerve root compression), burning (neuralgia, upper gastrointestinal inflammation of mucous membranes), tearing (dissecting aortic aneurysm, anal fissure), or vague (visceral disease). Temporal features (continuous: peritonitis, colicky stones, hernia; constant: cancer, migratory, emotional), factors that aggravate or relieve, the relation to other body functions (menstruation, defecation), and associated signs and symptoms (nausea, diarrhea, segmental distribution, spasm of rectus, abdominal distension) must be identified. A menstrual history should be obtained from all women. Any previous use of analgesics and other medications for associated symptoms should be noted.

B A complete physical examination is essential. Vital signs may suggest sepsis (fever, tachycardia, hypotension). Abdominal distension, hernias, stillness/reluctance to move (peritonitis), restlessness (ureteral stones), and concomitant sweating or pallor (or both) should be noted. Gentle palpitation of the abdomen should be performed with attention to any guarding (voluntary or involuntary) or the presence of rebound pain. Percussion may detect organomegaly, ascites (fluid wave) or masses and should be further evaluated with imaging. Careful auscultation notes silence or hyperperistalsis. A rectal or pelvic examination may be warranted.

C Clinical testing may require blood and urine sampling as well as radiography. Serum electrolyte as well as urine ketone and specific gravity tests suggest the degree of dehydration. Elevated white blood cell counts, especially with fever, suggest infection; and a low hematocrit suggests nonacute blood loss. Radiographs should include chest and abdominal views. An electrocardiogram (ECG) is warranted if there are cardiac risk factors. Additional tests include ultrasound (the focused assessment with sonography for trauma [FAST] examination, pelvic, or testicular]), computed tomography (CT) scan(s), or magnetic resonance imaging (MRI) scan(s) as indicated. Diagnostic laparoscopy may be indicated depending on results of the physical examination and clinical testing modalities.

D If the pain is not critical for monitoring the progression of a condition, initiate analgesia immediately. Nausea may be caused by pain, and adequate relief may be sufficient to treat it. Analgesics, especially opioids, do not mask pertinent findings, and a "constipating" effect may relieve pain secondary to peristalsis. Immobilization may offer temporary relief. Hydration must also be initiated early and the vital signs monitored. Transdermal opioids can be used for patients who are clinically stable and have prolonged nil per os (NPO) status.

E If surgery is required, infiltration of a local anesthetic by the surgeon or anesthetist at the end of the procedure is an effective alternative, especially in outpatients (e.g. wound infiltration for inguinal herniorrhaphy). A long-acting agent such as liposomal bupivacaine can reduce the need for analgesics and promote mobilization. Body wall somatic blocks can also be considered, including intercostal/subcostal, transversus abdominis plane (TAP), ilioinguinal/iliohypogastric, and rectus sheath blocks; however, these will only treat pain of the body wall and not visceral pain.

F Neuraxial anesthesia can provide excellent postoperative analgesia, reduce pulmonary complications, reduce ileus, and promote earlier mobility. Continuous epidural infusions can be maintained for several days with an opioid, local anesthetic, or both (for synergy). A local anesthetic provides sympathectomy to optimize perfusion, although orthostasis can occur and high concentrations may affect ambulation. Intraspinal opioids by epidural or intrathecal routes are effective for visceral pain, but can cause pruritus and urinary retention. A patient-controlled epidural analgesia (PCEA) device can be connected to an epidural catheter for more rapid breakthrough pain control. Epidural or intrathecal bolus of preservative-free morphine provides approximately 24 hours of analgesia. Delayed respiratory depression is possible.

G Administration of parenteral opioids is most efficacious when a patient-controlled analgesia (PCA) device is used. PCA pumps provide the patient with some control and independence. A "background" infusion can be added to provide continuous analgesia while the patient is sleeping. Opioids may complicate postoperative recovery by inducing or prolonging an ileus. "Balanced analgesia" can be provided by adding nonsteroidal anti-inflammatory drugs (NSAIDs) or acetaminophen to reduce opioid requirements, if allowable (i.e. no gastritis/hepatic disease). Antispasmodics (such as baclofen), antiepileptics (such as gabapentin), and antidepressants (such as duloxetine) can be used in select cases as well. Tricyclic antidepressants and α-2 agonists (such as clonidine) can also be used if analgesia is not adequate after other methods have been tried.

ACKNOWLEDGMENT

Kelly Knappe, MD, 2nd edition author.

SUGGESTED READING

Basurto Ona X, Rigau Comas D, Urrútia G. Opioids for acute pancreatitis pain. Cochrane Database Syst Rev. 2013;7:CD009179.

Castro-Alves LJ, Oliveira de Medeiros AC, Neves SP, et al. Perioperative duloxetine to improve postoperative recovery after abdominal hysterectomy: a prospective, randomized, double-blinded, placebo-controlled study. Anesth Anal. 2016;122:98-104.

Chen EH, Mills AM. Abdominal pain in special populations. Emerg Med Clin North Am. 2011;29:449-58.

Cowlishaw PJ, Scott DM, Barrington MJ. The role of regional anaesthesia techniques in the management of acute pain. Anaesth Intensive Care. 2012;40:33-45.

Falch C, Vicente D, Häberle H, et al. Treatment of acute abdominal pain in the emergency room: a systematic review of the literature. Eur J Pain. 2014;18:902-13.

Gallegos N, Hobsley M. Abdominal pain: parietal or visceral? J R Soc Med. 1992;85:379.

Gans SL, Pols SL, Stoker SL, et al. Guideline for the diagnostic pathway in patients with acute abdominal pain. Dig Surg. 2015; 32:23-31.

Hutchins J, Delaney D, Vogel RI, et al. Ultrasound-guided sub-costal transversus abdominis plane (TAP) infiltration with liposomal bupivacaine for patients undergoing robotic assisted hysterectomy: a prospective randomized controlled study. Gynecol Oncol. 2015;138:609-13.

Marsicano EE, Vuong GM, Prather CM. Gastrointestinal causes of abdominal pain. Obstet Gynecol Clin North Am. 2014;41:465-89.

Murphy KP, Twomey M, McLaughlin PD, et. al. Imaging of ischemia, obstruction and infection in the abdomen. Radiol Clin North Am. 2015;53:847-69, ix-x.

Prystupa A, Mróz T, Wojciechowska K, et al. Clinical approach to visceral pain in irritable bowel syndrome—pathophysiology, symptoms, and treatment. Ann Agric Environ Med. 2013;1:8-13.

Ragsdale L, Southerland L. Acute abdominal pain in the older adult. Emerg Med Clin North Am. 2011;29:429-48.

Taylor R Jr, Pergolizzi JV, Sinclair A, et al. Transversus abdominis block: clinical uses, side effects, and future perspectives. Pain Pract. 2013;13:332-44.

Viniol A, Keunecke C, Biroga T, et al. Studies of the symptom abdominal pain—a systematic review and meta-analysis. Fam Pract. 2014;31:517-29.

Wang DC, Parry CR, Feldman M, et al. Acute abdomen in the emergency department: is CT a time-limiting factor? AJR Am J Roentgenol. 2015;205:1222-9.

CHAPTER
30

Acute Pancreatic Pain

McKenny J, Wallisch BJ

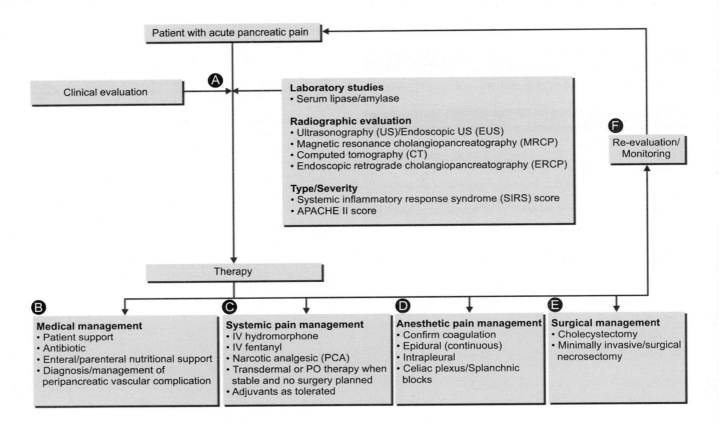

Acute pancreatitis (AP) is an acutely painful inflammatory process of the abdomen that has extensive local and systemic effects. In up to 90% of cases in the United States, the cause is related to either alcohol abuse or biliary tract disease. Common triggers of AP include infection, trauma, ischemia and genetic disorders. Additionally there are over 500 different drugs suspected of inducing pancreatitis including the angiotensin-converting enzyme (ACE) inhibitors, antibiotics, steroids, and acetaminophen. The Atlanta classification breaks AP into two broad categories: (1) interstitial edematous AP and (2) necrotizing AP. Interstitial edematous AP is characterized by acute inflammation of the pancreatic parenchyma and peripancreatic tissues without tissue necrosis. Conversely, necrotizing AP is characterized by acute inflammation and pancreatic necrosis. AP can be further classified as mild, moderate, or severe.

A Initial evaluation should seek to establish the clinical severity. Evaluation for fluid losses, signs of organ failure or shock and application of severity of disease classifications

systems such as the Acute Physiology and Chronic Health Evaluation II (APACHE II) score or systemic inflammatory response syndrome (SIRS) score will help guide the need for resuscitation and give an assessment of the necessary level of nursing care. A single serum amylase and lipase level is helpful in diagnosis but serial measurements will not provide level of severity or prognosis and cannot be used for guiding medical management. Routine computed tomography (CT) is not recommended at initial presentation unless there is diagnostic uncertainty as evidence of necrotizing pancreatitis is usually not evident until approximately 72 hours after the initial presentation of symptoms. Ultrasonography is less sensitive for detecting pancreatic abnormalities but more sensitive for detecting biliary calculi. Endoscopic retrograde cholangiopancreatography (ERCP), endoscopic ultrasonography (EUS) and magnetic resonance colonography (MRC) may be used to identify treatable causes of AP.

B Medical management of AP is directed at aggressive patient support to prevent morbidity and mortality in the early stages of severe AP. Patients with AP should be monitored closely for the first 24–48 hours, and those with severe AP will likely benefit from treatment in an intensive care setting or at a medical center that specializes in the AP. Maintaining tissue perfusion with aggressive volume resuscitation, respiratory support, transfusions in the face of anemia, prophylaxis against gastric ulcer and early enteral (preferably) or parenteral nutritional support are effective. Prophylactic antibiotics are not recommended in patients with AP, regardless of the type or disease severity.

C Pain management is most often accomplished with adequate fluid resuscitation and opioid analgesics. Patients often require the use patient-controlled analgesia (PCA) pumps with either fentanyl or hydromorphone. Both fentanyl and hydromorphone are preferred over morphine or meperidine due to lack of active metabolites that can accumulate in patients with renal impairment. In the recent past, meperidine was the preferred agent over morphine as it has less contractile action of the sphincter of Oddi; however, there are a no clinical studies supporting this theory or that such spasm would induce or aggravate pancreatitis or bile duct pathology. Meperidine has downsides as well in that its short half-life requires repeat doses that can lead to an accumulation of a metabolite (normeperidine) shown to produce neuromuscular side effects and induce seizure activity.

D Epidural opioids can provide excellent analgesia without biliary spasm. Epidural infusion of dilute local anesthetic provides pain relief; however, improved outcomes with the use of epidural analgesia versus intravenous opioid analgesia have not been established. AP and concomitant alcoholism can lead to an immunosuppressed state; therefore, placement of an indwelling catheter requires careful consideration. Intermittent or continuous celiac plexus block offers an effect alternative treatment for pain in AP in patients whom the conventional methods fail to provide proper pain relief.

E Surgical intervention during the acute phase is discouraged as there is lack of benefit and in fact risk of infecting a sterile phlegmon. An exception to this rule is when serious concomitant intra-abdominal pathology is suspected. ERCP is avoided during the early stages unless the patient has an obstructed common bile stone. EUS and MRC can be performed in select patients to determine the need for ERCP.

F Frequent monitoring for local, perivascular and systemic complications secondary to AP is vital as they carry a great risk of increase morbidity and mortality. Local complications include pancreatic pseudocyst, acute peripancreatic fluid collection, walled-off necrosis, and acute necrotic collections. These may require CT-guided fine-needle aspiration (FNA) for antibiotic delivery or drainage. Vascular complications are potentially devastating in the form of splanchnic venous thrombosis, pseudoaneurysm formation, and abdominal compartment syndrome. The stress of AP places patients at risk for exacerbation of concurrent underlying comorbidities and they should be followed closely.

ACKNOWLEDGMENT

Linda Tingle, MD, 2nd edition author.

SUGGESTED READING

Basurto Ona X, Rigau Comas D, Urrutia G. Opioids for acute pancreatitis pain. Cochrane Database Syst Rev. 2013;7:CD009179.

Bellocchi MC, Campagnola P, Frulloni L. Drug-induced acute pancreatitis. Pancreapedia: Exocrine Pancreas Knowledge Base. American Pancreatic Association; 2015.

Bradley EL 3rd. A clinically based classification system for acute pancreatitis. Summary of the International Symposium on Acute Pancreatitis, Atlanta, Ga, September 11 through 13, 1992. Arch Surg. 1993;128:586-90.

Heller AR, Ragaller M, Koch T. Epidural abscess after epidural catheter for pain release during pancreatitis. Acta Anaesthesiol Scand. 2000;44:1024-7.

Kennedy SF. Celiac plexus steroids for acute pancreatitis. Reg Anesth. 1983;8:39-40.

Tenner S, Baillie J, DeWitt J, et al. American College of Gastroenterology guideline: management of acute pancreatitis. Am J Gastroenterol. 2013;108:1400-15; 1416.

Working Group IAP/APA Acute Pancreatitis Guidelines. IAP/APA evidence-based guidelines for the management of acute pancreatitis. Pancreatology. 2013;13:e1-15.

Working Party of the British Society of Gastroenterology; Association of Surgeons of Great Britain and Ireland; Pancreatic Society of Great Britain and Ireland, et al. UK guidelines for the management of acute pancreatitis. Gut. 2005;54 (Suppl 3):iii1-9.

Obstetric Pain

King AL, Liles DR

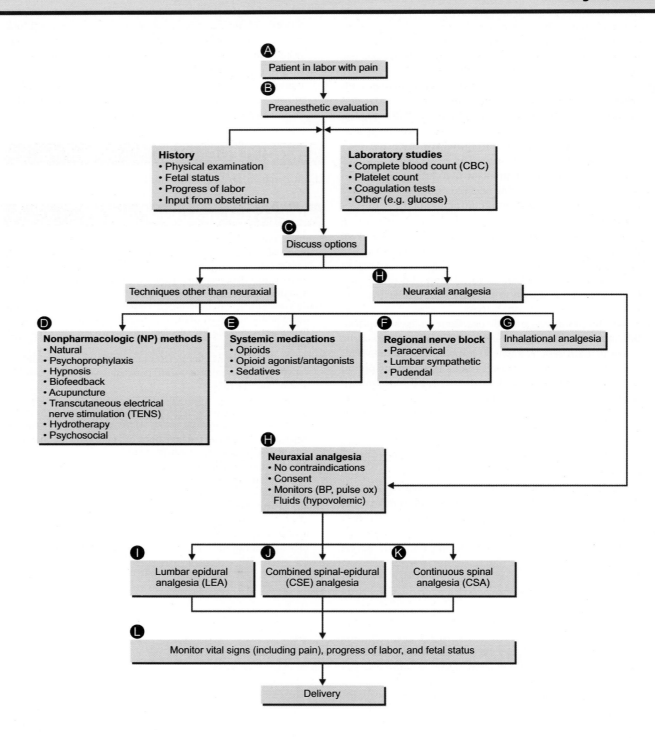

A Patient in labor with pain

B Preanesthetic evaluation

History
- Physical examination
- Fetal status
- Progress of labor
- Input from obstetrician

Laboratory studies
- Complete blood count (CBC)
- Platelet count
- Coagulation tests
- Other (e.g. glucose)

C Discuss options

Techniques other than neuraxial

H Neuraxial analgesia

D **Nonpharmacologic (NP) methods**
- Natural
- Psychoprophylaxis
- Hypnosis
- Biofeedback
- Acupuncture
- Transcutaneous electrical nerve stimulation (TENS)
- Hydrotherapy
- Psychosocial

E **Systemic medications**
- Opioids
- Opioid agonist/antagonists
- Sedatives

F **Regional nerve block**
- Paracervical
- Lumbar sympathetic
- Pudendal

G Inhalational analgesia

H **Neuraxial analgesia**
- No contraindications
- Consent
- Monitors (BP, pulse ox) Fluids (hypovolemic)

I Lumbar epidural analgesia (LEA)

J Combined spinal-epidural (CSE) analgesia

K Continuous spinal analgesia (CSA)

L Monitor vital signs (including pain), progress of labor, and fetal status

Delivery

Labor is usually a painful experience, although it varies considerably from patient to patient. An ideal anesthetic provides rapid pain relief which lasts throughout the labor and delivery period and has no adverse effect on the mother, fetus, or progress of labor.

Ⓐ Labor pain has two anatomic components. During the first stage of labor, pain results from cervical dilatation and distension of the lower uterine segment with contractions. Pain is transmitted primarily by small, unmyelinated, visceral afferent C fibers that pass through the paracervical region, hypogastric nerve/plexus, and lumbar sympathetic chain to terminate in the ventral and dorsal horn of the spinal cord from T10 to L1. During the late first and second stages of labor, pain also results from vaginal and perineal distension or injury during fetal descent. This pain is transmitted by thin, myelinated, A-δ somatic sensory nerve fibers traveling in the pudendal nerve (S2, S3, S4). Ascending spinal cord tracts transmit afferent nociceptive impulses to the cortex. Several techniques have been used to target the pain pathways at all points, from the most distal (e.g. paracervical and pudendal nerve blocks) to the most proximal (e.g. systemic medications, psychotherapy).

Ⓑ Perform a thorough preanesthetic evaluation on any patient requesting analgesia for labor and delivery, and include the obstetric diagnosis, fetal status, and progress of labor. Obtain pertinent laboratory information (e.g. platelets in pre-eclamptic patients).

Ⓒ Labor pain causes adverse physiological changes (e.g. hyperventilation, increased oxygen consumption, catecholamine release) that can be attenuated with analgesia. Discuss analgesic options and counsel the patient regarding associated risks and benefits. Education decreases anxiety and allows the parturient to give informed consent. Selection of the appropriate analgesic technique must be individualized based on patient preference and medical indications/contraindications.

Ⓓ Nonpharmacologic (NP) methods of pain control during labor have several mechanisms of action, including competitive sensory stimulation, alteration of the biologic response to pain, and amelioration of negative psychological issues. NP methods include natural childbirth, psychoprophylaxis (e.g. Lamaze), hypnosis, biofeedback, acupuncture, transcutaneous electrical nerve stimulation (TENS), hydrotherapy (e.g. warm water baths), and psychosocial support. These methods provide a safe alternative for all laboring patients.

Ⓔ Systemic medications, including opioids, opioid agonist/antagonists (e.g. nalbuphine), and opioid adjuncts/sedatives (e.g. ketamine), are available for use during labor, but they have limited analgesic efficacy for labor pain and may result in limited patient satisfaction. Opioids are the most commonly used systemic medications and are the best option if neuraxial analgesia (NA) is contraindicated, technically challenging, or unavailable. Opioids can be given by intermittent bolus or by patient-controlled analgesia (PCA). Shorter-acting opioids, such as fentanyl or remifentanil, are more effective when using PCA. Side effects in both the mother (i.e. nausea and vomiting [N/V], sedation, respiratory depression, disorientation, delayed gastric emptying) and baby (i.e. respiratory depression, low neurobehavioral scores) are dose-dependent. Neonatal respiratory depression also depends on the timing of opioid administration.

Ⓕ Regional nerve blocks represent another analgesic option for labor and vaginal delivery. Paracervical block provides analgesia during the first stage of labor. This block has the potential for severe complications (i.e. fetal bradycardia, distress, and death), and is contraindicated if fetal compromise is present. Lumbar sympathetic block can also provide analgesia for the first stage of labor. Pudendal nerve block is useful during the second stage of labor. Analgesia from these options is time-limited and dependent on choice of local anesthetic (LA).

Ⓖ Inhalational analgesia (e.g. nitrous oxide, volatile halogenated agents) combined with oxygen can be effective. Advantages include rapid onset and minimal neonatal depression. However, this technique is associated with several risks (i.e. loss of consciousness, vomiting, aspiration, laryngospasm, hypoventilation, hypoxia, cardiac arrhythmias). Nitrous oxide is the most common inhalational agent used for labor analgesia worldwide and is garnering renewed interest in the United States. Use of volatile halogenated agents should be carefully weighed as they notably cause dose-dependent uterine smooth muscle relaxation.

Ⓗ Neuraxial analgesia is the most effective method for providing analgesia during labor. In addition to excellent pain relief, NA decreases circulating catecholamine concentrations, maintains adequate maternal and fetal oxygenation with a decrease in maternal hyperventilation, and decreases the incidence of maternal and fetal acidosis. NA is contraindicated in patients with coagulopathy, hypovolemia, sepsis, infection at the needle entry site, increased intracranial pressure, and allergy to an LA. If NA is chosen, obtain informed consent, apply appropriate monitors on the patient, and administer intravenous fluids as necessary to correct hypovolemia. NA can be initiated whenever the patient desires analgesia regardless of cervical dilatation without prolonging the duration of labor. NA does not increase the rate of cesarean delivery; however, dense NA may prolong the second stage of labor and increase the rate of instrumented vaginal delivery. Side effects of NA include hypotension, nausea and vomiting, urinary retention, pruritus, fever, shivering, and delayed gastric emptying. Potential complications include inadequate pain relief, inadvertent dural puncture, postdural puncture headache (PDPH), back pain, nerve injury, infection, hematoma, respiratory depression, and high sensory/motor blockade.

Ⓘ Lumbar epidural analgesia (LEA) provides excellent pain relief throughout the course of labor and can be extended to provide anesthesia for an instrumented vaginal delivery or cesarean section. A continuous infusion of dilute LA (with the possible addition of lipid-soluble opioid to reduce the LA requirement) produces reliable analgesia with minimal motor blockade as well as a minimal effect on uterine activity and fetal well-being. The risks of inadvertent subarachnoid or intravascular injection due to catheter malposition are prevented by careful test dosing and interval aspiration.

J Combined spinal-epidural (CSE) analgesia for labor offers the advantages of both intrathecal medications (i.e. rapid onset) and LEA (i.e. placement of a catheter). With this technique, the intrathecal injection (opioid, LA, or both opioid and LA) takes place prior to threading an epidural catheter. A test dose must be administered before the LEA catheter is activated. The catheter can be used immediately or at a later time.

K Continuous spinal analgesia (CSA) can provide tightly controlled labor analgesia or be extended for surgical anesthesia; however, it is associated with a higher likelihood of PDPH. It is an option in the setting of unintentional dural puncture.

L Patients who have been given labor analgesia must be carefully monitored. In all patients, the progress of labor and the fetal status must be followed. Anesthetic requirements may change throughout labor, and some patients require assistance with pain management after delivery.

SUGGESTED READING

American College of Obstetricians and Gynecologists Committee on Obstetric Practice. ACOG committee opinion no. 339. Analgesia and cesarean delivery rates. Obstet Gynecol. 2006;107: 1487-8.

Anim-Somuah M, Smyth RM, Jones L. Epidural versus non-epidural or no analgesia in labour. Cochrane Database Syst Rev. 2011;(12):CD000331.

Jones L, Othman M, Dowswell T, et al. Pain management for women in labour: an overview of systematic reviews. Cochrane Database Syst Rev. 2012;(3):CD009234.

Likis FE, Andrews JC, Collins MR. Nitrous oxide for the management of labor pain: a systematic review. Anesth Analg. 2014;118(1):153-67.

Wong CA. Epidural and spinal analgesia/anesthesia for labor and vaginal delivery. In: Chestnut DH, Wong CA, Tsen LC, Ngan Kee WD, Beilin Y, Mhyre J (Eds). Chestnut's Obstetric Anesthesia: Principles and Practice, 5th edition. Philadelphia: Elsevier Saunders; 2014.

SECTION 3

Chronic Pain Syndromes

Brian T Boies

Myofascial Pain

Nagpal A, Bickelhaupt B

Diagnosis and treatment flow chart for MPS

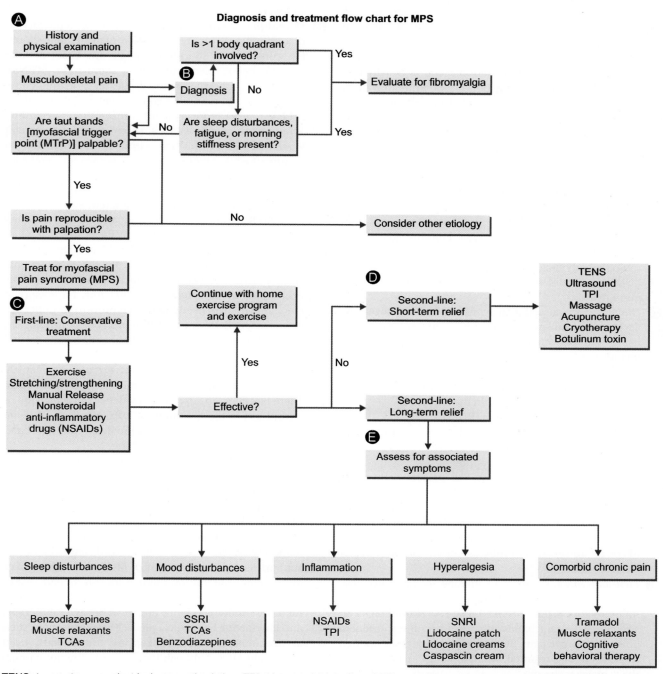

TENS, transcutaneous electrical nerve stimulation, TPI, trigger point injection, SSRI, selective serotonin reuptake inhibitor, SNRI, serotonin-norepinephrine reuptake inhibitor, TCAs, tricyclic antidepressants

Myofascial pain syndrome (MPS) is a broad term used to describe pain due to a muscular or tendinous etiology. It specifically requires the presence of myofascial trigger points (MTrPs), which are palpable contracted bands of muscle fibers. These taut bands produce localized, referred pain with deep pressure or aggravating movement. MPS can be distinguished from other muscular pain syndromes by the presence of taut skeletal muscle bands, reproducible, localized pain, autonomic symptoms, and absence of multiple pain generators.

A *Clinical Presentation:* Myofascial pain syndrome can be quickly diagnosed on history and a simple physical examination. MPS is commonly described as dull, deep-seated pain, felt in musculotendinous regions. The onset can be acute or chronic and is usually due to physical strain or long periods of immobilization, such as hospitalization. Associated symptoms may be present depending on the location of MPS. For example, if neighboring nerves are compressed or involved in the MTrPs, numbness and tingling may be present. With MTrP aggravation, autonomic symptoms such as vasodilation or piloerection can develop. Eventually MPS affects occupational participation and causes reversible muscle weakness, fatigue, and sleep disturbances. Multiple, coexistent MTrPs are not uncommon and can be mistaken for fibromyalgia. Fibromyalgia can be ruled out by the presence of tender myofascial points in multiple body quadrants and concomitant fatigue, sleep disturbance, and mood disorders (See Chapter 33 on Fibromyalgia).

B *Diagnosis:* Myofascial pain syndrome lacks a universally accepted diagnostic criterion and is instead diagnosed using clinical characteristics. These characteristics include the following:
- Localized, reproducible pain
- Taut, palpable band located within a muscle
- Localized tenderness within the taut band
- Restricted range of motion (ROM)
- Pain relieved by stretching the affected muscle or MTrP injections
- Palpation of transverse snapping

Myofascial pain syndrome will present with either restricted ROM or pain on movement regardless of ROM. Deep pressure will identify the hard, taut band and cause significant pain, reproducing the patient's primary symptoms. Deep pressure should be sustained over the MTrP for 10 seconds to fully assess for the presence of referred pain.

C *First-line Therapy:* First-line therapy includes exercise, stress reduction, manual therapy, and nonsteroidal anti-inflammatory drugs (NSAIDs). Exercise should focus on stretching the taut bands that have become shortened. This will improve pain, ROM, and mobility. Once optimal muscle length is restored, strengthening can be added to the exercise regimen.

Since the pathophysiology involves the central and peripheral nervous system, pharmacologic modalities are aimed at correcting for these dysfunctions. NSAIDs are commonly offered due to their accessibility, affordability, and well-studied side effects. However, there is limited literature for their efficacy in treating MPS.

Many of the above-mentioned therapies' effects can be augmented with manual release. Manual release focuses on stretching collagen tissue in and around the MTrP, also known as deep tissue cross friction massage. It is believed that this technique assists in restoring blood flow to the hypoxic tissue. After therapy, the patient should continue to stretch the affected muscle daily.

D *Second-line Therapy:* If the MPS pain is refractory to first-line therapy, more aggressive management should be considered. Short-term relief methods include transcutaneous electrical nerve stimulation (TENS), ultrasound, massage, manual massage, acupuncture, cryotherapy, botulinum toxin, trigger point injections (TPIs), and more potent analgesics. Regarding acupuncture, some studies show short-term benefit when compared with sham acupuncture, NSAIDs, or no treatment while other studies have shown no significant improvement compared to placebo. MTrPs and acupuncture needle sites frequently overlap, making the treatments' efficacies difficult to differentiate.

If MPS becomes refractory, a series of dry needling or TPIs can be offered. These are most effective when performed with manual release techniques. Dry needling is theorized to mechanically disrupt the dysfunctional activity of the motor end plate, eliciting a twitch response. It has been demonstrated to significantly improve pain compared to sham needling and has proven more effective in increasing ROM compared to placebo. Unfortunately, dry needling is highly dependent upon the technique and skill of the examiner.

Conversely, TPI treats MTrPs through mechanical stimulation and anesthetics, steroids, or botulinum toxin. There has been no supportive evidence for anesthetic or steroid use in the treatment of MPS. However, TPIs are frequently used due to their immediate pain relief and patient preference over dry needling.

Botulinum toxin acts through central and peripheral mechanisms to decrease pain by inhibiting release of acetylcholine (ACh) at the neuromuscular junction. Botulinum toxin is used off-label to treat MPS by treating MTrPs and disrupting nociceptive pain. Treatment of MPS with botulinum toxin has had mixed responses. Some investigators have found insufficient evidence to support its use for treatment of MPS while others have found significant improvement in short-term pain relief.

Long-term relief options for MPS include muscle relaxants, antidepressants, cognitive behavioral therapy, and long-acting benzodiazepines. Muscle relaxants, such as tizanidine and cyclobenzaprine, are regularly used in treating MPS. Although there is currently not enough evidence to support use of cyclobenzaprine in the treatment of MPS, it works well in treating musculoskeletal pain and can simultaneously function as a sleeping agent.

The α$_2$-adrenergic agonist, tizanidine, reduces the release of neurotransmitters in ascending pathways. It has been shown to significantly improve, pain, sleep, and disability in MPS.

Antidepressants have been gaining increasing popularity in pain treatment due to their dual effect on comorbid mood symptoms. Selective serotonin-norepinephrine reuptake inhibitors (SNRIs) are widely used to treat muscle pain and fibromyalgia, but have not been extensively studied in the treatment of MPS.

Lidocaine patches are easily applied agents with a low side effect profile. They are effective in the treatment of MPS although they do not generate as great of a pain reduction compared to needling. Other topical therapies such as capsaicin, lidocaine, and menthol creams can be provided for temporary, symptomatic relief.

E *Associated Symptoms:* As mentioned previously, the treatment of MPS should be individualized to each patient. Treatment goals of the patient, comorbid diseases, and myofascial-associated symptoms should all be considered. When insomnia is present, it is beneficial to consider benzodiazepines, muscle relaxants, or tricyclic antidepressants (TCAs), since their side effect profile includes somnolence. Some patients will have a concomitant mood disturbance, from the severity of the MPS itself or a coexisting disease. These patients should be considered for selective serotonin reuptake inhibitors (SSRIs), SNRIs, or TCAs due to their antidepressant and mood altering components. Coexistent inflammation of the MPS areas can be treated with NSAIDs and TPIs. In some patients, MPS can present with hyperalgesia. This sensation could be heightened in patients with pre-existing nerve damage, such as diabetes. This cohort can be given SNRIs, lidocaine creams, lidocaine patches, or capsaicin creams. It is not uncommon to have MPS patients who have comorbid chronic pain from other etiologies. These patients would benefit the most from tramadol, muscle relaxants, and cognitive behavioral therapy. It is important to understand that an effective treatment plan for MPS frequently involves multiple therapy modalities, tailored to the individual needs of the patient.

SUGGESTED READING

Borg-Stein J. Treatment of fibromyalgia, myofascial pain, and related disorders. Phys Med Rehabil Clin N Am. 2006;17(2):491-510.

Borg-Stein J, Iaccarino MA. Myofascial pain syndrome treatments. Phys Med Rehabil Clin N Am. 2014;25(2):357-74.

Cifu DX. Braddom's Physical Medicine and Rehabilitation, 5th edition. Philadelphia: Elsevier; 2016.

Giamberardino MA, Affaitati G, Fabrizio A, et al. Myofascial pain syndromes and their evaluation. Best Pract Res Clin Rheumatol. 2011;25(2):185-98.

Irnich D. Myofascial Trigger Points: Comprehensive diagnosis and treatment, 1st edition. Edinburgh: Elsevier-Churchill Livingstone; 2013.

Simons D, Travell J, Simons L. Myofacial pain and dysfunction: The trigger point manual, Vol. 1. Upper Half of Boyd. Baltimore: Williams & Wilkins; 1999.

CHAPTER
33

Fibromyalgia

Bautista A, Chang Chien GC, Candido KD

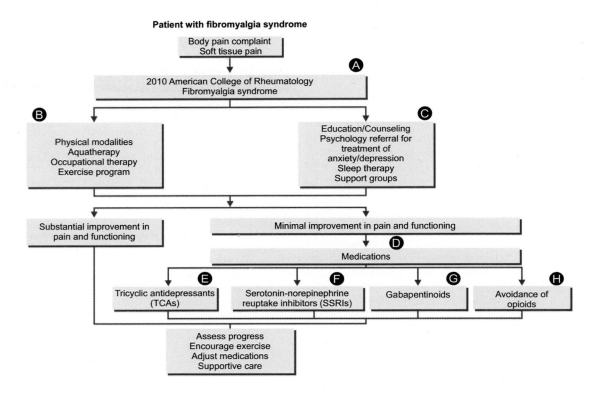

Patient with fibromyalgia syndrome

Fibromyalgia (FM) is a chronic condition associated with widespread musculoskeletal pain, fatigue, sleep disruption, a variety of somatic complaints, cognitive dysfunction, and psychiatric symptoms. It commonly affects women between ages of 20 years and 55 years. The etiology of this syndrome as well as the pathophysiology is still undefined. There is no evidence of tissue inflammation despite reported soft tissue pain affecting the muscles, ligaments and tendons.

A Typically, the diagnosis is primarily on the patient's complaints of "I am hurting all over." In the recent 2010 American College of Rheumatology (ACR) Classification Criteria, widespread pain index (WPI) greater than or equal to 7 and symptom severity (SS) scale score greater than or equal to 5 for at least 3 months with no other disorder that would otherwise explain the pain support the diagnosis of FM **(Table 1)**. Diagnostic testing should be kept to a minimum since no laboratory, radiographic nor pathologic testing is helpful in the diagnosis. Serologic testing for antinuclear antibody and rheumatoid factor should be reserved only for patients whose symptoms are highly suggestive of inflammatory or systemic rheumatic disease.

B Treatment of FM is challenging. The goal of treatment is primarily directed at reducing symptoms of fatigue, insomnia, chronic widespread pain and cognitive dysfunction. Patients usually respond best with an individualized and multidisciplinary treatment that involves the physician, physical medicine, rehabilitation and mental health specialists. Recent evidence suggests graded exercise training that includes aquatic, resistance, aerobic and mixed physical activity intervention improves pain and physical function while yoga, pilates and tai chi showed inconclusive evidences.

C It is important to educate patients in order for them to have a better understanding regarding their diagnosis and treatment, unknown pathogenesis, and most importantly their role for their own treatment. If possible, involvement of the patient's support group or family members is advocated. Patient education should include reassurance that their condition is a real illness and is not a figment of their imagination. However, the patient should be made aware that the condition is benign in nature. Patients should be told that good sleep hygiene and correction of

Table 1: Criteria for diagnosing fibromyalgia

1990 ACR criteria	2010 ACR criteria	
	Widespread pain index (WPI) score >=(0–19)	*Symptom severity scale (SS) >=5 (0–12)*

Widespread pain in combination with:
• Tenderness at >=11 out of 18 tender points
• Digital palpation with >=4 kg of force
	19 anatomical locations
	• Shoulder: Left and right
	• Upper arm: Left and right
	• Lower arm: Left and right
	• Jaw: Left and right
	• Neck
	• Buttock, hip, trochanter: Left and right
	• Upper leg: Left and right
	• Lower leg: Left and right
	• Upper back
	• Lower back
	• Chest
	• Abdomen
		A. Presence and severity (0–3) of fatigue, cognitive symptoms, waking unrefreshed
		B. General presence of somatic symptoms
		  • 0: No symptoms
		  • 1: Few symptoms
		  • 2: Moderate number of symptoms
		  • 3: A great deal of symptoms

	Symptom severity scale >=9 and WPI 3–6 are also acceptable	

ACR, American College of Rheumatology

poor sleeping habits and obtaining treatment for sleep disorders are necessary. Also, they should be encouraged to learn simple relaxation techniques and participate in mood and stress-reduction programs. Patients should also be counseled regarding the importance of exercise for reconditioning and temporary increase in myalgia during the initiation of the exercise program. Most importantly, they should be made aware that somatic symptoms may be remitting but the pain and fatigue generally persist.

D Some patients not responding to nonpharmacologic therapy alone may be started on medications that have been well studied and consistently effective for FM. These medications include antidepressants and selected anticonvulsants. For patients who have continued symptoms despite initial nonpharmacologic and maximum monotherapy dose, combination drug therapy is recommended based solely upon clinical experience. A low dose serotonin-norepinephrine reuptake inhibitors (SNRIs) ± tricyclic antidepressants (TCAs) or anticonvulsants in the evening have been studied and showed significant pain reduction and global improvement compared with each individual drug alone.

E Tricyclic antidepressants can be effective as an initial treatment for FM. Amitriptyline 25–50 mg single bedtime dose was found to be efficacious. The dose is usually lower than what is required to treat depression. Desipramine 5–10 mg can be a possible alternative and has generally fewer anticholinergic effects that include dry mouth, constipation, weight gain, and fluid retention among others. In some patients, the efficacy of TCAs may decrease over time.

F The SNRIs have been found to be effective as well for FM. Several systematic reviews regarding duloxetine 20–30 mg/day to a recommended dose of 60 mg/day and milnacipran 50 mg twice daily up to 100 mg twice daily have been found to demonstrate long-term benefits.

G Anticonvulsants have convincing evidence of efficacy for FM, including gabapentin 100 mg at bedtime to 1200–2400 mg/day and pregabalin 25–50 mg to 300–450 mg/day. Literature supports that it consistently reduced pain and improved sleep and quality of life especially in those unresponsive or intolerant to TCAs.

H Chronic medically-directed opioid therapy has not been proven effective in the treatment of FM. Analgesics, anti-inflammatory drugs, alternative antidepressants, and complementary and alternative therapies (acupuncture, tai chi or yoga) have limited evidence to substantiate its use for FM.

In summary, current evidence showed that a stepwise program emphasizing education, certain medications, exercise, and cognitive therapy should be recommended.

SUGGESTED READING

Bidonde J, Busch AJ, Bath B, et al. Exercise for adults with fibromyalgia: an umbrella systematic review with synthesis of best evidence. Curr Rheumatol Rev. 2014;10(1):45-79.

Fitzcharles MA, Ste-Marie PA, Goldenberg DL, et al. Canadian Pain Society and Canadian Rheumatology Association recommendations for rational care of persons with fibromyalgia: a summary report. J Rheumatol. 2013;40(8):1388-93.

Goldenberg DL, Burckhardt C, Crofford L. Management of fibromyalgia syndrome. JAMA. 2004;292(19):2388-95.

Wolfe F, Clauw DJ, Fitzcharles MA, et al. The American College of Rheumatology preliminary diagnostic criteria for fibromyalgia and measurement of symptom severity. Arthritis Care Res (Hoboken). 2010;62(5):600-10.

Wolfe F, Smythe HA, Yunus MB, et al. The American College of Rheumatology 1990 Criteria for the Classification of Fibromyalgia. Report of the Multicenter Criteria Committee. Arthritis Rheum. 1990;33(2):160-72.

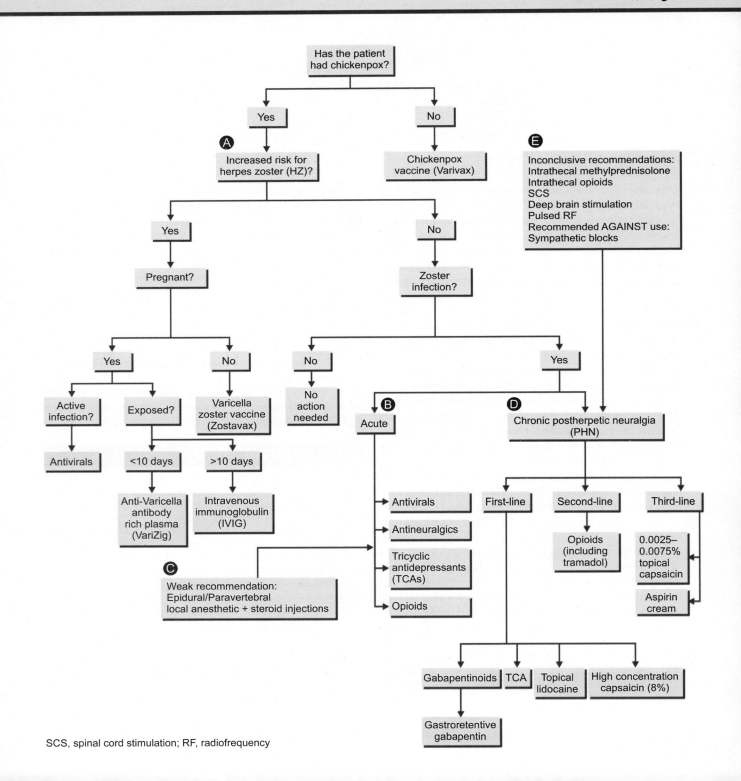

SCS, spinal cord stimulation; RF, radiofrequency

Initial exposure to the varicella-zoster virus (VZV) causes chickenpox. Once this common infection resolves, the virus becomes latent in the dorsal root ganglion (DRG), where it can reactivate in patients who experience immune-suppressing conditions. In this neural structure, viral replication causes intense inflammation, hemorrhaging and necrosis. Herpes zoster (HZ), shingles, is associated with significant morbidity given the severity of pain during the acute phase of infection. Chronic neuropathic pain after HZ, otherwise known as postherpetic neuralgia (PHN), occurs in approximately 20% of patients and is one of the most feared complications of the viral infection. Severe pain typically has a dermatomal distribution over the affected nerve and can be associated with burning, dysesthesia, pruritus, allodynia and/or anesthesia. Both acute HZ and PHN are associated with severe psychosocial dysfunction (anxiety and depression), impaired sleep, reduced appetite, and diminished libido, all of which can lead to social isolation and even suicide.

A While the use of the varicella vaccine has led to a significant decrease in the number of chickenpox cases and will eventually make shingles a relatively rare disease, the rate of shingles has increased over the past 2 decades. Luckily, development of the HZ vaccine has had a greatly positive impact on the disease and its consequences, decreasing the incidence of HZ by 51% and of PHN by 66% in those vaccinated. In patients at high-risk for severe disease who demonstrate lack of immunity to varicella (i.e. immune-compromised patients, premature infants, pregnant women), and for those whom the vaccine is contraindicated but have been exposed to the infectious disease, the Centers for Disease Control and Prevention (CDC) recommends prompt administration of varicella zoster immune globulin preparation ideally within 96 hours of exposure.

B Diagnosis of acute HZ is typically clinical, given the classic appearance of the rash. During the acute phase of infection, aggressive medication management to include tricyclic antidepressants (TCAs), gabapentinoids and opioids is the first-line treatment.

C Few randomized controlled trials have demonstrated that early use of epidural or paravertebral local anesthetic and steroid injections may decrease the development of PHN, and therefore, these injections should be limited to those cases in which more conservative measures have failed to provide adequate pain control.

D Once the rash has healed and PHN has developed, first-line drugs (as recommended by NeuPSIG, European Federation of Neurological Societies [EFNS], American Academy of Neurology [AAN]) are gabapentinoids, TCAs, topical lidocaine and high concentration capsaicin. Combination therapy has yielded better efficacy in the treatment of PHN.

E Interventional measures may offer additional therapeutic alternatives in the treatment of postherpetic neuralgia not responsive to aggressive conservative measures. Unfortunately, the lack of available good quality data allows only for weak recommendation for use of epidural steroids in acute HZ, while producing weak or inconclusive recommendations for pulsed radiofrequency (PRF), spinal cord stimulation (SCS), or intrathecal opioids (IO) and recommending against the use of intrathecal methylprednisolone and sympathetic blocks in the management of established PHN. Invasive treatments typically provide limited, partial and temporary relief of pain.

Clearly, multimodal treatment provides a more suitable approach to comprehensive pain management of intractable postherpetic neuralgia.

SUGGESTED READING

Attal N, Cruccu G, Baron R, et al. EFNS guidelines on the pharmacological treatment of neuropathic pain: 2010 revision. Eur J Neurol. 2010;17(9):1113-e88.

Centers for Disease Control and Prevention (CDC). (2013). Morbidity and Mortality Weekly Report (MMWR): Updated Recommendations for Use of VariZIG—United States, 2013. [online] Available from *www.cdc.gov/mmwr/preview/ mmwrhtml/mm6228a4.htm.* [Accessed January, 2017].

Dubinsky RM, Kabbani H, El-Chami Z, et al. Practice parameter: treatment of postherpetic neuralgia: an evidence-based report of the Quality Standards Subcommittee of the American Academy of Neurology. Neurology. 2004;63(6):959-65.

Dworkin RH, O'Connor AB, Kent J, et al. Interventional management of neuropathic pain: NeuPSIG recommendations. Pain. 2013; 154(11):2249-61.

CHAPTER 35

Complex Regional Pain Syndrome

Slogic KM, Guthmiller KB

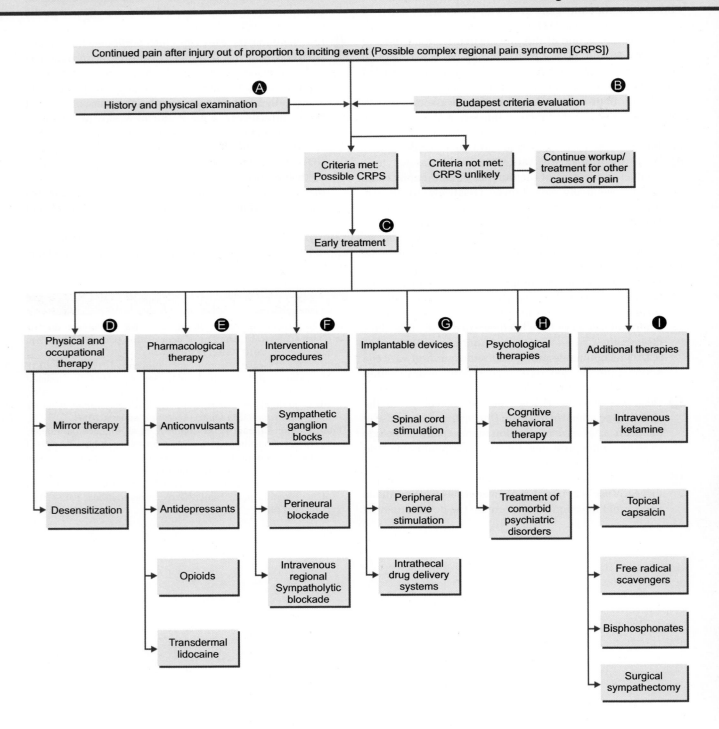

Table 1: Dyck's stages of severity for DSPN

	Grade 0	Grade 1a	Grade 1b	Grade 2a	Grade 2b
NC abnormality	None	>=95th percentile	>=95th percentile	>=95th percentile	>=95th percentile
Neurologic signs	None	None	Typical	With or without	Weakness of ankle dorsiflexion
DSPN symptoms	None	None	None	Positive	With or without

DSPN, diabetic sensorimotor polyneuropathy

As not all DSPN patients have pain, it is important to distinguish painful diabetic neuropathy, as defined by the International Association for the Study of Pain, "Pain arising as a direct consequence of abnormalities in the peripheral somatosensory system in people with diabetes." This type of neuropathy includes a subset of patients with DSPN but, as previously mentioned, contributes significantly to alterations in quality of life and incidence of disability in the population of diabetic patients. This, then, perhaps has some of the most significant impact on healthcare expenditure as related to diabetes when direct and indirect healthcare costs are taken into account. This diagnosis is based on the clinical description of pain in the setting of suspected or confirmed DSPN. Pain is typically described as burning but may also be stabbing, aching, and includes an element of anesthesia dolorosa. Hyperalgesia and allodynia may be seen on examination.

B The diagnosis of DSPN begins at an early stage with nerve conduction velocity testing, which may reveal abnormalities before clinical signs of the disease become apparent. This signals the clinician to aggressively control blood glucose, which may control, or even improve, the underlying the pathophysiology of the disease process.

If the diagnosis of DSPN is suspected and abnormalities are seen on nerve conduction velocity testing, the severity can then be assessed as described by Dyck **(Table 1)**.

C The exact pathogenesis of diabetic neuropathy remains under investigation. It is known that poor glycemic control is associated with early development of neuropathy. Glycemic control may stabilize and, in some cases, improve neuropathy in the earlier stages.

D The mainstay of treatment for diabetic neuropathy remains focused on symptomatic relief. First-line agents include tricyclic antidepressants (TCAs), used at lower dosing than traditionally used for antidepressant purposes. TCAs have effects at multiple sites as they inhibit the reuptake of serotonin and norepinephrine and act as antagonists at N-methyl-D-aspartate (NMDA) and alpha-adrenergic receptors. They do have a significant amount of anticholinergic side effects which limit their use, especially in the geriatric population.

E Serotonin-norepinephrine reuptake inhibitors (SNRIs) remain a more tolerable alternative treatment to TCAs in the treatment of neuropathic pain, including painful diabetic neuropathy. Duloxetine has been shown to improve symptoms in painful neuropathic syndromes, including painful diabetic neuropathy.

F Anticonvulsants also remain first-line treatment for diabetic neuropathic pain. These include gabapentinoids such as gabapentin and pregabalin as well as molecules such as carbamazepine and oxcarbazepine. Adverse effects of carbamazepine and oxcarbazepine can be significant, including immunosuppression, and require monitoring. The adverse effects of gabapentinoids are less severe but can still affect quality of life and include sedation, grogginess, and peripheral edema.

G Opioids remain second-line treatment for neuropathic pain. Tramadol, owing to its SNRI effects, may be effective in treating diabetic peripheral neuropathic pain. Tapentadol has similar effects and has more potent effects on μ-opioid receptors. Oxycodone has also been studied in the treatment of neuropathic pain conditions and found to be effective.

H Topical agents, including lidocaine, capsaicin, nitrate, and botulinum toxin have been studied with modest results in many studies. The great benefit of these agents is that systemic toxicity is largely limited.

I Interventional modalities for the treatment of painful diabetic neuropathy are still relatively new but have potentially promising results. These include transcutaneous electrical stimulation, acupuncture, sympathetic blockade and neurolysis, and dorsal column stimulation. However, due to the lack of large-scale controlled studies with these modalities, they have not advanced to first- or second-line treatment.

SUGGESTED READING

Dyck PJ. Detection, characterization, and staging of polyneuropathy: assessed in diabetics. Muscle Nerve. 1988;11(1):21-32.

Fradkin J, Rodgers GP. The economic imperative to conquer diabetes. Diabetes Care. 2008;31(3):624-5.

Lunn MP, Hughes RA, Wiffen PJ. Duloxetine for treating painful neuropathy, chronic pain or fibromyalgia. Cochrane Database Syst Rev. 2014;(1):CD007115.

Oliveira AF, Valente JG, Leite Ida C, et al. Global burden of disease attributable to diabetes mellitus in Brazil. Cad Saude Publica. 2009;25(6):1234-44.

Tesfaye S, Boulton AJ, Dyck PJ, et al. Diabetic neuropathies: update on definitions, diagnostic criteria, estimation of severity, and treatments. Diabetes Care. 2010;33(10):2285-93.

Tesfaye S, Stevens LK, Stephenson JM, et al. Prevalence of diabetic peripheral neuropathy and its relation to glycaemic control and potential risk factors: the EURODIAB IDDM Complications Study. Diabetologia. 1996;39(11):1377-84.

Treede RD, Jensen TS, Campbell JN, et al. Neuropathic pain: redefinition and a grading system for clinical and research purposes. Neurology. 2008;70(18):1630-5.

CHAPTER
37

Neuropathic Pain

Eckmann MS

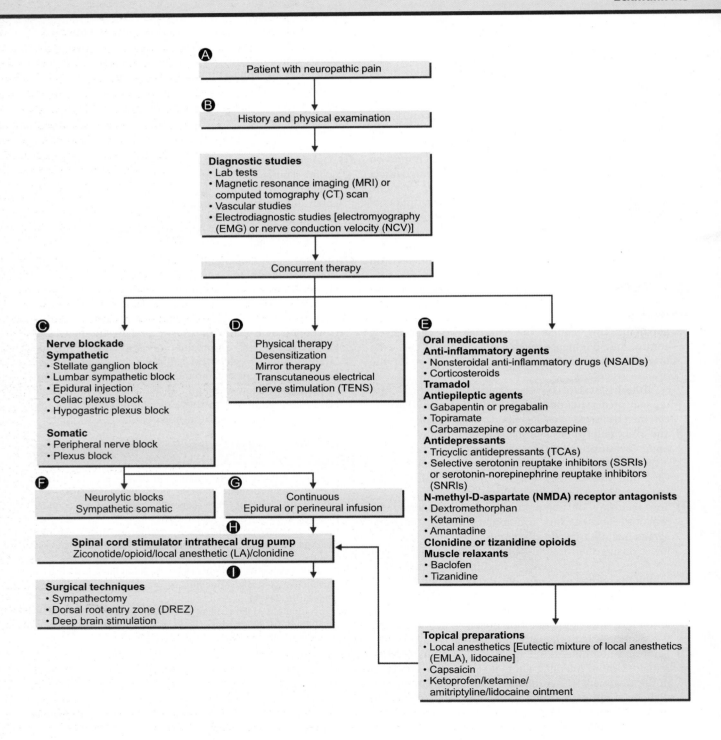

A Patient with neuropathic pain

B History and physical examination

Diagnostic studies
- Lab tests
- Magnetic resonance imaging (MRI) or computed tomography (CT) scan
- Vascular studies
- Electrodiagnostic studies [electromyography (EMG) or nerve conduction velocity (NCV)]

Concurrent therapy

C Nerve blockade
Sympathetic
- Stellate ganglion block
- Lumbar sympathetic block
- Epidural injection
- Celiac plexus block
- Hypogastric plexus block

Somatic
- Peripheral nerve block
- Plexus block

D
Physical therapy
Desensitization
Mirror therapy
Transcutaneous electrical nerve stimulation (TENS)

E Oral medications
Anti-inflammatory agents
- Nonsteroidal anti-inflammatory drugs (NSAIDs)
- Corticosteroids
Tramadol
Antiepileptic agents
- Gabapentin or pregabalin
- Topiramate
- Carbamazepine or oxcarbazepine
Antidepressants
- Tricyclic antidepressants (TCAs)
- Selective serotonin reuptake inhibitors (SSRIs) or serotonin-norepinephrine reuptake inhibitors (SNRIs)
N-methyl-D-aspartate (NMDA) receptor antagonists
- Dextromethorphan
- Ketamine
- Amantadine
Clonidine or tizanidine opioids
Muscle relaxants
- Baclofen
- Tizanidine

F
Neurolytic blocks
Sympathetic somatic

G
Continuous
Epidural or perineural infusion

H Spinal cord stimulator intrathecal drug pump
Ziconotide/opioid/local anesthetic (LA)/clonidine

I Surgical techniques
- Sympathectomy
- Dorsal root entry zone (DREZ)
- Deep brain stimulation

Topical preparations
- Local anesthetics [Eutectic mixture of local anesthetics (EMLA), lidocaine]
- Capsaicin
- Ketoprofen/ketamine/amitriptyline/lidocaine ointment

Neuropathic pain is described by the International Association for the Study of Pain as "pain caused by a lesion or disease of the somatosensory nervous system." This leads to grouping many varied, disparate pain processes, most with quite different etiologies, into the same general clinical description. The most common peripheral entities seen are diabetic neuropathy, peripheral neuropathy, postherpetic neuralgia (PHN), and human immunodeficiency virus-related neuropathy. Central causes are usually related to incomplete spinal cord injury, trigeminal neuralgia, and the poststroke condition. Central and peripheral syndromes are presented in **Box 1**. Generally, neuropathic pain can be characterized by several phenomena, including ectopic activity, peripheral and central sensitization, altered inhibitory control, and activation of non-neuronal cells. Peripheral nerve injury leads to release of intracellular contents and a subsequent cascade of further events which may include altered channel expression, inflammatory cell migration, upregulation sensitivity in the dorsal root ganglion (DRG), and excitatory stimulation from support cells such as microglia and astrocytes. Ectopic activity can result. Changes in signaling at receptors for N-methyl-D-aspartate (NMDA), calcitonin gene-related peptide, tachykinin neurokinin-1 (NK1), and the transient receptor potential cation channel subfamily V member 1 (TrpV1) may be instrumental in nociceptive initiation and propagation. "Central sensitization" often occurs at the level of the spinal cord in wide-dynamic-range neurons, producing prolonged symptoms, abnormal pain sensation, and expansion into noninvolved dermatomes. This is likely due to altered synaptic connectivity and recruitment of normally non-nociceptive pathways. Treatment of neuropathic pain ranges from nonpharmacologic to pharmacologic and interventional therapy. Generally, anti-neuropathic pain medications often have at most moderate efficacy; meanwhile, available evidence for interventional treatments best supports epidural steroid injections for PHN and radiculopathy as well as spinal cord stimulation (SCS) for failed back surgery syndrome and complex regional pain syndrome (CRPS). Therefore, treating persistent neuropathic pain continues to require individualized treatment in the hands of the experienced pain physician.

Ⓐ The history and physical examination comprise an important first step in identifying neuropathic pain. All precipitating factors should be elicited (e.g. trauma, tumor, surgery, infection). The evaluation concentrates on the signs and symptoms of nerve injury. Burning pain is one of the cardinal descriptions of neuropathic pain. Other symptoms include dysesthesias, hypersensitivity, numbness, lancinating pain, and sympathetic dysfunction. Dermatomal or sclerotomal patterns of sensory/motor/sympathetic changes should be evaluated. Quantitative sensory testing may be helpful in identifying and classifying nerve dysfunction. Hyperpathia, allodynia, or hypesthesia should be present. The differential diagnosis includes all processes that can cause neuropathy and peripheral vascular disease.

Ⓑ Laboratory studies should be performed to screen for the most common causes of peripheral neuropathy. Thyroid function tests and assays for vitamin B_{12}, folate, and homocysteine should be considered. Magnetic resonance imaging or computed tomography (MRI or CT) scans with contrast agents can locate cerebral and spinal cord lesions or plexus damage caused by tumor or infection infiltration or compression. Vascular studies (Doppler sonography, angiography) may be necessary to evaluate blood flow to rule out peripheral vascular disease. Electromyography or nerve conduction velocity (EMG or NCV) tests can help confirm large-fiber damage. Skin biopsies can confirm small fiber neuropathy. Autonomic function can be evaluated with the quantitative sudomotor axon reflex test (QSART).

Ⓒ Nerve blocks provide significant pain relief in many patients. While many agents such as local anesthetics, steroids, and clonidine have been used, the analgesia provided from nerve blocks should be leveraged to augment participation in physical therapy. Neuromodulation through application of pulsed radiofrequency (PRF) possibly extends duration of pain relief in certain neuropathic states of peripheral neuralgias and cervical radiculopathy. The site of injection depends on the location of the pain generator. Central lesions may produce unilateral pain and sympathetic dysfunction in the upper and lower extremities. Sympathetic blocks can be helpful in these cases. If bilateral lower extremity pain is noted, epidural or intrathecal injections or epidural infusions can provide bilateral coverage. Long-term (7–21 days) epidural infusions with bupivacaine and

---

Box 1: Causes of neuropathic pain

- Peripheral conditions
  - Diabetic neuropathy
  - Peripheral neuropathy
  - HIV-related neuropathy
  - Alcoholic neuropathy
  - Postherpetic neuralgia
  - Tumor compression or plexopathy
  - Cancer treatment (surgery or chemotherapy)
  - Complex regional pain syndrome
  - Phantom pain
  - Trauma
  - Trigeminal neuralgia
- Central conditions
  - Brain lesions (tumor or AVM)
  - Stroke or cerebral vascular accident
  - Multiple sclerosis
  - Spinal cord injury or lesions
  - Incomplete myelopathy
  - Radiculopathy
  - Failed back syndrome

HIV, human immunodeficiency virus; AVM, arteriovenous malformation

methylprednisolone can significantly decrease the pain of PHN. Weekly epidural injections (four injections) may provide the same level of pain relief. Compromise of the celiac plexus (pancreatic cancer) or the superior hypogastric plexus (pelvic tumors) can be treated by nerve block of the respective plexus. Neurolytic plexus injections are especially appropriate in these patients (see section F here).

Injury confined to specific dermatomes are best treated by specific peripheral nerve blocks. Iliohypogastric, ilioinguinal, or genitofemoral nerve blocks markedly reduce pain in patients suffering neuropathic pain following herniography. If peripheral nerve blocks are ineffective, sympathetic blocks should be considered, as described earlier. Somatic plexus blocks (brachial or lumbar) may be effective following trauma or after other damage to these areas, although they have reduced diagnostic value in suspected sympathetically maintained pain states.

D Physical therapy can provide desensitization and increased range of motion and function. A transcutaneous electrical nerve stimulation (TENS) unit may provide pain relief. In many cases, however, providing large-fiber afferent stimulation by TENS may worsen the pain if wide-dynamic-range spinal cord neurons are already sensitized. Specific pain conditions affecting one limb, such as CRPS or phantom limb pain, can respond to repetitive sessions of mirror therapy.

E Oral medications can be combined to provide effective pain relief in conjunction with nerve blocks and physical therapy. The use of anti-inflammatory agents should be attempted, as nociceptive activation occurs from prostaglandins. Tramadol may be used in patients with mild to moderate pain and has been shown to reduce allodynia significantly.

Tricyclic antidepressants (TCAs) are the "gold standard" of neuropathic pain treatment. Meta-analysis has shown significant pain relief. Unfortunately, the effect profile of these medications (central nervous system [CNS] changes, dry mouth, cardiovascular symptoms) limits their use to some extent. Amitriptyline is the standard bearer in most studies. Serotonin-norepinephrine reuptake inhibitors (e.g. duloxetine) have shown efficacy for conditions such as fibromyalgia and painful diabetic neuropathy.

Antiepileptic drugs have shown great promise, although they have unique side effects. Carbamazepine and oxcarbazepine are useful for conditions such as trigeminal neuralgia but require hematologic or metabolic monitoring. Gabapentin and pregabalin are moderately effective but can be associated with sedation and unwanted weight gain or peripheral edema. Zonisamide and topiramate are equally as effective and often contribute to weight loss. Clonidine, a central-acting α_2-agonist reduces peripheral sympathetic tone and has shown promise but may lead to orthostasis and physiologic dependence. Many patients believe that wearing the clonidine patch over the affected area is effective.

Neuropathic pain is thought to be opioid-resistant. Opioids may have a smaller therapeutic window for neuropathic pain over nociceptive pain; the long-term use of opioid therapy for chronic neuropathic pain is unproven and may lead to hyperalgesia among other problems. One study done with high-dose levorphanol showed some efficacy for pain; the average daily dose for pain relief was 9 mg, although some patients required up to 16 mg/day. Oral morphine equivalents for the doses of levorphanol used in the range from 135 mg/day up to 480 mg/day.

N-methyl-D-aspartate receptors can be blocked by several agents including ketamine, dextromethorphan, amantadine, magnesium, and methadone. Intravenous infusions of anesthetic and subanesthetic dose of ketamine show promise for refractory CRPS and possibly other forms of chronic pain. Ketamine is among the most potent NMDA blockers currently available, but oral bioavailability is poor. Oral dextromethorphan is a less potent NMDA blocker but also has less side effect burden. Oral amantadine has also been shown to be effective.

Systemic local anesthetics can reduce pain burden in both chronic pain states, possibly through blockade of inflammatory interleukins. Intravenous lidocaine can transiently reduce pain from refractory headaches and neuropathic pain associated with multiple sclerosis. Of note, lidocaine infusion may be useful for promoting earlier return of bowel function after abdominal surgery.

Baclofen is a gamma-aminobutyric acid (GABA) receptor agonist, predominantly working at the GABA-B receptor. It has been used successfully for neuropathic pain, especially trigeminal neuralgia. Tizanidine, another centrally acting muscle relaxant, has also shown promise as an adjuvant agent.

Substance P plays a role in neuropathic pain, and topical capsaicin may reduce pain by reducing existing pools of substance P in the neurons. High-dose (8%) capsaicin is shown to improve postherpetic neuralgia. Topical local anesthetics (eutectic mixture of local anesthetics [EMLA], lidocaine patch) can also be used but may be limited by their toxicity, including methemoglobinemia and tachyphylaxis.

F Neurolysis, for example, with neurolytic injection, radiofrequency ablation (RFA), or cryoablation, can be effective in carefully selected cases. RFA and cryoablation create well circumscribed but relatively small lesions. Neurolytic injections with caustic substances like phenol may cover larger nerves or plexuses. Neurolytic sympathetic blocks should be considered if sympathetic blocks provide significant short-term pain relief. Stellate ganglion neurolytic blocks are rarely performed because of the potential damage to nearby structures and because a permanent Horner's syndrome would occur. Neurolytic lumbar sympathetic blocks can be performed easily under fluoroscopy. Neurolytic celiac plexus or superior hypogastric blocks are especially effective for cancer-related pain, with success rates of 90% reported. The neurolytic medication should be mixed with a contrast agent to visualize its spread, so it can be limited to the sympathetic chain. This minimizes the risk of sensory or motor deficits.

Trigeminal neuralgia is a classic case where neurolytic injections or RFA have an excellent outcome. Gasserian ganglion injections can be dangerous if there is any spread into the surrounding cerebrospinal fluid. In peripheral causes of neuropathic pain, a neurolytic injection may be attempted if the nerve involved is predominantly sensory. The intercostal, iliohypogastric, and sural nerves are examples of nerves that can be ablated without clinically significant motor deficits. However, these injections, when performed with absolute alcohol or phenol, can cause significant trauma to tissues and even skin sloughing that requires treatment. Increased pain from partial denervation has been described, most commonly with absolute alcohol use. Neurolytic blocks may not reproduce the pain relief of the trial injection for a number of reasons, including the volume of medication used, so this risk must be explicitly stated to the patient.

G Indwelling long-term epidural catheter infusions have been effective for many types of neuropathic pain. One study has shown significant pain reduction in postherpetic neuropathy patients with a 3-week duration of local anesthetic and methylprednisolone epidural infusions. For CRPS, the use of local anesthetic with or without narcotic or clonidine has been highly effective. This therapy should be combined with physical therapy. In one study, pain reduction of 60–100% was measured in 95% of patients.

H If the following measures are not effective, more invasive procedures should be contemplated. SCS has been shown to provide excellent pain relief for CRPS and chronic lumbar radiculopathy or failed-back surgery syndrome. Patient satisfaction has been reported at 80% after 2.5 years and 63% after 4 years. SCS is cost-effective after approximately 2 years in appropriately selected patients who undergo proper screening. Intrathecal drug delivery devices may help patients with refractory neuropathic pain. Intrathecal ziconotide—the latest approved medication for intrathecal pain therapy—works through blockade of the N-type calcium channel, but it can cause hallucinations. Although intrathecal morphine can be complicated by long-term tolerance, addition of bupivacaine or clonidine can augment the durability of the therapy. Long-term high-dose morphine (>15 mg/day or >20 mg/mL) may lead to inflammation at the tip of the catheter (tip granuloma). Other medications can cause this as well. The addition of clonidine has been shown in animal studies to reduce the incidence of this side effect. Intrathecal baclofen has also been found to be effective in reducing dystonia symptoms in some patients.

I Surgical techniques are indicated if neurolytic techniques or interventional techniques have failed or are contraindicated. Success rates for surgical sympathectomy are usually reasonable if pain relief has been confirmed by sympathetic blocks before surgery. Success rates of up to 80% have been documented long-term. Postsympathectomy neuralgia has been seen in up to 40% of patients, although it is usually temporary. Thoracoscopy is used for upper extremity symptoms and allows a less invasive approach than traditional thoracotomy without the risk of Horner's syndrome. An open procedure is necessary for a lumbar sympathectomy and has a longer recovery phase. Deep brain stimulation has been shown to provide pain relief in recalcitrant cases. However, success rates over 30% have not been seen.

SUGGESTED READING

Aronoff GM. What Do We Know About the Pathophysiology of Chronic Pain? Implications for Treatment Considerations. Med Clin North Am. 2016;100(1):31-42.

Canadian Agency for Drugs and Technologies in Health. (2015). Gabapentin for Adults with Neuropathic Pain: A Review of the Clinical Efficacy and Safety. [online] Available from *www.ncbi.nlm.nih.gov/books/NBK304850*. [Accessed January, 2017].

Chua NH, Vissers KC, Sluijter ME. Pulsed radiofrequency treatment in interventional pain management: mechanisms and potential indications-a review. Acta Neurochir (Wien). 2011;153(4):763-71.

Denkers MR, Biagi HL, Ann O'Brien M, et al. Dorsal root entry zone lesioning used to treat central neuropathic pain in patients with traumatic spinal cord injury: a systematic review. Spine (Phila Pa 1976). 2002;27(7):E177-84.

Dworkin RH, O'Connor AB, Kent J, et al. Interventional management of neuropathic pain: NeuPSIG recommendations. Pain. 2013;154(11):2249-61.

Gilron I, Baron R, Jensen T. Neuropathic pain: principles of diagnosis and treatment. Mayo Clin Proc. 2015;90(4):532-45.

Koltzenburg M, Scadding J. Neuropathic pain. Curr Opin Neurol. 2001;14(5):641-7.

Mellegers MA, Furlan AD, Mailis A. Gabapentin for neuropathic pain: systematic review of controlled and uncontrolled literature. Clin J Pain. 2001;17(4):284-95.

Rowbotham MC, Twilling L, Davies PS, et al. Oral opioid therapy for chronic peripheral and central neuropathic pain. N Engl J Med. 2003;348(13):1223-32.

CHAPTER
38

Central Pain Syndrome

Arora SS, Galang E, Chang Chien GC

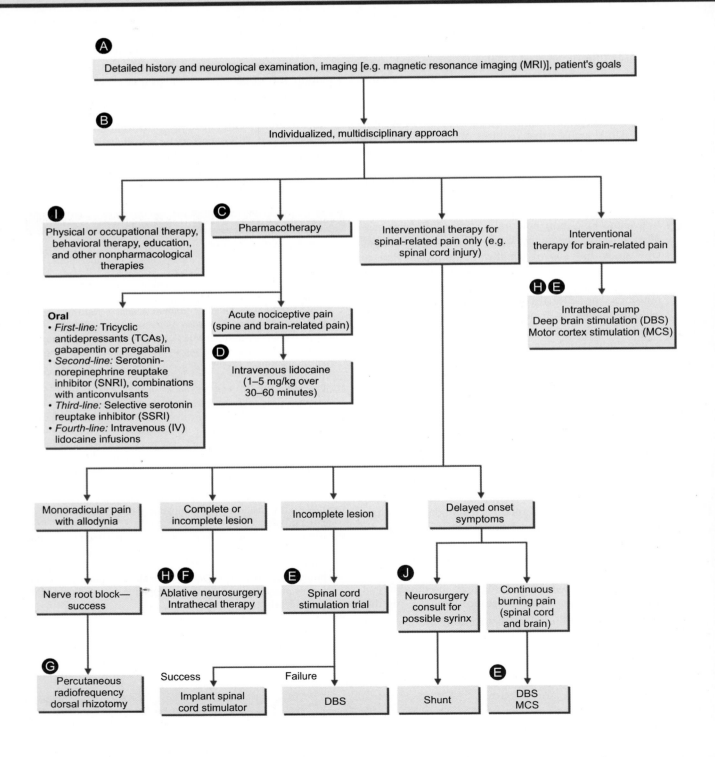

Central pain syndromes, a form of neuropathic pain, encompass a wide range of neurological disorders affecting the central nervous system (CNS). It presents with signs and symptoms that may vary in parallel populations and its pathophysiological mechanisms remain complex and poorly understood. As a result, it is one of the more difficult pain conditions to treat. The leading cause is stroke, followed by traumatic brain injury (TBI), spinal cord injury (SCI), phantom limb pain, and degenerative diseases of the CNS such as Parkinson's disease (PD) and multiple sclerosis (MS). Another example is fibromyalgia, which is now believed by most to represent the prototypical centralized pain state. Of note, people with centralized pain do not respond as well to mainstay treatments for peripheral nociceptive pain (e.g. opioids, injections, and surgery) as they do for centrally acting analgesics and nonpharmacological options.

A A detailed history and examination is the first step. Central pain can be categorized into spinal cord-related pain (e.g. trauma and motor vehicle accidents) and brain-related pain (e.g. vascular etiology). Symptoms are often reported days to weeks after a CNS lesion with cramping or crushing-like muscle pains and spasticity, poorly localized dysesthesias, hyperpathia, allodynia, well-localized shooting or lancinating pain, circulatory pain described as pins and needles that may be mistaken for neuropathic pain or poor circulation, and visceral pain expressed as bloating or burning pain with urinary urgency. Fear and anxiety may also aggravate symptoms. Imaging techniques (e.g. magnetic resonance imaging [MRI]) are useful in providing evidence for lesions in the CNS that may account for the patient's central pain or help distinguish it from other chronic pain states. Other tools and tests have been proposed, but have limited sensitivities and specificities due in part to the varied presentations of patients.

B Management is complicated and starts with the patient's goals for therapy focusing on each component of their pain. This is achieved through an individualized multidisciplinary approach utilizing pharmacotherapy, neuromodulation, behavioral therapy, physical therapy, and interventional therapy.

C Pharmacotherapy is primarily targeted at treating neuropathic pain. Oral medications that potentially act on the thalamus via noradrenergic and serotoninergic pathways, i.e. antidepressants, are the mainstay of treatment, with amitriptyline (a tricyclic antidepressant [TCA]) having the most evidence and, therefore, utilized as first-line therapy. Nortriptyline, also a TCA, has shown similar efficacy with less side effects. Anticonvulsants, most commonly gabapentin and pregabalin, are also effective for centralized pain. Lamotrigine has limited efficacy with only moderate benefit in those with incomplete SCI lesions. Other anticonvulsants have equivocal efficacy and, therefore, are not recommended as first-line therapy. The use of opioids in central pain is controversial. Furthermore, there is a concern for opioid-induced hyperalgesia and the possibility that it may actually potentiate hyperalgesia.

D Systemic intravenous (IV) lidocaine, shown to have antihyperalgesic and antiallodynic properties, is effective for both spontaneous and evoked pain due to spinal cord-related injuries. Although quite effective, lidocaine must be administered IV for central pain syndromes and, therefore, limits its practicality for everyday use. It may, however, be used for acute nociceptive pain.

E The invasive nature and expense associated with neuromodulation necessitate well-selected patients. In general, spinal cord stimulation (SCS) is more effective for spinal cord-related pain. When this fails, deep brain stimulation (DBS) is helpful. For the steady component of pain, such as continuous burning pain, DBS and motor cortex stimulation (MCS) may be effective.

F Ablative neurosurgery, including cordotomy, cordectomy, and dorsal root entry zone (DREZ) lesioning, are effective for the neuralgic component of spinal cord-related central pain in patients with complete or incomplete lesions. DREZ lesioning does not respond well to phantom or diffuse burning pain.

G Patients presenting with allodynia and monoradicular pain may benefit from percutaneous radiofrequency dorsal rhizotomy.

H Intrathecal pumps are useful for many pain conditions as well as spasticity. The most commonly administered medications are clonidine, bupivacaine and opioids. Intrathecal ziconotide is a nonopioid alternative with proven success, but it carries with it a significant side effect profile. Intrathecal baclofen, a gamma-aminobutyric acid (GABA) agonist, may be helpful in the treatment of pain and spasticity in poststroke, SCI, and MS pain.

I The most well-studied therapies are education, cognitive behavioral therapy, and exercise (e.g. physical and occupational therapy). Other options include biofeedback, hypnosis, and distraction techniques. Transcutaneous electrical nerve stimulation (TENS) is helpful for poststroke pain and incomplete SCI-related pain. Acupuncture, ultrasound, and massage have not been shown to be effect in the long-term.

J Patients with delayed onset symptoms following a SCI may complain of vague pain in an area where there is complete sensory loss, possibly due to the development of a syrinx. In this case, appropriate neurosurgical consultation is required to prevent further progression of the disease.

SUGGESTED READING

Brummett CM, Raja SN. Central pain states. In: Benzon H, Raja SN, Fishman S, Liu S, Cohen SP (Eds). Essentials of Pain Medicine, 3rd edition. Philadelphia: Elsevier Health Sciences; 2011. pp. 370-7.

McNicol ED, Midbari A, Eisenberg E. Opioids for neuropathic pain. Cochrane Database Syst Rev. 2013;(8):CD006146.

Nicholson BD. Evaluation and treatment of central pain syndromes. Neurology. 2004;62(5 Suppl 2):S30-6.

Wiffen PJ, Derry S, Moore RA, et al. Antiepileptic drugs for neuropathic pain and fibromyalgia - an overview of Cochrane reviews. Cochrane Database Syst Rev. 2013;(11):CD010567.

Phantom Pain

Salas MM, Goff BJ

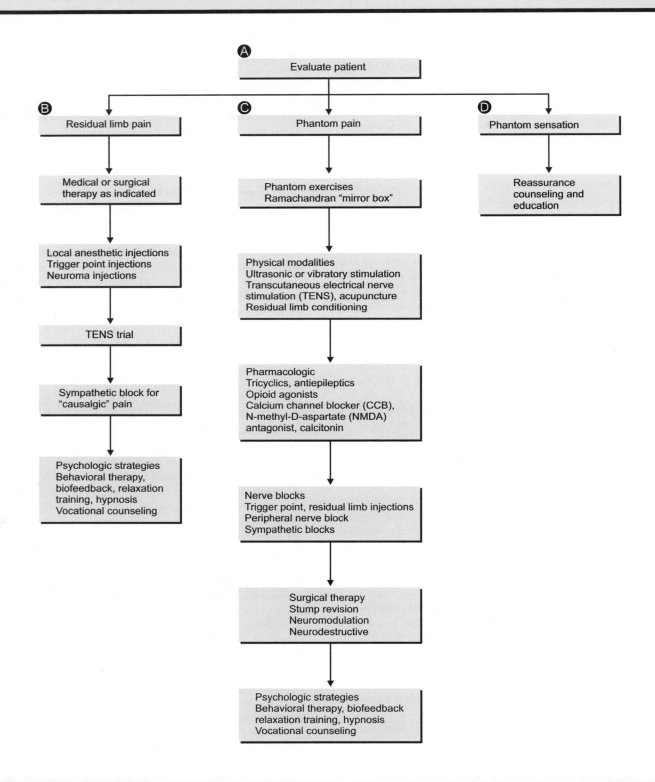

A Phantom pain occurs in any amputated body part. This includes limbs, breasts, nose, and genitalia, among other areas of the body. It is important to distinguish between three main and related entities: (1) residual limb (formerly referred to as a stump) pain, which is specifically located in, and does not extend beyond, the residual limb, (2) phantom pain, which is pain perceived as coming from the area of the amputated body part, and (3) phantom sensation, which is sensation information coming from the area of the amputated body part but, by definition, not painful. Whereas residual limb and phantom pain occur variably, phantom sensation is almost universal. As with all pain evaluations, the provider must elicit specifics of the syndrome including the intensity of the pain, its pattern of radiation, its character, temporal factors, exacerbating and remitting factors, and the response to previous therapy.

B The incidence of residual limb pain is approximately 10–25%. As mentioned earlier, the pain is specifically located in the residual part of the limb and does not extend beyond this. It may occur alone or along with phantom sensations. The pain may be continuous or intermittent, focal or diffuse, and triggered by stimulation or emotions.

Evaluation should begin with a careful examination of the residual limb for proper fitting of the prosthesis, as the residual limb may change in volume as muscle atrophies after amputation. Also, the patient should be evaluated for potential surgical or medical pathology (i.e. skin lesions, bone spurs, osteomyelitis, deep abscess, circulatory insufficiency, heterotopic ossification) **(Table 1)**. The provider should also palpate the residual limb for neuromas or trigger points which, if present, can be injected with local anesthetic for diagnosis. Transcutaneous electrical nerve stimulation (TENS) may provide good to excellent relief through localized vasodilatation, and it has been found that contralateral

stimulation is effective as well. Sympathetic blocks may be effective for burning pain. Psychological strategies such as biofeedback and relaxation training should be made available to patients with a significant emotional trigger. Repeated neuroma resection and progressive amputation for pain should be only cautiously considered; it is indicated primarily for infection or vascular insufficiency.

C Phantom pain is a well-recognized problem in amputees. Approximately 40–80% of amputees experience phantom pain at some point after their amputation, and it typically improves with time. Of those with phantom pain, approximately one-third has pain most of the time. When present, it usually develops within the first month and only rarely after the first year. Typical descriptors of phantom pain are cramping, burning, aching, hot, or cold character and may be associated with myoclonic jerks and contractions. A smaller portion of amputees describe the sensation of abnormal positions: extreme flexion or a tightly clenched fist with fingernails cutting into the palm. Some patients experience involuntary movements in their phantom limb, such as clenching spasms of the hand; voluntary unclenching can be difficult if not impossible to treat.

Several hypotheses have been proposed regarding the development of phantom pain, including peripheral, spinal, central, and psychological mechanisms. No single theory fully explains all of the clinical characteristics of this condition.

Experimental studies have shown that prior noxious conditioning may generate long-term changes in the central nervous system (CNS). It is argued that pain creates a nonerasable imprint in memory structures. Several clinical studies have suggested that phantom pain is more likely in patients who had pain prior to the amputation, and this is an argument for pre-emptive analgesia prior to amputation. This has also been an argument against prolonged limb salvage treatment when an early amputation might be a more functional option (with less chronic pain in the future). A history of phantom pain is a relative contraindication to regional anesthesia, as there are reports of pain recrudescence after spinal anesthesia.

There are several treatment options for phantom limb pain. If the patient has voluntary mental control of the missing limb, mentally exercising the former body part (phantom exercise) through isometric exercises can be helpful. This is referred to as mirror box therapy and conveys the visual illusion that the phantom limb has been "resurrected", enabling voluntary movements of the limb and relief of pain.

Additional physical therapy strategies include conditioning the residual limb and early prosthesis use. Ultrasonic and vibratory stimulation, residual limb percussion, heat, cold, and massage therapy, although rarely effective in and of themselves, should be considered as part of the treatment plan. Few reports in the Western literature address the role of acupuncture, but anecdotal evidence of its usefulness exists.

Table 1: Phantom pain: pathology, nerve injury, and central responses

- Local pathology
  - Surgical trauma or postoperative pain
  - Ischemia
  - Inflammation or stitch abscess
  - Skin infection or trauma
  - Bone spurs
  - Local scarring
  - Ill-fitting prosthesis
  - Osteomyelitis
  - Myofacial pain or trigger points
- Nerve injury and central responses
  - Neuromas
  - Major nerves
- Small nerves in skin and deeper structures
  - Autonomic system abnormality
  - CRPS I- and II-type symptoms
  - Spinal cord or central structures

CRPS, complex regional pain syndrome

Pharmacologic therapies include tricyclic antidepressants and antiepileptic drugs (AEDs), both of which have been thoroughly studied in models of neuropathic pain. Consider the AEDs for lancinating or shooting pain. Beta-blockers, calcitonin, and N-methyl-D-aspartate (NMDA) antagonists (through their diminution of CNS hyperexcitability) have had anecdotal success with phantom pain. Although classically considered to be ineffective, opioid analgesics (specifically methadone with its NMDA actions) have been shown to be effective in some patients.

Residual limb neuroma injections, peripheral nerve blockade, major conduction blocks, and sympathetic blocks have all been used to treat phantom limb pain. However, only 14% report a significant temporary change, and only 5% of patients demonstrate any permanent improvement or cure of pain. Consider sympathetic blocks in those with a causalgic description of the pain. Trigger points in the residual limb and on the contralateral side may be tried as well.

Surgical therapies include residual limb revision, neuromodulation (spinal cord stimulation and peripheral nerve stimulation), and neuroablation. For patients with palpable neuromas that are resected, only half show improvement. Neuromodulation may be considered in patients able to tolerate a minor surgical procedure. Neuroablation (dorsal rhizotomy, dorsal column tractotomy, anterolateral cordotomy, thalamotomy, cortical resection) have produced mixed results and have often resulted in more severe pain syndromes than the original phantom pain.

Psychological strategies such as biofeedback, relaxation training, and eye movement desensitization and reprocessing (EMDR) should be integral in the care of amputee patients with phantom limb pain.

D Phantom sensation is a non-painful, vividly detailed image of the former body part, described with definite volume and length. The sensation may be exteroceptive (surface sensations), kinesthetic (distortion of positional sensation), or kinetic (sensation of movement, willed or spontaneous). The phenomenon of "telescoping" involves gradual reduction of the phantom length and volume and is almost universal. The last part to disappear is the area with the highest cortical representation; for example, a patient with an upper arm amputation describes a phantom hand attached directly to the residual limb, with loss of all forearm sensation. The

incidence increases by age of amputee: 20% of patients 2 years old and younger have a phantom sensation compared to nearly 100% of patients older than 8 years of age. Most unwanted sensations gradually resolve within the first 24 months unless they become associated with pain. This sensation can be unwanted and/or frightening to an unprepared patient. Therefore, when feasible, preamputation counseling and education should occur, including arranging meetings with rehabilitated amputee patients if possible. Patients should be assured that these sensations are normal, natural, and not a sign of mental illness.

SUGGESTED READING

Broghi B, D'Addabbo M, Borghi R. Can neural blocks prevent phantom limb pain? Pain Manag. 2014;4(4):261-6.

Brunelli S, Morone G, Iosa M, et al. Efficacy of progressive muscle relaxation, mental imagery, and phantom exercise training on phantom limb: a randomized control trial. Arch Phys Med Rehabil. 2015;96(2):181-7.

Deconinck FJ, Smorenburg AR, Benham A, et al. Reflections on mirror therapy: a systematic review of the effect of mirror visual feedback on the brain. Neurorehabil Neural Repair. 2015; 29(4):349-61.

De Roos C, Veenstra AC, de Jongh A, et al. Treatment of chronic phantom limb pain using a trauma-focused psychological approach. Pain Res Manag. 2010;15(2):65-71.

Harvie D, Moseley GL. Exploring changes in the brain associated with recovery from phantom limb pain—the potential importance of telescoping. Eur J Pain. 2014;18(5):601-2.

Hommer DH, McCallin JP, Goff BJ. Advances in the treatment of phantom limb pain. Curr Phys Med Rehabil Rep. 2014;2(4): 250-4.

Hsu E, Cohen SP. Postamputation pain: epidemiology, mechanisms, and treatment. J Pain Res. 2013;6:121-36.

Karanikolas M, Aretha D, Tsolakis I, et al. Optimized perioperative analgesia reduces chronic phantom limb pain intensity, prevalence, and frequency: a prospective, randomized, clinical trial. Anesthesiology. 2011;114(5):1144-54.

Knotkova H, Cruciani R, Tronnier VM, et al. Current and future options for the management of phantom-limb pain. J Pain Res. 2012;5:39-49.

Lee IS, Jung WM, Lee YS, et al. Brain responses to acupuncture stimulation in the prosthetic hand of an amputee patient. Acupunct Med. 2015;33(5):420-4.

McCormick Z, Chang-Chien G, Marshal B, et al. Phantom limb pain: a systematic neuroanatomical-based review of pharmacologic treatment. Pain Med. 2014;15(2):292-305.

Ramachandran VS, Hirstein W. The perception of phantom limbs. The D. O. Hebb lecture. Brain. 1998;121(Pt 9):1603-30.

Spinal Cord
Injury-Related Pain

Averna J, Chang Chien GC, Saulino M

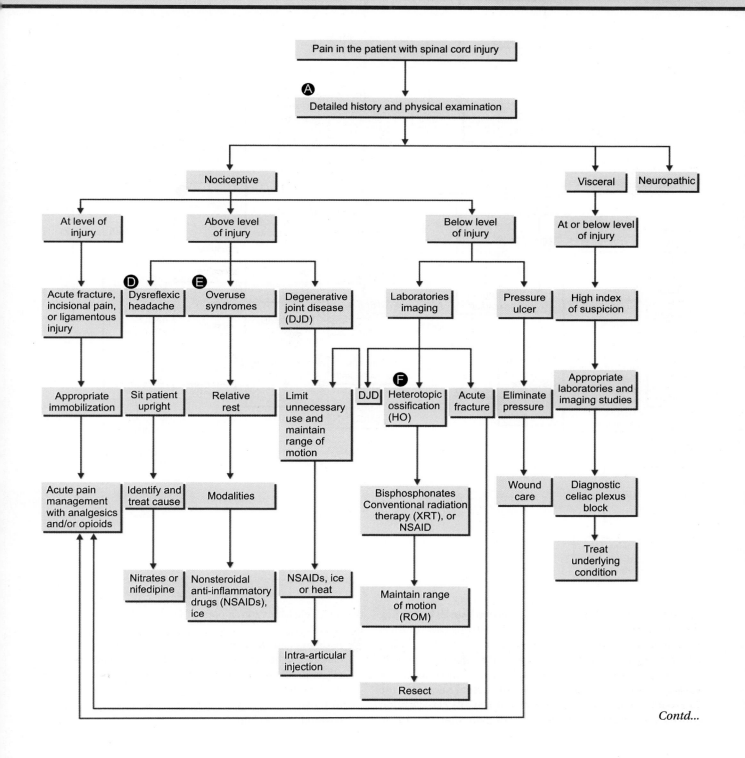

Contd...

Contd...

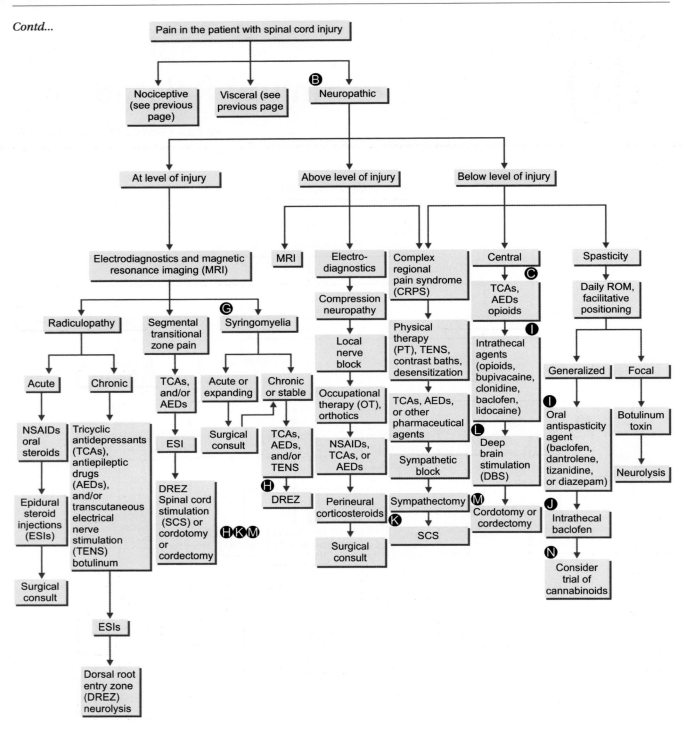

Treatment of spinal cord injury (SCI)-related pain is challenging for the treating physician and a devastating neurological condition for the patient. Appropriate treatment of SCI-related pain requires a comprehensive and multidisciplinary approach.

Many classification systems have emerged to better classify chronic SCI-related pain. One system known as the International Spinal Cord Injury Pain (ISCIP) classification provides a consensus classification of pain after SCI. Using the ISCIP classification, a patient's pain is divided into three tiers **(Table 1)**.

A A detailed history and physical examination assists in classifying the pain into general categories of nociceptive, visceral, or neuropathic type pain. Most aspects of nociceptive and visceral pain can be treated similarly to those without spinal cord injuries, and these are not covered in this chapter.

Table 1: International Spinal Cord Injury Pain (ISCIP) classification

Tier 1	Tier 2	Tier 3
Types of pain	*Subtypes of pain*	*Primary pain source or pathology*
Nociceptive pain	Musculoskeletal pain Visceral pain Other nociceptive pain	e.g. Spasm-related pain e.g. Constipation e.g. Pressure ulcer
Neuropathic pain	SCI-related pain At-level SCI pain Below-level SCI pain Other neuropathic pain	e.g. Cauda equina lesion or syringo-myelia e.g. Spinal cord lesion e.g. Post-thoracoto-my pain
Other pain (e.g. fibromyalgia)		
Unknown pain		

SCI, spinal cord injury

B Approximately 50% of SCI patients experience neuropathic pain, which is further divided into SCI-related pain at-level SCI pain or below-level SCI pain. The neurological level of SCI is commonly defined as the most caudal level with normal motor and sensory function. At-level pain is localized within two dermatomes above or below the neurological level of SCI, typically has an early onset and is also notoriously difficult to treat. Below-level SCI pain is more diffuse and onset can be delayed up to 12 months after injury. In a meta-analysis, gabapentinoids were effective in reducing neuropathic pain and other secondary outcomes after SCI at 6 months post-SCI.

C Antidepressants, in particular tricyclic antidepressants (TCAs), are considered second-line for SCI-associated neuropathic pain. Amitriptyline is the best studied with limited support for nortriptyline, and there is evidence to suggest increased efficacy when used in combination with anticonvulsants. A small randomized controlled trial (RCT) of duloxetine for central neuropathic pain (stroke or SCI) failed to show a reduction in pain intensity but did demonstrate changes in other aspects of these chronic pain syndromes, including allodynia. Opioids are effective in some patients with neuropathic SCI pain. However, long-term benefits are thwarted by chronic constipation, tolerance and dependence.

D Autonomic dysreflexia—noxious stimuli, or nociceptive pain, can result in this life-threatening emergency most often occurring in patients with a SCI above the T6 level. It is characterized by a reflexive hypertensive crisis with associated bradycardia, severe headache, flushing or sweating above the lesion in response to noxious stimuli below the neurological level of injury. Common triggers include restrictive clothing, ingrown toenails, bladder

distention or bowel impaction. Immediate management should include sitting the patient upright, removing all clothing and investigating the noxious source. Consider nifedipine or topical nitroglycerine paste to control hypertension while evaluating the source.

E Musculoskeletal pain is commonly seen in the paraplegic SCI patient secondary to overuse syndromes of the upper limbs. The upper limb, and shoulder joint in particular, bear the weight of the body for mobility, transfers and wheelchair propulsion. Muscle spasms can affect range of motion and exacerbate musculoskeletal pain. The treating physician should evaluate sudden increased spasticity for underlying pathology.

F Heterotopic ossification (HO), or the formation of new bone in soft tissue surrounding peripheral joints, is frequently diagnosed below the neurological level of SCI within the first 6 months after injury. HO most commonly affects the hip and can have associated decreased range of motion, increased muscle spasticity or periarticular swelling in addition to pain. Treatment of post-SCI HO includes bisphosphonates or radiation therapy; refractory cases may require surgical intervention.

G Delayed pain more than 1 year following the SCI could represent syringomyelia, or a cystic cavity within the cord typically at or above the neurologic level of injury. Treatment includes shunt placement and oral medications to help treat neuropathic-associated pain. Lesioning of the dorsal root entry zone (DREZ) can help dampen disinhibited polysynaptic pathways thereby reducing neuropathic pain in patients with continued pain despite syrinx collapse.

H Lesioning of the DREZ is proposed to reduce neuropathic pain by interrupting the abnormal neuroelectrical activity. It interrupts the sensory pathway by destroying neurons in the dorsal horn. Typically, this procedure is performed if other techniques to control pain have failed or are contraindicated. It is most effective for localized neuropathic segmental transitional zone pain, radicular at-level pain, or following failed shunt placement in the presence of syringomyelia.

I Spasmolytics are appropriate for pain associated with muscle imbalances from involuntary co-contraction. Oral baclofen, a gamma-aminobutyric acid-B (GABA-B) receptor agonist that works at spinal and supraspinal sites, is considered first-line despite there having been no formal, extensive studies on the drug. Tizanidine, a central alpha-2-adrenergic receptor agonist, has proven efficacy for spasticity and possibly for pain but has not formally been studied for either. Anticonvulsants like pregabalin, which binds the alpha-2-delta subunit of the voltage-dependent calcium channel, has demonstrated positive results in two randomized controlled trials; approximately 30% decrement in pain scores after 3–4 months with average dosing between 350 and 450 mg/day.

J Intrathecal therapies have demonstrated promising pain relief, but the intrathecal route is also associated with long-term side effects and tolerance, which has an impact on benefit. Intrathecal baclofen has been effective in the treatment of spasm-related pain and intrathecal morphine bolus displayed positive effects in a RCT for central pain.

K Spinal cord stimulation (SCS) may be effective in some patients with neuropathic SCI pain, although it is dependent on the type of injury and type of pain. At least partial preservation of sensation in the area of pain is normally required to obtain success. SCS may be more useful if the spinal cord lesion is incomplete according to some reports and appears to be more effective for at-level neuropathic SCI pain.

L Deep brain stimulation (DBS) can also be helpful, but is invasive. For the steady component of pain, such as continuous burning pain, DBS may be effective.

M Cordotomy and cordectomy may help to alleviate segmental transitional zone pain or unilateral below-level neuropathic central pain. They are typically reserved for end-stage cancer patients because of their potential serious complications.

N Cannabinoids have anecdotal evidence for treatment of SCI-related neuropathic pain but trials with synthetic cannabinoids have not been promising. Cannabis contains 60 or more cannabinoids, the most abundant of which are delta-9-tetrahydrocannabinol (THC) and cannabidiol (CBD). Dronabinol is a pure isomer of THC with conflicting data, more negative than positive with most common side effects being sedation and weight gain. A small RCT of dronabinol showed no relief in below-level neuropathic pain. Nabilone is an enriched THC preparation with minimal data to currently support its use but has been indicated for used with chemotherapy-related nausea and vomiting. Sativex is a fixed ratio of THC or CBD in an oral mucosal spray that is approved in Spain, United Kingdom, Canada and New Zealand for multiple sclerosis-related spasticity; effects on pain are somewhat variable and the most common side effects are fatigue and dizziness.

SUGGESTED READING

Finnerup NB, Norrbrink C, Trok K, et al. Phenotypes and predictors of pain following traumatic spinal cord injury: a prospective study. J Pain. 2014;15(1):40-8.

Hulsebosch CE, Hains BC, Crown ED, et al. Mechanisms of chronic central neuropathic pain after spinal cord injury. Brain Res Rev. 2009;60(1):202-13.

Jensen TS, Baron R, Haanpää M, et al. A new definition of neuropathic pain. Pain. 2011;152(10):2204-5.

Mehta S, McIntyre A, Dijkers M, et al. Gabapentinoids are effective in decreasing neuropathic pain and other secondary outcomes after spinal cord injury: a meta-analysis. Arch Phys Med Rehabil. 2014;95(11):2180-6.

Saulino M. Spinal cord injury pain. Phys Med Rehabil Clin N Am. 2014;25(2):397-410.

Siddall PJ, McClelland JM, Rutkowski SB, et al. A longitudinal study of the prevalence and characteristics of pain in the first 5 years following spinal cord injury. Pain. 2003;103(3):249-57.

Siddall PJ, Middleton JW. A proposed algorithm for the management of pain following spinal cord injury. Spinal Cord. 2006;44(2):67-77.

Siddall PJ, Yezierski RP, Loeser JD. Taxonomy and epidemiology of spinal cord injury pain. In: Yezierski RP, Burchiel KJ (Eds). Spinal Cord Injury Pain: Assessment, Mechanisms, Management, Progress in Pain Research and Management. Seattle: IASP Press; 2002. pp. 9-24.

Spasticity

Verduzco-Gutierrez M, Nguyen C, Mas MF

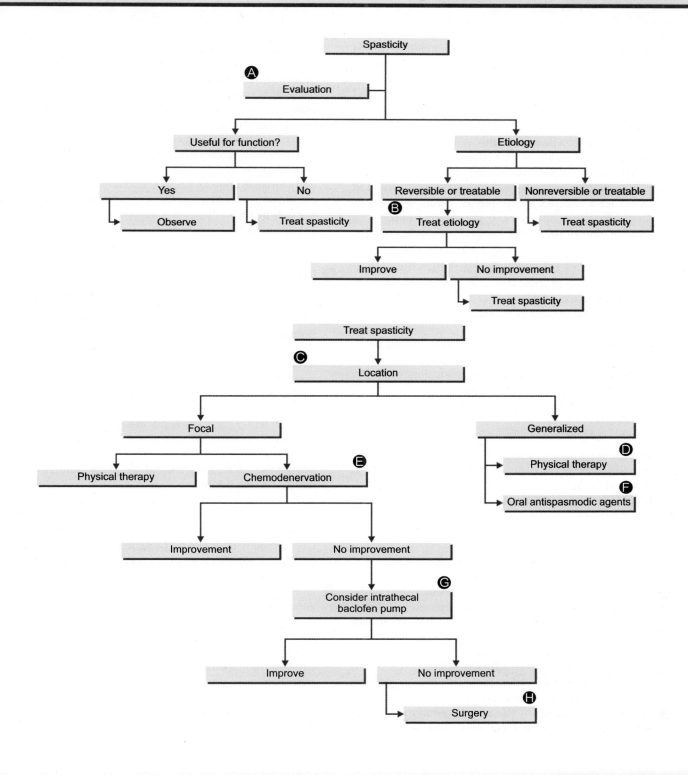

Spasticity is classically defined as an increase in velocity-dependent tonic stretch reflexes. It is a sign of involuntary muscle hyperactivity caused by upper motor neuron injury. Other signs of involuntary muscle hyperactivity include flexor and extensor spasms, clonus and co-contraction of antagonist muscles among others. These can all be categorized as "upper motoneuron muscle overactivity." Spasticity is commonly utilized as a term for all these signs; however, the clinician must be able to properly evaluate each one and recognize their differences as the treatment can potentially change.

A A comprehensive history and physical examination is imperative when evaluating for spasticity. It should include an analysis of the etiology of upper motor neuron injury and assessment of how it is affecting mobility, self-care and activities of daily living. The clinician should also be aware that spasticity can also be beneficial for patients, improving mobility and function in some cases. Proper evaluation must cover this as well, since "treating" the spasticity could in fact worsen mobility and/or independence. When monitoring chronic spasticity, it is important to compare with previous evaluation and assess for worsening of symptoms. If this is the case, then a thorough history must be repeated looking for deterioration of the initial cause or new injury. Scales such as the Modified Ashworth Scale and Tardieu Scale aid in objectively examining and monitoring spasticity.

Modified Ashworth Scale: Measures tone
0   No increase in muscle tone
1   Minimal increase in tone, "catch" and release at end of joint motion range
1+ Minimal increase in tone, "catch" at beginning range with minimal resistance less than 50% of range
2   Moderate increase in tone throughout range of motion (ROM), greater than 50% of range
3   Marked increase in tone with difficult passive ROM (PROM)
4   Affected limb rigid in flexion or extension

Tardieu Scale: measures spasticity
An assessment of resistance to passive movement at both slow and fast speeds.
0   No resistance throughout the course of the passive movement
1   Slight resistance with no clear catch
2   Clear catch at a precise angle
3   Fatigable clonus, less than 10 seconds
4   Nonfatigable clonus, more than 10 seconds

B In some cases, the etiology of spasticity can be reversible. For example, in spinal cord injury patients, spasticity can be the result of a treatable cause such as urinary tract infection, stool impaction, or infected skin ulcer. Patients with an acquired brain injury can have new spasticity caused by potentially treatable etiologies such as worsening hydrocephalus. In these scenarios, treating the reversible cause can improve or eliminate spasticity.

C The location of spasticity plays an important role in the subsequent management decisions. Spasticity can be confined to muscle groups in only one limb. This would warrant treatment considerations targeting these focal symptoms in order to decrease the possibility of systemic side effects. On the other hand, patients displaying generalized spasticity affecting multiple extremities and muscle groups benefit from more systemic treatment. These broader treatment options must be individualized to each patient judging the potential benefit of decreasing multiple focal interventions against the potential side effects of a more systemic approach.

D Physical therapy is here used as a broad term encompassing physical modalities and passive or active joint mobilization, among others. Cryotherapy has been proven to decrease the tonic stretch reflex activity, thus, decreasing spasticity and allowing for joint mobilization. Bracing and casting provide passive, constant mobilization that can increase joint range of motion. Active joint mobilization can be performed by a physical therapist and, potentially, by the patient after proper education. A weight-bearing program is imperative, and electrical stimulation is a modality currently being employed as well. Physical therapy and modalities should not only be seen as the initial management for spasticity, yet, should also be viewed as an essential adjunct for other treatment options such as the chemodenervation and oral antispasmodics.

E Chemodenervation is a commonly used tool in the treatment of focal spasticity. Generally, a substance is injected into the affected muscle or the perineurium of the nerve controlling said muscle or muscle groups. Botulinum toxin acts on the axon terminal blocking the release of acetylcholine and, thus, producing flaccid paralysis. There are two types of commercial botulinum toxin: (1) type A (onabotulinum toxin A, abobotulinum toxin A, incobotulinum toxin A) and (2) type B (rimabotulinum toxin B). The effects of botulinum toxin injection generally reach their peak at 2–3 weeks, eventually weaning off at 3 months. After a successful diagnostic block with lidocaine or other local anesthetic, phenol can be injected around the perineurium of the afflicted nerve producing myelin denaturation. This, in turn, decreases the overactivity of the affected muscle or muscle groups. These denaturing agents usually produce an immediate effect which can last for several weeks. Chemodenervation can be performed using anatomical guidance, electrical stimulation, electromyographical guidance, ultrasound, or a combination of these aids.

F Oral antispasmodic agents can be used to treat generalized spasticity. These can target different pathways that lead to muscle relaxation. Medications can be gamma-aminobutyric acid (GABA) agonists such as baclofen and benzodiazepines. Others can improve spasticity by targeting calcium release in the sarcoplasmic reticulum, as in the case of dantrolene. Clinicians must be wary of potential side effects from these systemic treatment options. For example, it has been reported that dantrolene can produce transaminitis. GABA agonists, such as baclofen, can produce sedation and potential cognitive impairment. The latter should be of particular importance for patients suffering from a stroke or an acquired brain injury.

G Patients who do not respond with other therapy interventions can be potential candidates for an intrathecal baclofen (ITB) pump. This is a method of delivering the GABA agonist, baclofen, directly into the spinal fluid, facilitating the delivery to the central nervous system while diminishing potential side effects of oral medications. Patients first undergo a trial to evaluate if they are candidates for this procedure. A small amount of baclofen (generally 50 μg) is injected into the spinal canal, similar to a lumbar puncture. Afterwards, the patient's spasticity is assessed throughout the course of several hours following the procedure. The clinician should monitor changes in spasticity using objective measures as detailed earlier. Side effects should also be noted, since these could eliminate the possibility of an ITB pump, despite spasticity improvement. If the trial is successful, the patient can be scheduled for a pump placement. The location of the catheter tip with regards to the spinal level can be influenced by the location of the patient's spasticity. Usually, catheter tips are located in the thoracic area, however, it is possible to position them in cervical regions in order to target upper extremity spasticity. An ITB pump must be closely followed by a clinician with proper training in its management. Patients can experience baclofen withdrawal and potential death making close supervision a priority.

H Surgical interventions for spasticity management can target the central nervous system, peripheral nerves or musculoskeletal system. Goals of surgery for spasticity can include: improving function, increasing active movement, pain relief, improved cosmesis and decreased reliance on systemic medications or chemodenervation. However, surgery cannot increase the force a muscle generates nor impart volitional control to a muscle. Timing for surgery is critical; it should not be performed in the early phases of rehabilitation where there is likelihood of improvement. As in other surgical procedures, medical stability is important for a patient to undergo surgery for spasticity management. Surgical interventions targeting spasticity include tendon lengthening procedures (to decrease stretch reflex), neurectomies and joint arthrodesis. Mobilization and weight-bearing following surgery is important to decrease risk of disuse osteopenia, although some surgeries do require a period of protection.

SUGGESTED READING

Brashear A. Botulinum toxin in the treatment of upper limb spasticity. In: Brashear A, Elovic EP (Eds). Spasticity: Diagnosis and Management, 2nd edition. New York: Demos Medical Publishing; 2011. pp. 131-40.

Haugh AB, Pandyan AD, Johnson GR. A systematic review of the Tardieu Scale for the measurement of spasticity. Disabil Rehabil. 2006;28(15):899-907.

Mayer NH. Managing upper motoneuroun muscle overactivity. In: Arciniegas DB, Bullock MR, Katz DI, Kreutzer JS, Zafonte RD, Zasler ND (Eds). Brain Injury Medicine: Principles and Practice, 2nd edition. New York: Demos Medical Publishing; 2012. pp. 821-49.

Meythaler J. Pharmacologic management of spasticity: oral medications. In: Brashear A, Elovic EP (Eds). Spasticity: Diagnosis and Management, 2nd edition. New York: Demos Medical Publishing; 2011. pp. 199-221.

Patrick E, Ada L. The Tardieu Scale differentiates contracture from spasticity whereas the Ashworth Scale is confounded by it. Clin Rehabil. 2006;20(2):173-82.

Pierson SH. Outcome measures in spasticity management. Muscle Nerve Suppl. 1997;6:S36-60.

Shingleton R. The role of physical and occupational therapy in the evaluation and management of spasticity. In: Brashear A, Elovic EP (Eds). Spasticity: Diagnosis and Management, 2nd edition. New York: Demos Medical Publishing; 2011. pp. 155-82.

Saulino M. Intrathecal baclofen for spasticity. In: Brashear A, Elovic EP (Eds). Spasticity: Diagnosis and Management, 2nd edition. New York: Demos Medical Publishing; 2011. pp. 229-42.

CHAPTER 42

Rheumatoid Arthritis

Eckmann MS

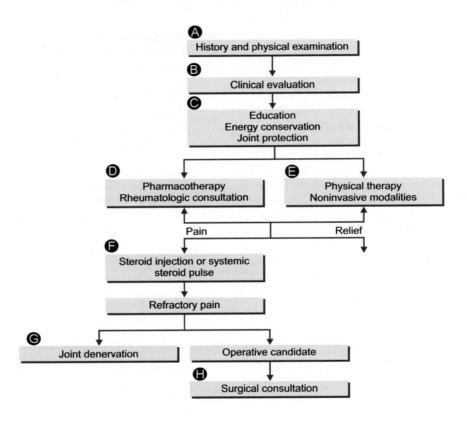

Rheumatoid arthritis (RA) is a systemic autoimmune disorder that stems from a breakdown in self-tolerance which can be promoted by environmental factors like smoking. Symmetric peripheral polyarthritis is the hallmark presentation. Erosion of articular surfaces is a prominent feature, and new bone formation and remodeling are noticeably absent (unlike osteoarthritis). Synovial proliferation is a common feature of RA. Additionally, extra-articular manifestations lead to multiple organ system involvement including accelerated cardiovascular disease, pulmonary fibrosis, endocrine, and exocrine disorders. Pain may vary with the stage of the illness and may arise from complications of therapy (e.g. steroid-associated avascular necrosis). Physical examination findings generally feature joint subluxation in advanced disease, as well as any signs of systemic disease such as rheumatoid nodules.

A Each joint should be carefully evaluated to assess joint effusion, synovial thickening, erythema, or warmth. Joint stability and deformity should also be noted. Number and size of joints involved are important for the American College of Rheumatology clinical classification criteria of RA **(Box 1)**.

B Evaluation should include the erythrocyte sedimentation rate (ESR), C-reactive protein (CRP), rheumatoid factor (RF), and anti-citrullinated protein antibody (ACPA) assays if there is clinical suspicion on examination. There is as much as a 5% false-positive rate associated with the RF alone. ACPA is highly specific for RA and associated with more aggressive disease. Radiographs show joint malalignment and subluxation, while bone scan or contrast magnetic resonance imaging (MRI) can demonstrate enhancement in areas of soft tissue or bony inflammation.

C Pain in RA patients is highly correlated with psychological stress relating to fears of debility, loss of self-image, and change in lifestyle. Education and counseling has been shown to reduce pain by up to 19% in this population. Energy conservation and joint protection techniques can help to reduce the severity and frequency of exacerbations while allowing relatively normal functioning.

D Nonsteroidal anti-inflammatory drugs (NSAIDs) are initial pharmacologic treatment for pain from RA, though they are limited by gastrointestinal (GI) and renal side effects. Current treatment strategy additionally incorporates early initiation of disease-modifying antirheumatic drugs (DMARDs). Through immune modulation, DMARDs such as hydroxychloroquine, sulfasalazine, methotrexate, and leflunomide slow RA progression. Biological DMARDs, such as etanercept and rituximab, are newer protein-based therapeutics against inflammatory cytokines. DMARDs may have adverse consequences regarding pregnancy and susceptibility to opportunistic infections. Systemic steroids are useful for intermediate-term treatment against inflammatory flare-ups but are not desirable for long-term treatment. Tramadol or opioid analgesics may be needed when satisfactory relief is not obtained. Rheumatology consult is warranted for complex pharmacological management of RA.

E Noninvasive modalities for treating RA pain have been attempted, including hydrotherapy, transcutaneous nerve stimulation, paraffin dips, diathermy, ultrasound application, fluidotherapy, hot packs, and ice. The success of these treatments was largely based on patient satisfaction. As with other forms of arthritis, physical therapy and bracing targeted at improving joint stability can be helpful.

F Intra-articular steroid injections can provide excellent results and specifically target and modulate the pathologic inflammatory response. By giving local injections, the deleterious systemic side effects are largely avoided. However, such procedures are not without risk of infection and atrophy, especially in structures already compromised by an autoimmune disease process.

G For patients who have continued suffering and are nonoperative candidates, long-term joint denervation can be achieved by image-guided destruction of articular nerve branches to some weight-bearing joints. Genicular nerves can be targeted by controlled diagnostic blocks followed by radiofrequency denervation or neurolytic injection without significant motor interruption of the knee joint. Similarly, the obturator and femoral articular branches can be targeted for refractory hip pain. Medial branches to the zygapophyseal joints of the lumbar, thoracic, and cervical spine can be also be disrupted.

H More than 90% of patients with severe, incapacitating RA have shown excellent pain relief following total hip or knee replacement. Surgery should be entertained as an option whenever the patient has intractable pain, severe deformity, or joint instability. Special attention should be paid to patients with atlanto-occipital joint instability as they may be candidates for cervical spine fusion.

SUGGESTED READING

Franco CD, Buvanendran A, Petersohn JD, et al. Innervation of the Anterior Capsule of the Human Knee: Implications for Radiofrequency Ablation. Reg Anesth Pain Med. 2015;40(4):363-8.

Gibofsky A. Overview of epidemiology, pathophysiology, and diagnosis of rheumatoid arthritis. Am J Manag Care. 2012;18(13 Suppl):S295-302.

Malik A, Simopolous T, Elkersh M, et al. Percutaneous radio-frequency lesioning of sensory branches of the obturator and femoral nerves for the treatment of non-operable hip pain. Pain Physician. 2003;6(4):499-502.

Quintana-Duque MA, Rondon-Herrera F, Mantilla RD, et al. Predictors of remission, erosive disease and radiographic progression in a Colombian cohort of early onset rheumatoid arthritis: a 3-year follow-up study. Clin Rheumatol. 2016; 35(6):1463-73.

Robinson V, Brosseau L, Casimiro L, et al. Thermotherapy for treating rheumatoid arthritis. Cochrane Database Syst Rev. 2002;(2):CD002826.

Stoffer MA, Schoels MM, Smolen JS, et al. Evidence for treating rheumatoid arthritis to target: results of a systematic literature search update. Ann Rheum Dis. 2016;75(1):16-22.

Osteoarthritis

Eckmann MS

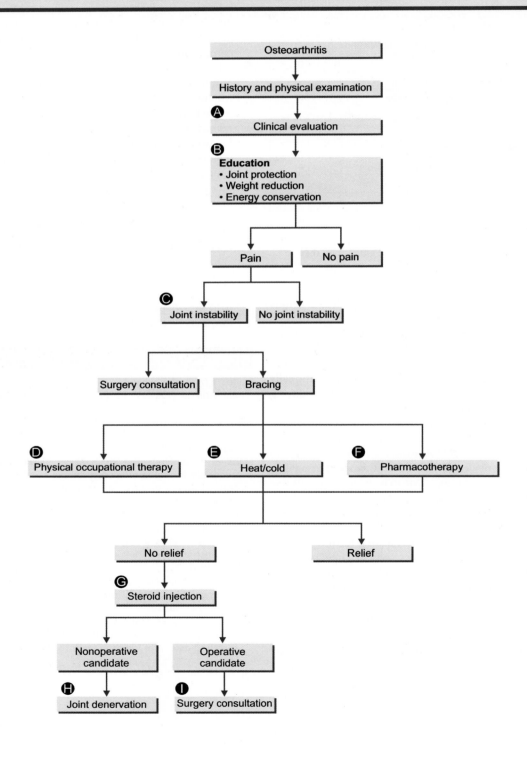

Osteoarthritis (OA) is the most common joint disease, affecting 80% of people over age 50. OA is a degenerative joint disease that stems from loss of joint protective structures; often cartilage fibrillation and catabolism or ligamentous injury initiate the cascade of accelerated joint wear. Ongoing low-grade inflammation from interleukin-1, tumor necrosis factor-alpha, prostaglandin E2, and nitric oxide leads to synovial inflammation and triggering of catabolism with dystrophic anabolism. The pathologic process results in further destruction of cartilage and bony overgrowth adjacent to the joint. Joint deformity without swelling of the distal interphalangeal joints and first metacarpal joints is often seen. Some familial heritabilities have been linked to the growth differentiation factor 5 (GDF5), asporin (ASPN), and double von Willebrand factor A genetic domains (DVWA).

A Clinical evaluation includes plain radiographs, which almost always show joint space narrowing. Osteophytes, subchondral cysts, and osteosclerosis may also be seen. Laboratory tests are of little value except when used to exclude systemic inflammatory arthritis. Crepitus and decreased range of motion are common findings. None of these diagnostic findings shows good correlation with pain.

B Education and lifestyle modification are keys to slowing progression of the disease and preventing exacerbations. Joint protection and energy conservation strategies can provide a great deal of symptomatic relief. Obesity has been shown to correlate with an increased incidence of hip and knee OA. Weight reduction can have a significant positive impact on disease progression.

C Joint instability exacerbates pain and can lead to weakness or falls, leading to further morbidity. Bracing may allow increased safety with weight-bearing and prevent further deleterious joint changes. When bracing is ineffective or impossible (especially in weight-bearing joints), surgery should be considered.

D Therapies are directed at maintaining functional range of motion, strengthening muscles crossing affected joints, and preventing debility. Increased muscle strength can improve joint stability.

E Heat and cold have each been shown to be effective for symptomatic pain relief. Neither modality has been shown to be superior. The modality chosen should be based on patient response.

F Nonsteroidal anti-inflammatory drugs (NSAIDs) and acetaminophen are the mainstays of OA pharma-cotherapy. NSAIDs are associated with the risk of gastrointestinal (GI) toxicity. Cyclooxygenase-2 (COX-2) selective inhibitors produce somewhat less GI toxicity and have considerably less antiplatelet activity. When satisfactory pain relief cannot be attained by the aforementioned, consideration may be given to using tramadol or opioid analgesics. Opioid schedule should be matched to activity and pain stimuli. Chronic opioid use necessitates a bowel program to prevent constipation. Direct GI specific opioid antagonists may have a role in refractory opioid-related constipation. Methotrexate and other immune modulators show promise for reduction of inflammatory factors in OA.

G Intra-articular steroid injection can be extremely effective for relieving pain, particularly if inflammation is present. The therapeutic window of steroid injection is limited by subsequent adrenal axis suppression and hyperglycemia following administration. Injected biologic agents such as autologous platelet-rich plasma, and viscosupplementation (hyaluronic acid-based lubrication), may be promising but remain unproven for consistent improvement in outcome.

H For patients who have continued suffering and are nonoperative candidates, long-term joint denervation can be achieved by image-guided destruction of articular nerve branches to some weight-bearing joints. Genicular nerves can be targeted by controlled diagnostic blocks followed by radio-frequency denervation or neurolytic injection without significant motor interruption of the knee joint. Similarly, the obturator and femoral articular branches can be targeted for refractory hip pain. Medial branches to the zygapophyseal joints of the lumbar, thoracic, and cervical spine can also be disrupted.

I Surgery can provide dramatic pain relief. Removal of structures affected by disease lead to prompt cessation of pain generation. Restoration of stability through ligament grafting slows OA progression. Hip and knee replacement procedures generally have good success, and multimodal analgesia can reduce the chance of postoperative chronic pain.

SUGGESTED READING

Buvanendran A, Kroin JS, Della Valle CJ, et al. Perioperative oral pregabalin reduces chronic pain after total knee arthroplasty: a prospective, randomized, controlled trial. Anesth Analg. 2010;110(1):199-207.

Franco CD, Buvanendran A, Petersohn JD, et al. Innervation of the Anterior Capsule of the Human Knee: Implications for Radiofrequency Ablation. Reg Anesth Pain Med. 2015;40(4): 363-8.

Goodwin JL, Kraemer JJ, Bajwa ZH. The use of opioids in the treatment of osteoarthritis: when, why, and how? Curr Rheumatol Rep. 2009;11(1):5-14.

Kalunian KC. Current advances in therapies for osteoarthritis. Curr Opin Rheumatol. 2016;28(3):246-50.

Malik A, Simopolous T, Elkersh M, et al. Percutaneous radio-frequency lesioning of sensory branches of the obturator and femoral nerves for the treatment of non-operable hip pain. Pain Physician. 2003;6(4):499-502.

McCarberg BH, Herr KA. American Academy of Pain Medicine. Osteoarthritis. How to manage pain and improve patient function. Geriatrics. 2001;56(10):14-7, 20-2, 24.

Takahashi H, Nakajima M, Ozaki K, et al. Prediction model for knee osteoarthritis based on genetic and clinical information. Arthritis Res Ther. 2010;12(5):R187.

CHAPTER
44

Back Pain in Pregnancy

Rosen M

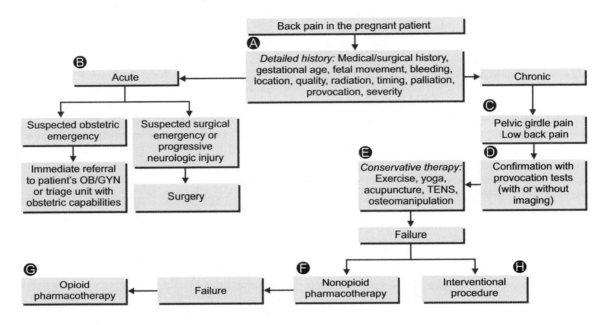

A Back pain and/or pelvic pain during pregnancy affect approximately 50–70% of women. Because back pain in pregnancy can be caused by any etiology found in the nonpregnant patient as well as obstetric-related causes, the most important step in management is accurate triage and diagnosis. Careful history and physical examination (H and P) are the mainstays of diagnosis. History should include gestational age. Imaging may be beneficial in diagnosing acute emergencies, and may occasionally aid in the diagnosis of nonemergent etiologies. Any suspicion of obstetric or acute etiologies of back pain should prompt immediate referral to the nearest triage department with obstetric capabilities.

B The first consideration must always be obstetric emergencies such as labor, contractions, placental abruption, or uterine rupture. Following this, and based upon H and P, the differential needs to include urinary tract infection, pyelonephritis/renal colic/renal calculi, chorioamnionitis, appendicitis, cholecystitis, pancreatitis, and costochondritis. Pregnant patients are at greater risk for acute musculoskeletal or neural injury due to changes in their center of gravity and pelvic relaxation. Other causes of back pain (aortic dissection, spondylolisthesis, disc herniation, and pubic symphysis diastasis) also need to be considered.

C Once acute etiologies of back pain have been evaluated, or if they are not suggested by H and P, nonemergent etiologies of back pain in pregnancy can be considered.

Postural changes and compensation of the body to the gravid uterus can lead to a wide array of symptoms. During pregnancy, the hormones relaxin, estrogen, and progesterone increase joint laxity. Anterior rotation of the pelvis pushes the center of gravity forward, forcing the pelvis to rotate around a changing fulcrum, and leads to hyperlordosis. This can lead to low back pain (LBP) and pelvic girdle pain (PGP). Hyperextension of the upper back can lead to rib pain and difficulty in breathing. The head extends backwards and the neck tilts forward, which can cause neck pain, headaches, upper back pain, carpal tunnel syndrome, and numbness/tingling in the hands. The gravid uterus exerts mechanical force anteriorly, which stretches and weakens muscles of the abdominal wall and places more strain on the lumbar muscles; and posteriorly, which can compress the aorta and vena cava, leading to vascular compromise of the neural structure. LBP can also be facet mediated.

Low back pain is defined as pain or discomfort in the lumbar region (below the costal margin and above the inferior gluteal folds), with or without radiation to the legs. PGP, which is a form of LBP that can be related to pregnancy, specifically refers to pain in the lumbosacral, sacroiliac, and symphysis pubis joints. It is often described as pain between the posterior iliac crest and the gluteal fold near one or both sacroiliac joints, can be associated with pubic symphysis pain, and can radiate into the anterior or posterior thigh. It is generally associated with prolonged postures or movement and has an intermittent course.

D Diagnosis is predicated upon pain provocation tests. Posterior pain provocation test has a sensitivity and specificity of 81% and 80%, respectively. The patient lies supine and the hip is flexed to 90°. Downward pressure is applied to the knee along the axis of the femur. A positive result is obtained when deep pain is produced in the gluteal region. The Patrick or FABER (Flexion, ABduction, External Rotation) test looks for pain to be elicited in the sacroiliac joints or the pubic symphysis. The patient lies supine with the hips flexed, the leg is externally rotated and ipsilateral heel is brought to the opposite knee. Other tests include the Active Straight Leg Raise Test, Modified Trendelenburg Test, Long Dorsal Sacroiliac Ligament Test, and Menell's test. Imaging can be utilized with the caveat that ionizing radiation can potentially be harmful to the fetus.

E Conservative treatments for PGP and LBP include exercise (both water and land-based exercise), pelvic belts, transcutaneous electrical nerve stimulation (TENS), spinal manipulation, acupuncture, and complementary medicine. Evidence is conflicting and difficult to categorize due to statistical heterogeneity, and the quality of evidence is generally low or moderate. A recent Cochrane review noted that low-quality evidence suggested that exercise reduces LBP (vs routine prenatal care) and that adding a rigid belt to exercise improved pain but not function. Moderate-quality studies showed that LBP and functional disability are improved with osteomanipulative therapy. Moderate- to low-quality studies have shown that PGP is reduced with exercise, that exercise decreased sick leave due to PGP in pregnancy, and that acupuncture improved PGP more than usual prenatal care. A small study showed that TENS was a safe and effective treatment of LBP, but more studies are needed.

F The Food and Drug Administration categorizes drug safety in pregnancy as A-D and X. Pharmacotherapy is generally limited to acetaminophen (which is category B in pregnancy) and opioids. Cyclobenzaprine is category B in pregnancy as well. Nonsteroidal anti-inflammatory drugs are generally category C in the first and second trimesters, and can be rated category D in the third trimester due to premature closure of the fetal ductus arteriosus.

G Hydrocodone, meperidine, methadone, morphine, oxycodone, hydromorphone, fentanyl, and hydromorphone are all opioids that have been used during pregnancy. However, they should not be used for extended amounts of time or in large doses near the time of delivery, and should be used as a measure of last resort.

H Interventional injections appear to be of low fetal risk and have demonstrated relief to women with PGP, but more studies are needed in this area. The American College of Obstetricians and Gynecologists (ACOG) recommends limiting fetal exposure to ionizing radiation during pregnancy, so ultrasound guidance should be used whenever possible. Surgical management should be reserved for emergent cases, such as when there is progressive maternal neurologic injury.

SUGGESTED READING

ACOG Committee on Obstetric Practice, Number 299. Guidelines for Diagnostic Imaging During Pregnancy. Obstet Gynecol. 2004; 104(3):647-51.

Bhardwaj A, Nagandla K. Musculoskeletal symptoms and orthopaedics complications in pregnancy: pathophysiology, diagnostic approaches and modern management. Postgrad Med J. 2014;90(1066):450-60.

Casagrande D, Gugala Z, Clark S, et al. Low Back Pain and Pelvic Girdle Pain in Pregnancy. J Am Acad Orthop Surg. 2015;23(9):539-49.

Keriakos R, Bhatta SR, Morris F, et al. Pelvic girdle pain during pregnancy and puerperium. J Obstet Gynaecol. 2011;31(7):572-80.

Pennick V, Liddle SD. Interventions for preventing and treating pelvic and back pain in pregnancy. Cochrane Database Syst Rev. 2013;(8):CD001139.

Smith MW, Marcus PS, Wurtz LD. Orthopedic issues in pregnancy. Obstet Gynecol Surv. 2008;63(2):103-11.

CHAPTER 45

Discogenic Back Pain

Chang Chien GC, Odonkor CA, Candido KD

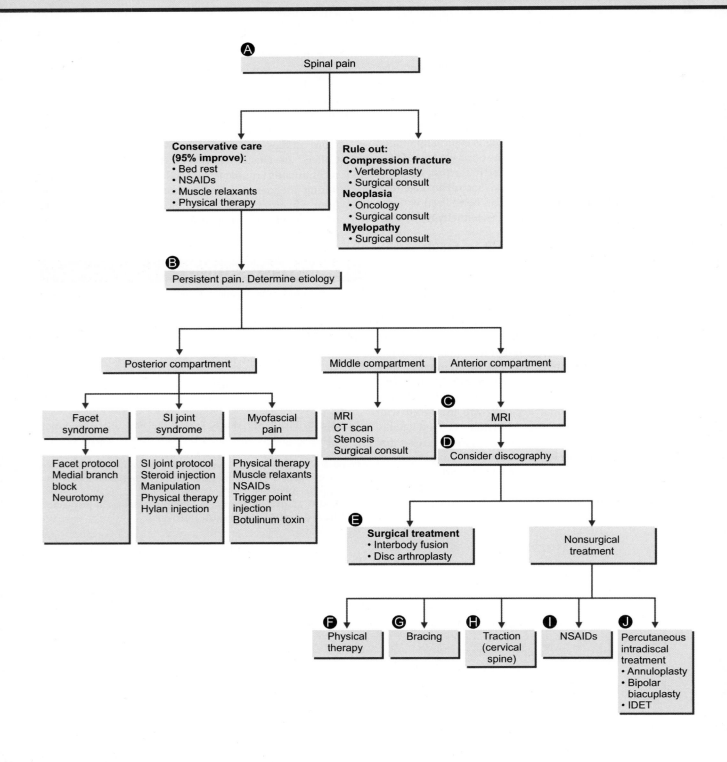

Discogenic pain refers to back pain arising from the disc itself. Discogenic low back pain (DLBP) is the most common disease of chronic low back pain, accounting for 39% of its incidence. Currently it is accepted that pain generation in DLBP is caused by disruption of the annulus fibrosus (AF), or the endplate.

The etiology of DLBP has not been definitively established, but it probably results from a compression injury causing an end-plate fracture. This injury triggers inflammatory degradation of the nucleus pulposus and eventually of the AF in the form of annular fissures.

The disc becomes painful as a result of chemical irritation of nerve endings in the outer annulus. The condition is characterized by alterations of the internal structure and metabolic functions of the intervertebral disc. Annular degeneration can be divided into three types: concentric fissuring, transverse tears, and radial tears.

The innervation of the normal disc is predominantly limited to the outer third of the AF. Disc innervation is mostly in the form of mechanoreceptors, which originate from plexuses along the anterior and posterior longitudinal ligaments. The posterior plexus receives its input from the sinuvertebral nerves and gray rami communicantes, while the anterior plexus receives contributions mainly from gray rami communicantes.

A A detailed history and physical examination can be helpful in determining the etiology of low back pain. Concerning signs and symptoms should be investigated, potentially with imaging, to rule out such diagnoses as compression fractures, neoplasms, and myelopathy. Once ruled out, conservative care can be initiated, as many improve with this alone.

B If pain persists, the practitioner must determine if the pain is coming from the posterior, middle, or anterior compartment of the spine. Discogenic pain arises from the anterior compartment and is typically nonradicular, axial back pain, and is aggravated by activities that increase the compressive forces on the spine such as lumbar flexion.

C Diagnostic evaluation by magnetic resonance imaging (MRI) plays an important, but not exclusive, role in the diagnosis of IDD. Correlation studies of MRI and cryomicrotome specimens have improved our understanding of annular fissures. Three types of annular tears have been described: type I, concentric outer annular tears; type 2, radial annular tears; type 3, transverse annular tears. These fissures can be demonstrated on MRI scans with the use of gadolinium. A high-intensity zone (HIZ) on T2 echography has been demonstrated to correlate with annular fissures and pain during discography. MRI scanning can be used as a screening tool prior to performing discography. An MRI of DLBP shows low-signal intensity of the disc on T2-weighted images, a HIZ at the rear of the disc, and end plate changes.

Degenerative diseases in the vertebral end plates as detected on MRI of the spine are classically referred to as Modic-type end plate changes. They are classified into three types based on MRI signal characteristics of T1- and T2-weighted images. Type I has low T1 and high T2 signals (represents bone marrow edema and inflammation) and indicates possible low-grade infection. Type II has high T1 and low to high T2 signal is thought to represent conversion of hematopoietic red bone marrow into yellow fatty marrow due to ischemia, whereas Type III has low T1 and low T2 signals and represents subchondral bony sclerosis. It has been suggested that subchondral marrow changes reflect reactive chemical inflammation in the vertebral end plates due to the diffusion of toxic substances from a degenerated disc. Modic changes are therefore considered a plausible secondary sign of DLBP. Clinically, the significance of degenerative disc disease on T2-weighted MRI scans and Modic changes at the end plate remains to be delineated. Some studies show no significant correlation between an MRI scan that is positive for vertebral end plate changes and concordant pain with provocative discography. Other biomechanical studies suggest that there is no direct correlation between degenerative changes to the disc and the adjacent vertebral bodies. Modic changes may, thus, demonstrate degenerative changes within the body and/or disc but so far have failed to clinically correlate with findings on provocative discography.

D Discography, a diagnostic procedure designed to ascertain whether a disc is intrinsically painful, is the single most important test for diagnosing IDD. It must be noted, however, that discography is a confirmatory test and must be performed only in conjunction with other diagnostic tools. Since its introduction, discography has been a controversial subject, and it has undergone some modifications. The introduction of discography utilizing manometry, has added a significant degree of objectivity to the procedure. The specificity of discography has been demonstrated in various studies. Discography is an accepted diagnostic test for evaluating the intervertebral disc. The diagnosis of IDD requires a demonstration of pain during discography associated with a grade 3 or more annular tear seen on the computed tomography (CT) scan after discography.

E A commonly recommended treatment for IDD is interbody fusion. This surgical approach may be satisfactory in well-selected patients, but it is associated with a high failure rate. Recently disc arthroplasty became a viable surgical option for discogenic back pain. Due to the short intraoperative duration and minimal blood loss, patients have shorter hospitalizations when compared to fusion surgery. Those who receive disc replacement may be rehabilitated faster and may return to work sooner than patients treated with fusion. Motion preservation with disc arthroplasty may decrease the incidence of adjacent level disease (transition syndrome) that occurs with fusion surgery. Overall, treating degenerative disc disease and discogenic pain with spinal fusion has remained controversial and the reported success is, at best, very modest. Clinical benefits may be obtained when the incriminating disc is confirmed by discography and subsequently removed. Further studies are therefore needed to evaluate the long-term effects of arthroplasty versus spinal fusion.

E There is evidence in the literature to support nonsurgical treatment for low back pain (excluding those with neurologic emergency) as most patients tend to recover without surgery. Exercise programs including abdominal wall and core muscle strengthening have shown definite therapeutic benefits for relieving DLBP. Physical therapy that helps to unload the joints also relieves discogenic back pain. Conversely, use of chiropractic treatment of chronic back pain (pain lasting >12 weeks) is of limited benefit and is no more therapeutic than the use of a placebo.

G Bracing, typically used for managing mechanical back pain has shown limited benefits for discogenic pain, based on several studies. In some cases, special orthosis with pneumatic pistons have been used for unweighting the lumbar spine with some therapeutic relief of discogenic pain.

H Traction has been used in the cervical spine for temporary relief of degenerative disc disease (DDD) and mild cervical disc herniations. However, the literature supporting its use for lumbar discogenic pain is limited given the technical challenges of performing traction in the lumbar spine.

I Several studies indicate the benefits of pharmacotherapy such as nonsteroidal anti-inflammatory medications as an adjunct to nonsurgical treatments such as physical therapy or spinal manipulation.

J Numerous nonsurgical percutaneous intradiscal treatments for IDD have been developed with varying degrees of success. These procedures are used to treat intradiscal (contained) versus extradiscal (extruded) herniations. The goal is to minimize volume of the disc to reduce intradiscal pressure and allow for disc remodeling. Nonvisualized procedures targeting the annulus include: annuloplasty, bipolar biacuplasty, and intradiscal electrothermal annuloplasty (IDET) involving insertion of a catheter into the disc to heat it up. IDET remains controversial due to suboptimal outcomes although some postulated that the procedure works by heat-induced contraction of collagenous tissue within the disc wall and thermal destruction of pain-sensitive fibers in the disc. Recently, biacuplasty has been shown to be a more effective treatment. Radiofrequency energy is applied to the painful disc via two thin probes placed in close proximity within the disc to ablate nociceptors in posterior aspect of the disc. Biacuplasty is reported to yield better pain outcomes compared to prior methods by avoiding adjacent tissue damage and ineffective intradiscal tissue heating.

SUGGESTED READING

April C, Bogduk N. High-intensity zone: a diagnostic sign of painful lumbar disc on magnetic resonance imaging. Br J Radiol. 1992;65(773):361-9.

Bao Q, Songer M, Pimenta L, et al. Nubac disc arthroplasty: preclinical studies and preliminary safety and efficacy evaluations. SAS J. 2007;1(1):36-45.

Borman P, Keskin D, Bodur H. The efficacy of lumbar traction in the management of patients with low back pain. Rheumatol Int. 2003;23(2):82-6.

Carragee EJ, Alamin TF. Discography: a review. Spine J. 2001;1(5):364-72.

Carragee EJ, Paragioudakis SJ, Khurana S. 2000 Volvo Award winner in clinical studies: Lumbar high-intensity zone and discography in subjects without low back problems. Spine (Phila Pa 1976). 2000;25(23):2987-92.

Carragee EJ, Tanner CM, Khurana S, et al. The rates of false-positive lumbar discography in select patients without low back symptoms. Spine (Phila Pa 1976). 2000;25(11):1373-80.

Cloward RB. Posterior lumbar interbody fusion updated. Clin Orthop Relat Res. 1985;193:16-9.

Coric D, Mummaneni PV. Nucleus replacement technologies. J Neurosurg Spine. 2008;8(2):115-20.

Crock HV. A reappraisal of intervertebral disc lesions. Med J Aust. 1970;1(20):983-9.

Davis TT, Delamarter RB, Sra P, et al. The IDET procedure for chronic discogenic low back pain. Spine (Phila Pa 1976). 2004;29(7):752-6.

Elfering A, Semmer N, Birkhofer D, et al. Risk factors for lumbar disc degeneration: a 5-year prospective MRI study in asymptomatic individuals. Spine (Phila Pa 1976). 2002;27(2):125-34.

Frymoyer JW, Wiesel SW. The Adult and Pediatric Spine. Philadelphia, PA: Lippincott Williams & Wilkins; 2004.

Hagg O, Fritzell P, Nordwall A, et al. Characteristics of patients with chronic low back pain selected for surgery: a comparison with the general population reported from the Swedish lumbar spine study. Spine (Phila Pa 1976). 2002;27(11):1223-31.

Jellema P, van Tulder MW, van Poppel MN, et al. Lumbar supports for prevention and treatment of low back pain: a systematic review within the framework of the Cochrane Back Review Group. Spine (Phila Pa 1976). 2001;26(4):377-86.

Kapural L, Mekhail N, Hicks D, et al. Histological changes and temperature distribution studies of a novel bipolar radiofrequency heating system in degenerated and nondegenerated human cadaver lumbar discs. Pain Med. 2009;9:68-75.

Kapural L, Vrooman B, Sarwar S, et al. Radiofrequency Intradiscal Biacuplasty for Treatment of Discogenic Lower Back Pain: A 12-Month Follow-Up. Pain Med. 2015;16(3):425-31.

Manchikanti L, Derby R, Benyamin RM, et al. A systematic review of lumbar disc decompression with nucleopalsty. Pain Physician. 2009;12(3):561-72.

McAfee PC, Fedder IL, Saiedy S, et al. SB Charite disc replacement: report of 60 prospective randomized cases in a US center. J Spinal Disord Tech. 2003;16(4):424-33.

Moneta GB, Videman T, Kaivanto K, et al. Reported pain during lumbar discography as a function of annular ruptures and disc degeneration. A re-analysis of 833 discograms. Spine (Phila Pa 1976). 1994;19(17):1968-74.

Park P, Garton HJ, Gala VC, et al. Adjacent segment disease after lumbar or lumbosacral fusion: review of the literature. Spine (Phila Pa 1976). 2004;29(17):1938-44.

Rahme R, Moussa R. The modic vertebral endplate and marrow changes: pathologic significance and relation to low back pain and segmental instability of the lumbar spine. AJNR Am J Neuroradiol. 2008;29(5):838-42.

Singh V, Derby R. Percutaneous lumbar disc decompression. Pain Physician. 2006;9(2):139-46.

van Tulder MW, Scholten RJ, Koes BW, et al. Nonsteroidal anti-inflammatory drugs for low back pain: a systematic review within the framework of the Cochrane Collaboration Back Review Group. Spine (Phila Pa 1976). 2000;25(19):2501-13.

Weishaupt D, Zanetti M, Hodler J, et al. Painful Lumbar Disk Derangement: Relevance of Endplate Abnormalities at MR Imaging. Radiology. 2001;218(2):420-7.

CHAPTER 46

Nonsomatic Pain

McGeary DD, McGeary CA

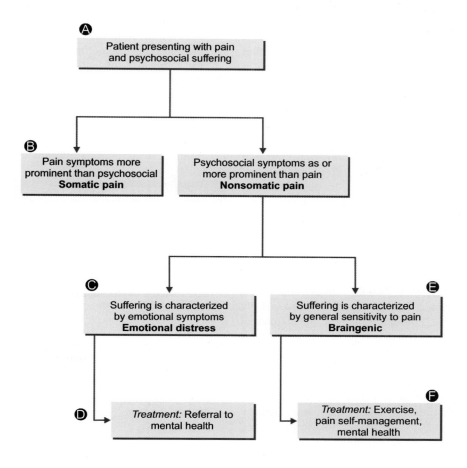

The term "nonsomatic pain" has been used interchangeably with other terms like "psychogenic pain" or "idiopathic pain" to describe pain experience for which there is no observable physiological substrate.

Ⓐ *Definition:* Though "nonsomatic" is not often applied to contemporary descriptions of chronic pain, this term is widely used in describing emotional symptoms that are likely to accompany pain (e.g., "nonsomatic depression"). In chronic pain populations, "nonsomatic" is generally believed to equate to pain-related suffering beyond physical pain and discomfort. Medical providers may be less likely to assess for nonsomatic pain symptoms because they are subjective, poorly defined, and do not have a clear physiological root. However, nonsomatic pain symptoms (e.g., depressed mood, negative thought patterns, and feelings of helplessness or worthlessness) can have a significant effect on pain-related coping,

functional activation, and response to treatment. Previously, nonsomatic pain was diagnosed as "Pain Disorder." Under new diagnostic criteria in the Fifth Edition of the Diagnostic and Statistical Manual of Mental Disorders, nonsomatic pain is now diagnosed as a "Somatic Symptom Disorder" (SSD) where pain is the primary complaint and is believed to be exacerbated by psychosocial factors.

Ⓑ *Differential Diagnosis:* Based on the SSD criteria, nonsomatic pain is best differentiated from somatic pain conditions by the presence and prominence of psychosocial distress as a component of the clinical presentation. For example, an individual presenting chronic low back pain with some disability and mild depression or anxiety symptoms may best be addressed as a "somatic" pain patient. However, if the patient presents with moderate to severe mood symptoms, or obvious signs of poor emotional or social adjustment due to pain, then they may qualify as a "nonsomatic pain" patient. It is important to note that nonsomatic pain is *not* exclusive of physical pain factors. Rather, "nonsomatic" pain is characterized by more prominent psychosocial factors that should be addressed for better overall pain management.

C *Emotional Distress Mechanism:* Because of the relevance of nonsomatic symptoms to mood experience, nonsomatic pain symptoms are of great interest in the differential diagnosis of depression and chronic pain. Both of these conditions share somatic symptoms (e.g., difficulty in sleeping, fatigue, and low energy) that can make it difficult to accurately assess depression in chronic pain patients. Although some have attempted to parse chronic pain and depression using nonsomatic measures of depression, these attempts have been largely unsuccessful. Regardless, those who attribute nonsomatic pain symptoms to psychological distress are likely to address this problem through a referral to mental health treatment. Although these referrals are likely to be beneficial to the patient, medical providers should take care to avoid indications that they believe the pain to be "unreal" or "illegitimate." There is sufficient evidence to show that patients with nonsomatic pain symptoms suffer significantly and treatment is warranted (especially in light of increased risk for suicide in these patients).

D *Treatment for Emotional Distress Nonsomatic Pain:* Due to the significant role of depression and anxiety processes under the "Emotional Distress" mechanism of nonsomatic pain, a referral to mental health is crucial for pain management with these patients. Data guiding the timing of this referral relative to other pain management strategies (e.g., treatment of pain before mood or vice versa) are inconclusive. However, some studies show a significant contribution of emotional distress to response to medical intervention for nonsomatic pain, so an early mental health referral is recommended.

E *Braingenic Mechanism:* Nonsomatic pain symptoms may also represent central pain processing abnormalities (i.e., central sensitization) that are a consequence of long-term pain experience. Under this hypothesis, some view nonsomatic or psychogenic pain as a sign of "braingenic pain" in which these symptoms are caused by brain-based changes in pain processing (similar to the mechanisms some attribute to widespread body pain phenomena like fibromyalgia). Braingenic nonsomatic pain may differ from emotional distress nonsomatic pain through a smaller role of emotional distress in pain presentation and a larger role of central sensitization to pain.

F *Treatment for Braingenic Nonsomatic Pain:* Under a "braingenic" conceptualization of pain, treatment would involve medication for neuropathic pain as well as other interventions (e.g., exercise, psychological treatment for pain management, and mood) that have been shown to be effective for neuropathic pain.

SUGGESTED READING

Elhai JD, Contractor AA, Tamburrino M, et al. The factor structure of major depression symptoms: A test of four competing models using the Patient Health Questionnaire-9. Psychiatry Res. 2012;199(3):169-73.

Nakamura M, Nishiwaki Y, Sumitani M, et al. Investigation of chronic musculoskeletal pain (third report): With special reference to the importance of neuropathic pain and psychogenic pain. J Orthop Sci. 2014;19(4):667-75.

Toda K. The terms neurogenic pain and psychogenic pain complicate clinical practice. Clin J Pain. 2007;23(4):380-1.

Toda K. The term "psychogenic pain" should be abolished or changed to "braingenic pain" (pain whose affected area is in the brain). Pain Pract. 2011;11(4):421.

Wilson KG, Mikail SF, D'Eon JL, et al. Alternative diagnostic criteria for major depressive disorder in patients with chronic pain. Pain. 2001;91(3):227-34.

CHAPTER
47

HIV-AIDS

Joves BC, Pangarkar SS

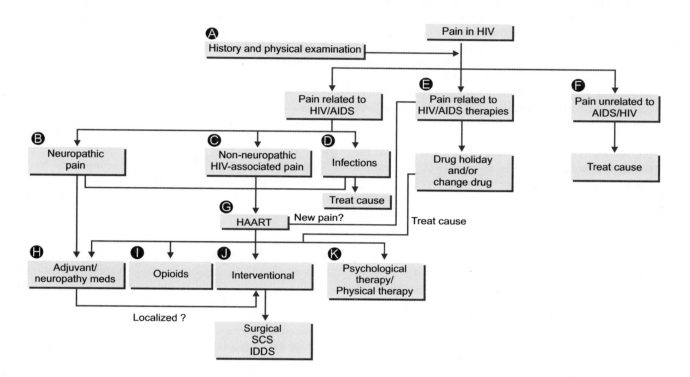

Human immunodeficiency virus (HIV) and acquired immunodeficiency syndrome (AIDS) remain worldwide epidemics affecting 36.9 million people today (Joint United Nations Programme on HIV/AIDS, 2014). New anti-retroviral therapies and mass availability have, however, changed the way the disease is viewed. As such, HIV is becoming a chronic medical illness with its treatment focus shifting to quality of life issues, including the debilitating pain.

The prevalence of pain in this population ranges from 30% to 90% and increases as the disease progresses. The World Health Organization has stated that "Palliative care is an essential component of a comprehensive package of care for people living with HIV/AIDS because of the variety of symptoms they can experience—such as pain …." Pain from HIV/AIDS is often compared to pain associated with cancer; however, it is less recognized and often undertreated.

Ⓐ A detailed history and physical examination are essential to diagnosing the cause of HIV-related pain. Patients can experience diverse pain syndromes including painful sensory peripheral neuropathy, headache, oral and pharyngeal pain, Kaposi's sarcoma, abdominal pain, chest pain, arthralgias, myalgias, and painful skin

conditions. These syndromes can be classified into three distinct categories: pain related to the disease itself or immunosuppression (~45%), pain related to treatment of the disease (15–30%), or pain unrelated to the disease (25–40%). As with many chronic pain states, however, the patient's pain is often multifactorial.

Ⓑ One of the most common pathologies affecting patients with HIV/AIDS is neuropathy. The HIV virus is highly neurotropic and can invade the central and peripheral nervous system throughout its disease course. This damage can occur from the disease itself, be immune-mediated, toxic, infectious, or from another medical comorbidity. Approximately 30% of patients with HIV develop a predominantly sensory neuropathy characterized by pain and numbness in the toes and feet. This is generally seen as a late manifestation of the disease process, but can occur at any time during the course of illness.

Ⓒ Many systems within the body can manifest pain syndromes from HIV and there are many potential causes. Headache is extremely common in HIV-infected patients, affecting up to 50%. The headache is usually of the tension variety, but can be caused by more serious conditions, such as HIV encephalitis, toxoplasmosis, or lymphoma. Rheumatologic conditions have also been reported in AIDS patients, including Reiter's syndrome, psoriatic arthritis, septic arthritis, vasculitis, Sjögren's syndrome, polymyositis, and dermatomyositis. Moreover, oropharyngeal ulcers are common sources of pain, as are skin lesion from extensive Kaposi's sarcoma.

D The HIV patients are prone to infection, especially when not treated with Highly Active Antiretroviral Therapy (HAART) therapy or on appropriate prophylaxis. This can include opportunistic infections such as toxoplasmosis, pneumocystis pneumonia, candidiasis, and cryptococcal meningitis, along with a higher incidence of typical infections seen in the community. Many of these can cause pain. For example, abdominal pain in AIDS patients may be related to infections such as cryptosporidiosis, and is accompanied by changes in bowel habits (more often diarrhea) and leading to organomegaly and obstruction. Treatment should be targeted towards the infective organism, as well as initiating HAART therapy, if not already started, to reduce recurrence.

E Treatment of HIV/AIDS can include modalities such as antiretrovirals, antimicrobials, Pneumocystis pneumonia (PCP) prophylaxis, chemotherapy, radiation therapy, surgery, and procedures such as bronchoscopies and biopsies. These treatments themselves can potentially cause pain and other side effects (such as azidothymidine [AZT] myopathy). If pain is from a medication side effect, consideration should be taken to change to another drug or initiate a drug holiday if no suitable alternative is available. If the medication or procedure cannot be avoided, or the side effect is allowed to continue in order to appropriately treat HIV/AIDS, pain should be treated as a chronic condition.

F Patients with HIV can also experience pain from sources unrelated to HIV, such as discogenic pain, diabetic neuropathy, or from any other somatic, visceral, or neuropathic source. Treatment for these conditions can be focused at the underlying cause, many of which can be found in other chapters in this textbook.

G When approaching HIV/AIDS-related pain, a multimodal and multidisciplinary approach should be used. The World Health Organization's approach to cancer pain has been utilized with success in patients with HIV/AIDS and has been recommended by the Agency for Health Care Policy and Research panel as well as other pain expert panels. The pharmacologic management of pain in AIDS patients should start with treatment of the underlying disease process with HAART. An individualized pain management plan should include judicious use of nonsteroidal anti-inflammatory drugs (NSAIDs), adjuvant medications, and opioids as needed.

H Adjuvant/neuropathic agents including antidepressants and anticonvulsants are considered first-line treatment for neuropathic pain. Initial treatment should include a trial of tricyclic antidepressants (TCAs), gabapentin or pregabalin. If TCAs are contraindicated, serotonin norepinephrine reuptake inhibitors (SNRIs) should be considered. Though data for neuropathic pain medications in this population is mixed, appropriate trial and titration of these agents should be considered prior to other therapies. Similarly, topical agents such as menthol or salicylate, capsaicinoids, and topical anesthetics may be employed.

I The HIV/AIDS pain is often managed with opioid-based therapies. Management generally includes use of long-acting opioids for basal pain control with short-acting medications for breakthrough. Data suggests that abuse of opioids may occur 25% of the time with dependence as high as 12%. As such, a practice that uses informed consents, random urine toxicology screens, and appropriate education may allow improved safety. Further, appropriate documentation of analgesia, adverse events, aberrant behavior, and activities of daily living should be made.

J Procedures such as nerve blocks or joint injections can be utilized if the patient has focal complaints. Nerve blocks may be particularly useful if localized neuropathic pain has developed. Other interventions, such as spinal cord stimulators (SCS), cordotomy, and intrathecal drug delivery systems (IDDS) are options for patients whose pain cannot be managed by other modalities.

K A variety of physical and psychological therapies may also prove useful. Physical interventions range from cutaneous stimulation (heat, cold, or massage) and transcutaneous nerve stimulation, to acupuncture. Patient education plays an important role in AIDS patients. Psychological interventions such as hypnosis, biofeedback, and reframing also play an important role.

SUGGESTED READING

Breitbart W, Rosenfeld BD, Passik SD, et al. The undertreatment of pain in ambulatory AIDS patients. Pain. 1996;65(2-3):243-9.

Cornblath DR, Hoke A. Recent advances in HIV neuropathy. Curr Opin Neurol. 2006;19(5):446-50.

Dinat N, Marinda E, Moch S, et al. Randomized, Double-Blind, Crossover Trial of Amitriptyline for Analgesia in Painful HIV-Associated Sensory Neuropathy. PLoS ONE. 2015;10(5):e0126297.

Finnerup NB, Attal N, Haroutounian S, et al. Pharmacotherapy for neuropathic pain in adults: a systematic review and meta-analysis. Lancet Neurol. 2015;14(2):162-73.

Frich LM, Borgbjerg FM. Pain and pain treatment in AIDS patients: A longitudinal study. J Pain Symptom Manage. 2000;19(5):339-47.

Hahn K, Arendt G, Braun JS, et al. A placebo-controlled trial of gabapentin for painful HIV-associated sensory neuropathies. J Neurol. 2004;251(10):1260-6.

Larue F, Fontaine A, Colleau SM. Underestimation and under-treatment of pain in HIV disease: multicentre study. BMJ. 1997;314(7073):23-8.

United Nations Programme on HIV/AIDS, World Health Organization. AIDS Epidemic Update. Geneva, Switzerland: UNAIDS Information Centre; 2007.

World Health Organization HIV-AIDS. Palliative Care. Geneva, Switzerland: World Health Organization; 2004.

Sickle Cell Disease

Vu AH, Pangarkar SS

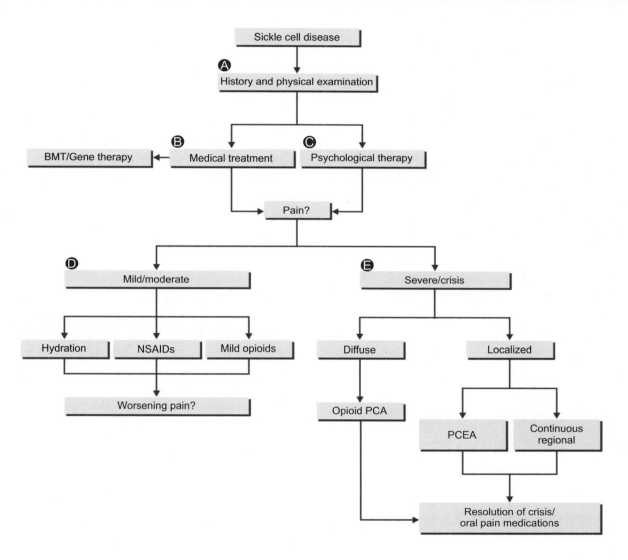

Sickle cell disease is prevalent in the Middle East, Mediterranean, Africa, and India. It results from a single gene mutation within the beta chain of hemoglobin A. This mutation results in the formation of hemoglobin S, which in the presence of low oxygen saturation, causes sickling of red blood cells and occlusion of blood vessels. This is often referred to as "Sickle cell crisis" and may be triggered by infection, dehydration, or other medical illness. Complications include chronic anemia, splenic infarction, renal/hepatic dysfunction, priapism, skin ulceration, bone necrosis, and cerebral infarction. Further, chronic splenic

injury may lead to autosplenectomy and leave the affected patient vulnerable to infections from encapsulated bacteria.

A A detailed history and physical examination must be obtained prior to treatment. Evaluation of the patient's baseline pain and the frequency and severity of pain crises must be obtained. Review of past hospitalization records and state prescription drug monitoring programs can be useful to determine prior doses and treatments to guide therapy. The mechanism of pain in this disorder is believed to be secondary to ischemia in various tissues and can be focal or generalized. The most common sites of pain are in the bones from bone marrow ischemia, and abdominal pain from visceral ischemia.

Ⓑ Hydroxyurea is commonly used and increases production of fetal hemoglobin, in turn decreasing circulating hemoglobin S. Presently, bone marrow transplantation (BMT) is being evaluated to improve outcomes; however, because of difficulty finding suitable donors and increased risks, BMT is still uncommon except at certain medical centers. Similarly, gene therapy is in early development but may be a treatment option in the near future. A hematology consult should be considered to investigate potential treatment options.

Ⓒ Manifestations of sickle cell disease begin at an early age and can interfere with childhood development, education, and employability. These factors may lead to socioeconomic circumstances that make healthcare burdensome along with psychologic impairment, anxiety, and depression. These negative thoughts about pain and coping have been found to correlate with increased pain and hospitalizations during acute crises, but generally do not affect the frequency of painful episodes. Caution should be exercised in managing patients who require frequent hospitalizations. The episodic nature of sickle cell disease can lead to resentment between hospital staff and patients if pain complaints are not taken seriously or if pain is insufficiently treated due to fear of overdose or drug abuse. Inadequately treated pain may lead to pseudoaddiction, drug seeking behavior, and poor outcomes due to mistrust between the patient and medical provider. Patients with significant organ failure and severe pain may be appropriate candidates for palliative care consultation. Goals of care, mental health, quality of life, and spiritual issues, along with functional restoration should then be addressed. Early discussions between patient and provider that emphasize education about the disease, its lifelong course, and the multidisciplinary approach to care may avoid some of these issues.

Ⓓ The majority of pain episodes can be managed with nonsteroidal anti-inflammatory drugs (NSAIDs), aceta-minophen, and mild opioids. Factors that worsen sickling of the red blood cells (dehydration, hypothermia, acidosis, hypoxia, hypercarbia, etc.) should be avoided or corrected to normal. If pain becomes severe, alternative treatments should be tried, as pain itself can worsen sickling.

Ⓔ Pain is the basis for 90% of hospital admissions in patients with sickle cell disease. While the majority of pain episodes can be managed with hydration, acetaminophen, and NSAIDs, severe episodes are often treated with opioids. In the hospital, parenteral morphine or hydromorphone is preferred due to speed of onset and ability to titrate these medications. Meperidine is not recommended in pain crises because of the active metabolite normeperidine, which can cause seizures, myoclonus, and agitation—especially in renal impairment. The use of patient-controlled analgesia (PCA) may also be effective in providing steady plasma concentrations compared to fixed intravenous (IV) bolus administration. It also offers autonomy over pain without waiting for "as needed" administration of medications. Additionally, patient-controlled epidural analgesia (PCEA) may be considered in patients with pain refractory to IV medications. Continuous regional anesthesia can also be considered in localized pain states, such as in priapism or extremity pain. The patient can be started on oral medications once the pain crisis has been controlled. After pertinent medical issues have been addressed, the patient may be discharged on a short course of appropriate medications.

SUGGESTED READING

Benzon HT. Essentials of Pain Medicine and Regional Anesthesia. Philadelphia: Churchill Livingstone; 2005. pp. 413-7.

Taylor LE, Stotts NA, Humphreys J, et al. A Review of the Literature on the Multiple Dimensions of Chronic Pain in Adults with Sickle Cell Disease. J Pain Symptom Manage. 2010;40(3):416-35.

Warfield CA, Bajwa ZH. Principles and Practice of Pain Medicine. New York: McGraw-Hill Scientific, Technical & Medical; 2004. pp. 533-9.

Chronic Abdominal Pain

Lai TT, Durning SJ, Boies BT

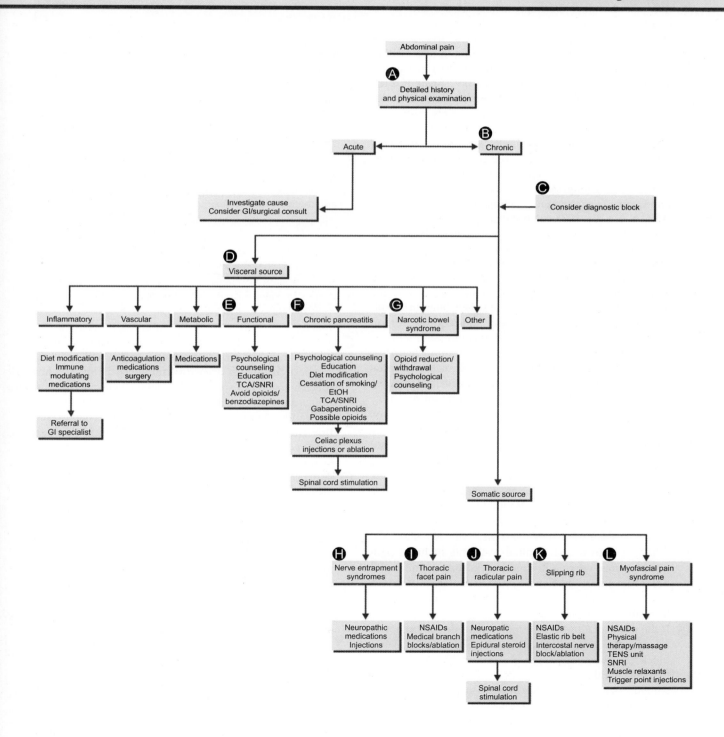

Abdominal pain is one of the most common complaints from patients, and this is often a challenge for physicians to evaluate and ultimately treat. Often abdominal pain can be benign, but it can also be the first symptom of serious and at times life-threatening pathologic processes.

Ⓐ The causes of abdominal pain can be numerous, so it is important to have an organized approach when evaluating these patients. An astute clinician can often narrow the differential with a thorough history of the abdominal pain. Patients can provide invaluable information, and the focus should be on the location of the pain, the temporal onset, the character of the pain, any inciting or relieving factors, and any family history of similar symptoms. Another key aspect is to investigate if there is any psychological component to the pain or lifestyle-related factors (i.e. stress related, anxiety provoked, etc.).

Imaging and laboratory studies should be reviewed. Pain originating from an organic cause can sometimes be visualized on computed tomography (CT), magnetic resonance imaging (MRI), or ultrasound imaging. An endoscopic retrograde cholangiopancreatography (ERCP) can be performed by a gastroenterologist to evaluate the pancreas. Laboratory studies, such as serum lipase/amylase, liver function tests, white blood cell counts, etc. can also be utilized to aid in diagnosis.

The first delineation for the evaluation of abdominal pain is the determination of acute versus chronic abdominal pain. Acute abdominal pain is often the result of a new intra-abdominal process, and requires workup to investigate an organic cause that could potentially be treatable by medications, surgery, or a more intensive workup by a gastroenterologist. In contrast, chronic abdominal pain is associated with a recurrent ongoing disease process or has an unknown organic cause.

Ⓑ The first branch point for chronic abdominal pain is the determination of whether the pain is coming from a somatic source (neuromuscular/musculoskeletal cause) or from a visceral source. A helpful physical examination finding called Carnett's sign can help determine the difference. To perform this maneuver, the patient lies supine and tenses the abdominal wall by lifting their head off the table or lifting both legs. If pain increases or remains constant (positive sign), pain is believed to originate from the abdominal wall; this includes pain from hernias, nerve entrapment syndromes, intercostal nerve root pain, trigger points, etc. If it decreases (negative sign), a visceral source is more likely (i.e. pain coming from abdominal organs).

Ⓒ If the cause of chronic abdominal pain is still unknown, a diagnostic block can also be performed. A celiac plexus block or splanchnic nerve blocks can be utilized as a diagnostic utility to help differentiate visceral versus somatic pain. If the block relieves a patient's pain, a visceral source is likely, whereas if the block does not relieve pain, a musculoskeletal or neuromuscular source is higher in the differential.

Box 1: Various causes of chronic abdominal pain
Inflammatory:
Appendicitis, celiac disease/gluten sensitivity, diverticular disease, eosinophilic gastroenteritis, inflammatory bowel disease (IBD), pelvic inflammatory disease, primary sclerosing cholangitis, sclerosing mesenteritis
Vascular:
Celiac artery syndrome, mesenteric ischemia, superior mesenteric artery syndrome
Metabolic:
Diabetic neuropathy, lead poisoning, porphyria
Neuromuscular:
Anterior cutaneous nerve entrapment syndrome, myofascial pain syndrome, slipping rib syndrome thoracic nerve radiculopathy
Other/miscellaneous:
Abdominal adhesions, abdominal neoplasms, anaphylaxis, angioedema, chronic pancreatitis, cannabis hyperemesis syndrome with cyclic vomiting, endometriosis, familial Mediterranean fever, gallstones, hernias, intestinal malrotation, intestinal obstruction, lactose intolerance, neurogenic abdominal pain, peptic ulcer disease, small intestinal and pelvic lipomatosis
Functional gastrointestinal disorders:
Biliary pain (gallbladder or sphincter of Oddi dysfunction), functional abdominal pain syndrome, functional dyspepsia, gastroparesis, irritable bowel syndrome, levator ani syndrome
Yarze JC, Friedman LS. Chronic Abdominal Pain. In: Sleisenger and Fordtran's Gastrointestinal and Liver Disease. Elsevier; 2016. p. 175-84.

Ⓓ Many sources of visceral abdominal pain, such as metabolic, inflammatory, oncologic, and vascular causes, are best treated by a gastroenterologist or by another specialist who can specifically treat the cause of the pain (inflammation, vascular insufficiency, surgical resection, etc.), and will not be discussed further in this chapter (see **Box 1** for list of conditions). While these must be ruled out or considered in the diagnosis, further discussion will be on syndromes more common to the pain specialist.

Ⓔ Functional abdominal pain syndrome (FAPS) is a distinct medical disorder characterized by continuous or near continuous recurrent abdominal pain which is poorly related to bowel habits and not well localized by patients. It is not caused by functional abnormalities in the gastrointestinal tract, but instead evidence points to central nervous system amplification of normal regulatory visceral signals. There may also be dysfunction of descending and cortical pain modulation circuits. Patients often have comorbid psychological problems, and this chronic abdominal pain can dominate their life. There are specific Rome III criteria for FAPS: continuous or almost continuous abdominal pain, no or only occasional relationship of pain with physiological events (eating, bowel movements, menses, etc.), some loss of daily functioning, and evidence of malingering or other organic gastrointestinal pathology which could account for the pain has been ruled out (criteria must be fulfilled for past 3 months with symptom onset 6 months prior to diagnosis).

Treatment of FAPS involves a "successful physician-patient-relationship" as it is crucial to understand a patient's understanding of the illness as well as the psychosocial background. Family interactions and cultural beliefs should be elucidated as these could all affect adherence to treatment strategies. It is important to impart a non-judgmental approach, validate to the patient that their illness is real and also impart to patient that treatments will improve their symptoms, but that they should not expect a "cure."

As for pharmacotherapy, nonsteroidal anti-inflammatory drugs (NSAIDs) show little benefit; narcotics and benzodiazepines can actually lower the pain threshold and possibly increase the pain sensitivity. Tricyclic antidepressants have shown promise in doses lower than those used for depression (to minimize anticholinergic effects). Selective serotonin reuptake inhibitors (SSRIs) or serotonin-norepinephrine reuptake inhibitors (SNRIs) may be safer, but there is less evidence for efficacy. Several of these drugs may also be beneficial in treating the often seen comorbid psychological diagnoses. Gabapentin and carbamazepine have not been shown to be effective. In addition to pharmacotherapy, patients will benefit from cognitive-behavioral treatment.

F Chronic pancreatitis encompasses a wide range of inflammatory diseases that eventually leads to pancreatic damage and failure of its function. The clinical triad consists of abdominal pain, exocrine pancreatic insufficiency, and diabetes. Pain is present in over 85% of patients, and is typically postprandial, associated with nausea and vomiting, and partially relieved by sitting forward. Diagnosis is made by history and physical examination, along with serum amylase and lipase evaluation, and can be aided by imaging such as CT, MRI, and ultrasound, possibly with biopsy.

Management of chronic pancreatitis should be undertaken as a team approach with pain specialists, gastroenterologists, and possibly surgeons. Nutrition, psychological counseling, patient education, dietary modifications, and lifestyle management are key components of its management, and endoscopic and surgical interventions can have a role in selected patients. Long-term opioid use is best avoided due to the development of tolerance and dependence, though tramadol may have some benefit with lower side effects than stronger opioids. Gabapentinoids, SNRI/SSRIs, and tricyclic antidepressants (TCAs) have been used to help with pain. Pancreatic enzyme-replacement therapy, octreotide, montelukast, and allopurinol have not been shown to be beneficial from a pain perspective, and antioxidants show mixed evidence. However, antioxidants and enzyme-replacement therapy are thought to be relatively free of side effects and are often tried. Alcohol and smoking cessation is important to reduce pain

and continued disease progression. Interventional techniques such as celiac plexus or splanchnic blocks can be utilized, and if successful, ablative procedures or spinal cord stimulation can be performed for longer lasting relief. Acute or progressive worsening of pain should be evaluated for any needed surgical or endoscopic intervention.

G An important differential diagnosis to consider in the chronic pain population is narcotic bowel syndrome (NBS). Abdominal pain is the defining symptom and is thought to be mediated by the central nervous system. It is important to rule out the potential side effects of chronic opioid therapy such as nausea, bloating, vomiting, abdominal distention, and constipation. Additionally, acute opioid withdrawal should be ruled out as well. NBS is diagnosed with the following criteria:

Chronic or frequently recurring abdominal pain that is treated with acute high-dose or chronic narcotics and at least three of the following:

- Pain worsens or incompletely resolves with continued or escalating dosages of narcotics
- Marked worsening of pain when the narcotic dose wanes and improvement when narcotics are reinstituted (*soar and crash*)
- Progression of the frequency, duration, and intensity of pain episodes
- Nature and intensity of the pain is not explained by a current or previous gastrointestinal diagnosis

Treatment and management should focus on the fact that NBS is a hyperalgesic condition resulting from the use of narcotic medications and can quickly degenerate into a negative patient-doctor interaction when the subject is broached. If NBS is unrecognized, it can frequently lead to escalation of narcotic therapy thus perpetuating the downward spiral of this condition resulting in frequent hospital admissions, emergency room visits, etc. The physician must have a high clinical suspicion in order to initiate early discussion of opioid wean. The ultimate goal for treatment is narcotic reduction or complete withdrawal and detoxification. Additionally, focus on long-term biopsychosocial treatment is needed to maintain prolonged results.

H Nerve entrapment syndromes are a known cause of abdominal pain, and of these, anterior cutaneous nerve entrapment syndrome (ACNES) is one that is frequently encountered. This is most commonly seen in females and is a "knife-like" pain located over the anterior cutaneous nerve on the anterior abdominal wall (unrelated to bowel function or meals) which is well-localized. ACNES is caused by the entrapment of the cutaneous branch of a sensory nerve from spinal levels T7-T12. Patients are often splinting to avoid tension on the musculature. Upon examination, pain can be produced with pressure on lateral wall of abdominis rectus which is where the nerve pierces the fascia of the abdominal wall. Clinical workup must exclude any bony pathology (fracture, malignancy, etc.) or gallbladder pathology which can cause referred pain, and further workup should be explored if any sign of these organic pathologies is noticed.

Initial treatment of ACNES should involve NSAIDs or cyclooxygenase-2 (COX-2) inhibitors, ice or heat, and possibly elastic rib belts. If further treatment is warranted, local anesthetic and steroid injection of the anterior cutaneous nerve and/or rectus sheath can be achieved. If relief is short-lived with steroids, neuroablative procedures may be considered.

Ⓘ Thoracic facet pain, while primarily causing pain over a segment of the thoracic spine, can refer over to the abdominal area as well, and should be considered in the diagnosis. If suspected, NSAIDs or other analgesics can be tried, but the pain should respond to thoracic medial branch blocks as well. If good response to the diagnostic blocks is obtained, radiofrequency ablation can be undertaken for more long-lasting relief.

Ⓙ Thoracic radiculopathy or radiculitis can cause pain that radiates into the abdomen. It is typically described as a burning, shooting, or electric-like pain that follows a dermatomal pattern. MRI can be used to evaluate for any disc pathology that could be causing nerve root irritation. Treatment consists of neuropathic medications like gabapentinoids, TCAs, and SNRIs, as well as interventional procedures, including epidural steroid injections. If relief is obtained but is of limited duration with a steroid injection, spinal cord stimulation can be considered.

Ⓚ "Slipping rib syndrome" is another source of somatic pain. This is usually found after trauma to costal cartilage during acceleration or deceleration injuries or blunt trauma to the chest. It is described as a sharp, typically unilateral pain in the subcostal region. Usually, the 10th rib is affected, but 8–9th ribs can be causative as well. Patients may be splinting to keep their thoracolumbar spine flexed. Upon examination, a "hooking maneuver test" demonstrates pain, clicking, and snapping when an examiner hooks the fingers under the rib cage and pulls outward gently while the patient is supine. Workup again must rule out bony pathology or underlying organic cause.

Treatment again should begin with NSAIDs, COX-2 inhibitors, and an elastic rib belt. Injections with local anesthetic and steroids near affected nerves can demonstrate good relief. If relief is short-lived after steroids, neuroablative procedures may be considered.

Ⓛ Myofascial pain and trigger points can also be found in the abdominal musculature. Palpation of these trigger points typically reproduces a patients pain and also causes a characteristic referral pattern of the pain for the muscle involved. Autonomic responses can also be seen with palpation of trigger points. Treatment can be focused on stretching and physical therapy, along with SNRIs, NSAIDs, and muscle relaxants. Trigger point injections, either with local anesthetics or dry needling, can also be helpful and can be performed under ultrasound guidance to avoid entry into the peritoneum.

SUGGESTED READING

Drossman D, Svigethy E. The narcotic bowel syndrome: a recent update. Am J Gastroenterol Suppl. 2014;2(1):22-30.

Majumder S, Chari ST. Chronic pancreatitis. Lancet. 2016; 387(10031):1957-66.

Mayer EA, Gupta M, Wong HY. A clinical perspective on abdominal pain. Wall & Melzack's Textbook of Pain. Churchill Livingstone: Elsevier; 2013. pp. 734-57.

Waldman SD. Abdominal wall pain syndromes. Pain Management. Churchill Livingstone: Elsevier; 2011. pp. 674-81.

Yarze JC, Friedman LS. Chronic abdominal pain. Sleisenger and Fordtran's Gastrointestinal and Liver Disease. Churchill Livingstone: Elsevier; 2016. pp. 175-84.

CHAPTER 50

Male Pelvic Pain

Mirchandani AA, Hwang S, Bonder JH

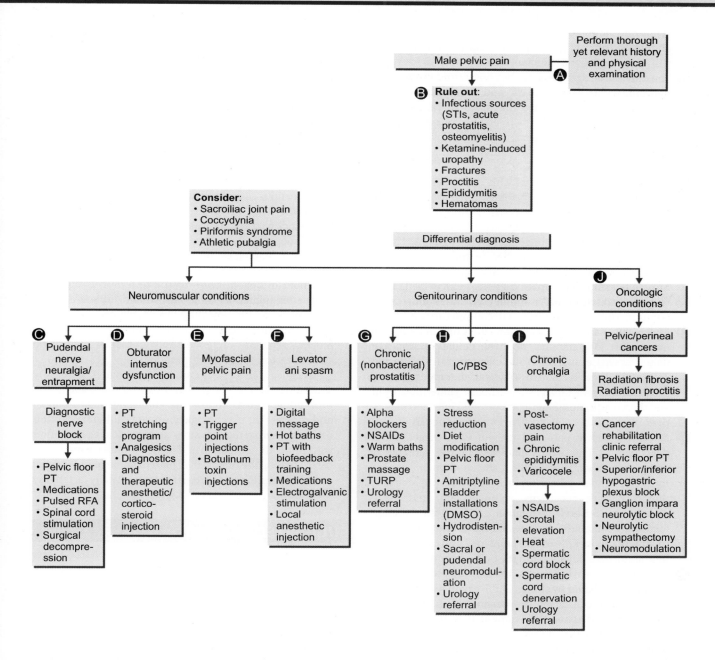

Male pelvic pain can include a wide variety of pain generators, which can be challenging for a clinician to identify and treat. For chronic male pelvic pain conditions, lifetime prevalence has been reported to be 2–14%. Often, diagnosis can be vague and requires consideration of the musculoskeletal, neurological, psychological, and genitourinary systems. For many conditions, diagnosis is obtained by exclusion and requires an experienced clinician to perform a relevant, yet thorough history and physical examination.

A The patient encounter should focus on obtaining all relevant genitourinary history pertaining to the chief complaint, including discussion regarding the nature of the pain and the various triggers. Prior treatments, surgeries, as well as bowel and bladder changes should be reviewed. Discussion should incorporate history of sexual function, sexual abuse, depression, anxiety, sexually transmitted infections, trauma, drug abuse, and occupational history. The patient's medical record and previous imaging should be reviewed. Physical examination should ensure optimal patient comfort and privacy. Conditions that may refer pain into the pelvic region should be ruled out. These include the sacroiliac joint, coccydynia, piriformis syndrome, and athletic pubalgia. Examination of the abdomen, external genitalia, perineal area, and rectum will further guide the clinician.

B The differential diagnosis can be compartmentalized into neuromuscular, genitourinary, and oncological sources. Other associated etiologies that need to be ruled out include (but are not limited to) infectious sources (sexually transmitted infections, acute prostatitis, osteomyelitis, etc.), ketamine-induced uropathy, fractures, proctitis, epididymitis, and hematomas.

C Pudendal neuralgia presents with unpleasant sensation of pain in the perineum, genitals, inner buttocks, and rectum. The pudendal nerve is susceptible to entrapment and can occur in cyclists. Palpation of the ischial spine may reproduce symptoms. Image-guided nerve blocks can be diagnostic or therapeutic. Further treatment may include pelvic floor physical therapy, medications (analgesics, muscle relaxants, neuropathic agents, etc.), pulsed radio-frequency ablation (RFA), spinal cord stimulation of the conus medullaris, and surgical decompression.

D Males with pain originating from the obturator internus may report long-standing perineal, penile, or testicular pain. Physical examination findings may be nonspecific. Treatment may include a physical therapy stretching program, along with analgesics. An image-guided diagnostic and therapeutic anesthetic/corticosteroid injection may be performed, if other conservative management fails.

E Myofascial pelvic pain will present with trigger points described as taut bands palpated in the muscles of the pelvic floor, hip girdle, and abdomen. Typical muscular tender points reported include puborectalis/pubococcygeus, coccygeus, sphincter ani, and rectus abdominis. Conservative treatment with physical therapy focusing on manual techniques should be initiated. Further treatment can include trigger point injections and possible botulinum toxin injections to the pelvic floor muscles.

F Levator ani spasm is described as dull, anorectal pain that can be exacerbated by sitting. Diffuse pain with palpation during transrectal digital examination of the levator ani can assist in diagnosis. Treatment may include digital massage, hot baths, physical therapy with biofeedback training, medications (analgesics, muscle relaxants, etc.), electrogalvanic stimulation, and local anesthetic injection.

G Chronic (nonbacterial) prostatitis is the most common form of prostatitis with symptoms lasting more than 3 months. It is thought to be due to atypical bacterial infection, nanobacterial dysfunction, or bladder sphincter dyssynergia. Patients may report lower urinary

symptoms, blood in semen or urine, genital pain, and sexual dysfunction. Treatment may include urology referral, alpha-blockers, nonsteroidal anti-inflammatory drugs (NSAIDs), warm baths, prostate massage, and transurethral resection of the prostate.

H Interstitial cystitis (IC)/painful bladder syndrome (PBS) typically presents with lower urinary tract symptoms particularly, frequency, urgency, and nocturia. Pain can be exacerbated with bladder filling and is relieved by voiding. Hunner's ulcers (areas of bleeding on the bladder wall) found on cystoscopy can aid in diagnosis of IC. If they are not present, PBS is diagnosed. Successful treatment is difficult and may include stress reduction, diet modification, pelvic floor physical therapy, amitriptyline, bladder installations of DMSO (dimethyl sulfoxide), hydrodistention, and sacral or pudendal neuromodulation.

I Chronic orchialgia will present with testicular pain lasting over 3 months. Etiologies include post-vasectomy pain, chronic epididymitis, and varicocele. Treatment should be tailored to the underlying etiology and the clinician should work in close conjunction with the urologist. Noninfectious causes that are refractory to NSAIDs, scrotal elevation, and heat, may benefit from a spermatic cord-block trial and if successful, may undergo spermatic cord denervation.

J Oncologic etiologies of pelvic pain can be seen in patients with pelvic and perineal cancers. These patients can benefit from referral to a multidisciplinary cancer rehabilitation clinic and should initiate a pelvic floor physical therapy program. Advanced treatments may include superior/inferior hypogastric plexus blocks, ganglion impar neurolytic blocks, neurolytic sympathectomy, and neuromodulation.

Because pelvic pain can be challenging, clinicians should develop robust patient-provider relationships by promoting regular follow up, managing expectations, and reassessing psychological impact of their condition regularly. A systematic history and physical examination will guide the clinician in diagnosis and treatment of care. Treating the male pelvic pain patient should involve a multidisciplinary approach and is usually a lengthy process.

SUGGESTED READING

Anderson RU, Sawyer T, Wise D, et al. Painful myofascial trigger points and pain sites in men with chronic prostatitis/chronic pelvic pain syndrome. J Urol. 2009;182(6):2753-8.

Andromanakos N, Kouraklis G, Alkiviadis K. Chronic perineal pain. Eur J Gastroenterol Hepatol. 2011;23(1):2-7.

Crofts M, Mead K, Persad R, et al. How to manage the chronic pelvic pain syndrome in men presenting to sexual health services. Sex Transm Infect. 2014;90(5):370-3.

Kavoussi PK, Costabile RA. Orchialgia and the chronic pelvic pain syndrome. World J Urol. 2013;31(4):773-8.

Mamlouk MD, vanSonnenberg E, Dehkharghani S. CT-guided nerve block for pudendal neuralgia: diagnostic and therapeutic implications. AJR Am J Roentgenol. 2014;203(1):196-200.

Potts JM, Payne CK. Urologic chronic pelvic pain. Pain. 2012;153(4):755-8.

Pelvic Pain in Women

Nagpal A, Hwang S, Bonder JH, Mirchandani AA

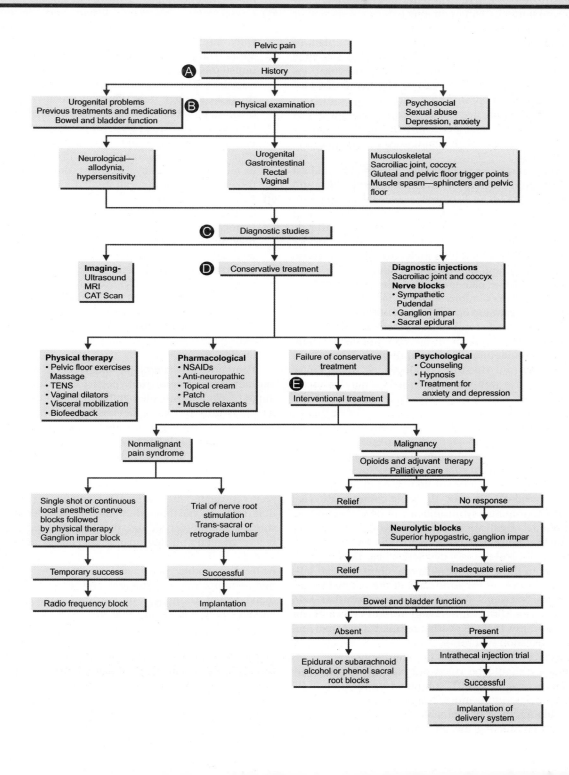

Pelvic pain is a very common pain syndrome, especially in women. The epidemiology of female pelvic pain is not well-studied, with prevalence estimates between 6% and 27%. It is important to appreciate that a diagnosis of pelvic pain can have a visceral and/or musculoskeletal etiology. Pain emanating from the nerves, muscles, and joints of the pelvic region, such as the sacroiliac joint, the pubic symphysis, the pelvic floor muscles, and the ilioinguinal/iliohypogastric nerves can refer into the lower abdomen, low back, hip, and buttocks. Differentiating between a visceral or musculoskeletal etiology is an essential step in the diagnostic pathway that will lead to an appropriate treatment plan. In a very high percentage of patients (10–50%), no causative factor can be established despite thorough investigations including imaging, laparoscopy, and hysterectomy. The lack of a clear diagnosis for chronic pain may lead to depression and anxiety. In addition, because of the sociocultural taboos associated with pelvic and perineal pain, patients have a tendency not to discuss it with health providers or with their support networks.

Ⓐ A thorough review of the patient's history and medical records should be performed. Prior investigations and treatments should be explored especially to ascertain that correctable gynecologic, genitourinary, and gastrointestinal conditions have been appropriately treated. Reviewing the patient's psychosocial history is essential because of a high incidence of sexual abuse history, anxiety, and depression. Although it may seem logical that these patients would then benefit from psychological interventions such as cognitive-behavioral therapy, this treatment option has not been well-studied.

Ⓑ Physical, neurologic, and musculoskeletal examination should specifically look for the possibility of referred pain from the sacroiliac joint, pubic symphysis, and the coccyx. The common musculoskeletal conditions which cause pelvic pain have well-known physical therapy protocols that have been shown to be efficacious. Examination of the genitalia should be performed to assess for erythema, lesions, and allodynia. Rectal and/or vaginal examination is performed to evaluate for tenderness, muscle spasm, or trigger points with reproduction of a patient's pain.

The examiner must rule out a gynecologic condition that may warrant a referral or be treated differently than a musculoskeletal disorder. The most common external genitalia neuropathic syndromes are pudendal neuralgia, dyspareunia, vaginismus, and vulvodynia. The primary chronic uterine pain conditions include endometriosis, adenomyosis, and primary dysmenorrhea. The definitive treatment of these conditions is oral contraceptive pills which can stave off the formation of the ectopic tissue, or surgical excision. The most common ovarian pain conditions are Mittelschmerz and ovarian cysts and less likely diagnoses include ovarian remnant syndrome and pelvic congestion syndrome.

Ⓒ *Diagnostics:* More ominous conditions such as malignancy should be ruled out with either magnetic resonance imaging (MRI), computed tomography (CT) scan, or pelvic ultrasound. Diagnostic local anesthetic nerve blocks may be valuable in establishing nerve pathways conducting the pain and also the possibility of sympathetically maintained pain. Transvaginal or transperineal pudendal nerve block may be helpful in diagnosing pudendal nerve entrapment syndrome. The pudendal block as performed by the pain management practitioner is more commonly transgluteal, under the guidance of either fluoroscopy or ultrasonography. Sacroiliac joint injections, ganglion impar blocks, coccygeal nerve blocks, and superior hypogastric plexus blocks may be utilized as further diagnostic injections.

Ⓓ *Conservative Treatment:* Pelvic and perineal pain due to nonmalignant conditions is best managed with multimodal and multidisciplinary conservative approaches. Pharmacological approaches include nonsteroidal anti-inflammatory drugs (NSAIDs), muscle relaxants, antidepressants, and anticonvulsant drugs to manage pain. Physical therapy, serial vaginal dilation, pelvic floor exercises, and biofeedback are very helpful in improving pelvic support and muscle spasms. Psychological counseling and adequate management of psychological comorbidities is likely to be beneficial in reducing pain and discomfort, though, as previously mentioned, this is not well studied.

Ⓔ *Interventional Treatment:* Local anesthetic nerve blocks of the pudendal nerve, sacral nerve roots, superior hypogastric plexus, ganglion impar, and trigger points may be very helpful in interrupting the pain cycle and facilitating physical therapy. Patients who have significant hypersensitivity may benefit from the application of a topical agent such as NSAIDs. Neurolytic block of the sacral nerve roots is not an option in patients who have intact bladder and bowel function. Stimulation of the sacral nerve roots may provide significant pain relief in neuropathic pain and in selected patients with interstitial cystitis.

Pain due to malignancy is managed with analgesics and adjuvants. Neurolytic hypogastric plexus and ganglion impar blocks may provide significant long-term pain relief. In patients who have lost bladder and bowel control, a neurolytic subarachnoid block may provide excellent pain relief. Patients with neurologically intact bowel and bladder function may be good candidates for an intrathecal drug delivery system after a successful trial.

In summary, chronic nonmalignant female pelvic pain represents an imminently treatable set of conditions that requires heightened attention. Musculoskeletal and somatic conditions should first be explored and treated before visceral and neuropathic diagnoses are entertained. Visceral and neuropathic pain conditions are best treated with neuropathic pharmacologic therapy, psychological interventions, physical therapy, and targeted interventional management. Ultimately, understanding the etiology of the patient's pain will ensure that the most optimal treatment paradigm is implemented.

SUGGESTED READING

Ahangari A. Prevalence of chronic pelvic pain among women: an updated review. Pain Physician. 2014;17(2):E141-7.

Burnett AI, Wesselmann U. Neurobiology of the pelvis and perineum: principles for a practical approach. J Pelvic Surg. 1999;5:224-32.

Cichowski SB, Dunivan GC, Komesu YM, et al. Sexual abuse history and pelvic floor disorders in women. South Med J. 2013;106(12):675-8.

Hooker AB, van Moorst BR, van Haarst EP, et al. Chronic pelvic pain: evaluation of the epidemiology, baseline demographics, and clinical variables via a prospective and multidisciplinary approach. Clin Exp Obstet Gynecol. 2013;40(4):492-8.

Hunter C, Dave N, Diwan S, et al. Neuromodulation of pelvic visceral pain: review of the literature and case series of potential novel targets for treatment. Pain Pract. 2013;13(1):3-17.

Kapural L, Narouze SN, Janicki TI, et al. Spinal cord stimulation is an effective treatment for the chronic intractable visceral pelvic pain. Pain Med. 2006;7(5):440-3.

Kucharski A, Nagda N. Pelvic pain. In: Warfield CA, Bajwa ZH (Eds). Principles and Practices of Pain Medicine, 2nd edition. New York: McGraw-Hill; 2004. pp. 359-68.

McDonald JS. Chronic pelvic pain. In: Copeland IJ, Jarell JF (Eds). Textbook of Gynecology. Philadelphia: WB Saunders; 2000. pp. 741-58.

Stuge B, Laerum E, Kirkesola G, et al. The efficacy of a treatment program focusing on specific stabilizing exercises for pelvic girdle pain after pregnancy: A randomized controlled trial. Spine (Phila Pa 1976). 2004;29(4):351-9.

Willard FH, Schuenke MD. The neuroanatomy of female pelvic pain. In: Bailey A, Bernstein C (Eds). Pain in Women: A Clinical Guide. New York: Springer; 2013. pp. 17-58.

SECTION 4

Cancer Pain

Brian T Boies

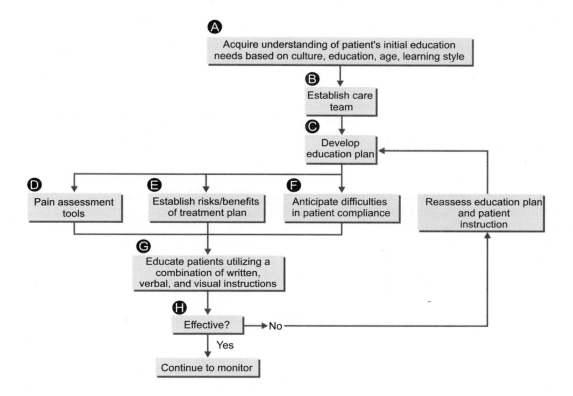

Patient education on pain management is an often-neglected aspect of a pain management program. Much information exists on patient misconceptions about pain management, and published articles describe attempts to correct these misconceptions. However, patient education is not a "one size fits all" program.

Ⓐ Educational programs for patients with cancer pain differ from those for patients with postoperative pain or chronic back pain. To complicate matters further, different populations of patients have different styles of learning. Some patients embrace computer-assisted learning, others prefer videotape instruction, or a printed instruction sheet, and still others require one-on-one instruction. Age, educational background, and culture influence learning as well.

Ⓑ Recent programs focus on physicians and nursing in the role of educators. As the frontline in hands-on patient care, oncology nurses often play a significant role in achieving the goal of positive health outcomes by addressing challenges that inhibit effective patient-provider communication and education.

Ⓒ There is overwhelming evidence that patients have misconceptions about the risks, benefits, and side effects of pain management therapies, and they need/want more information. Patient education alone cannot solve poor pain management practice, but poor patient education can certainly hinder effective strategies for obtaining pain relief.

Despite the problems of creating an effective educational program, there are several key features necessary for achieving one.

Ⓓ Patients must be taught an effective pain assessment tool to describe their pain and its intensity. The Verbal Rating Score, Visual Analog Scale, and Pediatric Faces assessment tool are just a few examples of pain assessment methods. No matter which tool is chosen, patients must be instructed on its effective use. For example, patients asked to rate pain on a scale of 1–10 sometimes respond, "It's an 11." Although descriptive in the sense that it is clear the patient is experiencing severe pain, it demonstrates a lack of understanding that there is no pain greater than 10. Education is best done before patients develop severe pain or at a time when pain has been brought under control.

E Patients must understand that controlling pain is not just a comfort measure but an important part of their recovery from illness. They should have an expectation of effective pain control. Knowing the physiological and psychological consequences of untreated pain can make patients more willing to request pain relief.

Patients should have an understanding of the common side effects and complications of their analgesic regimen. They should also learn how to avoid them if possible and manage them when they are unavoidable.

F Several difficulties arise in ensuring patient compliance to the treatment plan, many of which can be mitigated by proper education.

The educational program should debunk the myth that the use of opioids for pain treatment leads to addiction or can cause other serious harm. Patients have an exaggerated sense of the risks of opioid therapy, and they often refuse medication even when it is offered because of their fear of addiction or injury.

Patients should learn to request pain medication at the time of the onset of pain to avoid situations where the pain is out of control. Patients must understand that there is a delay from the time when the medication is administered until the onset of analgesia.

G How to deliver this information differs with the clinical setting and the population involved. It is unlikely that any one approach would work for all individuals all of the time.

The easiest method is a printed sheet given to a patient at the time of entry into the health system. However, a patient's ability to comprehend the printed material varies widely from one individual to another. Furthermore, giving the patient the material in no way ensures that the material is ever read and understood.

A more effective approach is to have a staff member review the printed material with the patient at the time it is distributed—this is often called coaching. This approach ensures that the patient has the material, has reviewed it at least once, and has had an opportunity to ask questions. The printed material is then available for future reference. Coaching interventions can be effective resources for helping cancer patients communicate about their pain concerns if they can be integrated within clinical routines, and it can lead to improved health outcomes.

Videos and computer-assisted instructions are also an option; but whether they work the same, better, or worse than a printed sheet is not known nor is the efficacy of one-on-one instruction.

H Knowing that there are problems with the delivery of information indicates the need for a feedback mechanism for an educational program. There must be some measure of the effectiveness of that program. Methods of feedback include having patients demonstrate the appropriate use of an analgesic device, such as a patient-controlled analgesia pump, or to recite back to the instructor the information received. Another form of feedback is a survey of the patient and staff after treatment to assess the patient's level of participation and effective use of analgesic therapy. This has the advantage of measuring the actual desired outcome: patient participation and degree of pain relief. It has the disadvantage, however, of being labor-intensive and time-consuming; moreover, it does not indicate whether poor pain relief is due to lack of education, poor staff performance, or other factors. No matter what feedback method is chosen, it must be used to guide the educational program continuously toward better patient outcomes.

SUGGESTED READING

Adam R, Bond C, Murchie P. Educational interventions for cancer pain. A systematic review of systematic reviews with nested narrative review of randomized controlled trials. Patient Educ Couns. 2015;98(3):269-82.

Dong S, Butow PN, Costa DS, et al. The influence of patient-centered communication during radiotherapy education sessions on post-consultation patient outcomes. Patient Educ Couns. 2014;95(3):305-12.

Hochstenbach LM, Zwakhalen SM, Courtens AM, et al. Feasibility of a mobile and web-based intervention to support self-management in outpatients with cancer pain. Eur J Oncol Nurs. 2016;23:97-105.

Jenerette CM, Mayer DK. Patient-Provider Communication: the Rise of Patient Engagement. Semin Oncol Nurs. 2016;32(2):134-43.

Luckett T, Davidson PM, Green A, et al. Assessment and management of adult cancer pain: a systematic review and synthesis of recent qualitative studies aimed at developing insights for managing barriers and optimizing facilitators within a comprehensive framework of patient care. J Pain Symptom Manage. 2013;46(2):229-53.

Sajjad S, Ali A, Gul RB, et al. The effect of individualized patient education, along with emotional support, on the quality of life of breast cancer patients - A pilot study. Eur J Oncol Nurs. 2016;21:75-82.

Salmon P, Young B. The validity of education and guidance for clinical communication in cancer care: evidence-based practice will depend on practice-based evidence. Patient Educ Couns. 2013;90(2):193-9.

Street R Jr, Slee C, Kalauokalani DK, et al. Improving physician-patient communication about cancer pain with a tailored education-coaching intervention. Patient Educ Couns. 2010;80(1):42-7.

van Weert JC, Bolle S, van Dulmen S, et al. Older cancer patients' information and communication needs: What they want is what they get? Patient Educ Couns. 2013;92(3):388-97.

Webb RJ, Shelton CP. The Benefits of Authorized Agent Controlled Analgesia (AACA) to Control Pain and Other Symptoms at the End of Life. J Pain Symptom Manage. 2015;50(3):371-4.

Zucca A, Sanson-Fisher R, Waller A, et al. Medical Oncology Patients: Are They Offered Help and Does It Provide Relief? J Pain Symptom Manage. 2015;50(4):436-44.

CHAPTER
53

Medical Management

Driver LC, Kim PY

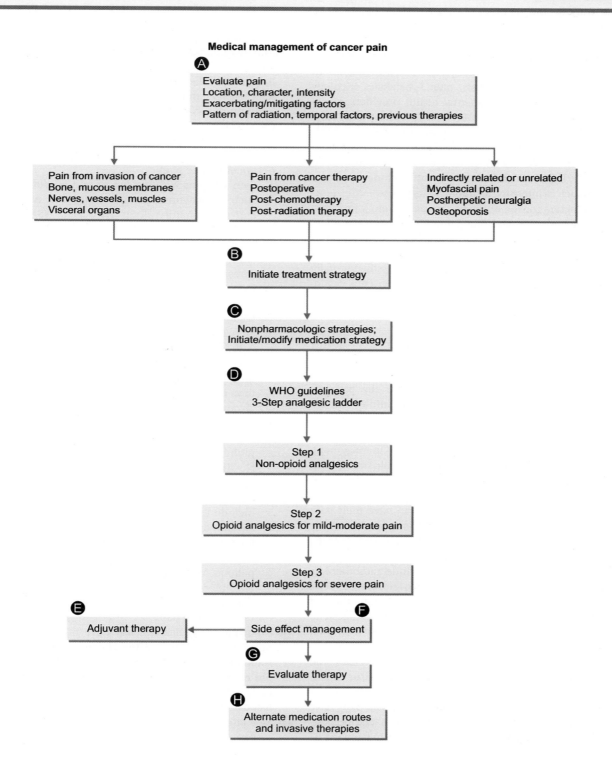

Medical management of cancer pain

A Evaluate pain
Location, character, intensity
Exacerbating/mitigating factors
Pattern of radiation, temporal factors, previous therapies

Pain from invasion of cancer
Bone, mucous membranes
Nerves, vessels, muscles
Visceral organs

Pain from cancer therapy
Postoperative
Post-chemotherapy
Post-radiation therapy

Indirectly related or unrelated
Myofascial pain
Postherpetic neuralgia
Osteoporosis

B Initiate treatment strategy

C Nonpharmacologic strategies;
Initiate/modify medication strategy

D WHO guidelines
3-Step analgesic ladder

Step 1
Non-opioid analgesics

Step 2
Opioid analgesics for mild-moderate pain

Step 3
Opioid analgesics for severe pain

E Adjuvant therapy

F Side effect management

G Evaluate therapy

H Alternate medication routes
and invasive therapies

Cancer pain is a dynamic condition, with an often complex presentation, which requires a thorough assessment and a multimodal approach to management. Cancer pain occurs in 25% of patients who are newly diagnosed, in 33% of patients undergoing treatment, and in 75% of those with advanced disease. Due to the high frequency of its occurrence, cancer pain should be treated aggressively and immediately. The benefits of effective treatment include facilitation of the diagnostic workup and treatment, improved functional status, and better quality of life, with increasing evidence suggesting improved survival rates.

Despite this evidence, cancer pain is undertreated for a variety of reasons. A comprehensive medical management team that includes oncologists, pain specialists, oncology nurses, physical therapists, mental health providers, social workers, and palliative care experts can provide optimal care.

A Cancer can produce any type of pain at any location. Evaluation should include pain classification (pain associated with tumor, associated with treatment and that unrelated to either), acute or chronic nature, and include characteristics such as intensity, location, pattern of radiation, temporal factors (onset, duration, frequency, etc.), provocative, exacerbating and mitigating factors, and the effect of previous control measures. Cancer pain syndromes vary by tumor type and are related to patterns of tumor growth and metastasis. The pain can be classified broadly as nociceptive (somatic, well-localized or visceral organ, poorly localized), or neuropathic (resulting from central nervous system or peripheral nerves; burning, lancinating).

Since all pain in the cancer patient is not necessarily from the tumor(s), and as such, pain may change character or break through a previously effective regimen. When choosing a treatment regimen, consider the patient's social status, health care access, comorbidities, and life expectancy, as well as the individual's desires and expectations. A comprehensive pain assessment and evaluation is integral to ensure adequate cancer pain management. There are a myriad of validated pain scales used—the Faces Pain Rating Scale being one that has broad utility in adults and children.

B About 90% of patients with cancer can have their pain adequately managed with oral medications, which is the most convenient route of administration. Oral therapy should be viewed as an integral part of the spectrum of many available strategies, which include radiotherapy, chemotherapy, surgery, physiotherapy, anesthetic blocks, and transcutaneous nerve stimulation, among others. It is important to (1) customize pharmacologic analgesia to the needs of the individual patient in terms of their pain and their preferred route of administration, (2) choose the appropriate drugs, (3) titrate the agent carefully, and (4) frequently reassess therapy, adjusting and/or substituting it as necessary.

C Nonpharmacologic interventions for cancer pain have been shown to be effective as part of a comprehensive pain management program. Since it is known that pain encompasses physical, psychosocial, and spiritual dimensions, use of nonpharmacologic interventions such as massage, heat-cold therapy, acupuncture, acupressure, and cognitive interventions (breathing, relaxation exercises, hypnosis, etc.) can be very useful as an adjunct to pharmacologic management.

D The World Health Organization (WHO) proposed a three-step analgesic ladder that provides a logical basis for the pharmacologic treatment of cancer pain. It has three points of entry, depending on the severity of pain, and allows progression between the various steps. Due to patient variability in the response to the various opioid agonists, sequential trials (or "opioid rotation"), may help identify the medication with the more favorable balance between the analgesic effects and the side effects. In addition, the National Comprehensive Cancer Network (NCCN) has expounded on the WHO guidelines and provides updated and more specific information on many aspects of the identification, treatment, and management of cancer-related pain.

1. Step 1 begins with the use of non-opioid analgesics such as acetaminophen, aspirin, and nonsteroidal anti-inflammatory drugs (NSAIDs). NSAIDs effectively alleviate mild cancer pain. They should be considered as an addition at any step in the analgesic ladder for bone pain, soft tissue infiltration, pressure sores, and any pain with an inflammatory component. Non-opioid analgesics are associated with ceiling effects, and exceeding the maximum dose range can result in organ toxicity.

2. Step 2 progresses to acetaminophen in combination with "weak" opioids (e.g., codeine, hydrocodone, oxycodone, and propoxyphene). Combination of short-duration medications may provide better analgesia than either drug alone. These medications should be given on a scheduled basis if a continuous baseline pain is present.

3. Step 3 introduces the potent opioids (e.g., morphine, hydromorphone, methadone, and fentanyl). No strong evidence speaks for the superiority of one opioid, however, unique pharmacologic profiles play a role in tailoring the analgesic regimen. Examples include transdermal fentanyl for patients unable to swallow or who are prone to constipation, methadone for patients with a neuropathic pain component, and hydromorphone with its nonactive metabolites for patients with impaired metabolism and clearance. Sustained-release formulations can be extremely effective. Remember to provide for both baseline and breakthrough pain.

E Adjuvant analgesics typically have primary indications other than cancer pain (**Box 1**), but they provide analgesia in many situations and may reduce the systemic opioid requirement. They should, therefore, be considered early in treatment. Agents given for other complaints are listed in **Box 2**.

F Side effect management is an essential aspect of therapy assessment. Uncontrolled side effects negatively affect

Box 1: Adjuvant analgesics

General analgesia potentiation

- Corticosteroids (prednisone, dexamethasone)
- Anxiolytics and muscle relaxants (clonazepam, diazepam, baclofen)
- SSRIs (paroxetine), SNRIs (duloxetine)
- α_2-Agonists (tizanidine, clonidine)
- Topical agents (capsaicin, local anesthetics)

Neuropathic drugs

- TCAs (amitriptyline, nortriptyline, desipramine)
- Anticonvulsants (gabapentin, pregabalin, oxcarbazepine, topiramate)
- Antidysrhythmics (mexiletine, tocainide)
- NMDA antagonists (ketamine, dextromethorphan)
- *Miscellaneous*: Baclofen, calcitonin

Bone pain

- NSAIDs (ibuprofen, naproxen, celecoxib, meloxicam)
- Bisphosphonates (pamidronate)
- Osteoclast inhibitors (calcitonin, radiopharmaceuticals)

NMDA, N-methyl-D-aspartate; SSRIs, selective serotonin reuptake inhibitors; SNRIs, serotonin-norepinephrine reuptake inhibitors; TCAs, tricyclic antidepressants

Box 2: Other agents and their indications

Constipation

- Stimulating agents (docusate, senna, bisacodyl)
- Osmotic agents (lactulose, magnesium citrate)
- Prokinetic agents (metoclopramide)
- Opioid antagonists (naloxone, naloxegol, methylnaltrexone)
- Miscellaneous: Octreotide, mestinon, hyoscine

Sedation

- Psychostimulants (caffeine, methylphenidate, dextroamphetamine)

Nausea

- Hydroxyzine, promethazine, ondansetron, haloperidol, metoclopramide, scopolamine, meclizine

Edema

- Diuretics

Insomnia

- Amitriptyline, hydroxyzine, trazodone, melatonin, mirtazapine

Pruritus

- Diphenhydramine, hydroxyzine, naloxone, nalbuphine

the quality of life. The key is to anticipate medication side effects and treat them proactively, promptly, and aggressively.

G Reassess the efficacy of therapy frequently. As the disease progresses, titrate medications appropriately. New-onset pain or breakthrough pain should direct the provider to look for new pathology or progression of the disease.

H If standard oral therapy fails, whether due to inadequate analgesia or intolerable side effects, consider invasive therapies. Interventional procedures for cancer pain include nerve conduction blockade, neuroablative techniques, and neuraxial analgesic delivery systems.

SUGGESTED READING

Brogan S, Junkins S. Interventional therapies for the management of cancer pain. J Support Oncol. 2010;8(2):52-9.

Chai T, Burton AW, Koyyalagunta D. Pain, Cancer. In: Encyclopedia of the Neurological Sciences, 2nd Edition. Oxford: Academic Press; 2014. pp. 731-3.

Goudas LC, Bloch R, Gialedi-Goudas M, et al. The epidemiology of cancer pain. Cancer Invest. 2005;23(2):182-90.

Grossman SA, Nesbit S. Cancer-related pain. In: Niederhuber JE, Armitage JO, Doroshow JH, Kastan MB, Tepper JE (Eds). Abeloff's Clinical Oncology, 5th edition. Philadelphia: Elsevier; 2014. pp. 608-19.

Hicks CL, vonBaeyer CL, Spafford PA, et al. The Faces Pain Scale-Revised: toward a common metric in adult and pediatric pain measurement. Pain. 2001;93(2):173-83.

Merskey H, Budgduk N. Classification of Chronic Pain. Descriptions of Chronic Pain Syndromes and Definition of Pain Terms, 2nd edition. Seattle, WA: IASP Press; 1994.

National Cancer Institute. (2016). PDQ® Supportive and Palliative Care Editorial Board, PDQ Cancer Center Pain. [online] NCI website. Available from *https://www.cancer.gov/about-cancer/treatment/side-effects/pain* [Accessed January, 2017].

National Comprehensive Cancer Network, Inc. (2014). NCCN Guidelines Version 1. Adult Cancer Pain. [online] NCCN website. Available from *https://www.nccn.org/professionals/physician_gls/f_guidelines.asp*.

Raslan AM, Burchiel KJ. Neurosurgical approaches to pain management. In: Benzon HT, Rathmell JP, Wu CL, Turk DC, Argoff CE, Hurley RW. Practical Management of Pain, 5th edition. Philadelphia: Mosby; 2014. pp. 328-34.

Ruben M, van Osch M, Blanch-Hartigan D. Healthcare providers' accuracy in assessing patients' pain: A systematic review. Patient Educ Couns. 2015;98(10):1197-206.

Saifan A, Bashayreh I, Batiha AM, et al. Patient- and family caregiver-related barriers to effective cancer pain control. Pain Manag Nurs. 2015;16(3):400-10.

Sharma V, de Leon-Casasola O. Cancer pain. In: Benzon HT, Rathmell JP, Wu CL, Turk DC, Argoff CE, Hurley RW. Practical Management of Pain, 5th edition. Philadelphia: Mosby; 2014. pp. 335-45.

Sheinfeld GS, Krebs P, Badr H, et al. Meta-analysis of psychosocial interventions to reduce pain in patients with cancer. J Clin Oncol. 2012;30(5):539-47.

Smith H, Argoff CE, McCleane G. Antidepressants as analgesics. In: Practical Management of Pain, 5th edition. Philadelphia: Mosby; 2014. pp. 530-42.

Stjernsward J, Colleau SM, Ventafridda V. The World Health Organization Cancer Pain and Palliative Care Program. Past, present and future. J. Pain Symptom Manage. 1996;12(2):65-72.

Svendsen KB, Anderson S, Arnason S, et al. Breakthrough pain in malignant and non-malignant diseases: a review of prevalence, characteristics and mechanisms. Eur J Pain. 2005;9(2):195-206.

van den Beuken-van Everdingen MH, Hochstenbach LM, Joosten EA, et al. Update on Prevalence of Pain in Patients With Cancer: Systematic Review and Meta-Analysis. J Pain Symptom Manage. 2016;51(6):1070-90.

Zucca A, Sanson-Fisher R, Waller A, et al. Medical Oncology Patients: Are They Offered Help and Does It Provide Relief? J Pain Symptom Manage. 2015;50(4):436-44.

CHAPTER 54

Metastatic Disease

Driver LC, Banik R

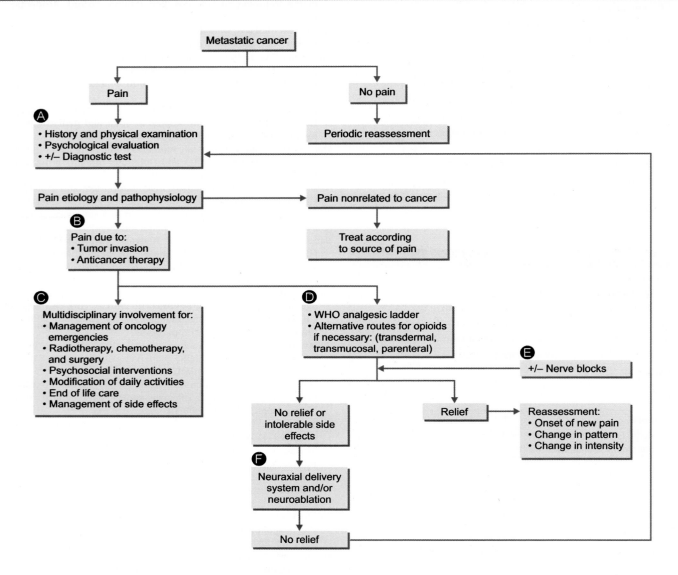

Cancer pain occurs in 33% or more of patients undergoing treatment and in 75–90% of those with advanced disease. Tragically, adequate cancer pain management remains a major healthcare problem. Minorities, women, and the elderly may be at even greater risk for undertreatment of pain.

A Cancer pain may be classified as nociceptive (somatic or visceral) or neuropathic, although psychological factors play an important role in individual perception. Pain assessment is a systematic clinical evaluation that

ends with a diagnosis that emphasizes on the etiology and pathophysiology of the pain complaint. The medical history emphasizes on pain characteristics (e.g., location, quality, duration, intensity, palliative, or provocative factors), cancer history and treatment, and psychological factors such as depression, fear, anxiety, and anger. In addition, patients with advanced cancer may also have generalized weakness, fatigue, and delirium. These symptoms affect pain perception, pain reporting, and the overall quality of life. The clinician should perform a physical examination of the painful sites and of the various systems with special attention to the neurologic and musculoskeletal systems. This systematic approach helps to identify the causes of pain in the cancer patient.

B Cancer pain results from direct tumor invasion, anticancer therapies, or causes not related to the cancer. Common cancer pain syndromes, such as bone metastasis, visceral pain, neuropathic pain, and mucositis, among others, can be identified, as can an oncologic emergency (e.g., spinal cord compression, cardiac tamponade, etc.).

C The involvement of specialists from multiple disciplines results in improved analgesia and other health outcomes. Discussing treatment decisions with the patient and family members is beneficial. Matching the options for optimal pain control depends on individual variations in needs, preferences, costs, and anticipated responses.

D Nonpharmacologic interventions for cancer pain have also been shown to be effective as part of a comprehensive pain management program. Since it is known that pain encompasses physical, psychosocial, and spiritual dimensions, use of nonpharmacologic interventions such as massage, heat-cold therapy, acupuncture, acupressure, and cognitive interventions (breathing, relaxation exercises, hypnosis, etc.) are very useful as adjunctive therapy to pharmacologic management.

Evidence for pharmacologic cancer pain control is outlined in the World Health Organization's (WHO) analgesic ladder. In addition, the National Comprehensive Cancer Network (NCCN) has broadened the guidelines and provides detailed, updated, and highly specific information on many aspects of the identification, treatment, and management of cancer-related pain. Both recommend initial administration of oral agents (non-opioids, opioids, adjuvants, etc.), however, the WHO focus is primarily reliant on pain intensity and to a lesser extent on the mechanism of the pain as determinants of therapy. The NCCN guidelines also include a multimodal approach to treatment including behavioral and psychosocial treatments as part of a comprehensive integrated pain management program.

1. Opioids are titrated to effect; there should be no predetermined maximum dose. The correct dose of an opioid is that which effectively relieves pain without inducing unacceptable side effects. The use of alternative routes of opioid administration (transdermal, transmucosal, parenteral delivery, etc.) depends on the patient's circumstances. Opioids are administered around the clock, with additional doses available for breakthrough pain.

2. Constipation is a common side effect in patients undergoing opioid therapy. These patients should receive prophylactic therapy with stool softener, often in combination with bulk agents, osmotic laxatives, or stimulant cathartics.

3. Other side effects of opioids, including tolerance, physical dependence, sedation, respiratory depres-

sion, nausea and vomiting, cognitive impairment, myoclonus, pruritus, and urinary retention, should be treated when they occur. Prophylaxis is not indicated. When tolerance to an opioid develops, another opioid can be substituted to provide better analgesia because the cross-tolerance among opioids is incomplete. However, it is recommended that the calculated dose be reduced by 25–50% to account for that incomplete cross-tolerance when converting from one opioid to another.

E For patients who do not respond to simple techniques, interventional approaches such as nerve blocks, neuroablative procedures, spinal cord stimulation, or implantation of drug delivery systems may be offered.

- Neural blockade with local anesthetics may be helpful for treating pain in a defined anatomic location. The patient is made aware that effective pain relief with a diagnostic block does not guarantee pain relief after a neuroablative procedure. Neuroablation can be accomplished by chemical, thermal, or surgical means. Deafferentation pain after a neuroablative procedure may be worse than the initial pain, however. Unwanted motor weakness or bladder/bowel dysfunction is a concern. Neuroablation does not always lead to cessation of opioid administration, but the dosage of the opioid should be reduced to avoid respiratory depression in case of significant pain relief.

- Drug delivery systems for chronic cancer pain management include epidural, spinal, and intraventricular systems. The spinal route for analgesia is widely employed. Consensus guidelines for initiation and management of intrathecal drug delivery systems exist to help guide their usage.

F The indication for neuraxial drug delivery and neuroablative procedures includes inadequate pain relief with oral analgesics, intolerable side effects of pharmacotherapy, and refractory neuropathic pain. These advanced modalities should be offered to the motivated, compliant patient in a setting that can provide readily available follow-up whenever indicated.

SUGGESTED READING

Auret K, Schug SA. Pain management for the cancer patient – current practice and future developments. Best Pract Res Clin Anaesthesiol. 2013;27(4):545-61.

Baumbauer KM, Young EE, Starkweather AR, et al. Managing Chronic Pain in Special Populations with Emphasis on Pediatric, Geriatric, and Drug Abuser Populations. Med Clin North Am. 2016;100(1):183-97.

Chai T, Burton AW, Koyyalagunta D. Pain, Cancer. In: Encyclopedia of the Neurological Sciences, 2nd edition. Oxford: Academic Press; 2014. pp. 731-3.

Deer TR, Prager J, Levy R, et al. Polyanalgesic Consensus Conference 2012: Recommendations for the management of pain by intrathecal (intraspinal) drug delivery: report of an interdisciplinary expert panel. Neuromodulation. 2012;15(5):436-64.

Grossman S, Nesbit S. Cancer-related pain. In: Niederhuber JE, Armitage JO, Doroshow JH, Kastan MB, Tepper JE (Eds). Abeloff's Clinical Oncology, 5th edition. Philadelphia: Elsevier; 2014. pp. 608-19.

He QH, Liu QL, Li Z, et al. Impact of epidural analgesia on quality of life and pain in advanced cancer patients. Pain Manag Nurs. 2015;16(3):307-13.

National Cancer Institute. (2016). PDQ® Supportive and Palliative Care Editorial Board, PDQ Cancer Center Pain. [online] NCI website. Available from http://*www.cancer.gov/about-cancer/treatment/side-effects/pain/pain-hp-pdq*. [Accessed January, 2017].

National Comprehensive Cancer Network, Inc. (2014). NCCN Guidelines Version 1. Adult Cancer Pain. [online] NCCN website. Available from *https://www.nccn.org/professionals/physician_gls/f_guidelines.asp*.

Saifan A, Bashayreh I, Batiha AM, et al. Patient- and family caregiver-related barriers to effective cancer pain control. Pain Manag Nurs. 2015;16(3):400-10.

Sayed D. The interdisciplinary management of cancer pain. Tech Reg Anes Pain Manag. 2013;17(4):163-7.

Sharma V, de Leon-Casasola O. Cancer Pain. In: Benzon HT, Rathmell JP, Wu CL, Turk DC, Argoff CE, Hurley RW (Eds). Practical Management of Pain, 5th edition. Philadelphia: Mosby; 2014. pp. 335-45.

Smith HS, Argoff CE, McCleane G. Antidepressants as analgesics. In: Practical Management of Pain, 5th edition. Philadelphia: Mosby; 2014. pp. 530-42.

Stjernsward J, Colleau SM, Ventafridda V. The World Health Organization Cancer Pain and Palliative Care Program. Past, present and future. J Pain Symptom Manage. 1996;12(2):65-72.

CHAPTER 55

Neurolytic Blocks

Driver LC, Patel MY

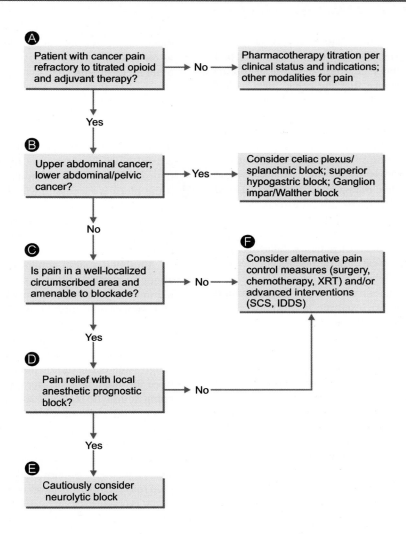

A Patient with cancer pain refractory to titrated opioid and adjuvant therapy? → No → Pharmacotherapy titration per clinical status and indications; other modalities for pain

↓ Yes

B Upper abdominal cancer; lower abdominal/pelvic cancer? → Yes → Consider celiac plexus/splanchnic block; superior hypogastric block; Ganglion impar/Walther block

↓ No

C Is pain in a well-localized circumscribed area and amenable to blockade? → No → **F** Consider alternative pain control measures (surgery, chemotherapy, XRT) and/or advanced interventions (SCS, IDDS)

↓ Yes

D Pain relief with local anesthetic prognostic block? → No →

↓ Yes

E Cautiously consider neurolytic block

Cancer pain is a dynamic, complex condition requiring a thorough assessment and a multimodal approach to management. Cancer pain occurs in 25% of patients who are newly diagnosed, in 33% of patients undergoing treatment, and in 75% of those with advanced disease. Simple, single-modal therapy with oral opioids fails to achieve adequate pain control in a significant number of patients. The interdisciplinary model for the management of cancer has long been a standard of practice, with collaboration among medical, radiation, and surgical oncologists. Unfortunately, some patients still do not achieve effective pain relief with oral or parenteral medication even when given large doses of parenteral opioids and

experience intolerable side effects. These patients may be candidates for neurolytic nerve blocks.

A Most patients who require a neurolytic block fall into three general categories. The first, most common group includes those who have tried oral and parenteral therapy but failed to achieve adequate pain relief or failed to get pain relief without intolerable side effects. It should be noted that all side effects should be aggressively managed, including the use of stimulants for severe sedation, aggressive antinausea medication, and potent osmotic agents for constipation. The second group of patients requiring a neurolytic block are those who have incident pain. An example is the patient with bone metastases who is comfortable at rest but cannot ambulate because weight-bearing produces severe pain. These patients are unlikely to achieve adequate relief for ambulation with oral opioid therapy. The third group of candidates for a neurolytic block includes patients with neuropathic pain. Painful neuropathy often responds poorly to opioids, even at high doses. For patients who do not respond, a neurolytic block may provide pain relief, although the idea that pain relief derived from further damaging an already injured nerve seems incongruous.

B Several neurolytic blocks have high utility. Neurolysis of the celiac plexus is extremely effective for alleviating pain due to pancreatic cancer or upper abdominal tumors. Some investigators believe that the celiac plexus block does not necessarily need to be reserved for those who fail opioid therapy. Moreover, because of the good side effect profile of the celiac plexus block and its relatively low risk of complications, it should be tried early in the course of this devastating malignancy. The hypogastric plexus block is extremely useful for managing refractory pain due to a pelvic malignancy. Prospective studies done in women with severe, unremitting pain due to a pelvic malignancy found that the hypogastric plexus block provided a significant degree of pain relief and low complication rates in most patients. Likewise, ganglion Impar/Walther block may be helpful for perineal pain.

C Not all patients with refractory cancer pain are candidates for a neurolytic block. An example is the patient with widely metastatic multiple myeloma in whom the large number of painful sites would greatly exceed the ability to anesthetize the affected area adequately.

Neurolytic blocks are best used in patients who have a well-defined anatomic location for their pain. This typically corresponds to a localized peripheral nerve distribution, and ideally one with a primarily sensory function. For example, head and neck cancers may be responsive to a block or neurolysis of the branches of the trigeminal nerve. Isolated chest wall pain may respond to intercostal nerve blockade or neurolysis. The advantage of blockade of the trigeminal and intercostal nerves is that, except for the third division of the trigeminal nerve, these nerves perform mostly sensory functions, so their block does not result in significant loss of motor function.

Blockade of other peripheral nerves is occasionally useful for pain control as well, but the degree of pain relief must be balanced against the loss of significant motor function. For example, neurolytic blockade of the brachial plexus would most often result in significant loss of motor function as well. This may be appropriate if the patient already has no function in these areas, but otherwise it may cause as much disability as the pain itself. Prognostic blocks would help answer this question and give the patient an idea of what the results of the neurolytic block might be. Patients may choose to have a somewhat painful, though functional extremity rather than having one that is numb and painless but totally nonfunctional.

D Once the anatomic site has been chosen, diagnostic blocks using local anesthetics may precede neurolytic blocks. The practitioner should also understand the limitations of prognostic blocks. A successful prognostic block with local anesthetic does not guarantee pain relief with a neurolytic procedure. There are several reasons for this. First, local anesthetics produce more intense blockade of a nerve condition than does a neurolytic procedure. Second, local anesthetics generally allow use of a larger volume of solution than one would be able to use with a neurolytic procedure. Third, the difference in the mechanisms of action of the local anesthetics compared to neurolytic agents may provide pain relief through other mechanisms, such as muscle relaxation or systemic effects. Therefore, the real value of prognostic blocks does not lie in identifying patients in whom success is guaranteed but in eliminating patients for whom the chance of success is negligible. In other words, a successful prognostic block does not guarantee pain relief, but an unsuccessful block can certainly identify patients for whom neurolytic blocks are *not* indicated.

E If the block is successful with local anesthetics, and the patient fully understands the risks of the neurolytic block, such as anesthesia dolorosa, loss of motor function, continued pain, etc., then it is reasonable to proceed with the procedure.

Another caveat to remember when talking to patients about a neurolytic block is that it seldom results in total elimination of the need for opioid therapy. Most patients with cancer pain must continue their oral medication if for no other reason than to prevent an abstinence syndrome. However, most patients continue to have some pain for which oral analgesics are needed, and if there is progression of the tumor, pain may recur, reaffirming the need for oral analgesic therapy. Patients who are undergoing neurolytic blockade solely for the purpose of eliminating oral analgesics have unrealistic expectations as to the effectiveness of these procedures. Patients should experience improved effectiveness of their medication at reduced doses and thus should also experience reduced side effects. The patient should also be counseled that pain may recur within several weeks to months, and additional procedures may be needed.

F Spinal cord stimulation (SCS) and intrathecal drug delivery systems (IDDS) are well-established techniques that have been utilized for over 25 years. IDDS have proven efficacy for a wide variety of intractable pain conditions and fewer adverse effects than systemic medical therapy in patients with refractory cancer-related pain. SCS is cost-effective and provides improved pain control compared with medical therapy in patients with a variety of refractory pain conditions including complex regional pain syndrome, painful diabetic neuropathy, and chronic radiculopathy. Patients who have intractable pain that has not responded to reasonable attempts at conservative pain care measures should be referred to a qualified interventional pain specialist to determine candidacy for these procedures.

SUGGESTED READING

He QH, Liu QL, Li Z, et al. Impact of epidural analgesia on quality of life and pain in advanced cancer patients. Pain Manag Nurs. 2015;16(3):307-13.

Mercadante S, Klepstad P, Kurita G, et al. Sympathetic blocks for visceral cancer pain management: A systematic review and EAPC recommendations. Crit Rev Oncol/Hematol. 2015;96(3):577-83.

National Cancer Institute. (2016). PDQ® Supportive and Palliative Care Editorial Board, PDQ Cancer Center Pain. [online] NCI website. Available from http://*www.cancer.gov/about-cancer/ treatment/side-effects/pain/pain-hp-pdq.* [Accessed January, 2017].

National Comprehensive Cancer Network, Inc. (2014). NCCN Guidelines Version 1. Adult Cancer Pain. [online] NCCN website. Available from *www.nccn.org/professionals/physician_gls/f_ guidelines.asp.*

Portenoy RK. Clinical strategies for the management of cancer pain poorly responsive to systemic opioid therapy: pain 2002—an updated review. In: Giamberardino MA (Ed). IASP Scientific Program Committee. Seattle: IASP Press; 2002.

Raslan A, Burchiel K. Neurosurgical approaches to pain management. In: Benzon HT, Rathmell JP, Wu CL, Turk DC, Argoff CE, Hurley RW (Eds). Practical Management of Pain, 5th edition. Philadelphia: Mosby; 2014. pp. 328-34.

Sayed D. The interdisciplinary management of cancer pain. Tech Reg Anesth Pain Manag. 2013;17(4):163-7.

Sharma V, de Leon-Casasola O. Cancer pain. In: Benzon HT, Rathmell JP, Wu CL, Turk DC, Argoff CE, Hurley RW (Eds). Practical Management of Pain, 5th edition. Philadelphia: Mosby; 2014. pp. 335-45.

Sheinfeld GS, Krebs P, Badr, H, et al. Meta-analysis of psychosocial interventions to reduce pain in patients with cancer. J Clin Oncol. 2012;30(5):539-47.

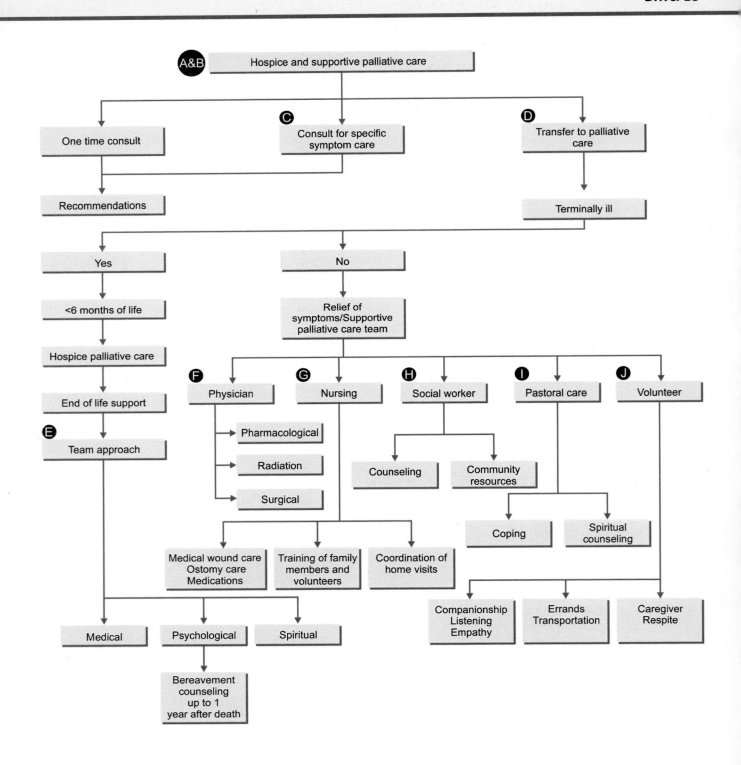

Ⓐ *Hospice Palliative Care:* In the United States, *hospice* is a care model that provides palliative care to terminally ill patients and supporting services to the patients and their families, 24 hours-a-day both at home and inpatient settings. Admission to hospice care is limited to patients who have a diagnosis that if untreated would be fatal within 6 months. Physical, emotional, spiritual, and social care are provided during the last stages of illness during the process of dying and during bereavement by a medically directed interdisciplinary team consisting of patient/family, professionals, and volunteers. Hospice care neither hastens nor delays the normal process of dying. Palliative bereavement support may be provided to the family for up to 1 year following the death of the patient.

Hospice in the United States includes a reimbursement program in which the patient must relinquish curative or life-prolonging therapy to qualify for the financial insurance benefit. The provider agrees to direct the treatment toward the relief of symptoms and forego life-prolonging and curative treatment. The patient must also agree to forego curative treatment or any other treatment in which prolongation of life is the goal rather than alleviation of symptoms. These restrictions include provision of all durable and disposable medical equipment, medications related to the terminal diagnosis, as well as visits by hospice professionals. The hospice is responsible for payment for all treatments, including invasive interventions such as radiation therapy, palliative chemotherapy, etc. The hospice is then reimbursed at a per diem compensation rate depending on the insurance carrier.

Ⓑ *Supportive Palliative Care:* Supportive palliative care emphasis is on patient-centered symptom control provided by an interdisciplinary care team, treating the patient/family as a unit of care, and may be appropriate at any stage of a serious illness in a variety of settings. Palliative care embraces the tenets of the hospice philosophy but is not confined by the regulations that define hospice programs in the United States, and is not restricted to patients who are dying or those enrolled in hospice programs. The goals of supportive palliative care are to relieve suffering and improve the quality of life by preventing, reducing, and relieving the symptoms of disease or a disorder without effecting a cure, even while running parallel to curative efforts. It provides an extra layer of support by addressing the physical, emotional, spiritual, and practical needs and goals of patients and those close to them, affirming life and providing support during recovery from a serious health crisis. It provides relief from pain and collateral symptoms that cause undue suffering in the patient and caregiving family. There is mounting evidence that palliative care can reduce medical costs in addition to helping a patient recover from a serious illness more quickly and easily, thus adding distinct value to the processes of providing care.

Ⓒ Consultation and referral to palliative care service is initiated when help is needed with symptom control. Pain is the most frequent cause of palliative care consultation. Other symptoms may include dyspnea, fatigue, weakness, nausea and vomiting, abdominal distension, ascites, constipation, bowel obstruction, diarrhea, anorexia, cachexia, urinary retention, incontinence of the bowel and bladder, skin breakdown, edema, anasarca, hiccups, depression, anxiety, delirium, and insomnia.

Ⓓ Co-management with or full transfer to the palliative care team may be a patient's best option, depending upon the diagnosis, prognosis, available resources, and other factors.

Ⓔ The team approach is integral to palliative care and treats all aspects of pain: physical, mental, or psychological, especially depression; social pain, especially communication with loved ones and attention to grief and bereavement; and spiritual pain, involving patients' and families' awareness of death, making peace, opportunity for growth, and finding life's deepest meaning. Since no one person has expertise in all areas, the palliative care team treats patients using an interdisciplinary approach that includes a physician, nurse, social worker, spiritual counselor or chaplain, other healthcare professionals, and volunteers. Success is measured by relief of suffering, not by termination of the disease or even prolongation of life.

Ⓕ The physician attends to physical symptoms using both pharmacological and nonpharmacological modalities.

Ⓖ The nurse acts as the case manager and coordinates all the services, including the ongoing assessments, and acts as triage for patients' needs. The nursing team does most of the hands-on care and has the most intimate relationship with the patient and the family, training the family members to take care of the patient with regard to medication management, feeding, ostomy care, catheter care, wound care, and even management of parenteral medications.

Ⓗ The social worker assesses social environment and other aspects of the patient, addressing problems such as loss of the patient's role in the family and in the community. In addition to connecting patients and their families to community resources, social workers also provide counseling. They teach patients how to link to life, work, and provide information about advance directives and medical durable power of attorney.

Ⓘ The pastoral care given by the spiritual counselor or chaplain assists in the relief of existential suffering and coordinates the bereavement support to the patient and the family while teaching them to cope.

Ⓙ Volunteers assist the patient and family by providing companionship, assistance with errands and transportation, occasional caregiver respite, and empathetic listening. Hospice volunteers undergo formal training before being involved with direct patient contact.

There are subtle as well as distinct differences between hospice palliative care and supportive palliative care. Many states have programs that are a blend of hospice care and palliative care that is done in the home with outpatient service support of the same professional care team. It is up to the patient and their caregiver/family to determine which program fits all of their needs while considering their goals of care, current physical and emotional status, and the requirements for their care.

SUGGESTED READING

Alexander K, Goldberg J, Korc-Grodzicki B. Palliative care and symptom management in older patients with cancer. Clin Geriatric Med. 2016;32(1):45-62.

Cagle JG, Zimmerman S, Cohen LW, et al. EMPOWER: An Intervention to Address Barriers to Pain Management in Hospice. J Pain Symptom Manage. 2015;49(1):1-12.

Coyle N, Glajchen M. Pain management in the home: using cancer patients as a model. In: Benzon HT, Rathmell JP, Wu CL, Turk DC, Argoff CE, Hurley RW. Practical Management of Pain, 5th edition. Philadelphia: Mosby; 2014. pp. 1040-8.

Kittelson SM, Elie MC, Pennypacker L. Palliative Care Symptom Management. Crit Care Nurs Clin North Am. 2015;27(3):315-39.

Lynch L, Simpson KH. Interventional techniques for pain management in palliative care. Medicine. 2015;43(12):705-8.

SECTION 5

Head and Neck Pain

Ameet Nagpal

ache Disorder; refer to this chapter for specific information. Cluster HAs are different from migraine HAs and this can often be determined with history alone. Cluster HAs are best known for the sympathetic symptoms and are usually accompanied by a feeling of restlessness or agitation. Men are affected more frequently than women. Cluster HAs attacks may occur several times daily for days to months over 2 weeks to 3 months. Fortunately, remission often lasts weeks to years. These patients may engage in headbanging or other activities as a means of distraction from the pain and symptoms.

Cluster HAs are diagnosed by at least:

- Five attacks
- Severe pain or very severe pain located in the unilateral orbital, supraorbital and/or temporal area lasting between 15 minutes and 180 minutes if untreated
- Sympathetic symptoms including:
  - Conjunctival injection and/or lacrimation
  - Ipsilateral nasal congestion and/or rhinorrhea
  - Ipsilateral eyelid edema
  - Ipsilateral abnormal forehead and facial sweating
  - Ipsilateral miosis and/or ptosis
  - A sense of restlessness or agitation.
- Attacks occur between one headache every other day to eight headaches per day.

Although rare, critical issues such as temporal arteritis, ocular trauma, and carotid cavernous fistulas should be ruled out before making a diagnosis of cluster HA.

B *Treatment and Prophylaxis:* For treatment of migraine HA, information about the number of HA, the intensity of the HA, and previous and ongoing interventions must be obtained. For more information, see Chapter 62 on Migraine Headache Disorder.

Given the abrupt onset and relatively brief duration of cluster HA (in comparison to migraine HA), nonoral routes of administration are preferred. First-line treatment of acute individual cluster HA includes 10–15 L/min of 100% oxygen, nasal or subcutaneous triptan, intramuscular or intranasal dihydroergotamine (DHE). Intranasal agents are most effective in the nostril ipsilateral to the HA.

Bridge treatments include high-dose prednisone or dexamethasone for several weeks or oral long-acting triptans, or DHE for short duration. These agents should be continued until the patient is HA-free for at least 2 weeks and then slowly tapered.

Preventive treatment may help to decrease attack duration and frequency. Useful daily agents include oral verapamil, sodium valproate, lithium, topiramate, or gabapentin. Preventive therapy should resume at the onset of the next attack.

SUGGESTED READING

Newman LC. Trigeminal Autonomic Cephalalgias. Continuum (Minneap Minn). 2015;21(4 Headache):1041-57.

Silberstein SD, Lipton RB, Goadsby PJ. Headache in Clinical Practice. Oxford: Isis Medical Media; 1998. pp. 41-90.

Swanson JW, Dodick DW, Capobianco DJ. Headache and other craniofacial pain. In: Bradley WG, Daroff RB, Fenichel GM, Marsden CD (Eds). Neurology in Clinical Practice, 3rd edition. Boston: Butterworth-Heinemann; 2000. p. 1832.

CHAPTER 59

Trigeminal Neuralgia

Boies BT, Thome CM

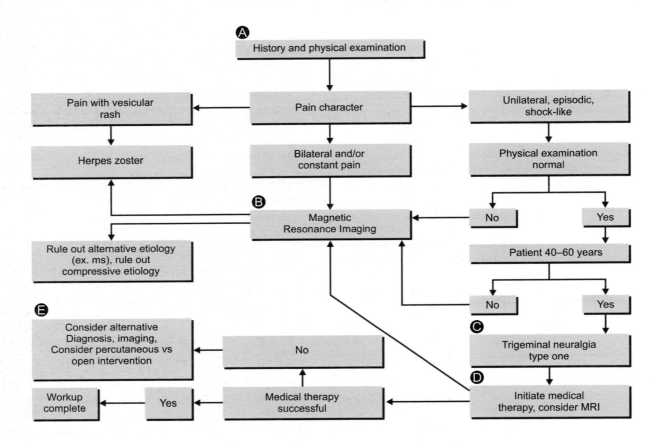

Trigeminal neuralgia (TN), also known as tic douloureux, is a facial pain syndrome characterized by brief, paroxysmal, intense, lancinating, or shock-like pain in the somatosensory distribution of the trigeminal nerve—the fifth cranial nerve (CN-V). Of the three branches of CN-V, the mandibular and maxillary divisions are affected more often than the ophthalmic.

A *History and Physical Examination:* The pain is typically exacerbated by minimal stimuli, including chewing, talking, brushing teeth, or cold wind over the face. These exacerbating factors are known as "triggering factors" and are an important component of the diagnosis of TN. The incidence of TN increases with advancing age, and it occurs most often in the sixth and seventh decades and rarely before the age of 40. TN is more common in females and more frequently involves the right side of the face. The condition is commonly unilateral, but bilateral cases have been reported. An important component

of the bilateral cases is that the pain is not synchronous between sides. The pain associated with TN is severe and among one of the most painful known conditions; cases of suicide have been reported secondary to the severity of the pain. Proper treatment needs to include psychological and social support in addition to analgesia.

The physical examination is typically normal in patients with TN. Symptomatic TN should be considered when sensory abnormalities, loss of corneal reflex, or facial muscle weakness are present. In the presence of an abnormal physical examination or presentation not consistent with classical TN, a magnetic resonance imaging (MRI) should be performed to evaluate for an alternative etiology.

B The diagnosis is primarily clinical, but an MRI of the brain without contrast with an MR angiogram of the brain can be justified in any patient with facial pain consistent with TN to confirm diagnosis and rule out alternative etiologies. If TN occurs in a patient younger than 40 years old, and/or the pain is bilateral, the possibility of multiple sclerosis should be considered. Multiple sclerosis is the most commonly associated disease.

The etiology of TN has classically been described as "unknown" or secondary to neurovascular compression in the prepontine cistern at the nerve root entry zone. The superior cerebellar and anterior inferior cerebellar arteries are commonly involved. Intracranial tumors, cysts, aneurysms, arteriovenous malformations, multiple sclerosis, and inflammatory diseases are other causes.

C *Nomenclature:* Recently the nomenclature of TN has changed, and variations of the condition have been categorized differently depending on the etiology and presentation. The International Headache Society has defined strict clinical criteria for the diagnosis of TN. To diagnose via this criteria, the pain must occur in one or more divisions of CN-V without radiation beyond the CN-V distribution, have at least three out of four of the following characteristics: (1) recurring, paroxysmal attacks lasting from a fraction of a second to 2 minutes, (2) severe intensity, (3) electric shock-like, shooting, stabbing, or sharp pain in quality, and (4) be precipitated by innocuous stimuli to the affected side of the face. In addition to these criteria, there cannot be any apparent neurologic deficit, and the pain cannot be attributed to another disorder.

Trigeminal neuralgia is now classified as type one and type two. TN type one, also known as classical or typical TN, is an idiopathic, episodic pain with the previously described clinical characteristics, lasting several seconds, with pain-free intervals between attacks. TN type two is more consistent with previously described atypical TN and is defined as idiopathic trigeminal facial pain that is aching, throbbing, or burning for more than 50% of the time and is constant in nature. TN type two typically manifests as a constant background pain with a more minor component of episodic sharp quality pain. Symptomatic TN is a term used to describe TN-like pain and presentation that is secondary to structural abnormality of the skull base, tumor compression, or multiple sclerosis. Trigeminal neuropathy simply refers to neuropathy in the distribution of the trigeminal nerve. Atypical facial pain is a diagnosis that shares many common features with TN and was used to describe facial pain with longer duration and a stabbing or aching quality. Patients with continuous, unilateral, aching pain that does not fulfill the diagnostic criteria for TN are often diagnosed with atypical facial pain or trigeminal neuropathy if neuropathic signs are present.

Occasionally, patients with connective tissue disease (Sjögren's disease, systemic lupus erythematosus, scleroderma) can present with trigeminal neuropathy. Usually, the serum antinuclear antibody (ANA) assay is positive.

D *Medical Treatment:* If all possible causes have been eliminated (including dental and temporomandibular joint disease), treatment is difficult; occasionally, tricyclic antidepressants can be useful. Herpes zoster can involve CN-V, usually in the ophthalmic division. The characteristic rash will eventually erupt. The pain is burning and constant and can persist after the rash has resolved (postherpetic neuralgia).

The initial treatment of choice of TN is medical therapy which consists of the following options: carbamazepine, oxcarbazepine, gabapentin, lamotrigine, baclofen, phenytoin, topiramate, clonazepam, pimozide, and valproic acid. Historically, carbamazepine has been known as the agent of choice. The side effects of carbamazepine are significant and include congestive heart failure, agranulocytosis, and bone marrow depression. Carbamazepine also has a Federal Drug Administration black box warning of potentially fatal dermatologic reactions. Oxcarbazepine is a popular alternative to carbamazepine as a first-line agent, but it still carries the important side effects of severe dermatologic disease and agranulocytosis. Routine monitoring of liver enzymes and blood count are important with administration of these agents.

Intravenous (IV) phenytoin can be used at the same time carbamazepine therapy is begun if the patient's pain is severe. Blood pressure and heart rate need to be closely monitored while the drug is being administered. Pain relief is often immediate and may last for several days until oral carbamazepine becomes effective.

E *Surgical Treatment*: If medical therapy fails, percutaneous or open surgical procedures should be considered. Most procedures are effective in providing short-term relief but most studies suggest that recurrence is likely within several years. The major advantages of percutaneous procedures are repeatability and the ability to perform the procedure in the outpatient setting, while the major disadvantages include associated sensory loss and recurrence of pain. Percutaneous approaches allow for chemical rhizotomy or neurectomy, balloon compression, radiofrequency ablation, and pulsed radiofrequency ablation. Approximately 8% of patients develop a dysesthetic pain syndrome (anesthesia dolorosa) following percutaneous rhizotomy. Open surgical procedures include microvascular decompression (Jannetta procedure), partial sensory rhizotomy, and neurectomy. Stereotactic radiosurgery (gamma knife, cyber knife) is a relatively new treatment for TN and has been used with success.

SUGGESTED READING

Jorns TP, Zakrzewska JM. Evidence-based approach to the medical management of trigeminal neuralgia. Br J Neurosurg. 2007; 21(3):253-61.

Montano N, Conforti G, Di Bonaventura R, et al. Advances in diagnosis and treatment of trigeminal neuralgia. Ther Clin Risk Manag. 2015;11:289-99.

Parmar M, Sharma N, Modgill V, et al. Comparative Evaluation of Surgical Procedures of Trigeminal Neuralgia. J Maxillofac Oral Surg. 2013;12(4):400-9.

CHAPTER 60

Temporomandibular Disorders

Talib HS, Phull RD

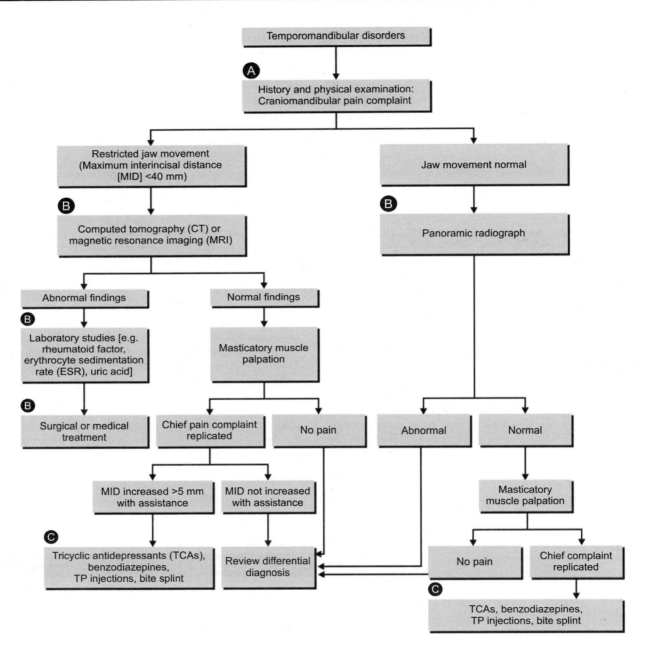

Temporomandibular disorder (TMD) is a term that refers to a variety of painful derangements of the temporomandibular joint (TMJ) and masticatory musculature. Because of the complex pain referral patterns, these disorders are commonly misdiagnosed. For example, masticatory myalgias can mimic odontalgias. In fact, many patients have undergone unnecessary endodontic therapy, or even dental extractions, as a result of misdiagnosed TMDs. Likewise, patients often seek treatment by otolaryngologists for TMDs that refer pain to the ear. Adding to the confusion, TMDs are commonly associated with subjective auditory symptoms (i.e. tinnitus, subtle hearing impairment), even though audiometric studies are typically normal.

The TMDs can be mimicked by other derangements of the head and neck. For example, patients suffering from cervical flexion-extension injuries often complain of pain in the preauricular and periorbital areas. Because common TMDs also refer pain to these areas, these patients may be misdiagnosed. For this reason, many clinicians believe that cervical flexion-extension injuries contribute to TMDs, although recent studies suggest that this is unlikely. It is interesting to note that the TMJ receives sensory innervation from the trigeminal nerve and from branches of cervical nerves (C2–5 in rodents).

Epidemiologic data indicate a female preponderance for common TMDs. In fact, some clinical reports indicate as high as a 9:1 female or male preponderance. Studies have implicated estrogens in the pathogenesis of some TMDs, although their significance has not been firmly established. For example, nerve growth factor (NGF), a neurotrophin involved in sensory and sympathetic nerve development, has been implicated in the genesis of some myalgias. The primary receptor for NGF is termed TrkA. The *TrkA* gene is positively regulated by an estrogen-response element. Clinical trials suggest that women are more susceptible to NGF-induced myalgias, presumably owing to the abundance of TrkA relative to their male counterparts.

Some TMDs are exacerbated by psychological stress. Clinical studies have provided evidence that jaw clenching increases in subjects subjected to stressful conditions. Most experts believe that this parafunctional behavior contributes to some TMDs by overuse of some masticatory muscles and by increasing or sustaining mechanical loads to the TMJs. However, another mechanism is suggested from studies that have confirmed that NGF is released from cellular stores, predominantly mast cells, in response to psychological stress.

Ⓐ *History and Physical Examination*: The patient typically presents with pain felt in the preauricular, temporal, periorbital, masseteric, or posterior cervical regions and the ear. The pain may vary in quality from a protracted aching sensation to an intermittent sharp, stabbing sensation. Patients may also complain of tinnitus, vertigo, or subtle hearing impairments that are not typically detected by audiometric studies. Pain from TMDs is commonly intermittent, with the intensity varying from day to day. Often patients experience periods of remission that can last days to weeks before recurrence. Patients suffering from TMDs may rarely report nausea with severe episodes of pain. Vomiting is extremely unusual. Scotomas and photophobia are not typically associated with TMDs.

Patients suffering from TMD or severe masticatory myalgias exhibit a reduction in the range of jaw movement. The maximum interincisal distance (MID), measured in millimeters from the incisal edges of the maxillary and mandibular central incisors at maximum opening, is commonly used to assess jaw movement. A normal MID for adults ranges from 45 mm to 60 mm. Recordings of 40 mm or less are viewed as abnormal in most cases. In addition,

some derangements of the TMJ (e.g. articular disc displacement, mass lesions) can interfere with the normal translational (i.e. forward) movements of the joint, resulting in jaw deviations that are clinically evident. Under normal conditions, the jaw opens and closes in a straight vertical movement observed in the frontal plane. However, TMJ derangements that restrict joint movement result in deviation of the jaw toward the affected side. Manual palpation of involved masticatory muscles (i.e. masseter, temporalis, medial pterygoid, and lateral pterygoid muscles) produces pain similar in quality and distribution to that described by the patient as the chief complaint.

Some TMJ disorders (e.g. osteoarthritis, rheumatoid arthritis, synovial chondromatosis) can result in irregular articular surfaces that may produce pops or clicks with jaw movements. These are easily detected with auscultation of the affected joint. In addition, articular disc interference can produce pops or clicks with jaw movements.

Ⓑ *Diagnostics*: Laboratory tests, including creatinine kinase assay, erythrocyte sedimentation rate, and C-reactive protein assay, are typically normal for usual TMDs. Magnetic resonance imaging, computed tomography, and panoramic radiographs of the TMJ can delineate a variety of joint diseases. Imaging should be normal in routine TMD aside from "wear and tear" age-related changes.

Ⓒ *Treatment*: Injection of a small volume (<0.25 mL) of a dilute solution of local anesthetic into the affected muscle sites provides temporary pain relief. Patients with TMDs who have undergone previous TMJ surgery may experience secondary pain, including sympathetically-mediated pain (i.e. complex regional syndrome). These patients typically complain of burning pain in the preauricular region of the operated joint and exhibit marked mechanical allodynia to light touch of this region.

Treatment protocols for common TMDs include tricyclic antidepressants (i.e. mixed serotonin-norepinephrine reuptake inhibitors, e.g. amitriptyline). Ironically, selective serotonin reuptake inhibitors (SSRIs), commonly administered to manage depression, can exacerbate some TMDs by inducing nocturnal bruxism. Drug-induced bruxism is observed in approximately 1–5% of patients taking SSRIs. Other treatments, including nonsteroidal anti-inflammatory drugs (for inflammatory joint derangements only), benzodiazepines (e.g. clonazepam, diazepam), muscle relaxants (e.g. cyclobenzaprine), opiates, trigger-point injections with local anesthetics or botulinum toxin, bite splints, or TMJ surgery may be indicated. Appropriate treatment protocols for managing sympathetically maintained pain is indicated in some patients.

SUGGESTED READING

Bays RA, Quinn PD. Temporomandibular disorders. In: Fonseca RJ, Bays RA, Quinn PD (Eds). Oral and Maxillofacial Surgery. Philadelphia: Saunders; 2000.

Kaplan AS, Assael LA. Temporomandibular Disorders: Diagnosis and Treatment. Philadelphia: Saunders; 1991. pp. 522-5.

Okeson JP. Management of Temporomandibular Disorders and Occlusion, 6th edition. UK: Mosby; 2008.

CHAPTER

61

Orofacial Pain

Talib HS, Phull RD

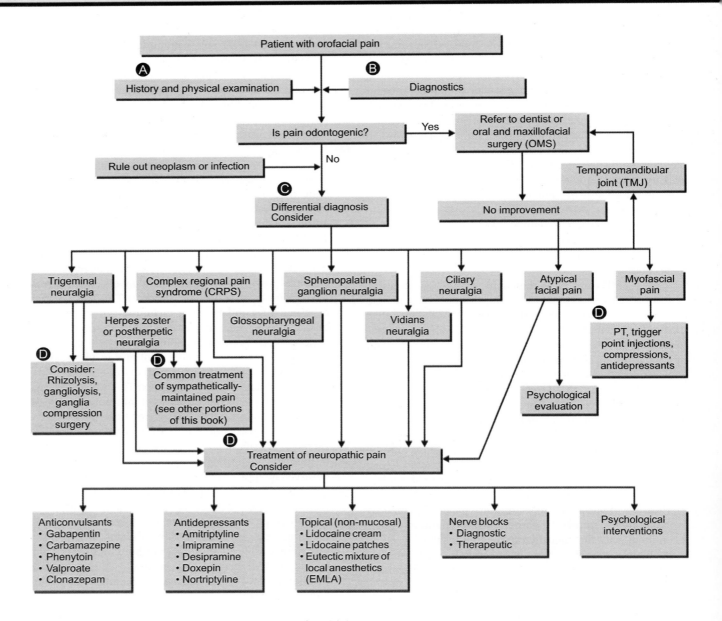

A Generally, the diagnosis of orofacial pain conditions can be readily determined with an appropriate history and physical examination. However, the presentations of many pain syndromes overlap and can also be mimicked by pathologic processes involving the primary pain generator, such as when tumor or infection invades nerve tissue and presents as a neuralgia.

B Testing may include radiography and, where indicated, computed tomography, magnetic resonance imaging, magnetic resonance angiography, or brain scans. An infectious etiology workup may include a complete blood count, erythrocyte sedimentation rate, and C-reactive protein studies. Psychological testing is recommended for individuals with chronic or recalcitrant pain.

C *Differential Diagnosis*: Dental or odontogenic pain is the most common form of orofacial pain. Tooth-related pain is the most common form, but others include pain arising from the pulp or periodontal structures. In such cases, the patient is referred to a dentist.

Orofacial cancer does not typically present as pain at its onset or during the early phases of the disease. If neurologic changes such as sensory loss are present in addition to the pain, there is increased likelihood of a destructive process such as malignancy or infection.

Temporomandibular joint (TMJ) disorders may have intra-articular or extra-articular origins. Pain is often a deep, aching pain involving the frontal or temporal head, preauricular region, or mandible.

Trigeminal neuralgia typically presents as a lancinating pain in the distribution of one or more branches of the trigeminal (V) nerve. The pain lasts seconds to minutes and is frequently unilateral. The pain usually involves a trigger stimulus such as talking, eating, chewing, or oral hygiene. It more commonly affects women and typically occurs after age 40. Earlier onset could be suggestive of possible multiple sclerosis.

Trigeminal neuropathic pain may result from acute herpes zoster (HZ). The pain is usually of a burning, tingling, or lancinating nature and may precede skin lesions by 2–3 days. If the pain persists for 1 month after the onset of skin lesions, the diagnosis becomes postherpetic neuralgia (PHN). This pain may be perceived as burning, tearing, or itching with a superimposed lancinating component. Sympathetic blocks (stellate ganglion) may alleviate the pain and, if employed early, may prevent or attenuate the PHN.

The complex regional pain syndrome manifests as superficial burning or aching pain in a diffuse nondermatomal pattern. Hyperpathia and allodynia are usually present along with possible vasomotor, sudomotor, and trophic changes.

Glossopharyngeal neuralgia involves episodic bursts of pain in the posterior tongue, pharynx, or soft palate. There may be trigger zones in these areas or posterior to the mandibular ramus. It is described as a stabbing pain precipitated by tongue movement, yawning, or coughing. The pain lasts about 30 seconds followed by a burning sensation that persists 2–3 minutes. It may be associated with bradycardia, syncope, or seizures due to involvement of the vagus nerve. The neuralgia may be diagnosed and the symptoms relieved by a local injection of anesthesia into the lateral pharyngeal wall.

Sphenopalatine ganglion neuralgia presents as a unilateral, constant boring pain in the lower half of the face below the eyebrows sometimes precipitated by sneezing. It is occasionally associated with rhinorrhea, lacrimation, conjunctival injection, and salivation. It may respond to sphenopalatine ganglion blocks (injected, topical).

Vidian neuralgia is similar to sphenopalatine neuralgia except it presents as severe paroxysmal attacks of pain involving the nose, face, eye, ear, head, neck, and shoulder; it often occurs at night. If an infection of the sphenoid sinus is present, see that it is treated, with an appropriate referral.

Ciliary neuralgia is a form of migraine caused by middle meningeal artery spasm. It presents as paroxysmal pain in one eye and the ipsilateral face, with accompanying rhinorrhea, nasal congestion, iritis, and keratitis. Immediate relief of ocular pain and keratitis or iritis may be obtained with cocainization of the anterior half of the lateral wall of the affected nostril (anterior ethmoidal nerve).

Atypical facial pain is a diagnosis of exclusion and may involve significant psychological factors. Patient denial of possible psychogenic factors and excessive use of the health care system are common. The pain may be bilateral and migratory. It is often perceived as a sensory loss but nondermatomal. Invasive treatments are usually avoided because of their poor success rates and the possibility of increasing the pain. Treatment should include psychological testing and intervention.

Orofacial pain of myofascial origin presents as persistent, deep, aching, poorly localized pain that involves facial muscles, often the muscles of mastication. The diagnosis is based on the presence of trigger points that reproduce the pain.

D Pharmacologic treatment of orofacial pain of neurogenic origin is similar to that for other neuropathic pain states. Anticonvulsants, antidepressants, opioids, and in some cases muscle relaxants (baclofen) are the most common medications used. Diagnostic and therapeutic nerve blocks are of limited utility.

SUGGESTED READING

Haasis JC. Alternative therapies. In: Tollison CD, Satterthwaite JR, Tollison JW (Eds). Practical Pain Management, 3rd edition. Philadelphia: Lippincott Williams & Wilkins; 2001. pp. 209-15.

Hsu FP, Israel ZH, Burgess JA, et al. Orofacial pain: differential diagnosis and treatment. In: Tollison CD, Satterthwaite JR, Tollison JW (Eds). Practical Pain Management, 3rd edition. Philadelphia: Lippincott Williams & Wilkins; 2001. pp. 359-73.

Loeser JD. Cranial neuralgias. In: Bonica JJ (Ed). The Management of Pain, 2nd edition. Philadelphia: Lea & Febiger; 1990. pp. 676-86.

CHAPTER 62

Migraine Headache Disorder

Das R, DiTommaso C

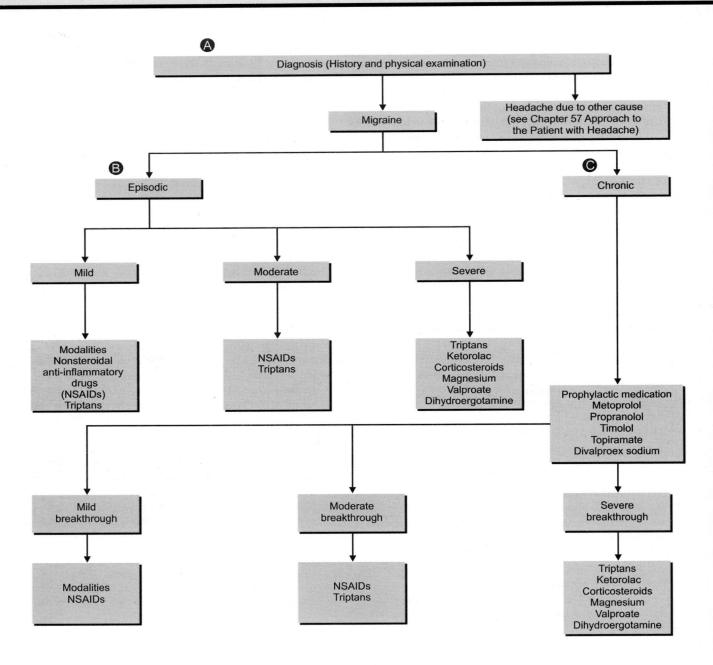

Migraine headaches (HA) are a painful HA disorder and some estimates report that migraine HA affect 14% of the population. Migraine HA affect the sexes differently, occurring in about 20% of women and 6% of men. The diagnosis of migraine depends on clinical history as there are no imaging studies or

biological markers with good specificity or sensitivity. Accurate diagnosis and treatment is essential for improving pain management, decreasing suffering, and lessening disability.

Ⓐ *Diagnosis (History and Physical Examination):* The International Classification of Headache Disorders (ICHD-2) requires specific criteria for diagnosis of migraine HA disorder. Per the criteria, migraine HA are diagnosed by a history of:

- At least five HA
- Duration of 4–72 hours (untreated)
- At least two of the following characteristics:
  - Unilateral location
  - Pulsating quality
  - Moderate to severe intense pain
  - Aggravated by routine physical activity
- At least one of the following characteristics:
  - Nausea and/or vomiting
  - Photophobia and phonophobia

The onset of migraine HA is typically between the first decades and third decades of life. For this reason, other secondary diagnoses should be pursued in patients over the age of 40 presenting with new onset of a severe HA.

Migraine HA may be subclassified by the presence or absence of an aura. Auras are a neurological disturbance that typically present as unilateral, fully reversible, and lasting anywhere from 5 minutes to 60 minutes. The most common aura is a visual phenomenon preceding or accompanying the HA but auras may also include any transient neurologic symptoms. During a visual aura, the symptoms are often described as an area of sparkling or flashing lights (scintillating) with an associated region of visual loss (constricting scotoma). Other auras include somatic sensory changes, motor weakness in hemiplegic migraine, or brainstem symptoms (vertigo, double vision, ataxia). Because of these neurological changes, initial evaluation should rule out more critical central nervous system pathology. For more information, see Chapter 57 on Approach to the Patient with Headache.

Ⓑ *Acute Episodic Treatment:* Nonpharmacologic treatments are attractive interventions in migraine HA due to the relatively safe profile and lack of interaction with other treatments. Nonpharmacologic treatments are too numerous to mention individually but some common interventions include hot and cold modalities, biofeedback, and/or sleep or resting in a dark, quiet area. Of note, cool compress modality has been especially helpful in several research studies. For more information regarding modalities, see Chapter 114 Physical Therapy and Chapter 115 Occupational Therapy.

For mild to moderate HAs, abortive agents, including nonsteroidal anti-inflammatory drugs (NSAIDs) may be effective. Aspirin, ibuprofen, naproxen, and diclofenac have supporting evidence for use in migraine; acetaminophen appears less effective. Oral antiemetics can be used for nausea. For more moderate HA, triptans are especially helpful. Of note, earlier treatment in the migraine attack tends to be more successful as opposed to use of abortive medications in later stage or when maximally severe.

Opiates and opiate-containing medications should be avoided for the habitual treatment of HA, given long-term dependency and risk of analgesic overuse. Butalbital combination analgesics use should be discouraged as well if possible.

For moderate to severe migraine or for milder HAs that have not responded to more conservative measures, acute first-line treatment includes HA-specific medication. First-line treatment is the triptan medications (e.g. sumatriptan, rizatriptan, zolmitriptan, almotriptan, frovatriptan, and naratriptan) and these medications are available in tablets, oral dissolving wafers, intranasal, subcutaneous or intramuscular forms. Intravenous, intramuscular, and per rectum antiemetics (such as metoclopramide or prochlorperazine) are useful in patients with severe migraine to control nausea and pain. Intravenous fluid hydration, ketorolac, corticosteroids, magnesium, valproate or dihydroergotamine (DHE) may also be considered for rescue therapy in patients with status migrainosus. Intranasal, intramuscular, or subcutaneous DHE can be utilized when the earlier measures have failed but monitor for paradoxical nausea. DHE is contraindicated is individuals with prior vascular disease.

Migraine HA may be worsened by medication overuse or "rebound" HA. Analgesics, prescribed triptans, or any medication taken more than 15 days per month, or combination medications taken more than 10 days per month can lead to medication overuse HA. Elimination of these medications may help to control or eliminate migraine or migraine-like HA.

Ⓒ *Chronic Migraine Treatment:* Current guidelines recommend prophylactic daily medication if HA occurs more than 15 times per month to decrease HA frequency and severity. There is level A evidence supporting the use of metoprolol, propranolol, timolol, topiramate, and divalproex sodium. These medications should be titrated to the highest tolerated dose for at least 6–8 weeks before the agent is deemed ineffective. Other consideration can be given to amitriptyline which has level B evidence and can be titrated up as tolerated to a dose of 100–150 mg/day.

Again, elimination of analgesics, prescribed triptans, or any medication known to precipitate rebound HA may help to control or eliminate migraine-like HA.

SUGGESTED READING

Becker WJ. Acute Migraine Treatment. Continuum (Minneap Minn). 2015;21(4 Headache):953-72.

Headache Classification Subcommittee of the International Headache Society. The International Classification of Headache Disorders, 2nd edition. Cephalalgia. 2004;24(Suppl 1):9-160.

Katsarava Z, Buse DC, Manack AN, et al. Defining the differences between episodic migraine and chronic migraine. Curr Pain Headache Rep. 2012;16(1):86-92.

Silberstein SD. Practice parameter: evidence-based guidelines for migraine headache (an evidence-based review): report of the Quality Standards Subcommittee of the American Academy of Neurology. Neurology. 2000;55(6):754-62.

Silberstein SD. Preventive Migraine Treatment. Continuum (Minneap Minn). 2015;21(4 Headache):973-89.

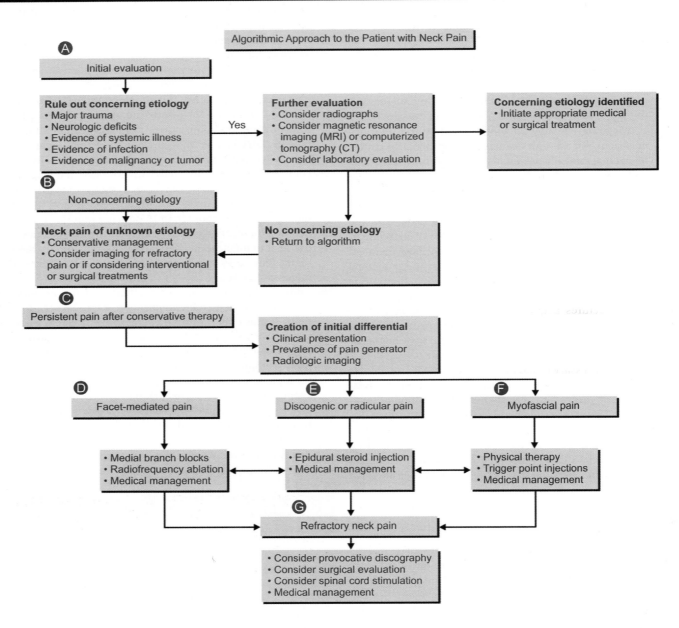

Neck pain is common in the adult population with a reported prevalence of 26–71% resulting in significant disability and economic costs. Neck pain may be reported as being axial in nature, or may occur with associated head or upper extremity pain see Chapter 57 Approach to the Patient with Headache and Chapter 65 Cervical Radiculopathy. Pain referred from the cervical spine may include intervertebral discs, facet

joints, atlanto-axial or atlanto-occipital joints, ligaments, fascia, muscles, or nerve roots. Given the complexity of the cervical anatomy and referral patterns, pain generator identification for persistent symptoms proves difficult.

Ⓐ Initial evaluation of the patient with neck pain is focused upon identifying acute or concerning pathology that include fracture or instability due to trauma, neurologic deficits from nerve injury or compression, oncologic etiologies, systemic illness, and infection. Evidence of such processes may necessitate neck imaging with a possible laboratory workup to guide further surgical and medical treatments. Imaging should begin with plain radiographs with escalation to magnetic resonance imaging (MRI) evaluation if there is evidence of systemic symptoms, neurologic changes, or myelopathic signs. Computerized tomography (CT) may also be use to better visualize osseous structures or in those for which MRI is contraindicated. Surgical management is considered necessary in patients with a surgical lesion who exhibit progressive motor abnormalities, sensory loss, or bladder/bowel dysfunction. Similarly, treatment of either neoplasm or infection may involve surgical intervention.

B Neck pain without concerning presentation should initially be treated with conservative measures such as anti-inflammatory medications, over-the-counter analgesic medications, activity modification, and physical therapy as the majority of episodes will improve with these modalities without the increased risk associated with procedural interventions or more potent prescription medications. Imaging of the neck and spine in patients without concerning presentation is not indicated unless pain remains refractory to conservative measures (3 months for plain radiographs or 6 months for MRI) or during consideration of interventional or surgical treatments.

C Persistent neck pain of unknown etiology should continue to be evaluated based upon clinical findings in conjunction with radiologic imaging. Prevalence of facet-mediated pain has been estimated at 45–55% and discogenic pain at 10–20%. This makes these two pain generators attractive initial targets for evaluation. Other targets may include bone pain (tumor or fracture), myofascial pain, lateral atlanto-axial joint pain, and neuritis of the upper cervical nerve roots. Less common neck pain generators may include mass effect due to tumors, syrinx, or spinal stenosis, but are typically accompanied by radicular symptoms.

D Given its prevalence, facet (zygapophyseal joint) arthropathy should be considered prior to a less common diagnosis. Depending upon the level of involvement, the symptoms may be referred into the head, shoulders, or upper extremities. Physical examination may be revealing for tenderness over the joints and pain may be exacerbated with loading. Arthritic changes or hypertrophy of the zygapophyseal joint on radiologic imaging is supportive. If this diagnosis is suspected, evaluation should continue with controlled medial branch blocks. Given the high rate of false positive testing, multiple blocks are recommended. Steroid may be added to nerve blocks for therapeutic purposes, although this is not substantiated

by literature. Additionally, limited evidence exists for efficacy with intra-articular injections. Definitive treatment following confirmatory blocks includes radiofrequency neurotomy.

E Degenerative changes in the cervical spine may include changes in the intervertebral discs to include desiccation or herniation. Herniation of the discs may result in nerve root compression and radicular symptoms in their respective dermatomes. Specifically, upper level cervical radicular complaints (C4 and above) may include pain in the neck and shoulders rather than in the upper extremities. Discogenic pain will often present as axial neck pain but may also refer to the shoulders or proximal upper extremities. Degeneration of the cervical intervertebral discs is often apparent on radiologic imaging but may also be typical of age-related changes. Initial interventional treatment for both radicular symptoms and discogenic pain include interlaminar epidural steroid injections. The efficacy and safety of transforaminal epidural steroid injections in the cervical spine have been questioned and are controversial. Epidural steroid injections should be completed when discogenic pain is more likely than facet-mediated pain by evaluation or upon failure of facet evaluation in identifying the pain generator.

F Myofascial neck pain presents as a deep aching sensation that is poorly localized and may be referred to adjacent structures. It is diagnosed by the presence of trigger points that reproduce pain.

G Upon failure of facet joint evaluation, epidural injections for discogenic or radicular pain, and myofascial treatments, more invasive evaluations may be considered. Provocative discography may allow for identification of the painful disc for surgical purposes, but criteria for testing is less described than that for the lumbar spine. Similarly, invasive percutaneous procedures to target the degenerative discs in the cervical spine such as intradiscal radiofrequency treatments or percutaneous decompression have limited evidence of efficacy. In chronic, nonresponsive pain, spinal cord stimulation may also be considered.

SUGGESTED READING

Falco FJ, Erhart S, Wargo BW, et al. Systematic review of diagnostic utility and therapeutic effectiveness of cervical facet joint interventions. Pain Physician. 2009;12(2):323-44.

Manchikanti L, Helm S, Singh V, et al. An algorithmic approach for clinical management of chronic spinal pain. Pain Physician. 2009;12:E225-64.

Manchikanti L, Singh V, Falco FJ, et al. Cervical medial branch blocks for chronic cervical facet joint pain: A randomized, double-blind, controlled trial with one-year follow-up. Spine. 2008;33(17):1813-20.

CHAPTER 64

Cervical Facet Joint Pain

Kroski WJ, Lautenschlager K

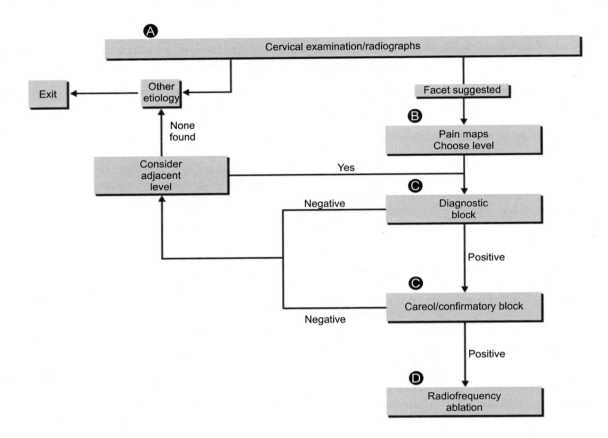

Cervical facet joints are paired synovial joints located along the posterior cervical spine between consecutive vertebrae from the C2 level to C7 level. From C3-4 to C6-7, each joint is innervated from above and below by medial branches of the dorsal rami that bear the same segmental number as the joint. Axial pain from facet joint degeneration accounts for 55–60% of the overall pain in the cervical spine. Severe facet arthrosis may cause myelopathy, and degenerative spondylolisthesis of the cervical spine.

Ⓐ The most common symptom associated with the cervical facet joint is unilateral neck pain not radiating past the shoulder. Pain in the cervical facet joint can have a specific radiation pattern. Rotation and extension may be limited or even painful. Stand-alone clinical examinations are neither diagnostic nor do they show good specificity for diagnosing cervical facet joint disease. Local pressure pain over the facet joints may indicate facet joint involvement, but this is not reliable for diag-

nosis. With the presence of degenerative changes in the cervical spine in asymptomatic patients, there is no relation between radiographic evidence of degeneration and pain. A thorough history and physical examination is necessary to exclude neurologic, infectious, or systemic etiologies of neck pain.

Ⓑ Pain maps may be used to deduce the likely segmental location of a painful facet joint, but these maps are not diagnostic of facet joint pain; the same pattern of referred pain can be caused by discogenic pain at the same segment. The C2-3 facet joint is uniquely innervated by the C2 and C3 medial branches as well as the third occipital nerve (TON). Typically, pain emanating from the C2-3 joint is experienced over the upper cervical region and occiput, and it may radiate into the forehead or orbit. Pain from C3-4 typically starts high in the neck but embraces the entire length of the posterolateral aspect of the neck. C4-5 pain is focused over the angle between the neck and the top of the shoulder girdle. Pain from C5-6 spreads to cover the scapular supraspinous and deltoid regions of the shoulder. C6-7 pain radiates over the blade of the scapula. Because cervical facet joint pain is common, it should be suspected in any patient with such distribution of pain, and a provisional diagnosis of facet joint pain can be entertained on epidemiologic grounds alone. Pain maps serve only to direct where definitive investigations should commence.

C Controlled diagnostic blocks under fluoroscopic guidance are the only means of confirming a diagnosis of cervical facet joint pain. The medial branches of the dorsal rami cross the middle of the ipsisegmental articular pillars, providing radiographically recognizable landmarks for diagnostic blocks. Each nerve can be anesthetized with as little as 0.3 mL of local anesthetic. Larger volumes risk compromising the target specificity of the block. The Spine Intervention Society (SIS) guidelines recommend a multilevel methodology with a screening test and multiple confirmatory blocks. In the current algorithm, only two blocks are performed provided the first block was positive, thus avoiding a screening block and repeat blocks for separate joints. Diagnostic blocks must be controlled in order to prevent a false diagnosis. The false-positive rate of single diagnostic blocks is anywhere from 27% to 63%. Placebo controls pose ethical and logistic problems and require a series of three injections to be valid. A practical, valid alternative is to use comparative local anesthetic blocks. On each of two occasions the patient undergoes a diagnostic block using different local anesthetic agents with different durations of action (i.e. lidocaine and bupivacaine). A positive response is one in which the patient obtains significant ($\geq$80%) relief of pain on each occasion with the duration of pain relief matching the expected duration of local anesthetic action. Such blocks can be performed on a double-blind basis to optimize validity.

D There is no evidence that intra-articular steroids are effective in treating facet-mediated pain in the cervical spine. One definitive, proven therapy for cervical facet joint pain is percutaneous radiofrequency medial branch neurotomy. A thermal radiofrequency lesion for medial branch denervation is performed at 80–85°C. Due to the mechanism of radiofrequency neurotomy, which is described as denaturing of the nerves, the pain returns when axons regenerate and repetition of the radiofrequency lesioning

may be required. The power of this therapy has been demonstrated in open trials and its validity has been supported in randomized, placebo-controlled, double-blind trials. The neurotomy involves coagulating the medial branches of the dorsal rami that innervate the painful joint. For this reason, the diagnostic protocol to locate a painful joint must involve medial branch blocks instead of intra-articular blocks. Medial branch blocks are thereby not only diagnostic but prognostic of a response to radiofrequency neurotomy. Recent systematic reviews for radiofrequency neurotomy show results were positive for short- and long-term pain relief for chronic cervical facet joint pain.

SUGGESTED READING

Aizawa T, Ozawa H, Hoshikawa T, et al. Severe facet joint arthrosis caused C7/T1 myelopathy: a case report. Case Rep Med. 2009;2009:481459.

Barnsley L, Lord S, Wallis B, et al. False-positive rates of cervical zygapophyseal joint blocks. Clin J Pain. 1993;9(2):124-30.

Bogduk N. International Spinal Injection Society guidelines for the performance of spinal injection procedures. Part 1: Zygapophysial joint blocks. Clin J Pain. 1997;13(4):285-302.

Coste J, Judet O, Barre O, et al. Inter- and intraobserver variability in the interpretation of computed tomography of the lumbar spine. J Clin Epidemiol. 1994;47(4):375-81.

Dwyer A, Aprill C, Bogduk N. Cervical zygapophyseal joint pain patterns. I: A study in normal volunteers. Spine (Phila Pa 1976). 1990;15(6):453-7.

Falco FJ, Erhart S, Wargo BW, et al. Systematic review of diagnostic utility and therapeutic effectiveness of cervical facet joint interventions. Pain Physician. 2009;12(2):323-44.

King, W, Lau P, Lees R, et al. The validity of manual examination in assessing patients with neck pain. Spine J. 2007;7(1):22-6.

Lord SM, Barnsley L, Wallis BJ, et al. Percutaneous radio-frequency neurotomy for chronic cervical zygapophyseal-joint pain. N Engl J Med. 1996;335(23):1721-6.

Manchikanti L, Abdi S, Atluri S, et al. An update of comprehensive evidence-based guidelines for interventional techniques in chronic spinal pain. Part II: guidance and recommendations. Pain Physician. 2013;16(2 Suppl):S49-283.

Manchikanti L, Boswell MV, Singh V, et al. Prevalence of facet joint pain in chronic spinal pain of cervical, thoracic, and lumbar regions. BMC Musculoskelet Disord. 2004;5:15.

Manchikanti L, Singh V, Rivera J, et al. Prevalence of cervical facet joint pain in chronic neck pain. Pain Physician. 2002;5(3):243-9.

Pellengahr C, Pfahler M, Kuhr M, et al. Influence of facet joint angles and asymmetric disk collapse on degenerative olisthesis of the cervical spine. Orthopedics. 2000;23(7):697-701.

CHAPTER 65

Cervical Radiculopathies

Hommer DH, Goff BJ

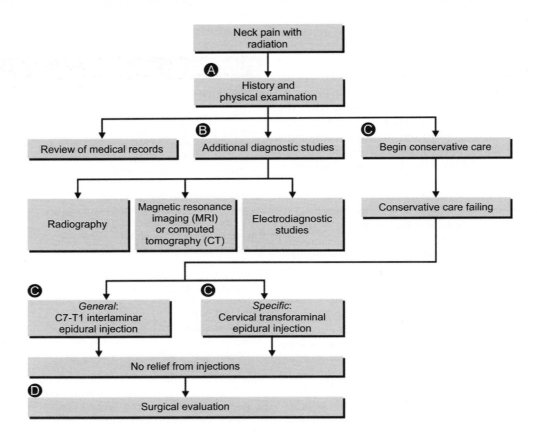

Cervical radiculopathy is typically associated with cervical spondylosis and/or intervertebral disc protrusion or, less commonly, disc herniation. Disc herniation can be chronic or acute due to trauma. Pain is caused by the irritation and compression of the cervical nerve root, producing radicular symptoms and signs in the upper extremity; most commonly in C6 and/or C7. Pain due to cervical radiculopathy usually begins in the middle of the neck and radiates to the shoulder and into the upper extremity in the distribution of the involved nerve root(s). Pain with active extension and rotation toward the affected side or passively with compression (Spurling sign) is consistent with radicular involvement. In-line traction to decrease the pain and compression of the head to reproduce the patient's pain may aid in diagnosis. The radicular pain may be associated with sensory, motor, and reflex changes in the upper extremity corresponding to the involved nerve root as shown in **Table 1**.

A *History and Physical Examination:* Pathology of other structures can simulate radicular pain. These include neck muscles, facet joints, cervical discs and/or the brachial plexus (due to inflammation or malignancy of the lung), as well as referred visceral pain. It is essential, therefore, to obtain a thorough history and perform a thorough neurologic examination, not only of the upper extremity, but also the lower extremity, because cervical spondylosis and disc herniation may be associated with compression of the spinal cord. Myelopathic symptoms (hyperreflexia, lower extremity weakness and/or spasticity, bowel or bladder changes) or progressive neurologic deficits should prompt immediate magnetic resonance imaging (MRI) of the cervical spine and prompt surgical referral.

B *Diagnostic Studies:* History and physical examination often suffice to diagnose cervical radiculopathy. Plain x-ray can be helpful to evaluate for zygapophyseal

Table 1: Manifestations of cervical root lesions

Nerve root	Pain radiation and sensory changes	Muscle weakness	Affected reflex
C4	Lower neck and trapezius	None	None
C5	Over the deltoid muscle	Deltoid, biceps, supraspinatus, infraspinatus	Biceps
C6	Upper lateral arm, lateral forearm, thumb, and index finger	Biceps, brachioradialis, wrist extensors	Brachioradialis
C7	Posterolateral arm and forearm, index and middle fingers	Triceps, wrist flexion	Triceps
C8	Medial arm and forearm, ring and small fingers	Finger flexors	None

arthritis, uncovertebral hypertrophy, and neuroforaminal narrowing; all of which can be associated with cervical radiculopathy. If conservative therapy does not result in relief and surgical or interventional procedures are being considered, MRI can be indispensable in correlating symptoms with imaging findings and providing a target for intervention. MRI findings must be interpreted with caution as false positive results are common. The MRI findings should correlate with the patient's signs and symptoms before engaging in surgical or interventional procedures. In patients with contraindication to MRI use, computed tomography (CT) scan can provide a sufficient but less sensitive evaluation of the cervical spine. Cervical myelography may be required to evaluate for cord compression in patients unable to have an MRI.

Electrodiagnostic studies such as electromyography (EMG) and nerve conduction velocity studies may be helpful in evaluating unclear cases of cervical radiculopathy; due to the discomfort of the studies, they should not be used in the early evaluation of clear cases of radiculopathy in which neurologic symptoms correlate with imaging findings. They are particularly helpful in evaluating for brachial plexopathy, median neuropathy, or ulnar neuropathy in combination with (double crush syndrome) or without associated cervical radiculopathy. In addition, they can be helpful in defining the level(s) of cervical radiculopathy to guide surgical intervention.

C *Treatment:* 95% of acute radicular pain usually resolves in 6–8 weeks. Use of oral steroids, nonsteroidal anti-inflammatory drugs (NSAIDs), transcutaneous electrical nerve stimulation (TENS) and other conservative measures can be beneficial. If the radicular pain continues and if there is no involvement of the spinal cord, epidural steroid injections can be very effective in relieving the symptoms in up to 60% of patients. The epidural steroids can be administered either through the interlaminar foramen or, much less frequently due to the additional risk, through the intervertebral foramen (transforaminal). This procedure should be performed by experienced physicians only because of the potential for serious complications such as spinal cord injury caused by needle trauma or injection of particulate matter into the radicular artery during a transforaminal epidural injection. Due to the embolic risk of particulate steroids, many interventional pain physicians use only non-particulate steroid for any transforaminal injection and for all injections into the cervical epidural space. As an alternative to the transforaminal approach, an epidural catheter advanced from a lower cervical or upper thoracic level can be selectively placed at the involved root level under fluoroscopy and may be a very safe and effective technique. If the patient obtains only temporary benefit from epidural steroid injections and if he or she is not a candidate for surgery, pulsed radiofrequency lesion of the cervical dorsal root ganglion may provide long-term pain relief, though evidence for this procedure is minimal.

D *Surgical Approach:* Surgical procedures are indicated if conservative therapy is not successful and the imaging studies indicate a clear-cut etiology or if there is significant spinal cord compression or progressive neurologic deficits. Anterior cervical discectomy with fusion and posterior foraminotomy are each commonly performed without convincing evidence to favor one over the other.

SUGGESTED READING

Bono CM, Ghiselli G, Gilbert TJ, et al. An evidence-based clinical guideline for the diagnosis and treatment of cervical radiculopathy from degenerative disorders. Spine J. 2011;11(1):64-72.

Corey DL, Comeau D. Cervical radiculopathy. Med Clin North Am. 2014;98(4):791-9.

Wong JJ, Côté P, Quesnele JJ, et al. The course and prognostic factors of symptomatic cervical disc herniation with radiculopathy: a systematic review of the literature. Spine J. 2014;14(8): 1781-9.

SECTION 6

Thoracic Pain

Larry C Driver

CHAPTER
66

Chronic Chest Wall Pain

Eckmann MS

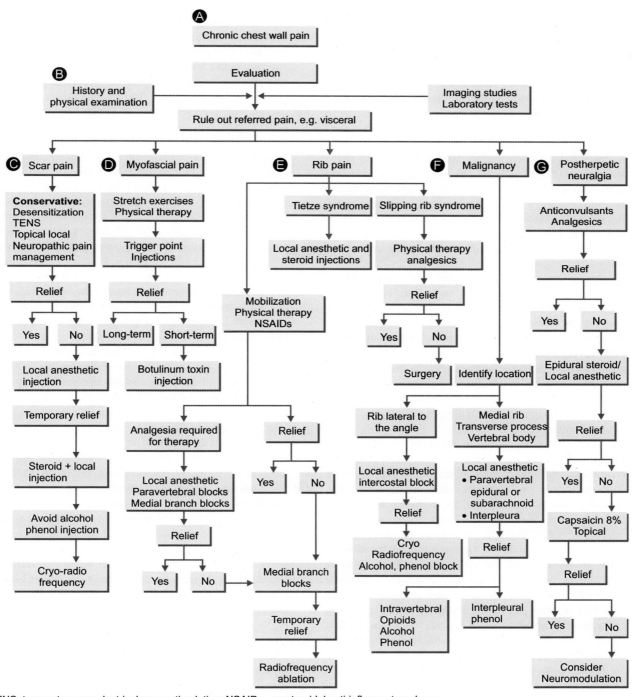

TENS, transcutaneous electrical nerve stimulation; NSAIDs, nonsteroidal anti-inflammatory drugs

A *Etiologies:* Chronic chest wall pain is a multidimensional pain syndrome. The pain can result from multiple etiologic factors including referred pain from thoracic viscera such as the heart, lungs and esophagus. The pain results most commonly from thoracotomy scar, postherpetic neuralgia, intercostal neuralgia, myofascial pain, rib, costochondral joints, and primary or secondary malignancy originating from the vertebral bodies or the ribs.

B *Evaluation:* A thorough history, physical examination, laboratory tests and imaging studies should be completed to rule out serious visceral disease or malignancy. The history and physical examination is very helpful in determining the etiologic factors responsible for pain production.

C *Scar Pain:* Palpation by picking up the scar between two fingers can localize the pain to the scar and neuromas can be found or stimulated. Usually there is decreased sensation to pinprick distal to the scar, together with allodynia and/or hyperpathia. Treatment consists of desensitization, topical local anesthetics, transcutaneous electrical nerve stimulation (TENS), antineuropathic drugs, and injection of the scar with local anesthetic and steroids. Cryoablation or radiofrequency lesion can provide long-term relief. Injection of alcohol or phenol is not recommended due to risk of skin breakdown and neuritis with increased pain. Postherpetic neuralgia is characterized by healed herpetic scars, allodynia, and hyperpathia.

D *Myofascial Pain:* Myofascial pain is characterized by the reproduction of pain on palpation of muscular trigger points, most commonly in the pectoralis major and minor, serratus anterior, trapezius, and latissimus dorsi muscles. Stretching of the muscles reproduces the patient's pain and local anesthetic injection of the trigger points relieves the pain. Although results in the literature are mixed, injection of botulinum toxin may be beneficial if physical therapy and exercises do not produce long-term pain relief, particularly if there is objective evidence of myoclonus.

E *Rib Pain:* The most common cause of rib pain is rib dysfunction with the involvement of the thoracic facet, costotransverse, and costovertebral joints. The syndrome is characterized by tenderness over the rib anteriorly, laterally, and posteriorly and over the corresponding thoracic facet joints. Pain is associated with deep breathing. The physical examination also reveals decreased motion of the rib with breathing on the affected side. Mobilization of the ribs with manual methods followed by physical therapy and exercises is likely to relieve the pain. Paravertebral local anesthetic blocks may be necessary to provide analgesia for mobilization. Occasionally thoracic medial branch blocks or ablation can provide pain relief in patients with a significant segmental spinal pain component.

Pain due to costochondritis (Tietze's syndrome) is usually felt over the anterior chest over the costochondral junction. Arthritis and swelling of the sternochondral joints can also cause chest wall pain. Palpation of the joints reproduces the patient's pain. Pain is relieved by intra-articular injection of local anesthetic and steroids; ultrasonographic or blind techniques are used. The xiphisternal joint may become painful, especially in later stages of pregnancy, and can be treated similarly.

Pain associated with slipping rib syndrome is usually seen among young people between 20 years and 40 years of age who complain of lower rib pain. The diagnosis is made by pulling up the lower edge of the rib cage and reproducing the clicking and the patient's pain (hooking maneuver). Patients usually respond to physical therapy, postural retraining and occasionally injection of local anesthetic and steroids. If the pain does not respond to conservative therapy, surgical resection of the ends of the ribs can be helpful.

F *Malignancy:* Pain secondary to malignancy is managed with opioids, adjuvants, radiation therapy, and surgical decompression as required. If the pain continues, neurolytic blocks may be beneficial. Secondary malignancy of the ribs with or without fracture can produce severe pain. Localized rib pain distal to the angle of the ribs can be relieved temporarily with local anesthetic blocks and on a long-term basis with neurolytic blocks using phenol, alcohol, or radiofrequency or cryoablation techniques. Intrathecal drug delivery systems employing spinal opioids can be effective. Primary or secondary malignancy involving the visceral structures in the thoracic cage or the vertebral canal or the vertebral bodies or the ribs medial to the angle can produce pain over the chest wall. Local anesthetic paravertebral blocks may be beneficial.

Phenol or alcohol neurolytic blocks should be avoided in the paravertebral area because of the possible spread to the epidural and subarachnoid space, resulting in serious complications including paralysis. Intrathecal phenol or alcohol is very effective in relieving pain confined to an area of fewer than three to four segments. If the pleural cavity is intact, interpleural injection of local anesthetic followed by the injection of 5–10% phenol in water or glycerin can provide significant long-term pain relief.

G *Postherpetic Neuralgia:* Advanced age and more significant segmental numbness portent worsened prognosis for the development of chronic pain from herpes zoster reactivation. Epidural steroid injections and local anesthetics in the affected dermatome may reduce nerve root inflammation and pain acutely. Intrathecal steroids have been reported to have sustained benefit but outcomes remain controversial. Capsaicin 8% topical therapy (best augmented by paravertebral or intercostal nerve block to control procedural pain) is the Food and Drug Administration (FDA)-approved treatment when pain persists despite rational multimodal systemic therapy including anticonvulsants. In extremely refractory cases, spinal cord stimulation may be considered.

SUGGESTED READING

Bonica JJ, Graney DO. General considerations of pain in the chest. In: Loeser JD (Ed). Bonica's Management of Pain, 3rd edition. Philadelphia: Lippincott Williams & Wilkins; 2001. pp. 1113-48.

Callstrom MR, Charboneau JW. Image-guided palliation of painful metastases using percutaneous ablation. Tech Vasc Interv Radiol. 2007;10(2):120-31.

Gregory PL, Biswas AC, Batt ME. Musculoskeletal problems of the chest wall in athletes. Sports Med. 2002;32(4):235-50.

Lu YF, Lin YC, Chen KH, et al. Image-guided intensity-modulated radiotherapy for refractory bilateral breast cancer in a patient with extensive cutaneous metastasis in the chest and abdominal walls. Onco Targets Ther. 2016;9:3025-30.

Mou J, Paillard F, Turnbull B, et al. Efficacy of Qutenza® (capsaicin) 8% patch for neuropathic pain: a meta-analysis of the Qutenza Clinical Trials Database. Pain. 2013;154(9):1632-9.

Soares A, Andriolo RB, Atallah AN, et al. Botulinum toxin for myofascial pain syndromes in adults. Cochrane Database Syst Rev. 2014;(7):CD007533.

Yanamoto F, Murakawa K. The effects of temporary spinal cord stimulation (or spinal nerve root stimulation) on the management of early postherpetic neuralgia from one to six months of its onset. Neuromodulation. 2012;15(2):151-4.

Postmastectomy Pain

Patel S, Soliman S

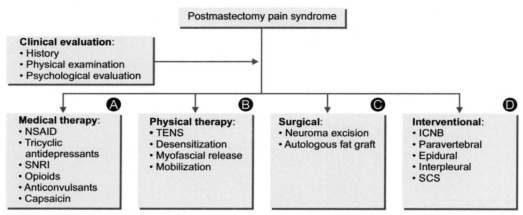

NSAID, nonsteroidal anti-inflammatory drug; TENS, transcutaneous electrical nerve stimulation; SNRI, serotonin-norepinephrine reuptake inhibitor; ICNB, intercostal nerve block; SCS, spinal cord stimulators

Postmastectomy pain syndrome (PMPS) is a known complication of the surgical treatment of breast cancer. It is a neuropathic pain condition that arises from damage to the axillary, intercostal, or intercostobrachial nerves during surgery. It is characterized as a sharp, burning, aching pain accompanied by lancinating pain in the distribution supplied by the injured nerve. It is aggravated by movement in 94% of women. The prevalence of PMPS ranges from 4% to 40%. Hyperesthesia, hyperalgesia, and hypoesthesia are present. A palpable neuroma may be present.

A Medical management includes a trial of oral analgesics, opioids, tricyclic antidepressants, and anticonvulsants used for neuropathic pain. Capsaicin cream has few side effects and may provide improvement. There are examples of medications being prior to surgery to prevent both acute and chronic pain. One example used to prevent postoperative acute pain occurs with postmastectomy pain. In a study on 150 patients comparing venlafaxine 37.5 mg/day to gabapentin 300 mg/day, it was found that both cause analgesia in days 2 through 10 postoperatively and the venlafaxine group had less pain even 6 months postoperatively. This medication was given for ten continuous days, starting with the night before surgery. In addition, patient's pain is likely to improve if the underlying psychosocial issues are also addressed. A recent study in which 611 postmastectomy patients were analyzed for psychosocial issues (including anxiety, stress, sleep, etc.), for treatment-related issues (including tumor size, recurrence, surgical complications, etc.), and for pain

levels (those with pain levels of ≥ 3/10 were considered) was performed. It was found that postmastectomy pain syndrome is very common, occurring in about one-third of the patients. On average, patients were analyzed about 3.2 years after surgery. It was found that pain severity and psychosocial issues are correlated. However, treatment-related factors were not associated with postmastectomy syndrome.

B Physical modalities such as transcutaneous nerve stimulation (TENS), myofascial release, thoracic facet joint or rib mobilization (or both), and stretching exercises may benefit if indicated.

C Surgical excision of palpable neuromas can result in complete pain relief. Also, a less known procedure to consider is an autologous fat graft. There is level two evidence that performing this will yield a significant reduction in pain. In one study of 113 patients with postmastectomy pain, 78 underwent this procedure. Many had significant pain relief and 28 of the 34 patients who were on analgesics were able to stop them. It is worth considering in patients suffering from this syndrome if less invasive alternatives have failed.

D A successful intercostal block with local anesthetic may be followed by pulsed radiofrequency lesioning or cryoablation of the intercostal nerve. Paravertebral blocks, epidural blocks, or interpleural blocks provide analgesia for desensitization techniques and mobilization. Spinal cord stimulation may be considered when more conservative interventions are unsuccessful.

SUGGESTED READING

Amr Y, Yousef A. Evaluation of efficacy of the perioperative administration of venlafaxine or Gabapentin on acute and chronic postmastectomy pain. Clin J Pain. 2010;26(5):381-5.

Belfer I, Schreiber K, Shaffer J, et al. Persistent postmastectomy pain in breast cancer survivors: analysis of clinical, demographic, and psychosocial factors. J Pain. 2013;14(10):1185-95.

Caviggioli F, Maione L, Forcellini D, et al. Autologous fat graft in postmastectomy pain syndrome. Plast Reconstr Surg. 2011; 128(2):349-52.

Crawford JS, Simpson J, Crawford P. Myofascial release provides symptomatic relief from chest wall tenderness occasionally seen following lumpectomy and radiation in breast cancer patients. Int J Radiat Oncol Biol Phys. 1996;34(5):1188-9.

Sloan P, Carpenter J, Andrykowski M. Post-mastectomy pain syndrome in women treated for breast cancer. Anesthesiolgy. 1997;87:751A.

Watson CP, Evans RJ, Watt VR. The post-mastectomy pain syndrome and the effect of topical capsaicin. Pain. 1989;38:177-86.

Wong L. Intercostal neuromas: a treatable cause of postoperative breast surgery pain. Ann Plast Surg. 2001;46:481-4.

Chronic Vertebral Pain

Ovsiowitz R, Pangarkar SS

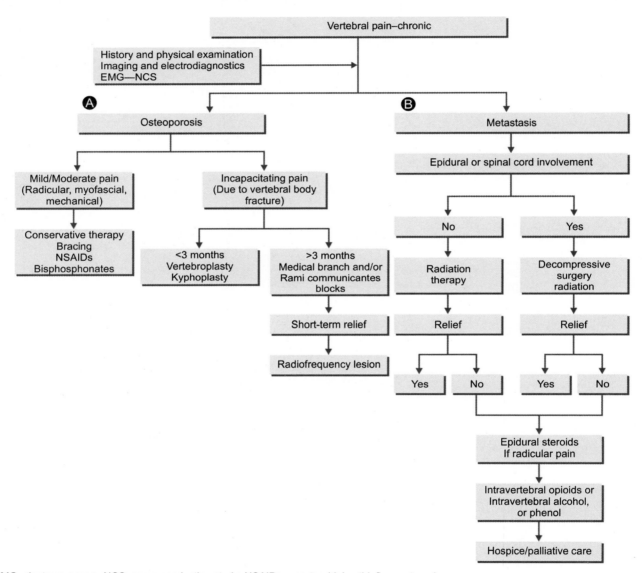

EMG, electromyogram; NCS, nerve conduction study; NSAIDs, nonsteroidal anti-inflammatory drugs

Vertebral pain generators included in this chapter are osteoporosis, bone fractures (traumatic fractures, compression fractures or pars fractures) and metastasis. Other vertebral pain generators, which are not discussed in this chapter, include spinal kyphosis or scoliosis, spinal instability, metabolic disorders (i.e. Paget's disease), infections (i.e. osteomyelitis/discitis), facet joint disorder, ligament strain, muscle strain, spinal stenosis, and sacroiliac joint dysfunction.

Ⓐ *Osteoporosis:* Vertebral bone pain can result from traumatic, compression or pathological fractures. Pathological fractures are more commonly related to osteoporosis (OP), which is more prevalent in older, postmenopausal Caucasian females with history of smoking, prior fractures, hyperthyroidism, heparin use, low bone mineral density (BMD) and chronic steroid therapy. OP predisposes individuals to develop chronic vertebral pain with or without fractures. Screening patients with risk factors by dual-energy x-ray absorptiometry may identify populations at high risk for fractures.

Conservative management of vertebral bone pain includes age appropriate calcium and vitamin D intake. Rehabilitation should include education, lumbar-extensor strengthening, weight-bearing exercises and modalities such as heat for pain relief. In the presence of fractures, the use of braces to limit spinal flexion may reduce the risk for additional fractures and provide comfort. Medications for pain and prevention include use of analgesics, bisphosphonates, selective estrogen receptor modulators, and calcitonin. Newer treatments with sclerostin inhibitors that enhance osteoblast function and improve bone mass are being studied. OP-related acute compression fractures are painful and can be managed with relative rest, bracing and analgesics. In cases of incapacitating pain, surgical consideration with vertebral augmentation (vertebroplasty and kyphoplasty) may be useful, though the evidence at this time is conflicting.

B *Mestasis:* Bone metastases to the vertebrae are common with breast, lung, thyroid, kidney and prostate cancers. There may also be extensive bony involvement in multiple myeloma. Onset of bone pain in patients with a history of cancer should prompt updated spine imaging to delineate bone, epidural and/or spinal cord involvement. In the absence of neurologic findings and compression, palliative radiotherapy may be helpful. In those patients with neurologic findings, neurosurgical decompression and stabilization followed by radiation therapy can provide relief. If pain persists or worsens, neurodestructive procedures using thermal or chemical agents can be employed in the epidural or intrathecal space. Use of implantable pain pumps may be considered in those patient's with a life expectancy greater than 3 months. Palliative care consultation should be offered in patients with terminal prognosis.

SUGGESTED READING

Benzon HT. Essentials of Pain Medicine, 3rd edition. Philadelphia: Elsevier; 2011.

Buchbinder R, Osborne RH, Kallmes D. Vertebroplasty appears no better than placebo for osteoporotic spinal fractures, and has potential to cause harm. Med J Aust. 2009;191(9):476-7.

Kallmes DF, Comstock BA, Heagerty PJ, et al. A randomized trial of vertebroplasty for osteoporotic spinal fractures. N Engl J Med. 2009;361(6):569-79.

Li X, Ominsky MS, Niu QT, et al. Targeted deletion of the sclerostin gene in mice results in increased bone formation and bone strength. J Bone Miner Res. 2008;23(6):860-9.

Loeser JD (Ed). Bonica's Management of Pain, 3rd edition. Philadelphia: Lippincott Williams & Wilkins; 2001.

Osteoporosis prevention, diagnosis, and therapy. NIH Consensus Statement. 2000;17:1-45.

CHAPTER
69

Rib Pain

Nick CT, Lautenschlager K

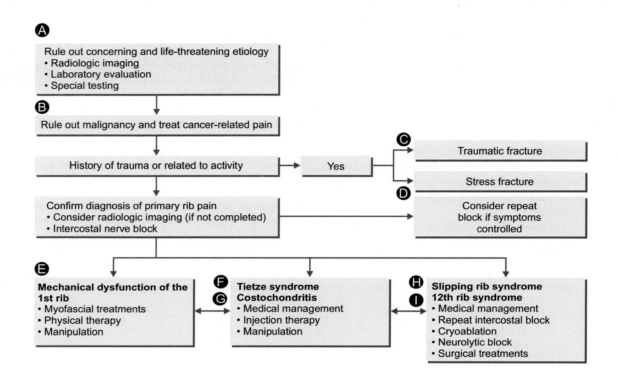

Rib pain can be associated with rib fractures secondary to trauma, stress fractures associated with activity, infiltration of bone or neural tissues by tumor, or a number of musculoskeletal disorders. Similarly, pain may be referred pain from the visceral structures of the chest or abdomen.

A Key to the diagnosis and treatment of rib pain is exclusion of more serious generators of chest pain to include a thorough investigation into cardiac (angina or myocardial infarction), pulmonary (pneumothorax or DVT), vascular (aortic dissection), or gastrointestinal etiologies. Once a thorough workup has been performed and life-threatening etiologies ruled out, rib pain can be categorized further.

B Thoracic chest wall tumors involving the ribs and intercostal nerves can be of primary or metastatic origin. Oral analgesics are appropriate for most patients, but a subset of patients requires more aggressive pain control strategies. Anterior chest wall tumors create pain responsive to intercostal nerve blocks as both a diagnostic and therapeutic tool. Chemical neurolysis of the intercostal nerve may subsequently be utilized for long-term pain control. Posterior chest wall tumors not

encroaching on the thoracic nerve are often responsive to both paravertebral blocks and subsequent neurolysis. When encroaching upon the thoracic nerve, pain from posterior tumors may be treated with thoracic nerve radiofrequency ablation or cryoablation. For refractory cases, epidural catheter, intrathecal infusion, spinal cord stimulation, and surgical neurolysis should be considered.

C Rib fractures secondary to blunt thoracic trauma represent a significant source of morbidity in trauma patients. Diagnosis is often made by identifying ecchymosis over the ribs, possible seat belt sign in motor vehicle accidents, pain with rib palpation or inhalation, or crepitus of the overlying skin. Chest radiographs are integral for locating rib fractures and identifying underlying pulmonary contusion, pneumothorax, or hemothorax. Children and elderly are at an increased risk for pneumonia, hypoxemia, atelectasis, and ultimately respiratory failure, making adequate pulmonary toilet and pain control essential. Modalities for pain control include initial analgesics such as opioids or nonsteroidal anti-inflammatory drugs (NSAIDs). Thoracic epidural catheters with opioids or local anesthetics and paravertebral blocks with or without catheters may provide prolonged relief into the posthospital period. Intercostal blocks and intrapleural blocks are shorter acting resulting in limited utility. Transcutaneous electric nerve stimulation (TENS) units have been utilized for rib pain secondary to fracture, but have not been validated for efficacy versus other modalities.

D Stress fractures of the ribs provide a different set of challenges for diagnosis and treatment compared to traumatic fractures. Risk factors include poor preactivity conditioning and extent of activity. Muscle fatigue in the thoracic cage can weaken the rib framework and predispose to fracture. Point tenderness and potential swelling at the site of fracture may be present. Recreation of the inciting activity can aid in diagnosis unless the stress fracture was caused by repetitive thoracic motion or intense weight-bearing activities. Activities associated with rib stress fractures include rowing, overhead throwing, weightlifting, and those with significant axial rotation of the thorax. Likely sites for potential fracture include the anterolateral first rib, the posterolateral fourth through ninth rib, and the posteromedial upper ribs. Although potentially missed on initial imaging, stress fractures appear within three weeks of injury for 50% of patients. Bone scintigraphy provides 100% sensitivity for detecting stress fractures, while magnetic resonance imaging (MRI) provides the highest combined sensitivity and specificity early in presentation while revealing soft tissue injuries. Initial treatment for rib stress fractures begins with grading of the fracture to determine the optimal strategy. Activity modification to avoid causative activity and physical therapy to educate proper technique are imperative. Immobilization or rest may be necessary based on symptom profile. If fractures are severe or symptoms fail to improve over 4–6 weeks, surgical intervention may be necessary. Pharmacological pain control can be achieved with oral medications such as acetaminophen or opioids for severe fractures.

E Mechanical dysfunction of the first rib has been associated with upper extremity conditions to include thoracic outlet syndrome and complex regional pain syndrome. Limited motion is noted with respiration on the involved side. Restoration of motion through manipulation and physical therapy has been shown to result in significant reduction of upper extremity symptoms.

F Tietze syndrome is represented by benign inflammation at the site of the costal cartilages causing painful swelling and tenderness. Unilateral involvement of the upper ribs is common. Likely etiologies include physical strain from injury, coughing, vomiting, or trauma. Tietze syndrome is most often self-limited and resolves within a matter of weeks to months. In addition to reassurance, symptoms can be relieved by rest, NSAIDs, heat application, or local steroid or lidocaine injections.

G Similarly, costochondritis presents with pain and tenderness at the costal cartilages but is distinguished by an absence of inflammation and swelling at the site. The diagnosis makes up nearly a third of emergency room complaints of chest pain. Review of the history elicits pain that can be experienced both at rest and with activity that is often exacerbated by heavy breathing. Etiologies proposed include a relationship with the seronegative spondyloarthropathies and repetitive movements of the rib cage. As with Tietze syndrome, costochondritis is usually self-limited and treatment modalities include reassurance, manual therapy, manipulation, and localized injection of local anesthetics or sulfasalazine.

H Slipping rib syndrome results from impingement of the intercostal nerve. Loosening of fibrous cartilage attachments between the costal segments of the lower ribs (8th–10th) allows a lower cartilaginous rib tip to curl under the adjacent rib above. On palpation, the cartilage and rib tip are easily manipulated allowing for manual release of the trapped rib tip with a "click". The "hooking maneuver" involves pulling on the painful cartilage with a finger reproducing the pain. Treatment includes reassurance and avoidance of positions that recreate the symptoms, local infiltration with local anesthetics or steroids, and radiofrequency ablation of intercostal nerves. Refractory cases may require resection of the implicated rib cartilage.

I Twelfth rib syndrome presents as referred pain to the lower abdomen, groin, and thigh. Pain can be reproduced with palpation of the twelfth rib and is due to a connection between the subcostal nerve and the L1 nerve. Diagnosis is confirmed with subcostal nerve blockade. Permanent relief has been achieved with blockade using injected steroid, cryoablation, or surgical excision of the painful rib.

SUGGESTED READING

Ayloo A, Cvengros T, Marella S. Evaluation and treatment of musculoskeletal chest pain. Prim Care. 2013;40(4):863-87.

Gadsden J, Warlick A. Regional anesthesia for the trauma patient: improving patient outcomes. Local Reg Anesth. 2015;8:45-55.

Gulati A, Shah R, Puttanniah V, et al. A retrospective review and treatment paradigm of interventional therapies for patients suffering from intractable thoracic chest wall pain in the oncologic population. Pain Med. 2015;16(4):802-10.

Karmakar MK, Ho AM. Acute pain management of patients with multiple fractured ribs. J Trauma. 2003;54(3):615-25.

Karmy-Jones R, Jurkovich GJ. Blunt chest trauma. Curr Probl Surg. 2004;41(3):211-380.

Keoghane SR, Douglas J, Pounder D. Twelfth rib syndrome: a forgotten cause of flank pain. BJU Int. 2009;103(5):569-70.

Miller TL, Harris JD, Kaeding CC. Stress fractures of the ribs and upper extremities: causation, evaluation, and management. Sports Med. 2013;43(8):665-74.

Stochkendahl MJ, Christensen HW. Chest pain in focal musculoskeletal disorders. Med Clin North Am. 2010;94(2):259-73.

SECTION 7

Low Back Pain

Ameet Nagpal

CHAPTER
70

Acute Low Back Pain

McKenny J, Wallisch BJ

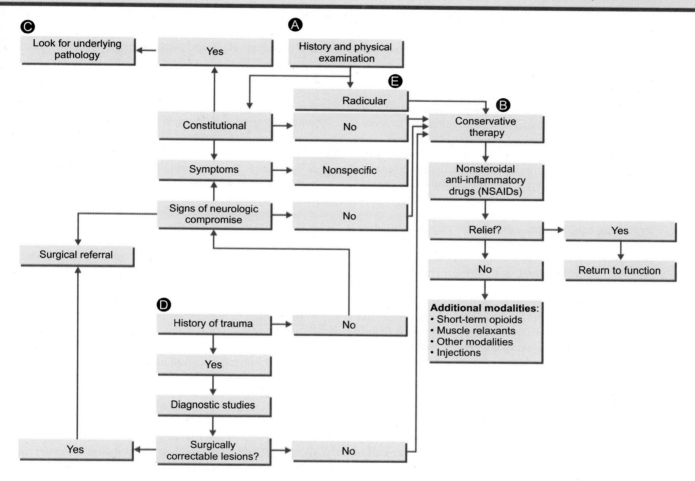

Acute low back pain, defined as pain lasting less than 4 weeks, is one of the most common medical disorders in the industrialized world. Most cases are nonspecific, self-limited and resolve with return to normal daily activities after conservative treatment. Recurrences, however, are common and affect up to 50–70% of patients. Predictors of disabling chronic low back pain at 1 year include maladaptive pain coping behaviors, functional impairment, poor general health status, presence of psychiatric comorbidities or nonorganic signs. In most cases, an accurate diagnosis can be obtained by a detailed history and physical examination. Laboratory studies, radiologic imaging, and electrodiagnostic testing are used to confirm the diagnosis or the pathology in difficult cases. Treatment strategies utilize a multimodal strategy that includes pain control measures, physical therapy, psychological counseling and patient education. Early return to functional activities is emphasized and achieved in most

patients. Serious disease or pathology mandating immediate surgical evaluation and intervention is uncommon and accounts for less than 1% of patients presenting to the primary care clinic with the chief complaint of lower back pain.

A An appropriate history and physical examination should be performed to determine whether the patient can be treated with conservative therapy or if he/she will require additional workup to rule out ominous conditions.

B Acute low back pain not associated with traumatic onset, systemic symptoms, or features of discogenic or posterior element injury or dysfunction suggests either nonspecific low back pain or an isolated soft tissue disorder. Myofascial pain is indicated by the presence of discrete trigger points in affected muscle groups. Fibromyalgia is identified by the presence of multiple tender points in classically described locations that overlie joint lines, bursae, and muscle bodies and may include symptoms of low back pain. In some patients, physical examination and secondary diagnostic studies are unremarkable, and the patient is given the diagnosis of nonspecific lower back pain. Conservative therapies are successful in resolving or controlling symptoms in most cases and initial monotherapy with a trial of short-term (2–4 weeks) nonsteroidal anti-inflammatory drug (NSAID) is indicated. Acetaminophen is a reasonable alternative to NSAIDs in patients suffering from acute low back pain who cannot tolerate or have contraindications to NSAID use. For patients with pain refractory to initial monotherapy use, the addition of a nonbenzodiazepine muscle relaxant such as cyclobenzaprine, methocarbamol, carisoprodol, baclofen, chlorzoxazone, metaxalone, orphenadrine or tizanidine may provide additional symptom relief, but should be limited to a 2- to 4-week period of use. The use of opioids is reserved for patients with refractory or severe pain and should be based on clinical judgment. It is advisable to limit these to short-term use (<2 weeks). The current evidence to support the use of these medications for acute low back pain is limited. Additionally, there is very limited evidence to support the effectiveness of antidepressants, systemic glucocorticoids, antiepileptics, topical agents, herbal therapies, exercise therapy, spinal manipulation, acupuncture, massage, heat, cold, paraspinal injections, yoga, muscle energy techniques, traction, lumbar supports, or mattress recommendations to treat acute nonspecific lower back pain.

C Back pain associated with constitutional symptoms, weight loss, changes in genitourinary or gastrointestinal function, abdominal of pelvic pain, night pain, or profound morning stiffness suggests an underlying medical disorder and demands appropriate evaluation with laboratory, imaging, and diagnostic studies. Common medical causes of low back pain include pancreatic disease, gallbladder disease, hepatitis, diverticular disease, colorectal cancer, kidney stones, pyelonephritis, endometriosis, pelvic inflammatory disease, cervical or uterine malignancy, pregnancy, aortic aneurysm, spinal neoplasm, prostatitis, prostate cancer, or inflammatory arthropathy.

D Back pain resulting from a high-energy injury or impact or the sudden onset of back pain in osteoporotic or elderly individuals must be evaluated for spinal fracture. Compression fractures with less than 50% loss of anterior column height, transverse process fractures, or spinous process fractures can be managed conservatively. Compression fractures with loss of more than 50% of anterior column height, or burst fractures, may be unstable and should be referred to a surgeon. Back pain that develops following lifting of flexion-rotation injuries may result from disruption or a tear of the disc annulus fibrosis or acute herniated nucleus pulposus (HNP). Back pain radiating into the lower extremities with or without neurologic loss may indicate acute lumbosacral radiculopathy secondary to spinal stenosis or acute HNP. Lumbar spinal stenosis is often multifactorial and most commonly caused by spondylosis, spondylolistheses or thickening of the ligamentum flavum. Acute bowel or bladder dysfunction with or without saddle anesthesia or radicular symptoms suggests cauda equina compromise. Prolapse of the intervertebral disc, ankylosing spondylitis, lumbar puncture, trauma, malignant/nonmalignant tumor and infection are potential causes of spinal cord or cauda equina compression and should be evaluated immediately with noncontrast magnetic resonance imaging (MRI) or computed tomography (CT) scan if patient is not a candidate for MRI. Back pain resulting from repetitive stress or sudden overload of the spine in neutral position or extension may be due to injury of the posterior elements, including the zygapophyseal (facet) joints or the pars interarticularis. Facet joint pain is often aggravated by standing or spinal extension. Low back pain following a shear injury to the pelvis of lower extremities may indicate an insult to the sacroiliac (SI) joint. Piriformis syndrome is a condition in which the sciatic nerve is compressed by the piriformis muscle.

E A history of radicular pain associated with the presence of dural tension signs (straight leg raise, Lasègue's sign, bowstring sign) suggests acute lumbosacral radiculopathy. L5 and S1 compression accounts for over 90% of the reported radiculopathies. Appropriate conservative care consists of offering NSAIDs, narcotic and non-narcotic analgesics, or muscle relaxants as well as epidural steroid injections. Physical therapy modalities (superficial heat, ultrasound application, electrical stimulation) are used to control pain and reactive muscle spasm and to decrease inflammation. Specific low back exercise protocols are implemented to strengthen the spinal musculature and stability. Spinal manipulation and massage benefit some patients. Home exercise programs and patient education in spinal biomechanics and lifestyle factors help prevent future episodes of back pain. Imaging studies (CT or MRI) and electrodiagnostic examination can be used to clarify the pathology in patients unresponsive to initial conservative care or those with neurologic deficits or known underlying pathology. Patients with intractable pain or progressive neurologic deficits should be referred for surgical evaluation and management.

SUGGESTED READING

Acute low back problems in adults: assessment and treatment. Agency for Health Care Policy and Research. Clin Pract Guidel Quick Ref Guide Clin. 1994;(14):iii-iv, 1-25.

Friedman BW, Dym AA, Davitt M, et al. Naproxen with cyclobenzaprine, oxycodone/acetaminophen or placebo for treating acute low back pain: a randomized clinical trial. JAMA. 2015; 314:1572-80.

Mehling WE, Gopisetty V, Bartmess-LeVasseur E, et al. The prognosis of acute low back pain in primary care in the United States: a 2-year prospective cohort study. Spine (Phila Pa 1976). 2012;37:678-84.

Sun JC, Xu T, Chen KF, et al. Assessment of cauda equina syndrome progression pattern to improve diagnosis. Spine (Phila Pa 1976). 2014;39:596-602.

Wertli MM, Eugster R, Held U, et al. Catastrophizing—a prognostic factor for outcome in patients with low back pain: a systematic review. Spine J. 2014;14(11):2639-57.

Chronic Low Back Pain

Jones JR, Day M

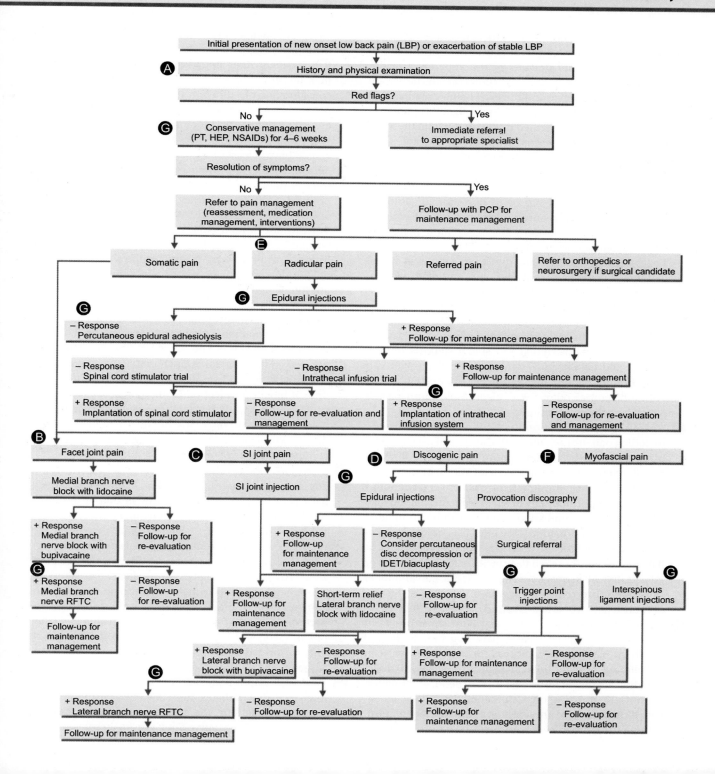

Low back pain (LBP) is one of the most common causes of pain and disability. It is estimated that 80% of the population will experience LBP in their lifetime. This translates into a large economic cost and billions of dollars spent each year in related healthcare costs secondary to management of LBP. Appropriate management of LBP can help minimize this economic impact.

The lumbar spine consists of five vertebrae separated by intervertebral discs. Lumbar facet joints are synovial joints which are paired and located dorsally. Each joint is formed by a superior and inferior articular process from the corresponding vertebrae. The medial branch of the dorsal ramus passes over the junction of the superior articular process and the transverse process to innervate the facet joint at the same vertebral level and the level below creating dual innervations at each facet joint. The sacroiliac (SI) joints are paired diarthrodial joints formed by the sacrum and the ilium on each side. The SI joints receive innervations anteriorly from the L5 to S2 ventral rami and sacral plexus. Innervation posteriorly is from the lateral branches of the L4 to S4 dorsal rami, with the predominant innervations from S1 to S3. The anterior longitudinal ligament, posterior longitudinal ligament, ligamentum flavum, and interspinous ligaments help to stabilize the spine. Paraspinal musculature maintains posture and creates movement in the lumbar spine.

Low back pain can originate from many sources. It can be divided into somatic pain, radicular pain, and referred pain. Somatic pain includes facet joint pain (prevalence of 40%), SI joint pain (prevalence between 2% and 38%), discogenic pain (prevalence of 26%), spinal ligament pain, and muscle pain. Radicular pain includes spinal nerve root radiculitis (prevalence of 13%), secondary to spinal stenosis or disc herniation, and post-surgery syndrome. Referred pain can originate from the abdominal and pelvic viscera. Often, the pain is multifactorial, but using an algorithmic approach can simplify the treatment decisions.

A *History and Physical Examination:* A thorough history, including pain history, medical history, and psychosocial history, should be obtained from the patient. Physical examination of the musculoskeletal and neuromuscular systems involving the low back and lower extremities should be performed. Any available imaging should also be reviewed. An impression and plan can be formulated based on this information. One must also be cognizant of the red flags for LBP and refer to an appropriate specialist if encountered. These red flags include age less than 20 or greater than 50 at onset, history of trauma, constitutional symptoms (fever/chills, night sweats, weight loss), history of cancer, pain worse at night, and neurologic deficits.

B *Facet Joint Pain:* Facet joint pain is the most prevalent source of chronic LBP. Facet pain is generally located axially in palmprint-sized areas for each level, but can be referred into the gluteal region or posterior thigh. Pain is exacerbated by extension, side bend, and rotation (positive Kemp's test) on examination. Diagnostic blocks with local anesthetic are accepted as the best technique to diagnose facet-mediated pain. Several studies have been performed comparing facet intra-articular injections to medial branch blocks prior to the definitive treatment with radiofrequency thermocoagulation (RFTC). While each technique has limitations, a double diagnostic medial branch nerve block (one with a short-acting local anesthetic and the second with a long-acting local anesthetic) is generally accepted as the confirmatory method prior to RFTC. The first medial branch nerve block should be performed at the painful levels on the painful side or bilaterally if appropriate with a short-acting local anesthetic such as lidocaine. An appropriate response to the injections is pain reduction of at least 50% for 1 hour. If the patient does not have an appropriate response, then he should be seen in clinic for a re-evaluation and consideration of a different somatic pain generator. If the patient does have an appropriate pain reduction, then a second diagnostic block should be performed with bupivacaine or ropivacaine at the same levels. The patient should have at least a 50% pain reduction for 4–6 hours.

C *Sacroiliac Joint Pain:* SI joint pain has a similar presentation to facet pain, but is usually more localized. Specialized physical examination tests (Patrick's test, Gaenslen's test, Fortin finger test, compression/distraction) are sensitive for SI joint pain, but not very specific. This is why multiple positive physical examination tests (at least 3) are generally needed to support the clinical diagnosis of SI joint pain. A diagnostic SI joint injection with local anesthetic and steroid should be performed initially for confirmation. If the patient gets lasting relief, then he can be followed in clinic for maintenance management. If the patient has good relief from the SI joint injection, but the duration of relief is not prolonged, then one can proceed to comparative lateral branch nerve local anesthetic blocks with lidocaine and bupivacaine similar to medial branch blocks for facet pain. There is no consensus on which nerves should be blocked for treatment of SI joint pain. Various combinations of the L4 medial branch, the L5 dorsal ramus, and the S1-3 lateral branches are commonly blocked.

D *Discogenic Pain:* Discogenic pain is secondary to degenerative changes of the disc. It presents as axial back pain which is exacerbated by flexion at the waist, prolonged sitting/standing, coughing, sneezing, and Valsalva maneuvering. Radiographic changes are variable, but circumferential and radial annular tears seen on magnetic resonance imaging (MRI) as a high-intensity zone (HIZ) and disc bulges, protrusions, extrusions are often seen in patients with discogenic pain. In past years, patients would often have provocation discography performed prior to a lumbar fusion, but this has fallen out of favor and currently provocation discography is only performed in rare patients at the request of the spine surgeon.

E *Radicular Pain:* Radicular pain involves pain in the low back that radiates into the lower extremity in a dermatomal pattern. The pain is caused by compression or irritation of the nerve root due to herniated discs, fibrosis, and foraminal stenosis. Patients will often have a positive straight leg raise or femoral nerve tension test.

F *Myofascial Pain:* Myofascial pain most often originates in the multifidi and supporting muscles of the spine and interspinous ligaments. Commonly, patients have myofascial pain secondary to other structural abnormalities like facet arthrosis, disc herniations, and spondylosis.

G *Treatment:* Without any red flags for back pain, the initial treatment plan should utilize conservative management. The patient should be referred to physical therapy for strengthening, range of motion, adaptive techniques, physical therapy modalities, and teaching of home exercises. The patients should be educated that physical therapy alone may not necessarily improve the pain and could exacerbate the pain while doing exercises initially, but will improve function and quality of life if continued regularly. A short course of a nonsteroidal anti-inflammatory drug (NSAID) and possibly muscle relaxants is also appropriate. The patient should be followed up in 6 weeks. The majority of benign LBP will subside with the initial treatments. If LBP persists, then the patient should be referred to a pain management physician for a reassessment with a thorough history, physical examination, and review of diagnostic imaging.

In the event of facet-mediated pain, the patient should then undergo a medial branch nerve RFTC at the corresponding levels. One can expect pain relief for 6–12 months after this procedure. For SI joint pain, a lateral branch RFTC can be performed for longer duration pain relief. In those patients with discogenic pain, they should initially undergo an epidural steroid injection. If the patient fails two fluoroscopically-guided epidural steroid injections, one could consider percutaneous disc decompression, or intradiscal electrothermal therapy (IDET)/biacuplasty. There has been little evidence to support the use of these various procedures and they are not often paid for by insurance companies; as a result, they are not often performed. If a patient is found to have radiculitis, then epidural injections should be pursued. Caudal, interlaminar, and transforaminal epidural injections are accepted techniques. However, some studies suggest that the transforaminal approach may be superior when a patient has abnormalities at one or two levels. Patients who do not respond to epidural injections may benefit from percutaneous epidural adhesiolysis, implantation of spinal cord stimulation, or an intrathecal infusion system. In cases of myofascial pain, if the primary pain generator is treated successfully, then often the myofascial pain will improve as well. However, if the myofascial pain persists, then trigger point injections or interspinous ligament injections should be pursued.

SUGGESTED READING

Ackerman WE 3rd, Ahmad M. The efficacy of lumbar epidural steroid injections in patients with lumbar disc herniations. Anesth Analg. 2007;104(5):1217-22.

Cohen SP, Raja SN. Pathogenesis, diagnosis, and treatment of lumbar zygapophysial (facet) joint pain. Anesthesiology. 2007;106:591-614.

Filippiadis DK, Kelekis A. A review of percutaneous techniques for low back pain and neuralgia: current trends in epidural infiltrations, intervertebral disc and facet joint therapies. Br J Radiol. 2016;89:20150357.

Gotfryd AO, Valesin Filho ES, Viola DC, et al. Analysis of epidemiology, lifestyle, and psychosocial factors in patients with back pain admitted to an orthopedic emergency unit. Einstein (Sao Paulo). 2015;13(2):243-8.

Koes BW, van Tulder M, Lin CW, et al. An updated overview of clinical guidelines for the management of non-specific low back pain in primary care. Eur Spine J. 2010;19(12):2075-94.

Manchikanti L, Helm S, Singh V, et al. An algorithmic approach for clinical management of chronic spinal pain. Pain Physician. 2009;12:E225-64.

Lumbosacral Radiculopathy

Haque AR, Pino CA

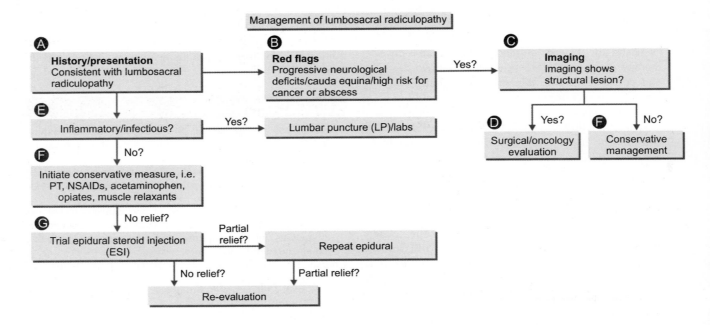

Management of lumbosacral radiculopathy

Lumbosacral radiculopathy originates secondary to either compression or impingement of a nerve root either at the level of the foramen or the lateral recess during its course from the spinal cord to its associated area of distribution. Due to this nerve impingement and its resultant inflammation, this insult to the nerve may progress to the point where it causes neurological symptoms such as numbness and weakness along the dermatomal distribution of the nerve. Radicular pain specifically describes the pain component that can emanate from a specific spinal nerve root along its distribution, independent of the existence of a radiculopathy. Nerves can be compromised by many sources such as surrounding bones, muscles, cartilage, or herniated discs that can eventually result in an inflammatory process leading to a multitude of symptoms.

ETIOLOGY

The most common causes of radiculopathy are spondylosis or herniated discs, where the nucleus pulposus extends beyond its boundaries due to a weakened outer rim of the annulus fibrosis, creating mechanical compression or inflammatory irritation of the exiting nerve root. These pathologies can be a result of acute injury, ongoing osteoarthritis, repetitive stress, or may occur spontaneously. Neoplastic causes such

as primary or metastatic tumors, infectious causes such as an epidural abscess, and inflammatory causes such as arachnoiditis and Paget's disease must also be taken into account when evaluating a patient with radiculopathy.

CLINICAL CONSIDERATIONS

A *History and Physical Examination:* When evaluating a patient, obtaining a thorough history is paramount. Patients suffering from radiculopathy have a varied time course that could range from an abrupt incident or trauma, that can be identified as the cause of their pain, to a more progressive and gradual course. The most common symptom of lumbosacral radiculopathy is usually a sudden onset of low back pain that gives way to a predominant symptom of leg pain overtaking the severity of the back pain. Some things to also take into account are certain actions that may exacerbate the pain such as sitting, coughing, or sneezing which may predictably reproduce the patient's radicular pain.

It is vital to perform a comprehensive physical examination when evaluating patients that present with acute low back pain and radicular pain. A thorough neurological examination must be performed in an attempt to further localize the patient's pain and to rule out any possible red flags that may indicate a need for acute intervention. Lower extremity reflexes, measures of strength, and levels of bilateral sensation must be gauged. Special note must be taken when performing provocative maneuvers such as straight leg raise tests and slump tests on whether they recreate the patient's baseline symptoms. A thorough musculoskeletal examination must also be undertaken to rule out any localized pain patterns, any pain pathology emanating from facet joint disease, or any myofascial origins.

B *Red Flags*: Particular attention must be paid when evaluating the patient to what some may refer to as alert signs or "red flags" that may be indicative of a more ominous pathology. Signs of fever, acute weight loss, chills, sudden neurological deficits, profound weakness, and saddle anesthesia may be signs that sway toward conditions such as tumors, infections, and cauda equina syndrome that require aggressive management. The patient population above the age of 50 is at a greater risk for such critical pathologies. Patients below the age of 20 have a higher risk of congenital and developmental etiologies.

C *Imaging*: Two common imaging studies that should be considered when evaluating a patient with lumbosacral radiculopathy are plain radiographs and magnetic resonance imaging (MRI). Plain x-rays can provide information on structural abnormalities, arthritic facet joints or instability at the vertebral levels responsible for the patient's symptoms. Pathologies concerning ruptured discs or any impingement of the nerve root cannot be adequately visualized with plain x-rays. Acute pain less than 6 weeks duration, in the absence of obvious red flags, rarely warrants any imaging studies. Obtaining an MRI, although not necessary in most cases, can help gather more information and further localize the patient's pathology. MRIs are significantly better at identifying nerve root impingements as well as distortions of spinal discs such as herniation. MRIs are indicated in circumstances such as progressive neurological deficits, any suspicion of possible cauda equina syndrome or malignancy. MRI can also help identify the level of pathology in concordance with physical examination and patient history which can help guide treatment options. It should be taken into account that most abnormalities found on MRIs do not necessarily correlate to obvious symptoms in the patient. Many asymptomatic patients have been found to have numerous incidental MRI findings without any pathological issues. Studies have demonstrated that 30–60% of adults may have completely asymptomatic disc bulges or minor herniation that do not require any intervention at all.

D For patients that have evidence of a lumbar disc herniation or compression of an exiting nerve root that correlates well with clinical findings, a surgical consult may prove beneficial to explore various surgical options that are available ranging from lumbar discectomy to surgical decompression of a symptomatic lumbar spinal nerve. Though surgical intervention is mostly elective in patients that have radicular pain with mild neurological abnormalities, more ominous signs such as cauda equina syndrome and progressive radiculopathy can hasten the need for urgent/emergent intervention. Radiculopathy from neoplastic origins is rare but diagnosis can be established by MRI. If there is evidence of primary versus metastatic lesions, an oncological evaluation should be garnered to further workup treatment options.

E In patients with suspicion for inflammatory or infectious cause of lumbosacral radiculopathy, a lumbar puncture and appropriate laboratory evaluation should be undertaken.

F In the face of normal MRI and no risk factors for inflammatory/infectious causes, conservative management should be initiated, to include a combination of physical therapy, nonsteroidal anti-inflammatory drugs (NSAIDs), acetaminophen, and muscle relaxants. Opioids should be reserved for refractory cases.

G In patients who have failed conservative therapy, an epidural steroid injection (ESI) should be performed. Prior to an ESI, an MRI should be performed to evaluate for the appropriate site of injection. If the patient's pain improves only partially, repeat ESIs may be performed. In those patients who do not receive analgesia from ESIs, consideration should be made for re-evaluation of the patient.

SUGGESTED READING

Abram SE. Treatment of lumbosacral radiculopathy with epidural steroids. Anesthesiology. 1999;91:1937-41.

Benzon HT, Rathmell JP, Wu CL, et al. Practical Management of Pain, 5th edition. Philadelphia, PA: Elsevier Mosby; 2014.

Deen HG Jr. Diagnosis and management of lumbar disc disease. Mayo Clin Proc. 1996;71:283-7.

Henschke N, Maher CG, Refshauge KM. Screening for malignancy in low back pain patients: a systematic review. Eur Spine J. 2007; 16:1673-9.

Murphy DR, Hurwitz EL, Gerrard JK, et al. Pain patterns and descriptions in patients with radicular pain: does the pain necessarily follow a specific dermatome? Chiropr Osteopat. 2009;17:9.

Powell MC, Wilson M, Szypryt P, et al. Prevalence of lumbar disc degeneration observed by magnetic resonance in symptomless women. Lancet. 1986;2:1366-7.

Tarulli AW, Raynor EM. Lumbosacral radiculopathy. Neurol Clin. 2007;25:387-405.

Spinal Stenosis

Wirthlin JD, Lai TT, Jorgensen AY

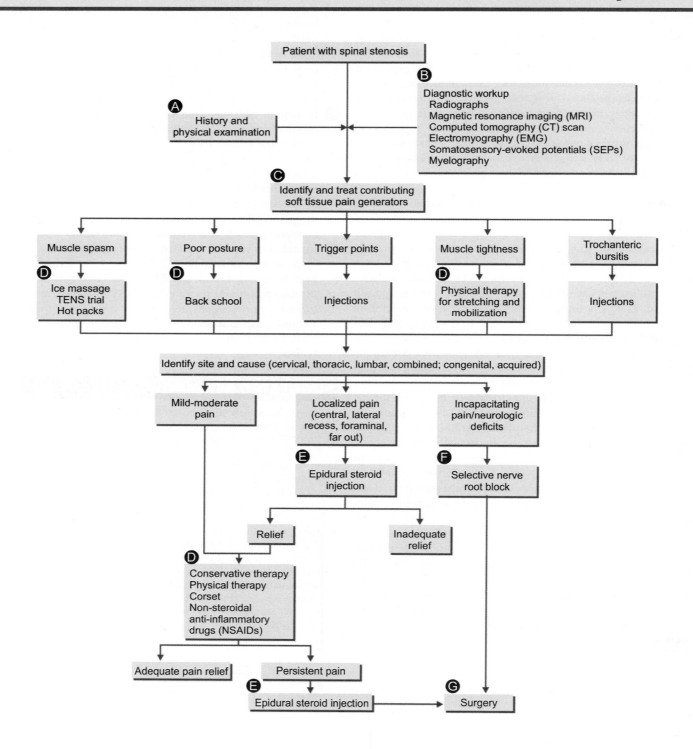

Spinal stenosis is the congenital or acquired narrowing of the spinal canal or foramina in either the lateral (apophyseal) or anteroposterior (AP) (laminar) direction resulting in compression on the spinal roots laterally and of the cauda equina anteroposteriorly. This narrowing can occur anywhere along the spinal column, from occiput to sacrum. Radiographic stenosis may not correlate with clinical symptoms, especially in the lumbar spine. The diagnosis of spinal stenosis is only established when symptoms of neurogenic claudication or cervical myelopathy are present. Stenosis in the cervical spine manifests with upper motor neuron signs and myelopathy, representing an injury to the spinal cord. Stenosis in the thoracic spine can also result in long tract signs and myelopathy. Stenosis of the lumbar spine (below L2) is a lesion of the nerve roots and presents with the classic constellation of findings of neurogenic claudication. It is not uncommon for patients with severe cervical stenosis and myelopathy to present without neck pain, although such patients with severe spondylosis and foraminal narrowing may also present with neck and arm pain. Pain in lumbar stenosis is likely caused by either ischemia of the nerve roots secondary to compression from either direct mechanical or indirectly from increased intrathecal pressure. Increased intrathecal pressure also may cause venous congestion and reduced venous drainage. Typical onset is during the fifth decade, although individuals with congenital stenosis may show symptoms as early as the third decade.

Most patients have a progressive presentation and are offered nonoperative management as first treatment strategy. Surgery is indicated for progressive intolerable symptoms or, more rarely, for the neurologically catastrophic initial presentations. In cervical stenosis, the neurologic catastrophe is a spinal cord injury. This typically occurs in the older patient with long-standing stenosis who presents after a hyperextension injury, such as a low energy fall or even a low velocity car accident without spine fracture. The classic pattern of spinal cord injury in this setting is a central cord syndrome. Early versus late decompression is controversial. However, since the cervical stenosis may contribute to continuing spinal cord injury surgical decompression is usually indicated.

In lumbar spinal stenosis, the theoretical neurologic catastrophe is conus medullaris syndrome from L1-2 and cauda equina syndrome below L2. This, however, is exceedingly rare. It seems that the nerve roots of the cauda equina are able to adjust to stenosis that occurs insidiously over long periods of time. The classic cause of cauda equina syndrome is a disc herniation and not the chronically developing degenerative changes that are the cause of most lumbar spinal stenosis.

Surgical strategy consists mainly of decompression (depending on the anatomical level and type of narrowing: laminectomy, foraminotomy, discectomy, corpectomy) with instrumentation and fusion should spinal stability and sagittal balance be at risk. For cervical spinal stenosis, the main objective of surgery is to halt disease progression.

Etiologies are progressive disc degeneration due to aging, trauma, or various other causes that result in disc desiccation, loss of height, and protrusion. Degenerative changes in the posterior elements such as facet joint osteophytes and ligamentum flavum hypertrophy contribute to the stenosis. As discs degenerate and collapse, there is associated infolding of the posterior ligamentum, so the process of stenosis is a combination of anterior and posterior degeneration. As in most spine surgeries, the timing of surgery is determined by the severity of patient symptoms and failure of nonoperative measures. Patients with stenosis and relatively mild symptoms may never require surgical management. For the vast majority of patients, surgery for stenosis falls firmly into the category of elective surgery.

Ⓐ *History and Physical Examination:* For lumbar spinal stenosis, the classic presenting symptoms include low back and leg pain, especially with prolonged standing, walking, or hyperextension. The lower extremity pain and paresthesias are usually relieved by flexion of the lumbar spine such as with the typical "grocery cart" sign (comfort from walking with lumbar spine flexed like hunched over a grocery cart). Unlike vascular claudication, this pseudoclaudication is less predictable in onset, slower to subside, and not relieved simply by standing. Physical examination is often normal, showing strong peripheral pulses (unless concomitant vascular disease exists) and minimal static tension signs such as straight leg raises.

Presenting symptoms of cervical stenosis may be those of myelopathy, with weakness, atrophy, hyperreflexia, and spasticity. Additional concerning upper extremity symptoms include loss of dexterity and fine motor control. Gait changes and subtle changes in bowel and bladder function should be assessed as these are additional signs of upper motor neuron injury. Often, asymptomatic cervical stenosis is encountered in the clinical setting during the workup of a symptomatic lumbar stenosis and degenerative disease. Physical examination is more often abnormal in cervical spondylotic myelopathy.

Ⓑ *Diagnostic Workup*: A diagnosis of spinal stenosis at any spine level relies on the clinical picture corresponding to changes identified by advanced imaging techniques, most importantly magnetic resonance imaging (MRI). Loss of T1 signal on MRI represents loss of myelin and injury to the spinal cord. Computed tomography (CT) can be added as an adjunct to better evaluate bony stenosis. Plain radiographs usually demonstrate spondylosis with loss of disk height, osteophytes, and sclerosis of the facet joints. CT, myelography, and MRI can further delineate the lesion, although far lateral stenosis is often missed with myelography. Degenerative lumbar stenosis most frequently involves the L4-5 and L5-S1 levels. In the neck, the C5-6 level is most commonly involved. Clinical diagnosis cannot be based on isolated radiographic findings. Each radiographic examination has its limitations; for example, false-negative rates of 10–25% have been reported with myelography. Electrodiagnostic studies may also aid in localization.

C Discomfort that stems from concomitant soft tissue disorders should be aggressively diagnosed and treated.

D *Conservative Treatment:* Most patients benefit from a trial of aggressive conservative therapy, which includes modalities such as physical therapy and the use of nonsteroidal anti-inflammatory drugs. The best results are achieved with a multidisciplinary team focused on returning the patient to productivity. See Flowchart for other conservative treatment options.

E Epidural blocks with or without steroids are a controversial topic; however, they may help delay the need for surgery, especially in older patients with radicular pain. In a comparative meta-analysis of epidural corticosteroid injections, treating radiculopathy (30 trials) and spinal stenosis (8 trials) showed small, unsustained, and poor results. Injections for radiculopathy were associated with immediate improvement in function, reduction in pain, and reduction of short-term surgery risk; however, the benefits are often short-lived without any effect on long-term surgery risk. Injections for spinal stenosis showed no clear effects but the power of this analysis is relatively weak with only 8 trials identified.

F Selective nerve blocks aid in diagnosing the symptomatic level(s) in patients with predominantly radicular symptoms, as multilevel stenosis is commonly seen. Limiting surgical decompression to symptomatic levels minimizes iatrogenic instability. One must always remember that radiographic stenosis often does not correlate well with symptom severity.

G Surgery is indicated in patients who have significant neurologic involvement, such as marked or progressive muscle weakness, gait changes, loss of dexterity, severe claudication symptoms, and progressive loss of bowel and bladder function. Acute onset cauda equina syndrome is rare, and requires emergent decompression. Consider surgery in patients who have failed to achieve pain relief through conservative treatment. The basic goal of surgery for spinal stenosis is to achieve decompression without compromising spinal stability.

SUGGESTED READING

Chou R, Hashimoto R, Friedly J, et al. Epidural corticosteroid injections for radiculopathy and spinal stenosis: a systematic review and meta-analysis. Ann Intern Med. 2015;163(5):373-81.

Ghobrial GM, Oppenlander ME, Maulucci CM, et al. Management of asymptomatic cervical spinal stenosis in the setting of symptomatic tandem lumbar stenosis: a review. Clin Neurol Neurosurg. 2014;124:114-8.

Hopp E. Spine: State of the Art Reviews: Spinal Stenosis. Philadelphia: Hanley & Belfus; 1987.

Lispon SJ, Branch WT. Low back pain. In: Branch WT (Ed). Office Practice of Medicine, 2nd edition. Philadelphia, WB Saunders; 1987. p. 875.

Loeser JD, Bigos SJ, Fordyce WE, et al. Low back pain. In: Bonica JJ (Ed). The Management of Pain, 2nd edition. Philadelphia: Lea & Febiger; 1990. p. 1468.

Melancia JL, Francisco AF, Antunes JL. Spinal stenosis. Handb Clin Neurol. 2014;119:541-9.

Wood GW. Other disorders of the spine. In: Crenshaw AH (Ed). Campbell's Operative Orthopaedics. St. Louis: Mosby; 1987. p. 3347.

CHAPTER 74

Ankylosing Spondylitis

Jorgensen AY, Lai TT, Galang E, Arora SS, Chang Chien GC

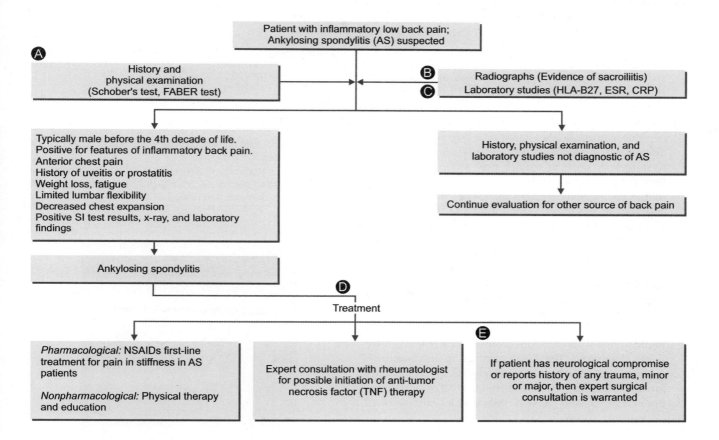

Ankylosing spondylitis (AS) is a chronic systemic inflammatory disease affecting primarily the sacroiliac (SI) joints and spine. The disease affects young adults between the second to fourth decades of life, and it has a 5:1 male predominance. It is likely passed down through genetic transference with an environmental component. AS commonly affects the low back starting in the SI joints and ascending to involve the lumbar, thoracic, and cervical spine. Diagnosis is mainly accomplished by a thorough history and physical examination. The hallmark sign is pain along the SI joints with or without restriction in range of motion depending on the severity. As the disease progresses, involvement extends to the hips with contractures and ankylosis. Radiographs may show erosion in the SI joints, but this may take 7–10 years of disease progression before it is evident on plain x-rays. Magnetic resonance imaging (MRI) will show evidence of AS, but exact MRI diagnostic criteria are still in development.

Late stages of AS result in structural changes to the spine with characteristic changes in alignment. As the disease progresses cephalad from the SI joints, the inflammatory processes effect the tendon insertions into the spine. Specifically, the classic disease progression involves ankylosis of the facet joints and inflammatory changes at the discovertebral junctions. The inflammation at the discovertebral junctions progresses to ossifications and ankylosis of the disc spaces. While the spinal ankylosis progresses, the spinal alignment tends to tip forward and the spine tends to fuse in kyphosis. With advanced changes, patients cannot maintain upright posture or horizontal gaze.

While the bony elements and discs of the spine are undergoing fusion as part of the AS process, they are also undergoing overall loss of bone density, i.e. osteoporosis. The spine fuses but also becomes structurally weaker. This is a problem because the fused spine needs to be structurally strong, but the AS process tends to weaken it. As a result, even minor low energy trauma can result in fracture. In the setting of an ankylosed spine, a single fracture will propagate anterior to posterior across the entire spine. A patient with a sudden new onset of pain after minor trauma may have a highly unstable fracture.

A *History and Physical Examination:* The patient will complain of low back pain that is chronic (>3 months). The onset is insidious without a history of an inciting event and usually before age 45. Pain and stiffness exacerbated by immobilization, usually worse at night or in the morning upon waking. Pain is usually eased by physical activity and exercise. On physical examination, tenderness may be elicited via palpation along the SI joint or the posterior-superior iliac spine. Physical examination findings may be normal early in the disease course. Other maneuvers for diagnosis of SI joint pain such as the Flexion, ABduction, External Rotation (FABER) test may be positive, but are also nonspecific. A reported history of iritis, uveitis, gastrointestinal infections (Crohn's or ulcerative colitis), or a family history of AS may also contribute to a diagnosis.

B *Diagnostic Imaging:* AS may not be ruled out with a negative radiograph since it may take 7–10 years of disease progression for evidence of sclerosis of the SI joints. Nevertheless, imaging studies may show characteristic findings that can confirm the diagnosis in the proper clinical setting. Radiographic changes are first noted in the SI joints and later in the lumbar spine, then the thoracic spine, and last in the cervical spine. The radiographic findings of sacroiliitis are typically symmetric and exhibit a "blurring" of the subchondral bone plate, followed by erosions and sclerosis of the adjacent bone. MRI can detect early signs of sacroiliitis that are negative on plain radiographs.

C Laboratory workup should include HLA-B27, C-reactive protein (CRP), and erythrocyte sedimentation rate (ESR). The ESR and CRP may or may not be elevated. HLA-B27 is found in 90% of patients with AS; however, a positive result is not diagnostic. The Assessment of Spondyloarthritis international Society (ASAS) developed specific criteria for the diagnosis and classification of AS with patients under age 45 who present with a chief complaint of chronic low back pain **(Fig. 1)**.

D *Treatment:* The initial treatment of AS is to reduce pain and stiffness with the goal of maintaining function. Treatment should begin with conservative therapy to include a regimented physical therapy program. Early referral to a physical therapist is advised. Extension based exercises are prescribed to prevent kyphosis and maintain flexibility, range of motion, and pulmonary function. Good seating, with appropriate back support, is helpful. A firm bed, sleeping on the back, and no more than one pillow may help to avoid cervicothoracic flexion contractures. If pain prevents effective therapy, the first line pharmacological treatment for AS is nonsteroidal anti-inflammatory drugs (NSAIDs). NSAIDs should be prescribed as initial therapy to relieve the pain associated with AS and have been shown to improve joint pain and morning stiffness. Local injection of corticosteroids may also be used to provide targeted relief. Facet joint injections or SI joint injections may provide temporary relief to facilitate physical therapy or daily exercise. Though there is limited evidence to support its use, a rheumatologist may initiate other immune-suppressing

ASAS classification criteria for axial spondyloarthritis (SpA) In patients with ≥ 3 months back pain and age at onset <45 years	
Sacroiliitis on imaging* plus ≥1 SpA feature#	HLA-B27 plus ≥2 other SpA features#
#SpA features • Inflammatory back pain • Arthritis • Enthesitis (heel) • Uveitis • Dactylitis • Psoriasis • Crohn's/colitis • Good response to NSAIDs • Family history for SpA • HLA-B27 • Elevated CRP	*Sacroiliitis on imaging • Active (acute) inflammation on MRI highly suggestive of sacroiliitis associated with SpA • Definite radiographic sacroiliitis according to modified New York criteria

Fig. 1: The Assessment of Spondyloarthritis International Society (ASAS) criteria for classification of axial spondyloarthritis (to be applied in patients with chronic back pain and age at onset of back pain <45 years)
Source: Sieper J, Rudwaleit M, Baraliakos X, et al. The Assessment of Spondyloarthritis International Society (ASAS) handbook: a guide to assess spondyloarthritis. Ann Rheum Dis. 2009;68 (Suppl 2):ii1-44.

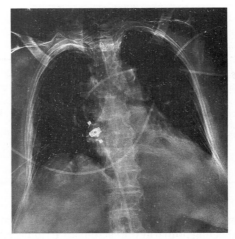

Fig. 2: Anteroposterior chest radiograph of a 70-year-old female patient after fall at home with pain in the back and the right ankle. This patient was neurologically intact. She was also diagnosed with a right ankle fracture, and additional imaging of the spine was performed

medications such as disease-modifying antirheumatic drugs (DMARDs) or tumor necrosis factor (TNF) blockers.

E Surgery may be considered, such as total hip arthroplasty for flexion contracture and ankylosis. Spinal surgery may be indicated for fracture or pseudoarthrosis. Traumatic fracture pattern may be difficult to appreciate on plain x-rays. These patients should undergo CT scan or MRI to rule out a fracture, and if a fracture is found it may be highly unstable and require surgical fixation. A missed fracture in AS is likely to result in a neurologic injury if not surgically stabilized **(Figs. 2-4)**. Spinal osteotomy is

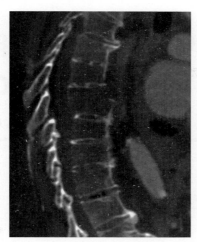

Fig. 3: Computed tomography (CT) scan of chest showing unstable three-column fracture of the T8 level. Fractures can often be difficult to discern on regular x-rays. Full appreciation of the fracture and diagnosis often depends on advanced imaging

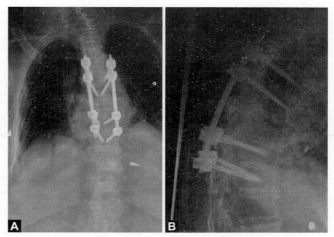

Figs 4A and B: Patient after surgical stabilization of the fracture

indicated for correction of disabling deformity. The classic spinal deformity in late stages of AS is a progressively stooped posture from kyphosis of the cervical, thoracic, and lumbar spine. This can be exacerbated by flexion contracture of the hips. In these advanced cases, a combination of total hip arthroplasty to correct the hip flexion contracture and spinal osteotomy to correct the stooped forward posture of the spine and restore horizontal gaze and upright posture may be required.

SUGGESTED READING

Bennett AN, Marzo-Ortega H, Rehman A, et al. The evidence for whole-spine MRI in the assessment of axial spondyloarthropathy. Rheumatology (Oxford). 2010;49(3):426-32.

Kubiak EN, Moskovich R, Errico TJ, et al. Orthopaedic management of ankylosing spondylitis. J Am Acad Orthop Surg. 2005;13(4): 267-78.

Marzo-Ortega H, McGonagle D, Bennett AN. Magnetic resonance imaging in spondyloarthritis. Curr Opin Rheumatol. 2010; 22(4):381-7.

Poddubnyy D, Gaydukova I, Hermann KG, et al. Magnetic resonance imaging compared to conventional radiographs for detection of chronic structural changes in sacroiliac joints in axial spondyloarthritis. J Rheumatol. 2013;40(9):1557-65.

Sieper J, Rudwaleit M, Baraliakos X, et al. The Assessment of Spondyloarthritis International Society (ASAS) handbook: a guide to assess spondyloarthritis. Ann Rheum Dis. 2009;68 (Suppl 2):ii1-44.

Sudoł-Szopińska I, Kwiatkowska B, Włodkowska-Korytkowska M, et al. Diagnostics of sacroiliitis according to ASAS criteria: a comparative evaluation of conventional radiographs and MRI in patients with a clinical suspicion of spondyloarthropathy. Preliminary results. Pol J Radiol. 2015;80:266-76.

CHAPTER 75

Failed Back Surgery Syndrome

Levin D, Anitescu M

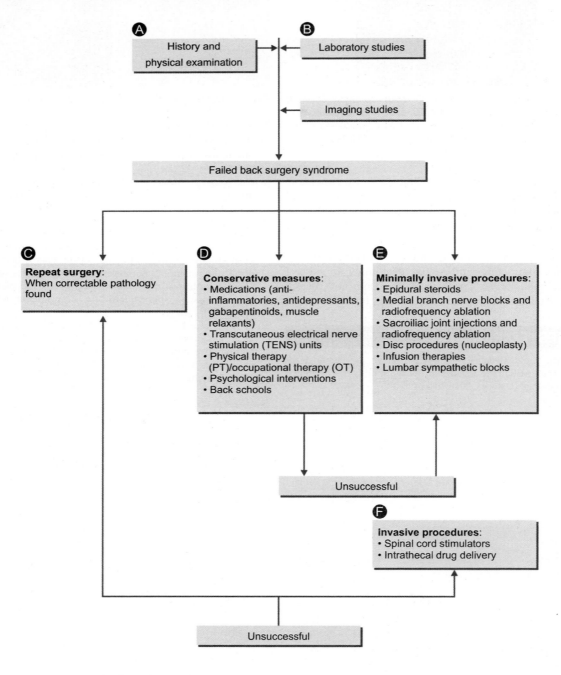

Failed back surgery syndrome (FBSS), also known as failed laminectomy syndrome, postlumbar surgery syndrome, or failed back syndrome, is a condition characterized by persis-tence of pain following spine surgery. The pain may manifest as persistence of preoperative symptoms, can be secondary to intraoperative events or a result of postoperative changes.

Among the causes are suboptimal patient selection for surgery, incorrect surgical diagnosis, poor surgical technique, failure to achieve surgical goals and recurrent pathology. A vast array of pathologies lead to FBSS which may stem from any anatomical region of the vertebral column, including bony abnormalities, joint problems, muscular changes, neural disorders and psychological difficulties. The most common are foraminal stenosis, internal disc disruption syndrome, pseudoarthrosis and neuropathic radicular pain. Management of pain in FBSS depends on the identification and treatment of the underlying pathophysiology; there are no controlled studies defining algorithms to guide diagnosis and treatment. A basic algorithm should include a pain history and targeted physical examination. Any red flags or surgically correctable factors should be identified to prompt early surgical referral. If a decision against the need for surgical intervention is made, an interdisciplinary approach to conservative management is indicated. If pain persists, the algorithm advances to interventional options, the choice of which is determined by symptomatology. Lastly, invasive procedures, such as spinal cord stimulation, intrathecal drug delivery systems and ultimately revision surgery complete the algorithm.

Ⓐ *History and Physical Examination*: The history includes previous surgical diagnosis, the number and types of previous surgery, medication use, the extent of disability and psychological screening. The work and home environment also are considered. A comprehensive treatment plan taking into account these factors is required for a good outcome. The physical examination rules out serious pathology and identifies the source of pain. Waddell's signs, such as superficial or non-anatomic tenderness, overreaction to stimuli or reports of pain during evaluations that are not designed to be painful assess nonorganic physical findings. Vital signs, posture, gait and function are evaluated. The lumbar spine is inspected and palpated, noting surgical scars, vertebral alignment, points that elicit pain, step-offs and indentations indicative of spondylolisthesis. Range of motion, muscle power and sensation are ascertained to note radiating pain associated with movement. Special tests, such as the femoral stretch test, straight leg raise and Lasègue's sign nerve tension are performed. Lastly, a combination of sacroiliac joint (SIJ) provocative tests rule out the SIJ as the source of pain.

Myofascial pain syndrome (MFPS) usually coexists with almost all failed laminectomy syndrome. Early treatment may alleviate many symptoms and allow therapy to progress more rapidly.

Ⓑ Diagnostic studies should first focus on mechanical causes for pain that are unrelated to the prior spine surgery. Abdominal or pelvic inflammatory disease, infectious or malignant lesions such as a psoas abscess, pancreatic cancer and spinal cord neoplasms or vertebral metastatic lesions can be ruled out with laboratory studies and appropriate imaging.

Imaging conventionally begins with standing plain radiographs with flexion and extension of the spine to evaluate alignment, degeneration and stability. These studies, however, are limited for identifying soft tissue pathology. Magnetic resonance imaging (MRI) further delineates the soft tissue pathology of epidural fibrosis, residual disc herniation, stenosis, discitis and pseudomeningocele. MRI produces sharper images of soft tissues, but computed tomography (CT) is more effective in imaging bony abnormalities. A CT myelogram is recommended for patients with contraindications to MRI.

Interventional diagnostic investigations are indicated when etiology cannot be definitively determined by noninvasive imaging. Such procedures include lumbar medial branch blocks (help diagnosis of facet joint pain), SIJ blockade (targets SIJ pain), selective nerve root block (isolates a specific spinal level as the source of pain), and provocative lumbar discography (identifies intervertebral disc pathology). Further details regarding these procedures can be found throughout Section 9.

Ⓒ Repeat operations are performed only if there is overwhelming evidence of a surgically correctable lesion. Examples include spinal stenosis, retained disc material or a recurrent disc at the site of previous surgery, a new herniated nucleus pulposus, or instability or a pseudarthrosis at the site of a previous fusion. This condition may be diagnosed by CT or MRI but requires confirmation by lateral flexion-extension radiography, as motion is not always the cause of pain. One study that evaluated repeat operations in patients with failed laminectomy found that greater than 79% of 67 patients had some pain relief and 43% discontinued narcotic use. Of these, 12% experienced good relief of pain, and the complication rate was 13%. Approximately 50% of patients with epidural fibrosis showed a poor result after repeat surgery. The best outcomes after repeat surgery were associated with four factors: (1) a pain-free interval of more than 1 year after the initial surgery, (2) a complete myelographic block, (3) a true disc herniation, and (4) evidence of instability.

Ⓓ *Conservative Treatment*: Although algorithms for treatment exist in the literature, no single algorithm has proven superior. Of the data available from large systemic reviews, most pertain to chronic low back pain (CLBP). With respect to controlled trials pertaining to FBSS, data are scarce. There is agreement in the literature, however, that pain management in FBSS should be interdisciplinary, tailored to the individual patient and guided by diagnostic studies discussed above. The objectives of directed therapy are primarily functional restoration and improvement in quality of life and activities of daily living.

Conservative medical management (CMM) includes pharmacologic treatment, physical therapy and psychological therapy. Nonsteroidal anti-inflammatory drugs (NSAIDs) should be given an adequate trial of at least 8 weeks before changing or discontinuing medications. If one class of NSAIDs fails, one from another class is substituted. In 2007, the American Pain Society and American College of Physicians published guidelines containing good evidence to support the use of antidepressants and fair evidence that acetaminophen, tramadol, benzodiazepines and gabapentin are effective for pain relief. Selective norepinephrine and serotonin reuptake inhibitors (SNRIs) and tricyclic antidepressants (TCAs) are also efficacious in achieving analgesia. Opioids can help as a short-term regimen, but their efficacy as a long-term medication has not been proven and should not be used routinely in FBSS.

Several large systemic reviews have demonstrated the efficacy of exercise therapy, although no evidence exists that any one program is superior. Transcutaneous electrical nerve stimulation (TENS) is often effective in decreasing pain in MFPS, degenerative joint disease, and nerve root irritation and should be attempted if any of those pain generators are suspected.

"Back school" should be started in patients when no further interventional therapy is planned. This school involves operant conditioning, behavior modification, physical or occupational therapy, and often drug detoxification.

Psychological interventions, such as cognitive behavioral therapy (CBT), are a component of the multidisciplinary care plan. Biofeedback, relaxation techniques, and hypnosis also may be useful. A recent review concluded that multidisciplinary biopsychosocial rehabilitation programs resulted in better outcomes for long-term pain and disability compared to usual care or physical treatments.

E *Interventional Treatment*: Although lumbar epidural steroid injections (LESIs) have commonly been used to treat both CLBP and FBSS, the efficacy of such treatment is controversial and technique-dependent. Caudal, interlaminar and transforaminal methods have been employed. In general, epidural fibrosis, altered anatomy and instrumentation decrease the success rate and increased the complication rate of LESIs in FBSS; the success rate can be partly improved by using fluoroscopic guidance for placement of the injection.

Minimally invasive procedures targeting the facet joint (source of pain in up to 16% of FBSS patients) are used in patients with predominantly axial pain. These include intra-articular injection and medial branch block. Following two diagnostic positive medial branch nerve blocks, radiofrequency ablation of the nerve has been shown to be effective.

For patients with evidence of significant epidural fibrosis, adhesiolysis may be performed. This technique involves placement of a catheter into the epidural space and an injection is targeted based on epidurography. Several studies have examined efficacy of various injectates, including normal saline, hypertonic saline and hyaluronidase. Conclusive evidence of superiority of any injectate has yet to be demonstrated. Epidural adhesiolysis also may be achieved endoscopically, providing the advantage of direct visualization of epidural fibrosis. No randomized, controlled trials comparing endoscopic and percutaneous techniques exist.

When patients with FBSS are diagnosed with SIJ dysfunction, steroid deposit into the joint can be of benefit. In refractory cases, radiofrequency denervation of the SIJ innervation can be attempted.

Lastly, several minimally invasive procedures exist to relieve discogenic pain from annular fibrosis, such as thermal treatments, as well as procedures to relieve disc pressure, including nucleoplasty and mechanical decompression. Patients with central pain syndromes may suffer persistent neuropathic pain from nerve entrapment because of epidural scarring and fibrosis. These patients may benefit from intravenous infusions with lidocaine or ketamine. If pain is sympathetically mediated, lumbar sympathetic blocks can be tried.

F If conservative management fails, more invasive therapies may be considered: spinal cord stimulator (SCS) implantation, peripheral nerve stimulation, intrathecal analgesic delivery implant systems and revision surgery. SCS requires an electrode to be placed within an epidural space. The stimulator is traditionally thought to function by means of the "gate control theory" and gamma-aminobutyric acid (GABA)-mediated inhibition, although further research has demonstrated components of supraspinal modulation. Patients with FBSS and neuropathic leg pain demonstrated benefit from SCS of greater than 50% relief of leg pain at 6-, 12- and 24-month follow-up. SCS is not without risk. Evolving technologies in spinal cord stimulation, including high-frequency stimulation and burst stimulation, have shown promise in improving efficacy in terms of pain reduction as well as expanding the breadth of application beyond only radicular back pain, while at the same time removing unpleasant paresthesias from the equation. Peripheral nerve stimulation has also been used as a less invasive form of neuromodulation, but few data support its efficacy. Similarly, good evidence is lacking to support the use of intrathecal analgesic delivery implant systems in patients with nonmalignant pain. This technique should be reserved for situations in which all other strategies have failed.

SUGGESTED READING

Abdi S, Datta S, Trescot AM, et al. Epidural steroids in the management of chronic spinal pain: a systematic review. Pain Physician. 2007;10:185-212.

Anitescu M, Amish P, Simon A. (2009). Benefit of functional anesthetic discography, a double-blinded, prospective surgery outcome study. [online] Available from http://*www.asaabstracts. com/strands/asaabstracts/abstract.htm;jsessionid=604AE91212 2181067F93F1AB86E1270F?year=2009&index=3&absnum=474.* [Accessed January, 2017].

Anitescu M, Leung D. (2008). Functional anesthetic discogram (FAD), an improved technique for evaluation of intervertebral disc. [online] Available from http://*www.asaabstracts. com/strands/asaabstracts/abstract.htm;jsessionid=EAED45D55 97B461023CAC71647125FDC?year=2008&index=3&absnum=36.* [Accessed January, 2017].

Avellanal M, Diaz-Reganon G, Orts A, et al. One-year results of an algorithmic approach to managing failed back surgery syndrome. Pain Res Manag. 2014;19:313-6.

Bogduk N. Practice Guidelines for Spinal Diagnostic and Treatment Procedures, 1st edition. San Francisco: International Spine Intervention Society; 2004.

Chan CW, Peng P. Failed back surgery syndrome. Pain Med. 2011; 12(4):577-606.

Chou R, Huffman LH. Medications for acute and chronic low back pain: a review of the evidence for an American Pain Society/American College of Physicians clinical practice guideline. Ann Intern Med. 2007;147:505-14.

de Vos CC, Bom MJ, Vanneste S, et al. Burst spinal cord stimulation evaluated in patients with failed back surgery syndrome and painful diabetic neuropathy. Neuromodulation. 2014;17(2):152-9.

Dreyfuss P, Schwarzer AC, Lau P, et al. Specificity of lumbar medial branch and L5 dorsal ramus blocks. A computed tomography study. Spine (Phila Pa 1976). 1997;22(8):895-902.

Fredman B, Nun MB, Zohar E, et al. Epidural steroids for treating "failed back surgery syndrome": is fluoroscopy really necessary? Anesth Analg. 1999;88:367-72.

Gilron I, Bailey JM, Tu D, et al. Morphine, gabapentin, or their combination for neuropathic pain. N Engl J Med. 2005;352:1324-34.

Gilron I, Bailey JM, Tu D, et al. Nortriptyline and gabapentin, alone and in combination for neuropathic pain: a double-blind, randomised controlled crossover trial. Lancet. 2009;374:1252-61.

Guyer RD, Patterson M, Ohnmeiss DD. Failed back surgery syndrome: diagnostic evaluation. J Am Acad Orthop Surg. 2006;14:534-43.

Hoffman BM, Papas RK, Chatkoff DK, et al. Meta-analysis of psychological interventions for chronic low back pain. Health Psychol. 2007;26:1-9.

Horton WC, Daftari TK. Which disc as visualized by magnetic resonance imaging is actually a source of pain? A correlation between magnetic resonance imaging and discography. Spine (Phila Pa 1976). 1992;17(6 Suppl):S164-71.

Hussain A, Erdek M. Interventional pain management for failed back surgery syndrome. Pain Pract. 2014;14(1):64-78.

Kamper SJ, Apeldoorn AT, Chiarotto A, et al. Multidisciplinary biopsychosocial rehabilitation for chronic low back pain: Cochrane systematic review and meta-analysis. BMJ. 2015;350:h444.

Kapural L, Yu C, Doust MW, et al. Novel 10-kHz high-frequency therapy (HF10 therapy) is superior to traditional low-frequency spinal cord stimulation for the treatment of chronic back and leg pain: the SENZA-RCT randomized controlled trial. Anesthesiology. 2015;123(4):851-60.

Khadilkar A, Odebiyi DO, Brosseau L, et al. Transcutaneous electrical nerve stimulation (TENS) versus placebo for chronic low-back pain. Cochrane Database Sys Rev. 2008;(4):CD003008.

Kumar K, Taylor RS, Jacques L, et al. Spinal cord stimulation versus conventional medical management for neuropathic pain: a multicentre randomised controlled trial in patients with failed back surgery syndrome. Pain. 2007;132(1-2):179-88.

Kumar K, Taylor RS, Jacques L, et al. The effects of spinal cord stimulation in neuropathic pain are sustained: a 24-month follow-up of the prospective randomized controlled multicenter trial of the effectiveness of spinal cord stimulation. Neurosurgery. 2008;63(4):762-70.

Lee F, Jamison DE, Hurley RW, et al. Epidural lysis of adhesions. Korean J Pain. 2014;27:3-15.

Nath S, Nath CA, Pettersson K. Percutaneous lumbar zygapophysial (facet) joint neurotomy using radiofrequency current, in the management of chronic low back pain: a randomized double-blind trial. Spine (Phila Pa 1976). 2008;33:1291-7.

North RB, Kidd D, Shipley J, et al. Spinal cord stimulation versus reoperation for failed back surgery syndrome: a cost effectiveness and cost utility analysis based on a randomized controlled trial. Neurosurgery. 2007;61(2):361-9.

Ragab A, DeShazo RD. Management of back pain in patients with previous back surgery. Am J Med. 2008;121:272-8.

Rodrigues FF, Dozza DC, Oliveira CR, et al. Failed back surgery syndrome: casuistic and etiology. Arq Neuropsiquitr. 2006;64(3B):757-61.

Rowlingson J. Epidural steroids in treating failed back surgery syndrome. Anesth Analg. 1999;88:240-2.

Slipman CW, Shin CH, Patel RK, et al. Etiologies of failed back surgery syndrome. Pain Med. 2002;3(3):200-14.

Vad VB, Bhat AL, Lutz GE, et al. Transforaminal epidural steroid injections in lumbosacral radiculopathy: a prospective randomized study. Spine (Phila Pa 1976). 2002;27:11-6.

Van Goethem JW, Parizel PM, Jinkins JR. Review article: MRI of the postoperative lumbar spine. Neuroradiology. 2002;44:723-39.

Zhang TC, Janik JJ, Grill WM. Mechanisms and models of spinal cord stimulation for the treatment of neuropathic pain. Brain Res. 2014;1569:19-31.

Zucco F, Ciampichini R, Lavano A, et al. Cost-effectiveness and cost-utility analysis of spinal cord stimulation in patients with failed back surgery syndrome: results from the PRECISE study. Neuromodulation. 2015;18(4):266-76.

Lumbar Facet Joint Pain

Benedetti EM, Garg S

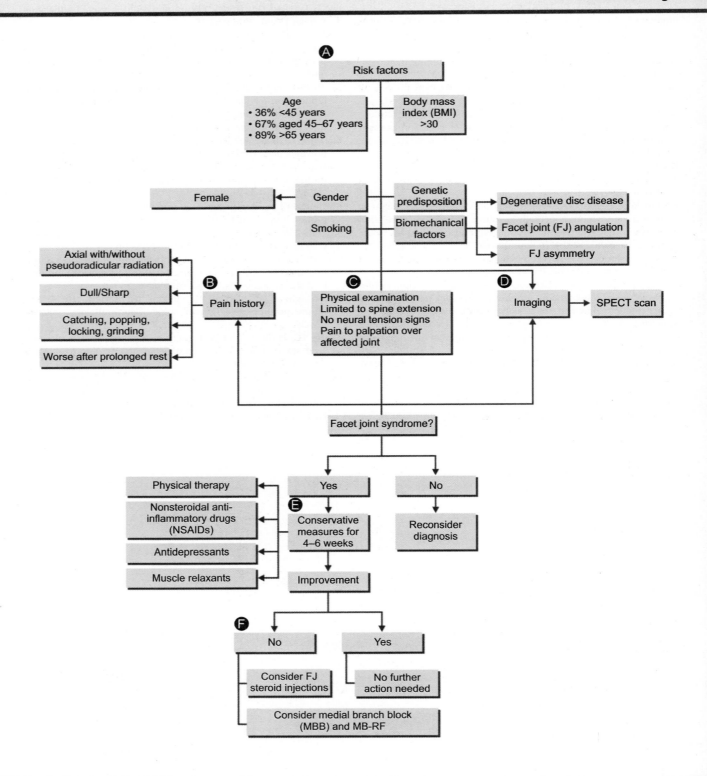

Although low back pain is typically considered to be multifactorial, it is estimated that facet arthropathy accounts for up to 40% of all cases of low back pain, 15% of work injury-related back pain, and 16% of cases of postlaminectomy syndrome. The zygapophyseal joints are true synovial joints and are located in the posterolateral aspect of the lumbar vertebral column. Formed between the inferior articular process of the upper vertebra and the superior articular process of the lower vertebra, in the lumbar region, they are located obliquely and inclined nearly to a vertical orientation. Their surface is curvilinear, being a limiting factor for rotation. These paired joints, in conjunction with the intervertebral disc, form one spinal motion unit and on their integrity lies the stability of the segment.

A *Risk Factors:* Risk factors for chronic low back pain include increasing age, weight (body mass index [BMI] >30), female gender, genetic factors, and smoking. Factors that affect spine biomechanics, including degenerative disc disease (load distribution) and facet tropism (angulation, alignment and symmetry), are thought to be major factors in the development and progression of facet joint osteoarthritis (FJOA). The decreasing paraspinal mass, especially with aging, compromises the vertebral column stabilization and allows poor segmental biomechanics, further adding to joint degeneration.

B *History:* Pain arising from the facet joints is usually described as localized over low back region with some degree of radiation into the lower extremities, predominantly into the buttocks and posterior thighs but possibly extending below the knee and into the calves (pseudoradicular radiation pattern). It is not, however, routinely associated with paresthesias. Characteristically, the pain is described as dull and achy but can be sharp in quality. It is typically associated with "catching," "locking," "grinding," and "popping" with motion and axial pain tends to predominate over the lower extremity discomfort. Prolonged standing, rotation, extension, and walking tend to exacerbate pain (induced by facet loading). Rest may improve pain temporarily, but after a more prolonged period of repose, pain on initiation of motion tends to become severe. Paraspinal muscle contracture is commonly coexistent.

C *Physical Examination:* No physical examination maneuver is pathognomonic for facet joint syndrome. Mechanical tests targeted to load the facet joints induce disc, ligamentous and neural traction as well. Pain on palpation over the affected articulation, and pain worsening with spine extension and/or extension-rotation is typically, however, considered to be a positive marker. Strength of the paraspinal muscles is commonly preserved and no neural tension signs are identified on examination.

D *Imaging:* Lack of clinical-radiological (x-ray, computed tomography (CT), magnetic resonance imaging [MRI]) correlation is significant. Single-photon emission CT (SPECT) scans may be used to identify facets with 99mTc-methylene diphosphonate (MDP) uptake, identifying those joints with increased activity, so as to decrease the number of injections performed. However, radiotracer activity may not correlate with the clinical presentation, making it a cost-ineffective alternative.

Computed tomography imaging demonstrates moderate or severe facet joint osteoarthritic changes in 36% of adults aged less than 45 years, 67% of adults aged 45–64 years, and 89% of those aged 65 years and older in the absence of low back pain. Studies have not shown a positive correlation between the severity of MRI abnormal findings and the presence of low back pain.

E *Conservative Measures:* Conservative treatment modalities for at least a trial of 4–6 weeks are of paramount importance and include core strengthening and education on body mechanics. Anti-inflammatory medications, muscle relaxants and antidepressants may be used as part of a multimodal approach.

F *Invasive Treatment:* Facet joints have a complex and dual innervation. Afferents from each joint travel via the medial branch of the primary dorsal ramus. Each joint receives innervation from two adjacent medial branches, one at the same level and one from the level above. The anatomical landmark used to target the medial branch in the lumbar spine is the junction of the transverse process and the superior articular process (except at the L5 level where the medial branch is found at the junction of the superior articular process of S1 and the sacral ala). Fluoroscopically-guided local anesthetic medial branch blocks are still proposed by some as the gold standard for diagnosing FJOA. Diagnosis, however, cannot be reliable after using single blocks when their rate of false positives is as high as 40%. Despite the widespread use of facet interventions, intra-articular facet joint injections, regardless of the technique, whether periarticular or intracapsular, have limited evidence (Level III) while lumbar medial branch neurotomy has Level II evidence for short- and long-term efficacy (see Chapter 133 Medial Branch Blocks and Chapter 136 Radiofrequency Ablation).

SUGGESTED READING

Boswell MV, Manchikanti L, Kaye AD, et al. A best-evidence systematic appraisal of the diagnostic accuracy and utility of facet (zygapophysial) joint injections in chronic spinal pain. Pain Physician. 2015;18:E497-533.

Brinjikji W, Luetmer PH, Comstock B, et al. Systematic literature review of imaging features of spinal degeneration in asymptomatic populations. AJNR Am J Neuroradiol. 2015;36(4):811-6.

Cohen P, Huang JH, Brummett C. Facet joint pain—advances in patient selection and treatment. Nat Rev Rheumatol. 2013;9(2):101-16.

Gellhorn AC, Katz JN, Suri P. Osteoarthritis of the spine: the facet joints. Nat Rev Rheumatol. 2013;9(4):216-24.

Manchikanti L, Kaye AD, Boswell MV, et al. A systematic review and best evidence synthesis of the effectiveness of therapeutic facet joint interventions in managing chronic spinal pain. Pain Physician. 2015;18(4):E535-82.

Nachemson AL. Newest knowledge of low back pain. A critical look. Clin Orthop Relat Res. 1992;(279):8-20.

Schwarzer AC, Wang SC, Bogduk N, et al. Prevalence and clinical features of lumbar zygapophysial joint pain: a study in an Australian population with chronic low back pain. Ann Rheum Dis. 1995;54(2):100-6.

Van Zundert J, Vanelderen P, Kessels AG. Re: Chou R, Atlas SJ, Stanos SP, et al. Nonsurgical interventional therapies for low back pain: a review of the evidence for an American Pain Society Clinical Practice guideline. Spine (Phila Pa 1976) 2009;34:1078-93. Spine (Phila Pa 1976). 2010;35(7):841; author reply 841-2.

Sacroiliac Joint Pain

Kroski WJ, Hommer DH

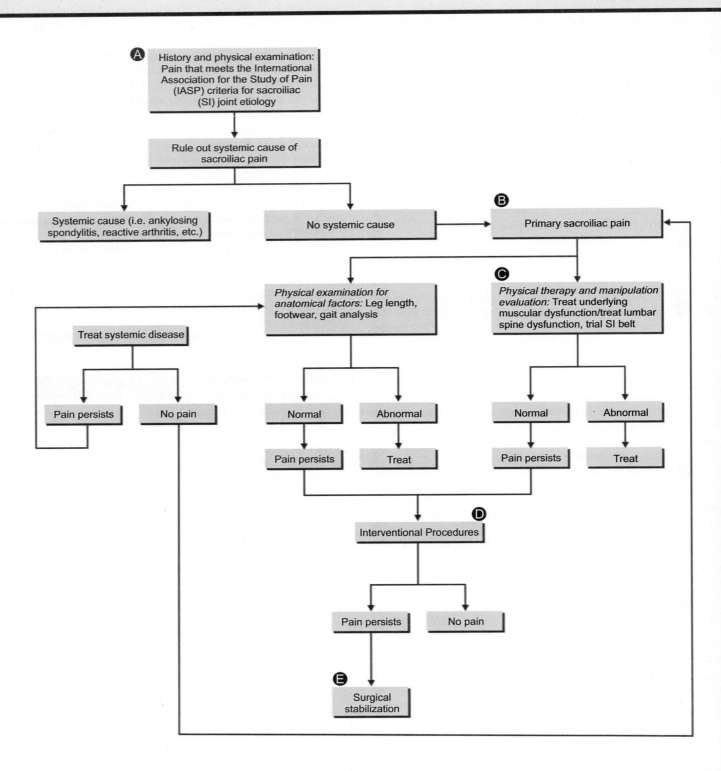

The sacroiliac joint (SIJ) is the largest axial joint in the body and is characterized as a large, diarthrodial synovial joint, which differs from others in that it has fibrocartilage in addition to hyaline cartilage. Only the anterior, inferior one-third of the joint is a true synovial joint. The SIJ is composed of well-developed ligaments and irregular articular surfaces to help limit motion and add stability as well as to serve as a site for muscle attachment. The SIJ has a complicated and ambiguous innervation. Many investigators believe the fibers from L4 to S3 comprise the major innervation to the posterior SIJ. More recent cadaveric studies suggest a contribution from S4, which innervates the sacroiliac ligaments in up to 59% of individuals, and a branch of the superior gluteal nerve that enters the long posterior sacroiliac ligament in 42% of cadavers. Another recent cadaver study suggested that 90% of the innervation of the posterior sacroiliac complex arises from the lateral branches of the primary dorsal rami of S1, S2, and S3. The novel discovery of these anatomical features has gained attention with the possibility of using radiofrequency ablation (RFA) to treat the affected nerves supplying the joint.

The SIJ can be a significant source of low back pain with a prevalence varying from 15% to 30% in patients with low back pain. In patients with persistent low back pain, magnetic resonance imaging (MRI) studies have found that SIJ disease is presented in approximately 20% of patients. In normal, healthy subjects, studies have shown noxious stimulation of the joint evokes low back pain, which can radiate into the gluteal region and upper posterior thigh.

Ⓐ *History and Physical Examination:* The diagnosis of SIJ disease is typically based on clinical symptoms, physical examination, degenerative changes seen on imaging studies, and diagnostic interventional procedures. The International Association for the Study of Pain (IASP) has proposed a set of diagnostic criteria for the diagnosis of SIJ pain: (1) pain must be present in the region of the SIJ, (2) stressing the SIJ by clinical tests reproduces pain, and (3) selectively infiltrating the symptomatic joint with local anesthetic relieves the pain. It is important to note that this criterion is set forth for mechanical disorders of the SIJ and fails to encompass sacroiliitis, ankylosing spondylitis, or other seronegative spondyloarthropathies. These more ominous systemic diseases should be ruled out and treated appropriately prior to assuming that the patient is suffering from primary SIJ pain. SIJ pain may be caused by multiple etiologies making the diagnosis difficult and a universally accepted "gold standard" for diagnosis does not exist.

Ⓑ Primary SIJ disease is frequently the result of an accident or a traumatic injury, but can also result from an unguarded or unexpected movement, e.g. a chronic strain in the workplace, or repetitive activity such as swinging a golf club. Studies have shown up to 80% of patients with low back pain materializing from SIJ dysfunction (SIJD) also have malalignment of the pelvis owing to unilateral pelvic anterior tilt. Pain in the SIJ often leads to alterations of the gait cycle. Individuals with a leg length discrepancy (LLD) appear to be at an increased risk for SIJD due to abnormal mechanical alignment and high loads passing through the SIJ. Removing or correcting these stresses may relieve the problem.

Ⓒ *Conservative Treatment:* The SIJD is influenced by muscle force and ligament tension and can be utilized to resist SIJ shear forces. Foot mechanical features are important in order to modify the movement of abnormal lower extremities associated with SIJD. Foot orthotics can be useful as clinical intervention tools. In particular, the heel height appears to enhance the muscle activity of the erector spinae, enabling it to fire faster and control increased lumbar flexion, eventually increasing lumbar lordosis. Stability can be attained through alteration of specific anatomic features which influence friction and tension of both muscles and ligaments crossing the SIJ. The erector spinae, hamstrings, and gluteus muscles appear to be most important for the stability of the SIJ. A physical therapy program which includes manipulation can greatly benefit the shear forces across the SIJ in patients with SIJD. Gluteus muscle weakness, accompanied with shortening of the hamstrings, should be a main focus during physical therapy. Manipulation techniques used may involve high-velocity, low-amplitude thrust techniques or muscle energy techniques; a form of precise contract-relax stretching which mobilizes the joint. Alone, manipulation may be sufficient to resolve many SIJ problems and should be considered. An SIJ belt worn tightly around the pelvis just below the level of the iliac crest and above the pubic symphysis while weight-bearing can be useful in hypermobile patients, providing stability by compressing the SIJ.

Ⓓ If conservative therapy fails, several interventional procedures are available to diagnose and treat SIJD. SIJ local anesthetic blocks have been promoted as the best available tool to identify painful SIJs as the source of low back pain. The benefit for dual block over a single block is unclear. This should not be confused with lateral branch blocks, which may anesthetize both the SIJ as well as the posterior ligamentous structures. Injection of corticosteroids into the SIJ is also a common procedure performed for the treatment of SIJ pain. Cooled radiofrequency neurotomy is a recent therapeutic treatment for SIJD and is supported only by observational studies at this time but appears to be better supported than conventional radiofrequency neurotomy.

Ⓔ Surgical intervention may be required when pain is intractable or disabling, and when all other possibilities have been excluded. A review of 16 peer-reviewed journal articles that included 430 patients receiving open or minimally invasive SIJ fusion concluded that surgical fusion could be beneficial but given the general lack of evidence of efficacy, serious consideration should be given to non-surgical treatments before attempting surgery. Underscoring this admonition, the same review found major complication rates were as high as 20%.

SUGGESTED READING

Arnbak B, Jensen TS, Egund N, et al. Prevalence of degenerative and spondyloarthritis-related magnetic resonance imaging findings in the spine and sacroiliac joints in patients with persistent low back pain. Eur Radiol. 2016;26(4):1191-203.

Barton CJ, Coyle JA, Tinley P. The effect of heel lifts on truck muscle activation during gait: a study of young healthy females. J Electromyogr Kinesiol. 2009;19:598-606.

Bird AR, Payne CB. Foot function and low back pain. Foot. 1999; 9:175-80.

Cho BY, Yoon JG. The effect of gait training with shoe inserts on the improvement of pain and gait in sacroiliac joint patients. J Phys Ther Sci. 2015;27(8):2469-71.

Cohen S, Chen Y, Neufeld NJ. Sacroiliac joint pain: a comprehensive review of epidemiology, diagnosis, and treatment. Expert Rev Neurother. 2013;13(1):99-116.

Cohen SP. Sacroiliac joint pain: a comprehensive review of anatomy, diagnosis, and treatment. Anesth Analg. 2005;101(5):1440-53.

Cole AJ, Dreyfuss P, Stratton SA. The sacroiliac joint: a functional approach. Clin Rev Phys Rehabil Med. 1996;8:125-52.

Cox R, Fortin J. The anatomy of the lateral branches of the sacral dorsal rami: implications for radiofrequency ablation. Pain Physician. 2014;17:459-64.

Forst SL, Wheeler MT, Fortin JD, et al. The sacroiliac joint: anatomy, physiology and clinical significance. Pain Physician. 2006;9:61-7.

Fortin JD, Dwyer AD, West S, et al. Sacroiliac joint: pain referral maps upon applying a new injection/arthrography technique. Part 1: Asymptomatic volunteers. Spine (Phila Pa 1976). 1994;19:1475-82.

Han D. Muscle activation of paraspinal muscles in different types of high heels during standing. J Phys Ther Sci. 2015;27:67-9.

Lippitt AB. Recurrent subluxation of the sacroiliac joint: diagnosis and treatment. Bull Hosp Jt Dis. 1995;54:94-102.

Maigne JY, Aivaliklis A, Pfefer F. Results of sacroiliac joint double block and value of sacroiliac pain provocation tests in 54 patients with low back pain. Spine (Phila Pa 1976). 1996;21:1889-92.

Massoud Arab A, Reza Nourbakhsh M, Mohammadifar A. The relationship between hamstring length and gluteal muscle strength in individuals with sacroiliac joint dysfunction. J Man Manip Ther. 2011;19(1):5-10.

McGrath MC, Zhang M. Lateral branches of dorsal sacral nerve plexus and the long posterior sacroiliac ligament. Surg Radiol Anat. 2005;27:327-30.

Schwarzer AC, Aprill CN, Bogduk N. The sacroiliac joint in chronic low back pain. Spine (Phila Pa 1976). 1995;20:31-7.

Van Wingerden JP, Vleeming A, Buyruk HM, et al. Stabilization of the sacroiliac joint in vivo: verification of muscular contribution to force closure of the pelvis. Eur Spine J. 2004;13:199-205.

Zaidi HA, Montoure AJ, Dickman CA. Surgical and clinical efficacy of sacroiliac joint fusion: a systematic review of the literature. J Neurosurg Spine. 2015;23:59-66.

SECTION 8

Upper Extremity Pain

Miles Day

referred for surgical repair. Studies report mixed results for return to sport success in athletes who undergo MCL repair, and MCL repair should not be offered as an elective procedure for enhanced sport performance.

D Common posterior elbow pain etiologies include posterior impingement, olecranon bursitis, triceps tendinopathy (see Chapter 83 Tendinopathy: Upper Extremities), and crystal arthropathy. For posterior impingement, underlying osteoarthritis should be considered. Management typically includes physical therapy and taping/bracing. If conservative measures fail, surgical intervention can be considered for removal of impinging posterior bone or soft tissue. For olecranon bursitis, treatment typically starts with anti-inflammatory medications, rest and compression. If these measures fail, aspiration of bursa contents followed by injection of corticosteroid and local anesthetic can be performed. However, prior to any injection of a corticosteroid, physicians must be aware of the possibility of an infectious etiology. Poor relief after injection may require surgical excision of bursa.

BONE AND JOINT

E When evaluating bone or joint pain complaints in the elbow, fractures or dislocations must be considered and possibly ruled out with radiographs if history or examination warrants.

F Rheumatoid arthritis (RA) is the most common type of elbow arthritis, followed by post-traumatic osteoarthritis (OA), while primary OA is uncommon. Crystal arthropathies including gout and pseudogout should also be considered. Imaging and joint aspiration can assist with diagnosis. All elbow arthritic pathologies are typically first treated conservatively with appropriate medical management and physical therapy. Patients with refractory RA or advanced OA who continue to have symptoms can be referred for surgical intervention.

G The most common fracture around the elbow is the radial head fracture, and most are minimally displaced or non-displaced and difficult to appreciate on radiographs. Immobilize with a removable device, and commence range of motion exercises early. Complete healing can be expected in 6–8 weeks.

H Any fractures involving the supracondylar humerus, and fractures that are displaced more than 2 mm, unstable, or preventing elbow extension should be evaluated for surgical repair.

I Posterior dislocation is the most serious acute injury to the elbow due to its potential neurovascular complications. First, assess for distal pulses, and if pulses are present, obtain imaging prior to reduction. If pulses are absent, urgent reduction is necessary. If pulses remain absent after reduction, urgent surgical intervention is necessary. Radiographs that reveal a nondisplaced or minimally displaced fracture can be managed with a sling. Displaced or large fractures involving the coronoid or capitellum require surgical repair.

A common complication after any elbow injury, either an acute injury or degenerative disease, is elbow contracture. To prevent elbow stiffness and loss of function, compliance to therapeutic exercise or range of motion prescriptions are paramount. Aggressive physical therapy and progressive splinting are the first lines of therapy for contracture, and surgical debridement techniques are a later line of therapy.

SUGGESTED READING

Brukner P, Khan K. Clinical Sports Medicine. Australia: McGraw Hill; 2012.

Dones VC 3rd, Grimmer K, Thoirs K, et al. The diagnostic validity of musculoskeletal ultrasound in lateral epicondylalgia: a systematic review. BMC Med Imaging. 2014;14:10.

Erickson BJ, Harris JD, Chalmers PN, et al. Ulnar collateral ligament reconstruction: anatomy, indications, techniques, and outcomes. Sports Health. 2015;7(6):511-7.

Miller MD, Thompson SR, Hart JA. Review of Orthopaedics, 6th edition. Philadelphia: Elsevier; 2012.

CHAPTER 80

Wrist and Hand Pain

Patel S, Soliman S

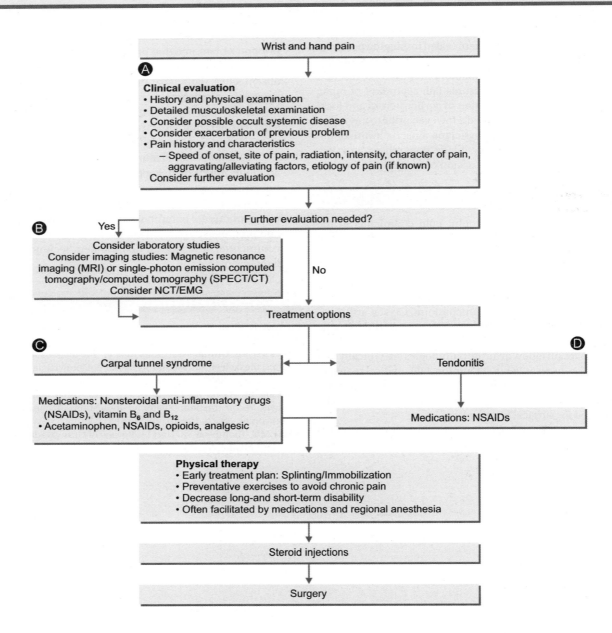

Pain in the wrist and hand is not an unusual problem, especially in the younger population as people perform repetitive tasks which can lead to carpal tunnel. For the most part, however, hand pain is largely unexplained. From an 8000-person study, it was determined that only about 20–25% of hand pain has a determinant as to the cause of the pain, leaving a large section of hand pain completely unexplained. Besides the idi-

opathic causes of hand pain, the major determinants of hand pain and their respective frequency include female sex (frequency of 58.3%), age more than or equal to 70 years (30.8%), manual occupation (29.4%), and radiological hand osteoarthritis (28.3%).

Ⓐ The wrist and hand have complex anatomy that goes beyond the course of this text. Briefly, the wrist consists of the radius, ulna, carpal, and metacarpals (the bases). For this type of pain, a thorough history and physical examination must be obtained. Important aspects to note include trauma or surgery to the area, similar involvement in other areas of the body (if musculoskeletal), repetitive or provocative motions in the area, timing of the pain, as well as if workers compensation is being sought. Any examination should first begin with inspection of both hands and note any visual differences. Take note of any atrophy which can signal neurological complication. Range of motion should include flexion of 80°, extension of 70°, as well as pronation and supination of 90°. Vascular examination should be included with a minimal of radial and ulnar palpation and capillary refill. Sensory and motor testing should focus on each nerve including the median, radial, and ulnar nerves. Palpation should be used to examine the osseous and nonosseous structures.

B Oftentimes a good history and physical examination can lead to the cause, or potential treatment of wrist and hand pain. When this is not enough, or if there is concern for a possible fracture, x-ray imaging is often employed. If this is negative, further imaging may be required as the wrist and hand are composed of very small, complex structures. In someone with chronic pain, one can consider either a magnetic resonance imaging (MRI) or a single-photon emission computed tomography/computed tomography (SPECT/CT) scan. Although an MRI is recommended by the American College of Radiology for someone with negative x-rays and chronic wrist pain, a SPECT/CT has been shown to yield a much higher specificity (1.0 for CT vs 0.2 for MRI), although a lower sensitivity (0.71 for CT and 0.86 for MRI). Additionally, for nerve damage, electrodiagnostic studies must be considered.

C One of the many complaints of hand pain will likely be carpal tunnel syndrome. Carpal tunnel syndrome, which involves the median nerve of the wrist, is the most common compressed nerve in the body, accounting for about 0.2% of all outpatient office visits in 2006 and is estimated to be present in 3.8% of the population. It has a prevalence rate of up to 9% in females and 6% in males. Oftentimes, the areas of discomfort and pain go beyond the distribution of the median nerve, however. The patient may report numbness, tingling, and clumsiness in the hand, often worse at night. If suspected, a nerve conduction study might be in order. The aims of this include (1) confirming median nerve damage, (2) quantifying the severity of damage, and (3) defining the neuropathophysiology. Ultrasound has also been used in diagnoses and has shown to have about the same sensitivity as electrodiagnostic studies. Treatment includes steroid injections,

nonsteroidal anti-inflammatory drugs (NSAIDs), vitamins B$_6$ and B$_{12}$, splinting, and surgery. Regarding duration of treatment, a study review indicates that strong and moderate evidence existed to support the use of nonsurgical procedures including splinting, steroid injections, ergonomic keyboards, and ultrasound for short and medium term treatments. Steroid injections and oral steroids are the only treatments to have shown any long-term relief. High-dose steroids showed greater medium-term relief but the same long-term relief.

D Given the complexity of the wrist and hand, there are numerous treatment options depending on the underlying cause. For a tendonitis, conservative measures should first be attempted. This includes immobilization and possibly NSAIDs. If this is not sufficient, corticosteroid injections may be done knowing that this can acutely make the tendon weaker. If no significant relief occurs, a surgical consult may be in order. The surgery performed often depends on whether the pathology is in a vascular or avascular area, with the former involving repair and the latter involving debridement. The scope of the surgeries performed is vast and beyond the scope of this text. Important, however, is confounding factors such as depression which may affect outcomes. A recent study noted that for minor hand surgery such as for carpal tunnel syndrome, psychosocial factors such as depression play a "notable proportion of the variation" in pain after surgery.

SUGGESTED READING

Dahaghin S, Bierma-Zeinstra S, Reijman M, et al. Prevalence and determinants of one month hand pain and hand related disability in the elderly (Rotterdam study). Ann Rheum Dis. 2005;64(1):99-104.

Huellner MW, Bürkert A, Schleich F, et al. SPECT/CT versus MRI in patients with nonspecific pain of the hand and wrist–a pilot study. Eur J Nucl Med Mol Imaging. 2012;39(5):750-9.

Huisstede B, Hoogvliet P, Randsdorp M, et al. Carpal tunnel syndrome. Part I: Effectiveness of nonsurgical treatments—a systematic review. Arch Phys Med Rehabil. 2010;91(7):981-1004.

Ibrahim I, Khan W, Goddard N, et al. Carpal tunnel syndrome: a review of the recent literature. Open Orthop J. 2012;6:69-76.

Vezeridis P, Yoshioka H, Han R, et al. Ulnar-sided wrist pain. Part I: anatomy and physical examination. Skeletal Radiol. 2010; 39(8):733-45.

Vranceanu A, Jupiter J, Mudgal C, et al. Predictors of pain intensity and disability after minor hand surgery. J Hand Surg Am. 2010;35(6):956-60.

Watanab A, Souz F, Vezeridis P, et al. Ulnar-sided wrist pain. II. Clinical imaging and treatment. Skeletal Radiol. 2010;39(9): 837-57.

Werner R, Andary M. Electrodiagnostic evaluation of carpal tunnel syndrome. Muscle Nerve. 2011;44(4):597-607.

CHAPTER 81

Entrapment Syndromes: Upper Extremities

Bhavaraju-Sanka R

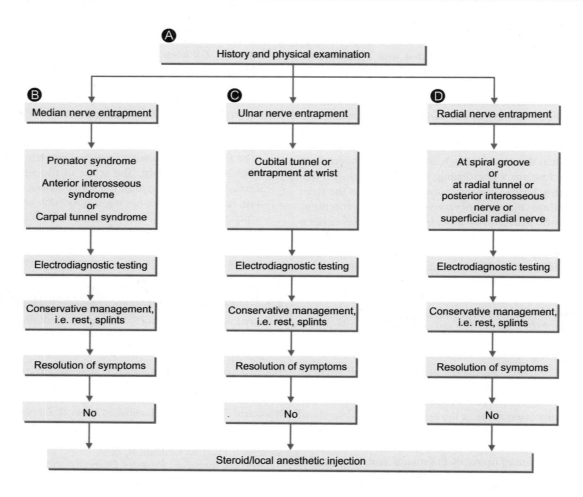

Entrapment syndromes are neuropathies that are caused by compression of peripheral nerves. The nerve can be compressed at any site, but it is more common at specific anatomical sites where the nerve travels through a fibro-osseous or fibrocartilaginous structure or a muscle.

A *History and Physical Examination:* The patients commonly present with symptoms of pain, paresthesia or weakness distal to the entrapment. Clinical history, neurological examination and electrodiagnostic studies can help localize the site of entrapment. Recently, imaging techniques can also help with lesion localization.

B *Median Nerve Entrapment Neuropathies:* The median nerve is formed from branches from the median (C5/6/7) and lateral cord (C8/T1) of the brachial plexus. It has no branches until it reaches the elbow where it supplies

pronator teres, flexor carpi radialis and flexor digitorum superficialis before giving a pure motor branch, the anterior interosseous nerve. It continues in the forearm to go through the carpal tunnel to supply the muscles of the hand (lumbricals I and II, abductor pollicis brevis, lateral half of flexor pollicis brevis and opponens pollicis) and provide sensory supply to the three and half digits.

Median nerve entrapment can be seen commonly at three sites:

1. *Pronator Teres Syndrome:* It is a relatively rare disorder caused by compression of the median nerve between the ulnar and the humeral heads of pronator teres muscle **(Fig. 1)**. Trauma, muscle hypertrophy, persistent median artery or anomalous fibrous band between pronator teres and flexor digitorum super-

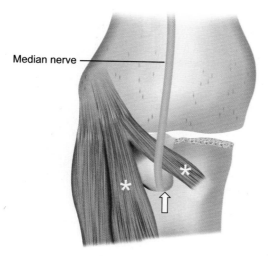

Fig. 1: Proximal median nerve in the anterior elbow
Stars: Two heads of pronator teres; Open arrow: Flexor digitorum superficialis

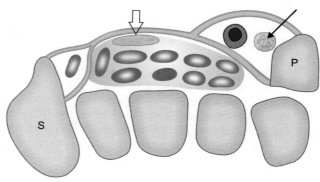

Fig. 2: Carpal tunnel and Guyon's canal at the level of pisiform bone
Open arrow: Median nerve; Arrow: Ulnar nerve; S: Scaphoid; P: Pisiform

ficialis can predispose to this entrapment syndrome. The syndrome is associated with strenuous activities involving frequent pronation/supination of the forearm or weight lifting. Patients present with pain in the forearm near pronator teres muscle along with numbness in the ventral aspect of forearm and wrist. Pain and paresthesias can be elicited by maneuvers like resisted pronation of the forearm with extended elbow or resisted flexion of index/middle finger at proximal interphalangeal joint. The loss of sensation on the thenar eminence differentiates this from carpal tunnel syndrome. Weakness is uncommon but spares pronator teres.

Electrodiagnostic studies show normal distal latency with mild slowing of conduction velocity in the forearm. Injection of corticosteroids in pronator teres may be diagnostic by relieving the pain. Definitive treatment is by surgical exploration and decompression.

Proximal median nerve compression can also be seen at the ligament of Struthers, a fibrous band between the supracondylar process and an anomalous spur on the anteromedial aspect of humerus. The nerve can be compressed proximal to the branch to pronator teres along with brachial artery above the elbow. Examination shows weakness and electrographic changes affecting flexor carpi radialis and pronator teres muscles. Similar presentation can be seen with compression by accessory bicipital aponeurosis.

2. *Anterior Interosseous Nerve Syndrome:* Anterior interosseous nerve (AIN) syndrome or Kiloh-Nevin syndrome is caused by injury or compression of anterior interosseous nerve. The nerve can be compressed due to fracture, mass or hematoma. As it is a pure motor nerve, the clinical presentation involves weakness without sensory deficits. Patients often complain of

pain in the elbow and forearm region. The weakness affects pronator quadratus, flexor pollicis longus and flexor digitorum profundus I/II. These three muscles can be evaluated by asking the patient to make an OK sign (pronate forearm, flex distal phalanges of thumb, index fingers to make an "O"). The patients will form a triangle (pinch sign) instead of a circle. Routine median nerve studies fail to show any electrographic abnormalities. Needle examination shows selective denervation of AIN innervated muscles. The treatment is surgical decompression but some of the lesions may be related to neuritis and spontaneous recovery is seen within 6–12 months.

3. *Carpal Tunnel Syndrome:* Carpal tunnel syndrome (CTS) is the most prevalent mononeuropathy with a lifetime risk of approximately 10%. It affects 3–6% of general population. The median nerve passes with nine digital flexor tendons in the carpal tunnel formed by carpal bones on the floor and transverse ligament on the roof **(Fig. 2)**.

Women are more commonly affected than men (3:1) with peak incidence in fifth or sixth decade. The symptoms usually start in the dominant hand and are often bilateral. Idiopathic CTS is seen in patients with congenitally small carpal tunnel or with repetitive movements of the wrist. Other predisposing conditions include pregnancy, endocrine disorders like hypothyroidism or acromegaly, immune disorders like lupus, rheumatoid arthritis or sarcoidosis, systemic disorders like diabetes or renal failure, infections, etc. Masses like ganglion cysts, lipoma, neurofibroma or hematoma can also cause compression of the nerve.

Clinical presentation includes paresthesias in the hand that often awaken the patient from sleep. The pain can often radiate to the elbow or shoulders, mimicking high median neuropathy or cervical radiculopathy. The compression can affect the vasomotor nerve fibers causing color changes, sweating, and swelling of the hand. Examination shows reduced sensation in the median three and half digits with weakness of the abductor pollicis brevis muscle. The sensory changes spare the thenar eminence. Tinel's sign (paresthesia in the distribution of the nerve caused by tapping the nerve) can be elicited at the carpal tunnel. Passive flexion of the wrist can cause or worsen paresthesias in 30–120 seconds (Phalen's sign).

Electrodiagnostic studies show slowing of sensory conduction across the transverse carpal ligament early in the condition. Later motor studies show prolonged distal latency and reduced motor amplitudes. Needle examination can show denervation in abductor pollicis brevis. Treatment includes splinting with a neutral splint, corticosteroid injections and surgical decompression. Surgical decompression is often affective but 7–30% of the patients can have residual or recurrent symptoms.

Conservative measures have a success rate of 60% in patients who have only one risk factor (age >50 years, Phalen's test at 30 seconds, symptoms for more than 10 months, constant paresthesias, associated trigger fingers). Those patients who have three risk factors have a failure rate of 93%, and those with four or more have a 100% failure rate. In patients who have thenar softening atrophy or whose symptoms persist for at least 6 months despite conservative measures, surgery should be considered.

C *Ulnar Nerve Entrapment Neuropathies:* Ulnar nerve is a continuation of medial cord of brachial plexus and has supply from (C7) C8 and T1 nerve roots. After entering the forearm it passes through cubital tunnel and supplies flexor carpi ulnaris and flexor digitorum profundus III/IV. In the distal forearm, it gives rise to dorsal ulnar cutaneous branch that supplies the medial aspect of the dorsum of the hand. It then enters the hand through Guyon's canal and gives a superficial branch that supplies the skin of the hypothenar eminence, medial one and hand digits. The deep muscular branch supplies adductor digiti minimi, opponens digiti minimi, flexor digiti minimi, adductor pollicis, flexor pollicis brevis (medial half), palmar and dorsal interossei and lumbricals III and IV.

The common sites of ulnar entrapments are at the elbow (cubital tunnel) or wrist (Guyon's canal).

- *Cubital Tunnel Syndrome:* It is the second most common entrapment neuropathy seen in humans. Ulnar nerve can get compressed in the retroepicondylar groove or at the humeroulnar aponeurotic arcade (arcuate ligament) between the two head of flexor carpi ulnaris **(Fig. 3)**. Repeated trauma at the epicondyle due to dislocation of the nerve, compression by abnormal fascial bands, soft tissue masses predispose to this neuropathy. Frequent use of the hand with elbow in flexed position can narrow the tunnel and exacerbate the symptoms.

The initial presentation includes numbness and paresthesias in the fifth digit and ulnar half of the fourth digit. Weakness and atrophy is prominent in the first dorsal interosseous muscle. Patient can develop partial claw hand due to contractures of flexor digitorum profundus III/IV. Examination shows sensory changes in the dorsal and palmar aspects of the ulnar hand

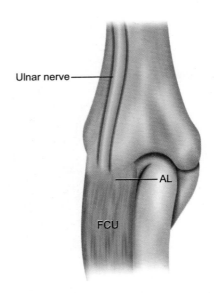

Fig. 3: Posterior view of ulnar nerve at elbow
FCU, flexor carpi ulnaris; AL, arcuate ligament

below the wrist. Weakness and wasting can be seen in first dorsal interossei and other ulnar innervated hand muscles, flexors of the distal phalanx of digits III/IV and flexor carpi ulnaris.

Nerve conduction studies show slowing of velocity (drop by 10 m/sec) across the cubital tunnel. There may also be a drop in the motor amplitude above the level of compression. Inching study with stimulation of the nerve at multiple points across the elbow can help localize the site of compression by showing a drop in amplitude (25% drop considered diagnostic). The sensory studies to the ring finger and dorsum of the hand (dorsal ulnar) may show abnormalities. Studies performed with elbow flexed have a better yield in detecting abnormalities. Denervation may be seen in all ulnar innervated muscle.

Treatment is usually conservative. Avoiding repeated trauma to the nerve like frequent or prolonged flexion of the elbow and resting the elbow on hard surfaces are recommended. Surgical treatment is considered for patients who fail conservative treatments or have a severe neuropathy. It includes decompression of the nerve and/or anterior transposition. Functional improvement is better if operated early in the course. If there is significant motor deficit, there is a 30% chance of persistent deficits.

- *Entrapment at Guyon's Canal:* Ulnar nerve enters the hand through Guyon's canal, a fibro-osseous tunnel in the anteromedial aspect of the wrist **(Fig. 2)**. The transverse carpal ligament forms the roof of the canal while hypothenar muscles and flexor retinaculum forms the floor. It is bound medially by pisiform bone with pisohamate ligament and laterally by the hook of hamate. It contains the ulnar artery and the nerve. Compression of the nerve here can be due to a space occupying lesion, anomalous muscle, aneurysm of ulnar artery or trauma. Inside the canal, the nerve bifurcates to the superficial sensory and deep motor branches.

Compression of the nerve before the bifurcation (Type 1) causes sensory and motor symptoms. Sensory changes involve the palmar surface of the medial hand, fifth and half of fourth digit. Sensation to the dorsum of the hand, which is supplied by the dorsal ulnar cutaneous nerve is preserved. Weakness is seen in all ulnar-innervated muscles in the hand. If the compression affects purely the deep branch (Type 2), there is no sensory deficit. The weakness affects all ulnar innervated hand muscles except palmaris brevis.

Motor nerve conduction studies to adductor digiti minimi or first dorsal interossei show reduced amplitude and/or prolonged latency. In type 1 lesions, the sensory responses are also affected with prolonged latencies and reduced amplitude. The studies also show sparing of involvement of dorsal ulnar cutaneous response.

Surgical decompression usually relieves the compression.

D *Radial Nerve Entrapment Syndromes:* The radial nerve is a continuation of the posterior cord of the brachial plexus and receives innervation from C5 to C8 nerve roots. Before entering the spiral groove, it supplies the three heads of triceps and anconeus muscles. In the spiral groove, it winds around the humerus posteriorly and enters the medial aspect of the arm. It gives the posterior antebrachial cutaneous nerve in the groove. After emerging from the spiral groove, it supplies brachioradialis and extensor carpi radialis longus. It enters the forearm between the brachialis and brachioradialis lateral to biceps muscle at the level of the lateral epicondyle. Here, it bifurcates into superficial radial nerve (sensory branch) and posterior interosseous nerve (motor branch) **(Fig. 4)**. The posterior interosseous nerve supplies supinator, abductor pollicis longus, extensor carpi radialis longus and brevis, extensor carpi ulnaris, extensor digitorum communis, extensor digiti minimi, extensor pollicis longus and brevis, and extensor indicis. The superficial radial nerve surfaces in the distal third of the forearm and supplies the lateral aspect of the dorsum of the hand.

Radial nerve compression can occur proximally in the axilla from improper use of crutches can cause weakness in all the radial innervated muscles with sensory changes in posterior arm, posterior forearm and lateral aspect of the dorsum of hand.

- *Compression at the Spiral Groove:* The radial nerve can be compressed in the spiral groove from trauma (supracondylar humeral facture) or from prolonged pressure from inactivity (Saturday night palsy) in intoxicated circumstances. Weakness is seen in all radial innervated muscles except the triceps (causes wrist and finger drop). Sensory loss is seen in the whole radial nerve distribution.

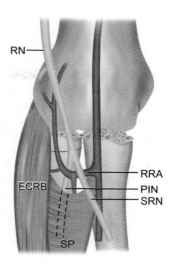

Fig. 4: Radial nerve at the elbow. Proximal edge of the supinator muscle forms the arcade of Frohse
RN, radial nerve; SRN, superficial radial nerve; PIN, posterior interosseous nerve; RRA, recurrent radial artery; ECRB, extensor carpi radialis brevis; SP, supinator muscle

Nerve conduction studies show slowing across the spiral groove. Conduction block may also be seen. If the compression is severe or prolonged, axon loss may occur. In these situations, distal sensory studies show reduced amplitude and needle examination shows neuropathic changes in radial innervated muscles except triceps. Pressure palsies show recovery spontaneously in 6–8 weeks, but may be slower and incomplete if associated with axon loss.

- *Radial Tunnel Syndrome:* It is the most common site of radial nerve entrapment. The tunnel is located at the proximal forearm. It is about 2 cm long and extends between the distal humerus (radiocapitellar joint) and the supinator muscle. It is bound medially by brachialis and biceps tendon and laterally by extensor carpi radialis longus and brevis, which also form the roof.

Compression can affect the radial nerve or the posterior interosseous nerve at five possible sites. Proximally at the origin of extensor carpi radialis longus or by a fibrous band in the muscle, at the thickened fascia proximal to the radiocapitellar joint, at leash of Henry by radial recurrent vessels, at arcade of frohse at proximal border of supinator or at the distal border of supinator muscle. Masses, edema, inflammation, repeated hand/wrist movements or trauma can predispose to compression.

Patients present with deep achy or burning pain, distal to the lateral epicondyle with radiation to proximal forearm. Pain is exacerbated with wrist extension or pronation of forearm. Point of tenderness can be located 3–4 cm distal to the lateral epicondyle within the extensor muscles.

Sensory loss can sometimes be seen in the distribution of superficial radial nerve and weakness may affect the extensors of wrist and fingers.

Conservative treatments like avoiding repetitive movements of the wrist, nonsteroidal anti-inflammatory agents, splinting or injection of corticosteroids into the radial tunnel can help relieve the symptoms.

- *Entrapment of Posterior Interosseous Nerve:* This terminal motor branch can be compressed as it enters the supinator muscle or inside the muscle. This can be associated with rheumatoid arthritis, trauma, mass lesions, and hereditary neuropathies like Charcot-Marie-Tooth disease type 1.

Patient presents with pain over the lateral aspect of proximal forearm or elbow. Weakness can be seen in extensors of the wrist and the forearm sparing the supinator muscle. There are no sensory changes.

Nerve conduction studies show slowing of motor conduction across the site of compression. Superficial radial nerve study shows a normal response. Needle examination shows neuropathic changes in extensors of the wrist and forearm.

Surgical decompression of the nerve usually results in recovery.

- *Superficial Radial Nerve Entrapment:* Isolated compression of this nerve can be seen at the wrist due to tight wristbands or handcuffs. It causes a condition also called cheiralgia paresthetica. Motor conduction studies are normal with sensory studies showing prolonged latency and reduced amplitude. Examination shows sensory loss in the lateral aspect of the dorsum of the hand with no weakness. Recovery is spontaneous with removal of the offending agent.

SUGGESTED READING

Don Q, Jacobson JA, Jamadar DA, et al. Entrapment neuropathies in the upper and lower limbs: anatomy and MRI features. Radiol Res Pract. 2012;2012:1-13.

Kimura J. Electrodiagnosis in Diseases of Nerve and Muscle: Principles and Practice, 3rd edition. Oxford University Press; 2001.

Wheeless III CR. Wheeless' Textbook of Orthopedics, 2014. [online] Also available *http://www.wheelessonline.com*.

CHAPTER
82

Bursitis: Upper Extremity

Bouffard KJ, Marshall B

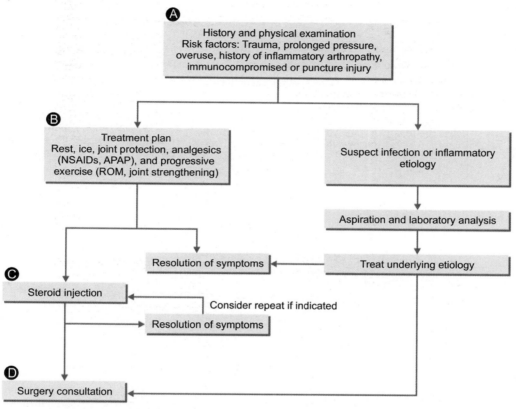

APAP, N-acetyl-p-aminophenol; NSAIDs, nonsteroidal anti-inflammatory drugs; ROM, range of motion

Bursae are thin, sac-like, fluid-filled structures which are enclosed by synovium and are commonly located between muscles to reduce friction as they glide over each other or on top of prominent bony protrusions to facilitate the movement of muscle or tendon across these structures or to protect them from direct trauma. Bursitis, or irritation of these structures, can result from inflammatory or noninflammatory processes. Common causes of bursitis include direct trauma, prolonged pressure, overuse or highly intensive activity, infection, and gout or inflammatory arthritis. Bursitis can present as an acute syndrome usually characterized by pain with focal tenderness, swelling, and possible discomfort with associated decreased joint range of motion (typically due to pain with further compression of the affected bursa). It can also present as a chronic syndrome in which swelling and thickening of the bursa predominates with relatively modest associated pain and tenderness.

Aspiration and laboratory analysis of the bursal fluid is indicated in cases where septic, gouty, or inflammatory bursitis is suspected. Imaging is typically not required though with deeper bursae, concern for alternative pathology, or to guide aspiration/injection, magnetic resonance imaging (MRI) or ultrasound may be helpful. Management can vary based on the location and etiology of the bursitis **(see Table 1)** but generally with the notable exception of septic or inflammatory bursitis, the condition is self-limited and the goal of the clinician should be to relieve the immediate symptoms with ice, nonsteroidal anti-inflammatory drugs (NSAIDs), joint protection, and possibly corticoid steroid injection (CSI) as well as prevent disability with exercises to maintain range of motion (ROM) and strengthen surrounding musculature. Rarely, bursitis will continue to persist despite these measures and may require surgical excision or evacuation. A general clinical algorithm of the diagnosis and

Table 1: Common sites of bursitis in the upper extremity

Bursa	Pathophysiology	A: History	A: Physical	B, C, D: Treatment
Scapulothoracic	Abnormal dynamics between anterior surface of scapula and rib cage	Repetitive overhead or reaching activities with increasing scapular pain and "snapping" Often can be thin, kyphotic patients with poor muscular development	Scapulothoracic crepitus, pain over superiomedial angle, scapular asymmetry or winging Occasionally soft tissue masses may precipitate, higher propensity for malignancy in older patients should prompt earlier use of diagnostic imaging	RIJA* May benefit from early PT for postural and scapulothoracic training If unimproved consider careful corticoid steroid injection (CSI) given possibility of pneumothorax Surgery indicated in refractory cases
Subacromial/ Subdeltoid	Compression of the tissues in the subacromial space, systemic inflammatory disorders (e.g. rheumatoid arthritis [RA], polymyalgia rheumatica)	Shoulder pain worsened with overhead activity Common referral pattern to deltoid insertion Often disrupts sleep or report inability to sleep on effected side	Not clinically distinct from impingement syndrome (will have positive Neers, Hawkins testing) and often associated with pathology of rotator cuff	RIJA* PT for posture and shoulder girdle strengthening is helpful Consider diagnostic and therapeutic CSI if no evidence of complete rotator cuff tear If does not improve with conservative measures should consider advanced imaging and surgical consultation as appropriate
Olecranon	Usually direct and/or repetitive trauma but also common site for septic, rheumatic and gouty bursitis	Focal pain and swelling over olecranon process of ulna	Elbow extension worsens pain in elbow effusion but unchanged in bursitis	RIJA* Low threshold for aspiration with analysis given superficiality and relatively high risk on nonaseptic etiology Corticosteroid injection and surgery should be reserved for highly resistant cases given the high incidence of infection

Note: *Rest, Ice, Joint protection, Analgesia (NSAIDs, Acetaminophen)

management of suspected bursitis is presented in this chapter's flow chart.

SUGGESTED READING

Cuccurullo S. Physical Medicine and Rehabilitation Board Review, 3rd edition, 2015.

Harrison AK, Flatow EL. Subacromial impingement syndrome. J Am Acad Orthop Surg. 2011;19(11):701-8.

Sayegh ET, Strauch RJ. Treatment of olecranon bursitis: a systematic review. Arch Orthop Trauma Surg. 2014;134(11):1517-36.

Warth RJ, Spiegl UJ, Millett PJ. Scapulothoracic bursitis and snapping scapula syndrome: a critical review of current evidence. Am J Sports Med. 2015;43(1):236-45.

CHAPTER 83

Tendinopathy: Upper Extremities

Bouffard KJ, Caldwell M

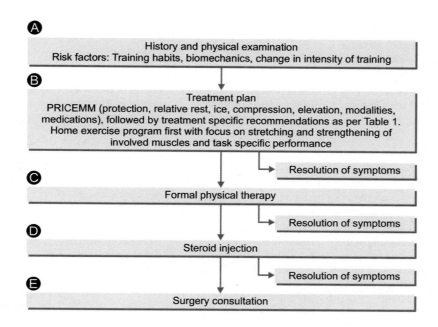

A
History and physical examination
Risk factors: Training habits, biomechanics, change in intensity of training

B
Treatment plan
PRICEMM (protection, relative rest, ice, compression, elevation, modalities, medications), followed by treatment specific recommendations as per Table 1. Home exercise program first with focus on stretching and strengthening of involved muscles and task specific performance

→ Resolution of symptoms

C
Formal physical therapy

→ Resolution of symptoms

D
Steroid injection

→ Resolution of symptoms

E
Surgery consultation

Tendinopathy is a clinical syndrome characterized by tendon thickening and chronic localized pain that can be caused by acute trauma or more commonly by overuse. The pathophysiology of tendinopathy is important to understand when treating the patient. When inflammation of a tendon occurs as the primary cause of tendinopathy, this is referred to as tendinitis. When minimal to no inflammation is present, as is often seen in chronic tendinopathy, the term tendinosis is more appropriate and is considered a failed healing response.

The difference between the two is very important for management as acute tendonitis is treated differently than chronic tendinosis.

The upper extremity tendons that are commonly affected are displayed in an easily accessible table format, in a proximal to distal fashion, discussing causes/risk factors, patient history, physical examination findings and treatment options **(Table 1)**. Risk factors, expanded below per individual tendon, consist of advancing age, prior tendon injuries and

Table 1: Common tendinopathy of upper extremity				
Tendinopathy	*Risk factors/cause*	*A: History*	*A: Physical Examination*	*B, C, D, E: Treatment*
Rotator cuff tendinopathy (typically the supraspinatus tendon or subscapularis tendon)	Advancing age, high body mass index (BMI), frequent overhead activities, male = female incidence	Pain with overhead activity, often in throwing, swimming or overhead shots in racquet sports. Pain free with activities at less than 90° of abduction. Night pain is common	Tenderness over the supraspinatus tendon, often at its insertion into the greater tuberosity of the humerus. Pain with abduction between 70° and 120° (supraspinatus) or pain with internal rotation (subscapularis). Impingement tests often positive	PRICEMM* Eccentric exercises to correct glenohumeral instability and shoulder weakness Stretching of posterior capsule Nitric oxide donor therapy or single corticosteroid injection If calcific, consider lithotripsy

Contd...

Contd...

Tendinopathy	Risk factors/cause	A: History	A: Physical Examination	B, C, D, E: Treatment
Biceps tendinopathy	Large volume of weight training. Very rare to occur without other pathology causing it. Typically caused from secondary shoulder impingement (scapular/shoulder instability, rotator cuff tendinopathy/tears, or labral tears)	Pain in anterior shoulder may radiate into deltoid. Recent large volume of weight training	Point tenderness over the bicipital groove. Pain with passive stretching of the biceps	PRICEMM Bicep treatment alone is not useful. Direct treatment at the underlying pathology Consider injection into tendon sheath for diagnostic purposes
Flexor/Pronator tendinopathy (Also called medial epicondylitis/Golfer's elbow) *(typically the pronator teres tendon)*	Excessive activity of the wrist flexors	Local pain at medial elbow. Often golfer or pain with tennis forehand	Pain at or below the medial epicondyle with pain on resisted wrist flexion and/or resisted forearm pronation	PRICEMM Stretching of tendon and eccentric wrist flexion exercises for strengthening Corticosteroid injection decreases pain but can lead to delayed recovery and greater recurrence
Lateral elbow tendinopathy (Also called lateral epicondylitis/tennis elbow) *(typically the extensor carpi radialis brevis tendon)*	Age > 40 years old, BMI > 30, and positioning of the affected joints in demanding ranges (wrist extension/gripping)	Local lateral elbow pain, with or without spread to forearm that occurs with minor everyday activities or repeated sport/job activities. Gradual onset of pain. Recent changes in training/duties/equipment	Pain in mid tendon or insertion of tendon. Pain reproduced with resisted wrist extension or middle finger extension	PRICEMM Address grip strength deficit and coordination of supination and pronation. Consider splint at wrist Stretching of tendon and eccentric exercises of wrist extension Corticosteroid injection decreases pain but can lead to delayed recovery and greater recurrence Nitric oxide donor therapy or platelet-rich plasma
de Quervains tenosynovitis (inflammation of synovium of abductor pollicis longus and extensor pollicis brevis tendons)	Caused by repetitive and continued strain of the tendons, more common in women	Complaints of pain and swelling over the radial dorsal area. Often pain with ulnar deviation activities (such as hammering a nail or lifting a child)	Local tenderness and swelling over the course of the tendons especially at radial styloid process. Crepitus can be felt. Finkelstein's often positive	PRICEMM Stretching and gradual eccentric strengthening of tendons Injection into tendon sheath Splinting rarely useful without injection as well

Note: *PRICEMM= protection, relative rest, ice, compression, elevation, modalities, medications

improper biomechanics. Physical examination is often pertinent for tenderness along the prospective tendon, though location of pain within the tendon varies depending on the location of the tendinopathy. There is typically pain with tendon loading. Imaging can also be useful for diagnosis, often by ultrasound or magnetic resonance imaging, as it can reveal tendon thickening, hypoechoic areas, or even partial tendon tears. Often, treatment is directed at correcting the predisposing biomechanical factors with a conservative approach. Acutely, protection, relative rest, ice, compression, elevation, modalities, and medications (PRICEMM), including nonsteroidal anti-inflammatory drugs (NSAIDs), are reasonable, but often rest and NSAIDs do not reduce symptoms. Corticosteroid injections can be useful in difficult cases, but with caution not to inject the tendon directly, which can lead to rupture. Without resolution of symptoms to conservative measures, surgical consultation can be considered.

SUGGESTED READING

Brukner P, Khan K. Clinical Sports Medicine, 4th edition, 2011.

Churgay CA. Diagnosis and treatment of biceps tendinitis and tendinosis. Am Fam Physician. 2009;80(5):470-6.

Cuccurullo S. Physical Medicine and Rehabilitation Board Review, 3rd edition, 2015.

Goel R, Abzug JM. de Quervain's tenosynovitis: a review of the rehabilitative options. Hand (N Y). 2015;10(1):1-5.

Khan KM, Cook JL, Bonar F, et al. Histopathology of common tendinopathies. Update and implications for clinical management. Sports Med. 1999;27(6):393-408.

Maffulli N, Wong J, Almekinders LC. Types and epidemiology of tendinopathy. Clin Sports Med. 2003;22(4):675-92.

Ortega-Castillo M, Medina-Porqueres I. Effectiveness of the eccentric exercise therapy in physically active adults with symptomatic shoulder impingement or lateral epicondylar tendinopathy: A systematic review. J Sci Med Sport. 2016;19(6):438-53.

Scott A, Ashe MC. Common tendinopathies in the upper and lower extremities. Curr Sports Med Rep. 2006;5(5):233-41.

Wilson JJ, Best TM. Common overuse tendon problems: A review and recommendations for treatment. Am Fam Physician. 2005; 72(5):811-8.

SECTION 9

Lower Extremity Pain

Miles Day

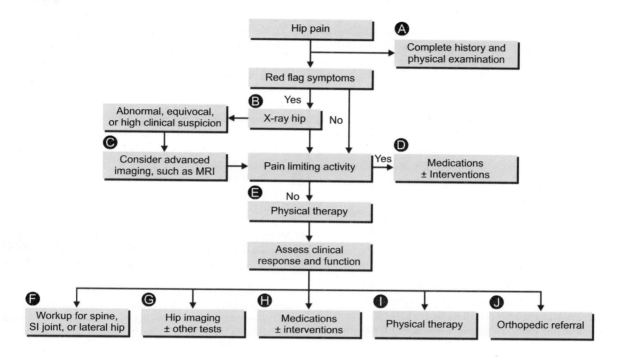

Hip pain is a common musculoskeletal complaint that can have multiple potential etiologies. Given the high prevalence of and treatment costs for musculoskeletal conditions, it is important to find effective methods to evaluate and manage common causes of hip pain. The chapter and the flow diagram are based on evidence-based evaluation and management of intra-articular causes of hip pain.

Ⓐ Detailed *history and physical examination* are critical given the multiple potential etiologies of hip pain and coexisting conditions that may contribute. Systemic causes of hip pain should be considered including rheumatological (osteoarthritis, rheumatoid arthritis, seronegative enthesopathy and arthropathy, and gout), infectious, and inflammatory conditions. Additionally, extra-articular and referred pain from the lumbosacral spine or sacroiliac joint must also be considered during evaluation. Specifics of the flow diagram are outlined below.

Ⓑ *X-ray:* The presence of risk factors requiring imaging is the initial step in evaluation. History of intravenous drug use, inability to bear weight, trauma, and concern for malignancy or fracture including low bone density typically requires an X-ray. Sedimentation rate, C-reactive pro-

tein, and complete blood count are laboratory tests that can also be obtained with concern for infection or malignancy.

Ⓒ *Advanced Imaging:* If the X-ray is negative or indeterminate, advanced imaging including magnetic resonance imaging (MRI) may be required to evaluate for conditions including infection or presence of bone stress injury. Referral to an orthopedic surgeon for management or infectious disease specialist may be necessary with fracture or infection.

The presence of fracture on X-ray directs further management. High-risk fractures including the tension side of the femoral neck or displaced fracture require non-weight-bearing status and urgent surgical referral.

Non-displaced fractures involving the lesser trochanter or compression side of the femoral neck require initial non-weight-bearing status and close clinical follow-up with repeat imaging to ensure bony healing given risk for progression.

Ⓓ *Pain Control:* Without red flag symptoms, initial management of hip pain is guided by functional limitations in pain and mobility. With the presence of activity-limiting pain, a 2–4-week trial of pain medications (typically nonsteroidal anti-inflammatory medications or acetaminophen) can be used to reduce pain. However, potential side effects, including hepatic, gastrointestinal, cardiac, and renal toxicity, limit use of these medications routinely or for prolonged treatments and must be considered on an individual basis. With severe hip pain, failure to have improvements in pain with oral medications, or contraindications to oral medications, interventional treatments may be considered. Intra-articular injection of anesthetics can aide in the diagnosis, while corticosteroids provide pain reduction in the setting of hip osteoarthritis. Data on hyaluronic acid is inconclusive. Emerging treatments with orthobiological agents including stem cell therapy and platelet-rich plasma may also hold promise, although research is limited and heterogenicity in responses currently limits widespread use.

E *Physical Therapy:* Addressing functional limitations through physical therapy is a mainstay treatment for most etiologies of hip pain. The goals of physical therapy include addressing the underlying biomechanical contributors to the etiology of hip pain, patient education, and developing a home exercise program to optimize function and reduce pain. Modalities such as direct heat or ultrasound, ice, electrical stimulation, and massage can be helpful adjuncts for treatment, although these should not take the place of developing an effective home exercise program.

After 4–8 weeks of physical therapy, the patient should be reassessed for improvements in function and pain. If the patient has no response to treatment, additional diagnostic workup may be required to evaluate for referred sources of hip pain, including sacroiliac-joint-mediated pain or spine-referred etiologies.

F With incomplete response to treatment, additional diagnostic tests may be required to evaluate for other non-intra-articular hip sources of pain.

G If clinical suspicion is that the source is likely intra-articular, X-rays would be reasonable to obtain. In the setting of suspected labral pathology or chondral injury, magnetic resonance direct arthrography with contrast dye has been proposed as the most effective imaging modality although high-resolution 3-Tesla MRI also holds promise.

H Alternatively, injections can be useful to confirm the etiology of pain as intra-articular. For example, an intra-articular injection of a long-acting anesthetic such as ropivicaine can be administered and pain relief monitored following the procedure to determine whether pain is likely from an intra-articular process such as labrochondral pathology. Intra-articular injections require image guidance due to the high miss rate of non-image-guided procedures.

I Following evaluation with advanced imaging, diagnostic procedures, and excluding referred sources of hip pain, additional physical therapy may be prescribed to address residual symptoms.

J Referral to an orthopedic surgeon may be considered for surgical consultation with failure to reach patient goals of pain control and function.

SUGGESTED READING

Naraghi A, White LM. MRI of labral and chondral lesions of the hip. AJR Am J Roentgenol. 2015;205(3):479-90.

Zhang W, Nuki G, Moskowitz RW, et al. OARSI recommendations for the management of hip and knee osteoarthritis: part III: Changes in evidence following systematic cumulative update of research published through January 2009. Osteoarthritis Cartilage. 2010;18(4):476-99.

Knee Pain

Patel S, Horrocks A

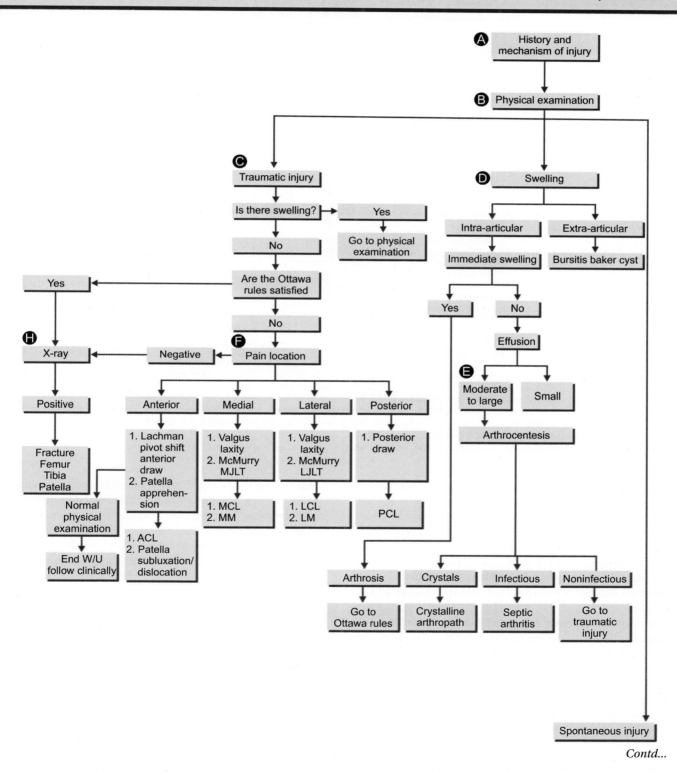

Contd...

Contd...

```
                    ┌─────────────────────┐
                    │  Spontaneous injury │
                    └─────────────────────┘
                               │
                    ┌─────────────────────┐
        ┌───────────┤   Is there swelling │
        │           └─────────────────────┘
   ┌─────────┐                 │
   │   Yes   │                 │
   └─────────┘            ┌─────────┐          ┌─────────┐
        │                 │   No    │─────────▶│   Yes   │
┌──────────────────┐      └─────────┘          └─────────┘
│ Go to physical   │           │                    │
│ examination      │  ┌────────────────────┐    ┌──────────────┐  ┌──────────────┐
└──────────────────┘  │ Rheumatologic Sx,  │    │  Lab work    │  │  Lab work    │
                      │ family history,    │    │  negative    │  │  positive    │
                      │ generalized Sx     │    └──────────────┘  └──────────────┘
                      └────────────────────┘                            │
                               │                              ┌──────────────────┐
                         ┌─────────┐                          │  Rheumatologic   │
                         │   No    │                          │  diagnosis       │
                         └─────────┘                          └──────────────────┘
                               │
      Ⓖ  ┌────────────────────────┐
          │ OA Clinical criteria met │◀────
          └────────────────────────┘
               │            │
          ┌─────────┐  ┌─────────┐
          │   No    │  │   Yes   │
          └─────────┘  └─────────┘
               │
      Ⓕ  ┌──────────────┐
          │ Pain location│
          └──────────────┘
```

Anterior	Medial	Lateral	Posterior
1. Patella femoral grind 2. ACL laxity 3. Quadriceps tendon TTP tenderness 4. Prepatella point tenderness 5. Patella femoral	1. MJLT McMurry 2. Virus laxity 3. Mobile nobularity 4. Anterior/medial; tibial pain 5. MJLT	1. LJLT McMurry 2. I and B tenderness 3. Valgus laxity 4. LJLT	1. Posterior draw 2. Popliteal fullness
1. PFPS 2. ACL Sprain 3. Quadricep tendonitis 4. Prepatella bursitis 5. Patella femoral OA	1. MM injury 2. MLL sprain 3. Plica 4. Pes anserine bursitis 5. Medial compartment OA	1. LM 2. LCL sprain 3. I and B tendonitis 4. Lateral compartment OA	1. PCL injury 2. Bakers cyst

LCL, lateral collateral ligament; MCL, medial collateral ligament; MJLT, medial joint line tenderness LJLT, lateral joint line tenderness; PFPS, patella femoral pain syndrome; PCL, posterior cruciate ligament; ACL, anterior cruciate ligament; TTP, tenderness to palpation; MM, medial meniscus; LM, lateral meniscus; I&B, Iliotibial band; OA, Osteoarthritis

Knee pain is a common presenting complaint in patients of all ages. It is present in approximately 20–25% of the general population and commonly occurs secondary to trauma, sport-related activities, overuse syndromes, and degenerative changes. Musculoskeletal-related injuries account for nearly 21% of visits to primary care office, with knee pain ranking second only to low back pain in that category. The most common etiology of knee pain are strains and sprains (42%), osteoarthritis (OA) (34%), meniscus (9%), collateral ligament (7%), cruciate ligament (4%), gout (2%), fracture (1.2%), rheumatoid arthritis (0.5%), infectious arthritis (0.3%), and pseudogout (0.2%). In people older than 55 years of age, the most common cause of disability related to knee is pain secondary to OA.

Ⓐ When formulating a differential diagnosis, the history and physical examination are key components that fur-ther direct the physical examination, laboratory testing, and imaging. Important information to obtain includes the following: how the injury occurred, any trauma, previous injury, "pop" or "tearing" sound or sensation (common with ligament or meniscus injury), swelling, hyperthermia, ecchymosis, visual deformity, or atrophy. Most injuries can be separated into spontaneous occurring pain and post-traumatic pain.

Ⓑ Physical examination involves inspection of the knee and leg, general alignment, evaluation of gait, ability to bear weight, palpable bony or soft tissue deformities, scars, position of the patella, and systemic involvement. Ligament and meniscus injuries are best diagnosed with a good musculoskeletal examination and special provocative tests, and the severity can range from mild sprain to complete tear. The Lachman test, pivot shift test, and anterior draw assess anterior cruciate ligament (ACL) injuries. Joint line pinpoint tenderness and reproduction of pain with the McMurray test suggest meniscus injury. Posterior draw assesses posterior cruciate ligament (PCL) integrity. Pain to palpation of the patella facets and patella instability/apprehension support the diagnosis of patella subluxation/dislocation. Range of motion of the knee, audible or palpable crepitus, and point tenderness over anatomic structures should be documented, and help narrow the differential diagnosis.

C Traumatic injuries commonly lead to ligament, meniscus, and/or bone injuries. Valgus and varus stress to the knee usually leads to medial collateral ligament (MCL) injury and lateral collateral ligament (LCL) injury, respectively. Hyperextension and twisting injuries can lead to ACL and meniscus injury. Posterior translation of the tibia and dashboard impact can lead to PCL.

D The presence and location of swelling may suggest particular diagnoses. Extracapsular swelling may indicate prepatellar bursitis when anterior, or popliteal cyst when posterior. Intracapsular effusion can occur with multiple injuries and is nonspecific. They can range from small to large, and moderate to large intracapsular effusion should be considered for an arthrocentesis. Immediate swelling following an injury suggests a hemarthrosis, and is associated with fracture, patella dislocation, and ligament and/or peripheral meniscus tear.

E A warm, erythematous, and swollen knee with no history of trauma suggests septic or crystal-induced arthritis. Arthrocentesis will provide a sample for cell count, Gram stain, culture, and crystal. A cell count greater than 50,000 per mm^3, with more than 75% neutrophils is consistent with an infectious source. Urate (gout) and calcium pyrophosphate dihydrate crystals (pseudogout) can be identified by microscopy.

F The location of pain is important in formulating a diagnosis. For example, anterior knee pain is usually secondary to patella femoral pain syndrome (PFPS); medial knee pain from medial plica syndrome, pes anserine bursitis, medial compartment OA, MCL, or medial meniscus injury; lateral knee pain may be iliotibial band, lateral compartment OA, LCL, or lateral meniscal injury; posterior knee pain may include popliteal (Baker's) cyst and PCL injury.

G The American College of Rheumatology's clinical criteria for OA includes at least three of the following: age greater than 50 years, stiffness for less than 30 minutes, crepitus, bony tenderness, bony enlargement, and no palpable warmth.

H Radiographs should be obtained if the pain occurs secondary to a fall or blow to the knee, and has at least one of four characteristics: age greater than 55 years, tenderness at the fibular head or patella, inability to bear weight, and lack of 90° of flexion (Ottawa rules). Radiography is helpful in assessing OA and osteochondral lesions. The Kellgren Lawrence radiographic criteria for OA included the presence of osteophytes, sclerosis, joint space narrowing, and cystic subchondral bone. If ligament or meniscus injury is suspected, magnetic resonance imaging (MRI) can help with diagnosis and has been shown to decrease diagnostic time, reduce the cost of additional diagnostic procedures, and improve quality of life for the first 6 weeks after an injury.

Other causes of knee pain include quadriceps tendon rupture, rheumatologic diseases (rheumatoid arthritis and Reiter's syndrome), avascular necrosis, neoplasm, and referred hip pain.

Treatment is directed to the underlying diagnosis. In general, conservative therapy consisting of nonsteroidal anti-inflammatory drugs (NSAIDs), physical therapy, modalities, bracing/casting, immobilization, and injections (steroid, anesthetic, and/or hyaluronic acid) is indicated. Genicular nerve radiofrequency ablation has been shown to decrease chronic knee pain in patients with severe OA when more conservative therapies have failed. Some injuries may require referral for further evaluation and treatment, or surgical intervention.

SUGGESTED READING

Calmbach WL, Hutchens M. Evaluation of patient presenting with knee pain, Parts I and II. Am Fam Physician. 2003;68(5):907-12, 917-22.

Choi WJ, Hwang SJ, Song JG, et al. Radiofrequency treatment relieves chronic knee osteoarthritis pain: A double-blind randomized controlled trial. Pain. 2011;152:481-7.

Hamer AJ. Pain in the hip and knee. Br Med J. 2004;328:1067-9.

Jackson JL, O'Malley PG, Kroenke K. Evaluation of acute knee pain in primary care. Ann Intern Med. 2003;139(7):575-88.

Karrasch C, Gallo RA. The acutely injured knee. Med Clin North Am. 2014;98(4):719-36.

Kozol RA, Konen J, Fromm D. When to Call the Surgeon: Decision Making for the Primary Care Provider. Philadelphia: FA Davis Company; 1999. pp. 204-20.

Foot and Ankle Pain

Tenforde AS, Kennedy DJ

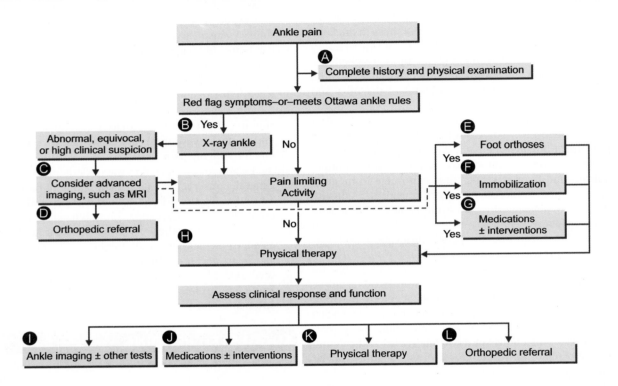

The complex anatomy and multiple potential contributors to pain in the foot and ankle region can be a challenge for clinicians and may require customized treatment with coexisting conditions.

A Initial evaluation includes obtaining complete history and physical examination. Pain descriptors and associated functional limitations are important to elicit to guide management. Infection, rheumatological conditions (including crystal arthropathy, rheumatoid arthritis, etc.), peripheral neuropathy, and referred sources of pain (including lumbosacral radiculopathy) can contribute to foot and ankle complaints. Details of a full examination are beyond the scope of this chapter. In general, a standard assessment of foot and ankle complaints to include evaluation of gait and balance to understand the functional demands of the foot and ankle is recommended. Additionally, aspects of the kinetic chain, including the spine, hip, and knee should be evaluated as indicated. Specifics of the flow diagram are outlined below.

B *X-ray:* Most conditions of the foot and ankle can be evaluated and managed initially without imaging. In the setting of trauma, or concerns for fracture, significant ligament injury, syndesmotic injury or arthritis, plain film X-rays with weight bearing should be obtained. The presence of "red flag symptoms" such as weight loss, unexplained fevers, chills, night sweats, night pain, or other systemic symptoms concerning for inflammatory, infectious, or neoplastic etiologies prompts obtaining an X-ray. In setting of acute trauma, imaging should be obtained in patients with positive Ottawa ankle rules. These include: (1) Ankle X-rays with pain in the malleolar zone with inability to bear weight, tenderness over the distal 6 cm of the lateral and/or medial malleolus, or (2) designated foot X-rays for pain in the malleolar zone with inability to bear weight, tenderness over the tarsal navicular or at the base of the fifth metatarsal.

C *Advanced Imaging:* With negative X-ray films and clinical concern for injuries including bone stress injuries, deltoid ligament injury, or significant tendon or other ligament tearing, magnetic resonance imaging (MRI) may be ordered to help guide management.

D *Orthopedic referral* for fractures at high-risk locations, advanced tendon, and joint conditions may be appropriate.

Vascular claudication is defined as discomfort, fatigue, or pain occurring in a specific limb muscle group during effort due to exercise-induced ischemia. It identifies the symptomatic subset of patients with lower extremity peripheral arterial disease (PAD). Vascular claudication is usually due to atherosclerotic lower extremity PAD but less common causes include emboli, radiation arteritis, thromboangiitis obliterans, popliteal entrapment, fibromuscular dysplasia, and trauma. The site of arterial stenosis often correlates with the specific leg symptoms. Occlusive disease in the iliac arteries produces hip, buttock, and thigh pain whereas disease in the femoral and popliteal arteries is often associated with calf pain. Tibial artery disease may produce calf pain, and rarely, foot pain and numbness.

Ⓐ The clinical history and examination should focus on features that distinguish vascular claudication from other causes of exertional leg pain with a focus on the location, pain characteristic, effects of exercise and rest, and effect of body position. The clinical history should also include risk factors for atherosclerotic disease including smoking, diabetes, hypertension, and dyslipidemia. The examination should focus on assessment of peripheral pulses, bruits, and nonhealing ulcers.

Ⓑ Exertional aching or cramping pain that is promptly relieved by rest is characteristic. The pain is usually nonradiating and is not affected by position changes including sitting or squatting.

Ⓒ The differential diagnosis of exertional leg pain other than PAD includes severe venous obstructive disease, lumbar disease and spinal stenosis, chronic compartment syndrome, osteoarthritis, and inflammatory muscle diseases.

Ⓓ Resting ankle-brachial index (ABI) should be obtained in all patients with claudication symptoms and should be followed by post-exercise ABI if normal. ABI less than or equal to 0.90 confirms the diagnosis. For normal (0.91–1.30) and supranormal (>1.30) values, additional diagnostic testing, such as toe-brachial index, duplex ultrasound, and segmental pressure examination should be used to confirm the diagnosis of PAD.

Ⓔ Goals in the management of vascular claudication include cardiovascular risk reduction and alleviation of symptoms. To reduce adverse cardiovascular events associated with lower extremity PAD, lifelong treatments should include smoking cessation, adequate control of hypertension and diabetes. High-intensity statin therapy is recommended for all patients with PAD thought to be of atherosclerotic origin. Similarly, antiplatelet therapy with aspirin (75–325 mg daily) or clopidogrel (75 mg daily) as an alternative to aspirin is recommended for all patients. Oral anticoagulation is not indicated.

Ⓕ Strategies to alleviate claudication symptoms include exercise, pharmacotherapy, and revascularization. Patients with low ABI, significant exertional symptoms, and no to mild comorbidities are expected to benefit the most.

A program of supervised exercise training is recommended as an initial treatment modality for patients with intermittent claudication. Supervised exercise training should be performed for a minimum of 30–45 minutes, in sessions performed at least three times per week for a minimum of 12 weeks.

Cilostazol, a phosphodiesterase type 3 inhibitor, should be considered in all patients with lifestyle limiting claudication (in the absence of heart failure symptoms) to improve symptoms and walking distance. The clinical effectiveness of pentoxifylline as therapy for claudication is marginal and not well established.

Ⓖ For patients with lifestyle limiting symptoms who have had inadequate response to exercise and pharmacotherapy or in those whose revascularization has a very favorable risk-benefit ratio, a revascularization intervention is recommended. Revascularization options include endovascular or surgical approach. Initial strategies will usually rely on endovascular techniques, and surgical options are reserved for patients with unfavorable anatomy for endovascular approach. Comparable efficacy can usually be achieved with less risk by an endovascular approach. Common endovascular techniques include percutaneous angioplasty with balloon dilation, stenting, atherectomy, laser, and cutting balloons.

Surgery is infrequently needed to treat claudication and it should be considered only after an appropriate trial of exercise and/or claudication pharmacotherapy has been utilized and in whom an endovascular option is expected to be less effective and the cardiovascular risk of surgical revascularization is low. Surgical strategy is determined by the site of occlusion and includes inflow (aortoiliac disease) and outflow (infrainguinal disease) procedures. For the outflow procedures, bypasses should be constructed with autogenous veins when possible.

Ⓗ For the small subgroup of patients with refractory symptoms deemed unsuitable for any revascularization, a successful trial of spinal cord stimulation using an epidural lead can be followed by implantation of a spinal cord stimulation system to provide pain relief.

SUGGESTED READING

Hirsch AT, Haskal ZJ, Hertzer NR, et al. ACC/AHA 2005 Practice Guidelines for the management of patients with peripheral arterial disease (lower extremity, renal, mesenteric, and abdominal aortic): a collaborative report from the American Association for Vascular Surgery/Society for Vascular Surgery, Society for Cardiovascular Angiography and Interventions, Society for Vascular Medicine and Biology, Society of Interventional Radiology, and the ACC/AHA Task Force on Practice Guidelines (Writing Committee to Develop Guidelines for the Management of Patients With Peripheral Arterial Disease): endorsed by the American Association of Cardiovascular and Pulmonary Rehabilitation; National Heart, Lung, and Blood Institute; Society for Vascular Nursing; TransAtlantic Inter-Society Consensus; and Vascular Disease Foundation. Circulation. 2006;113(11):e463-654.

Rooke TW, Hirsch AT, Misra S, et al. 2011 ACCF/AHA Focused Update of the Guideline for the Management of patients with peripheral artery disease (Updating the 2005 Guideline): a report of the American College of Cardiology Foundation/American Heart Association Task Force on practice guidelines. Circulation. 2011;124(18):2020-45.

Ubbink DT, Vermeulen H. Spinal cord stimulation for non-reconstructable chronic critical leg ischaemia. Cochrane Database Syst Rev. 2013;(2):CD004001.

CHAPTER 89

Entrapment Neuropathies: Lower Extremity

Bhavaraju-Sanka R

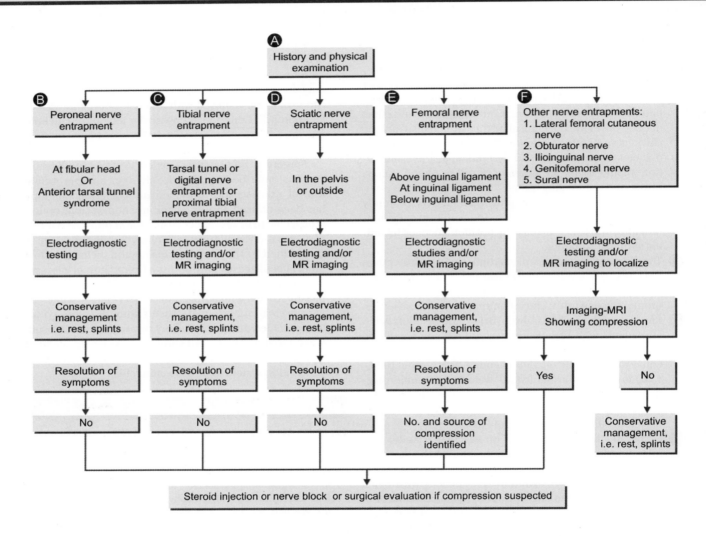

A History and physical examination

B Peroneal nerve entrapment

C Tibial nerve entrapment

D Sciatic nerve entrapment

E Femoral nerve entrapment

F Other nerve entrapments:
1. Lateral femoral cutaneous nerve
2. Obturator nerve
3. Ilioinguinal nerve
4. Genitofemoral nerve
5. Sural nerve

At fibular head Or Anterior tarsal tunnel syndrome

Tarsal tunnel or digital nerve entrapment or proximal tibial nerve entrapment

In the pelvis or outside

Above inguinal ligament At inguinal ligament Below inguinal ligament

Electrodiagnostic testing

Electrodiagnostic testing and/or MR imaging

Electrodiagnostic testing and/or MR imaging

Electrodiagnostic studies and/or MR imaging

Electrodiagnostic testing and/or MR imaging to localize

Conservative management i.e. rest, splints

Conservative management, i.e. rest, splints

Conservative management, i.e. rest, splints

Conservative management, i.e. rest, splints

Imaging-MRI Showing compression

Resolution of symptoms

Resolution of symptoms

Resolution of symptoms

Resolution of symptoms

Yes

No

No

No

No

No. and source of compression identified

Conservative management, i.e. rest, splints

Steroid injection or nerve block or surgical evaluation if compression suspected

---

A Entrapments syndromes are neuropathies that are caused by compression of peripheral nerves. The nerve can be compressed at any site but it is more common at specific anatomical sites where the nerve travels through a fibroosseous or fibrocartilaginous structure or a muscle.

Entrapment neuropathies of the lower extremity are much less common than those of the upper extremity. The nerves commonly affected are discussed below:

B *Common Peroneal Neuropathy:* This is the most common entrapment neuropathy of the lower limb and presents with foot drop. The common peroneal nerve originates from the sciatic nerve at the level of popliteal fossa **(Fig. 1)** and consists of fibers derived from L4, L5, and S1

nerve roots. It supplies the short head of biceps and travels superficially around the head of fibula. Here it enters the lateral aspect of the leg and divides into the superficial and deep peroneal nerves. The superficial peroneal nerve supplies peroneus longus and brevis muscles. The nerve travels between these muscles and divides into medial and intermediate dorsal cutaneous nerves. These sensory branches travel anterior to the extensor retinaculum and supply the lower anterolateral aspect of the leg and dorsum of the foot. The deep peroneal nerve innervates tibialis anterior, extensor hallucis longus, extensor digitorum longus, extensor digitorum brevis, peroneus tertius, and extensor digitorum brevis. It also supplies the

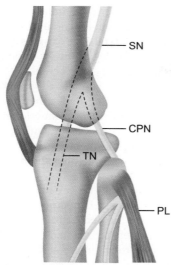

Fig. 1: Common peroneal nerve at the level of popliteal fossa
SN, sciatic nerve; CPN, common peroneal nerve; TN, tibial nerve;
PL, peroneus longus

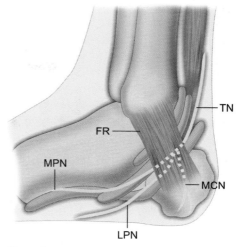

Fig. 2: Tarsal tunnel
TN, tibial nerve; MCN, medial calcaneal nerve; MPN, median plantar
nerve; LPN, lateral plantar nerve; FR, flexor retinaculum

skin over the first web space between the first and second toes.

Peroneal Neuropathy at the Fibular Head: The nerve here is very superficial, making it more prone to injury or compression. Common causes include habitual leg crossing, prolonged squatting or sitting in kneeling positions, synovial cyst, ganglion cysts, trauma like supracondylar fracture or knee dislocation or proximal tibial fractures. The deep peroneal is more vulnerable to injury. Patients present with foot drop with eversion weakness and sensory loss in the distribution of the affected nerve(s). Isolated injury to deep peroneal nerve causes dorsiflexion weakness with normal eversion. Sensory loss is limited to the first web space. If superficial peroneal nerve is affected then the weakness is noted in foot eversion with much large sensory loss affecting lower anterolateral leg and dorsum of the foot.

Nerve conduction studies show reduced motor amplitude when recorded from extensor digitorum brevis. Slowing of conduction velocities may be seen across the fibular head. Superficial peroneal nerve sensory amplitudes may be reduced. Needle examination shows denervation in all the peroneal innervated muscles except short head of biceps.

Treatment can be conservative avoiding the precipitating activities. Surgical treatment may be needed for compression from mass lesions or other traumatic neuropathies. The common peroneal nerve may be blocked by palpating the head of the fibula and inserting a 25-gauge 0.5-inch needle at a point just below the fibular head until a paresthesia is elicited or the needle contacts bone. The needle is then withdrawn 1 mm, and 5 mL of 1% preservative-free lidocaine is injected.

Anterior Tarsal Tunnel Syndrome: It is a rare disease caused by entrapment of the deep peroneal nerve at the ankle. Patients present with pain on the dorsum of the foot and examination shows sensory changes in the first web space. Weakness and atrophy affects extensor digitorum brevis muscle. Nerve conduction studies show prolonged distal latency at the ankle.

C *Tibial Neuropathy:* Tibial nerve arises from the sciatic nerve at the popliteal fossa. It descends in the posterior compartment deep to soleus and supplies gastrocnemius, soleus, tibialis posterior, flexor hallucis longus, and flexor digitorum longus. It enters the foot by passing through tarsal tunnel **(Fig. 2)**, the space between medial malleolus and flexor retinaculum. Here it divides into its terminal branches, medial, and lateral plantar nerves. The medial plantar nerves innervate abductor hallucis, flexor digitorum brevis, and flexor hallucis brevis. It supplies sensation to the medial anterior two-thirds of the sole, plantar skin of first three toes and half of the fourth toe. The lateral plantar nerve supplies abductor digiti minimi, flexor digiti minimi, abductor digiti minimi, and interossei. It supplies sensation to the lateral half of fourth toe, fifth toe, and lateral sole.

Tarsal Tunnel Syndrome: It is caused by entrapment of the tibial nerve at the tarsal tunnel. Common causes include ganglion cysts, other space-occupying lesions, post-traumatic fibrosis due to fractures, or dilated/tortuous veins. Patients have burning pain and dysesthesia of the foot with sensory deficit in the sole. Weakness is seen in the intrinsic foot muscles. Nerve conduction studies show prolonged tibial motor latency. Medial and/or lateral plantar sensory studies may show prolonged latencies or reduced amplitudes, but these studies are unreliable due to changes expected with age.

Interdigital Nerve Compression: The medial and lateral plantar nerves divide into interdigital nerves at the level of metatarsal base. Chronic compression of these terminal branches under the metatarsal heads gives rise to a

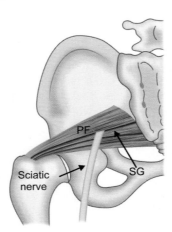

Fig. 3: Sciatic nerve passing inferior to PF
PF, pyriformis muscle; SG, superior gemellus muscle

painful syndrome called Morton's neuroma. It can also be seen with hyperextension of the toes as seen with use of high heels, or hallux valgus deformity or congenital malformations or rheumatoid arthritis. Patients complain of pain in the foot with nocturnal discomfort. Magnetic resonance imaging can identify the neuroma as an enhancing teardrop-shaped soft tissue mass with intermediate signal on both T1- and T2-weighted images.

Proximal Tibial Neuropathy: Proximal injury is very rare as it is a deep nerve. It can be seen as it travels beneath the tendinous sling at the origin of soleus muscle. Patients complain of pain in the calf with paresthesia in the sole of the foot. Needle examination shows denervation of gastrocnemius and soleus muscles.

D *Sciatic Neuropathy:* Sciatic nerve originates from the upper division of sacral plexus from the union of L4 to S2 nerve roots. It exits the pelvis through the greater sciatic foramen at the inferior border of pyriformis muscle **(Fig. 3)**. The peroneal and the tibial portions of the nerve exist as separate fascicles in the thigh and become separate branches at the popliteal fossa. The tibial component supplies long head of biceps, semitendinosus, and semimembranosus. The peroneal component supplies the short head of biceps.

Compressive lesions that affect the sciatic nerve affect the peroneal component more often than the tibial component.

Sciatic neuropathy is often seen due to neoplastic infiltrations from surrounding structures in the pelvis. Neuromas, neurofibromas, pelvic abscesses, fracture of pelvis, hip, or femur, ischemia due to aortic occlusion, compression from gravid uterus. Misdirected intramuscular injections and trauma are some of the other causes. Pyriformis syndrome is a controversial condition attributed to compression of the nerve by pyriformis muscle. The patient presents with pain at the site with weakness that spares the gluteus medius, minimus, and tensor fascia lata. Gluteus maximus is affected.

E *Femoral Neuropathy:* The femoral nerve is formed at the vertebral canal by anterior rami of L2 to L4. The nerve passes along the lateral edge of psoas muscle to enter the anterior part of the leg. It travels underneath the inguinal ligament where it exists lateral to the femoral artery and vein. The nerve supplies iliopsoas before entering the thigh. After passing under the inguinal ligament it sends sensory branches to the anterior thigh and supplies pectineus, sartorius, and the quadriceps femori muscles before becoming the purely sensory saphenous nerve. The saphenous nerve supplies the medial aspect of the thigh, leg, and foot.

Compression of the nerve can occur in the pelvis from tumors, psoas abscess, hematoma, or lymphadenopathy. Direct trauma to the nerve can be seen with fractures or femoral artery catheterization. Prolonged lithotomy position can cause stretch injury at the inguinal ligament. A complete lesion of the nerve causes weakness of hip flexion and knee extension. Sensory loss can be variable. Partial lesions can affect single head of quadriceps. Lesions at or below the inguinal ligament spare the iliopsoas muscle. Electrodiagnostic studies show prolonged distal latency, reduced amplitudes with denervation in the affected muscles.

Patients with diabetes can develop mononeuropathy of the femoral nerve, which starts with severe burning pain in the anterior thigh followed by weakness of all the muscles innervated by femoral nerve. It can also affect other L2 to L4 innervated muscles. Diabetic lumbosacral radiculoplexopathy or diabetic amyotrophy is proposed to be a vasculitic process. It is a self-limiting condition but steroids have been used to hasten the recovery.

F1 *Lateral Femoral Cutaneous Neuropathy:* Also called meralgia paresthetica, is a pure sensory neuropathy. The nerve is the first sensory branch of the lumbar plexus and receives fibers from L2/L3 roots. It runs along the lateral border of psoas muscle. It enters the thigh through a tunnel formed by lateral attachment of the inguinal ligament and the anterior superior iliac spine. It supplies sensation to the skin over the anterolateral and posterolateral thigh. The nerve is injured at the anterosuperior iliac spine by compression from tight belts, clothes, prolonged postoperative hip flexion for pain relief, sudden weight gain/ loss. Diagnosis is based on sensory changes in the anterolateral thigh with normal motor examination. Treatment is conservative but neurolysis with transposition can be considered for intractable symptoms.

The lateral femoral cutaneous nerve block is performed by inserting a 25-gauge 0.5-inch needle to 1 inch medial to the anterosuperior iliac spine, inferior to the inguinal ligament. It is inserted perpendicular to the skin until it pops through the deep fascia. Local anesthesia (5–7 mL) is deposited in this area in a fan-shaped manner.

F2 *Obturator Neuropathy:* Obturator nerve arises from the anterior divisions of L2 to L4 nerve roots within the psoas muscle. It passes through the obturator canal and gives anterior and posterior branches. Anterior branch supplies adductor longus, brevis, and gracilis. The posterior branch innervates obturator externus and half of adductor magnus. The sensory branch supplies medial aspect of the upper thigh and sends anastomoses to saphenous nerve.

Selective damage to obturator nerve can be seen during pregnancy or labor due to pressure from the uterus or from pelvic fractures, obturator hernia repairs, prolonged urological surgeries causing compression in the obturator canal and cancers. Injury causes weakness in adductors, external and internal rotators of the thigh. Patients also complain of pain in the groin radiating to the medial thigh. Denervation is seen in adductor muscles.

F3 *Ilioinguinal Neuropathy:* Arising from L1/L2 nerve roots it supplies sensation to the upper and medial parts of the thigh. It innervates the transversalis and internal oblique muscles. The nerve may be injured accidentally during surgery. Patients complain of pain in the groin region. Pressure medial to the anterosuperior iliac spine causes pain radiating to the crural region.

F4 *Genitofemoral Neuropathy:* Arising from L1/L2 nerve roots, it branches into lumboinguinal and external spermatic nerves. Lumboinguinal nerve supplies the skin over the femoral triangle. External spermatic nerve supplies the cremasteric muscle and skin of the upper inner thigh, scrotum, or labium. Injury is from trauma or surgical adhesions. Patients complain of pain in the inguinal region with sensory loss over the femoral triangles. Cremasteric reflex is lost.

F5 *Sural Neuropathy:* Sural nerve originates from the union of medial sural cutaneous branch of the tibial nerve and the sural communicating branch of common peroneal nerve below the popliteal fossa and travels between the medial and lateral heads of gastrocnemius muscle. It travels behind the lateral malleolus to enter the dorsolateral aspect of the foot. It receives supply from L5, S1, and S2 nerve roots (mostly S1). It is a sensory nerve supplying sensation to the skin over the posterolateral aspect of distal leg and lateral aspect of the foot.

Isolated compression and trauma to the nerve is rare but can be seen due to ganglions, stretch injury, trauma from combat boots or iatrogenic from biopsy.

Patients can present with paresthesia on the affected region with loss of sensation on the posterolateral distal leg and dorsolateral foot.

SUGGESTED READING

Dong Q, Jacobson JA, Jamadar DA, et al. Entrapment neuropathies in the upper and lower limbs: Anatomy and MRI features. Radiol Res Pract. 2012;2012:230679.

Kimura J. Electrodiagnosis in Diseases of Nerve and Muscle: Principles and Practice, 3rd edition. New York: Oxford Press; 2001.

Wheeless CR III. (2014). Wheeless' Textbook of Orthopedics. [online] wheelessonline website. Available from *www.wheelesonline.com* [Accessed January, 2017].

Tendinopathy: Lower Extremities

Bouffard KJ, Caldwell M

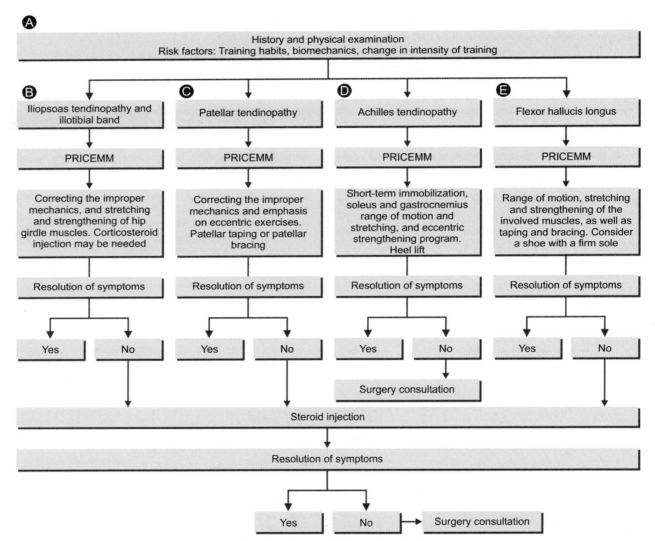

PRICEMM; protection relative rest, ice, compression, elevation, modalities, and medications

Ⓐ Tendinopathy is a clinical syndrome characterized by tendon thickening and chronic localized pain that is likely from a number of etiologies, including acute trauma or overuse. The pathophysiology of tendinopathy is important to understand when treating the patient. When inflammation occurs of a tendon, this is referred to as tendinitis. When minimal to no inflammation is present, the term tendinosis or chronic tendinopathy is more appropriate, and may even be considered a failed healing response. The

difference between the two is very important for management as acute tendonitis is treated differently than chronic tendinosis. Khan et al. created a classification system that theorizes tendinitis and is followed by tendinosis: (1) Acute tendonitis alone (resolves in 2–3 days), (2) chronic tendinosis with acute tendonitis, and (3) chronic tendinosis alone (typically resolves in 2–6 months).

There are tendons that are commonly affected and displayed in an easily accessible format, in a proximal to distal fashion, discussing causes/risk factors, patient history, physical examination findings, and treatment options. Physical examination is often pertinent for tenderness along the prospective tendon, though location of pain within the tendon varies depending on the location of the tendinopathy. Imaging can also be useful for diagnosis, often by ultrasound or magnetic resonance imaging, as it can reveal tendon thickening, hypoechoic areas, or even partial tendon tears. Often treatment is directed at correcting the predisposing biomechanical factors with a conservative approach. Protection, relative rest, ice, compression, elevation, modalities, and medications (PRICEMM), including nonsteroidal anti-inflammatory drugs (NSAIDs), are reasonable acutely. Eccentric exercises are most useful to reduce pain and improve strength, but may not be better than other modalities. Steroid injections are options for chronic tendinopathy, with exception of the Achilles tendon in which rupture can occur after injection. Without resolution of symptoms to conservative measures, surgical consultation can be considered.

B *Iliopsoas Tendinopathy and Iliotibial Band Tendinopathy (also known as "Snapping Hip Syndrome"):* Risk factors include repetitive friction of the muscle tendon unit with weak lateral gluteal muscles, improper biomechanics and inflexibility, often excessive running in same direction. History is consistent frequently with a runner often who reports audible snapping of hip or clicking with or without pain during basic movement or ambulation. Physical examination pertinent for tenderness over the respective tendon. There is snapping that occurs with hip provocative maneuvers. Obers maneuver is often positive (with regards to iliotibial band tendinopathy). Treatment includes PRICEMM, correcting the improper mechanics, and stretching and strengthening of hip girdle muscles. Corticosteroid injection may be needed if no improvement with conservative management.

C *Patellar Tendinopathy:* Risk factors include overuse from high quadriceps loading activities, decreased hamstring and quadriceps flexibility, and external tibial torsion. History is often positive for frequent jumping, squatting, or kneeling. There is reported pain in inferior pole of patella and often pain is diminished during activity. On examination, pain is reproducible with palpation over the inferior or superior pole of the patellar tendon. The decline squat test often reproduces patient's pain. Treatment consists of PRICEMM, correcting the improper mechanics, and emphasis on eccentric exercises and could consider patellar taping or patellar bracing.

D *Achilles Tendinopathy:* Risk factors include repetitive eccentric overload, improper mechanics such as hyper-pronation, poor strength with inflexibility in hamstring and gastrocsoleus complex, and male gender. History is consistent with frequent running or jumping activities with possible recent change in intensity or duration of training. Often reported pain in the back of the ankle associated with swelling and thickening of the tendon. Physical examination is consistent with pain 2–6 cm above the tendon insertion on the calcaneus and often posterior ankle swelling with crepitus at the tendon. Treatment with PRICEMM, short-term immobilization, soleus and gastrocnemius range of motion and stretching, and eccentric strengthening program. Heel lift is helpful as well to offload the tendon. Injections are not recommended due to risk of tendon rupture.

E *Flexor Hallucis Longus Tendinopathy (commonly referred to as Dancer Tendinopathy):* Risk factors consist of improper biomechanics and repetitive push-off at the first toe. History often is a dancer that reports pain during plantar flexion. Physical examination is consistent with tenderness along the tendon at the posteromedial aspect of the great toe, as well as pain with active plantar flexion and passive dorsiflexion. Treatment consists of PRICEMM, range of motion, stretching and strengthening of the involved muscles, as well as taping and bracing. Consider a shoe with a firm sole.

SUGGESTED READING

Cook JL, Purdam CR. Rehabilitation of lower limb tendinopathies. Clin Sports Med. 2003;22(4):777-89.

Cuccurullo S. Physical Medicine and Rehabilitation Board Review, 3rd edition. New York: Demos Medical Publishing; 2015.

Fredericson M, Wolf C. Iliotibial band syndrome in runners: innovations in treatment. Sports Med. 2005;35(5):451-9.

Khan K, Cook J. The painful nonruptured tendon: clinical aspects. Clin Sports Med. 2003;22(4):711-25.

Khan KM, Cook JL, Bonar F, et al. Histopathology of common tendinopathies. Update and implications for clinical management. Sports Med. 1999;27(6):393-408.

Maffulli N, Wong J, Almekinders LC. Types and epidemiology of tendinopathy. Clin Sports Med. 2003;22(4):675-92.

Scott A, Ashe MC. Common tendinopathies in the upper and lower extremities. Curr Sports Med Rep. 2006;5(5):233-41.

Simpson MR, Howard TM. Tendinopathies of the foot and ankle. Am Fam Physician. 2009;80(10):1107-14.

Wasielewski NJ, Kotsko KM. Does eccentric exercise reduce pain and improve strength in physically active adults with symptomatic lower extremity tendinosis? A systematic review. J Athl Train. 2007;42(3):409-21.

Wilson JJ, Best TM. Common overuse tendon problems: A review and recommendations for treatment. Am Fam Physician. 2005;72(5):811-8.

CHAPTER
91

Bursitis: Lower Extremity

Bouffard KJ, Marshall B

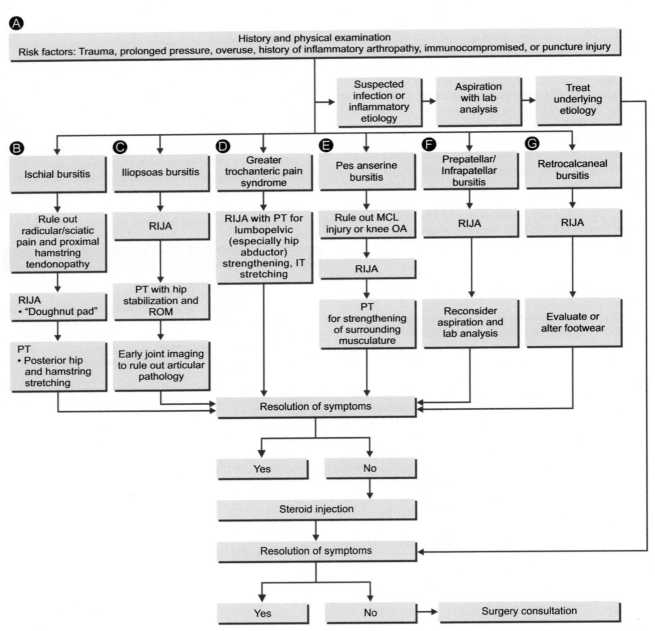

RIJA, rest, ice, joint protection analgesics (NSAIDs), acetaminophen; PT, physical therapy; ROM, range of motion; IT, iliotibial; MCL, medial collateral ligament; OA, osteoarthritis

Bursae in the lower extremity are typically located on top of prominent bony protrusions to facilitate the movement across these structures or protect from direct trauma.

A Acute bursitis is characterized by focal tenderness, swelling, and discomfort with associated decreased joint range of motion. Chronic bursitis has prominent swelling or thickening with relatively modest associated pain and tenderness.

General management, with the exception of septic or inflammatory bursitis, should aim to relieve the immediate symptoms with rest, ice, joint protection, and analgesics including nonsteroidal anti-inflammatory drugs (NSAIDs) or acetaminophen (RIJA) with consideration of corticoid steroid injection (CSI) or physical therapy (PT) in more resistant cases. Rarely bursitis will continue to persist despite these measures and may require surgical excision or evacuation.

B Ischial bursae are located between the gluteus muscles and ischial spine and are uncovered and at risk for direct injury with hip flexion (i.e. sitting) which gave the nickname of "Weavers" or "Tailors bottom". Pain is worse with sitting with focal tenderness at the ischial spine. Pain in proximate structures including the sciatic nerve and hamstring insertion may emulate symptoms and should be excluded on examination. Typically RIJA including offloading with a "doughnut" pad and posterior hip and hamstring stretching are effective and CSI should be used conservatively given proximity to sciatic nerve.

C Iliopsoas bursae are located between the anterior hip joint and iliopsoas muscle. Bursitis here is often associated with articular pathology (osteoarthritis [OA], rheumatoid arthritis [RA], septic, etc.) or hip flexor overuse. Patients will report groin pain worsened by activity and may have audible hip "snapping" which can be recreated with the "snapping hip" maneuver. Examination often mimics articular pathology which may be present concurrently. Treatment starts with RIJA but the clinician should consider early advancing imaging (magnetic resonance imaging [MRI], ultrasound [US]) to exclude alternative hip pathology (labral tear, synovitis, and avascular necrosis). If conservative measures fail, patient is likely to benefit from CSI.

D Greater trochanteric pain syndrome has taken the place of the traditional diagnosis of trochanteric bursitis for lateral hip pain, as a majority of cases are a result of gluteus medius/minimus tendinopathy, occasionally associated with a secondary bursitis whereas primary trochanteric bursitis is rare and usually microbial. The pain is near/on the greater trochanter and is worsened by ambulation, stair ascension or direct pressure (i.e. sleeping on affected side). Greater trochanteric tenderness with gluteus medius weakness evident by manual testing or positive Trendelenburg is typical, but many have positive Ober's or FABER's tests as well. Early treatment should include RIJA as well as PT for lumbopelvic, hip, and thigh strengthening with iliotibial (IT) band stretching. CSI can then be performed if symptoms persist and surgery should be considered in cases that persist more than 1 year despite conservative care or in the presence of significant gluteus tears on MRI.

E Pes Anserine bursae are located between the medial tibial plateau and conjoint tendon or approximately 6 cm distal to medial joint line. Bursitis here is commonly caused by abnormal gait or medial knee OA. Pain is focal and usually worse at night. Closely related pain etiologies should be ruled out with valgus stress test (medial collateral ligament injury) and X-ray (knee OA). Conservative treatment includes RIJA with limits on squatting, crossing legs, or repetitive bending and CSI is indicated if not improved with conservative care.

F Prepatellar and infrapatellar bursae are located above and below the patella, respectively, and are susceptible to direct trauma from repetitive kneeling (*Housemaids knee*) or infection. Pain is focal and worse with direct pressure. Examination is notable for improvement of pain in full extension, whereas knee effusions would prefer modest flexion. Treatment is typically RIJA but one should have a low threshold for aspiration given prevalence of septic etiology. CSI indicated in refractory cases.

G Retrocalcaneal bursitis is typically from overuse or repetitive trauma but can be inflammatory. History may include recent footwear alteration (often high-heels) and focal pain at posterior heel. Haglund deformity (increased prominence of the posterosuperior aspect of the calcaneus) may be present. RIJA with appropriate fitting footwear (included cessation of high-heel use) is typically effective and CSI should be used sparingly due to risk of Achilles rupture.

SUGGESTED READING

Cuccurullo S. Physical Medicine and Rehabilitation Board Review, 3rd edition. New York: Demos Medical Publishing; 2015.

Fearon AM, Scarvell JM, Neeman T, et al. Greater trochanteric pain syndrome: defining the clinical syndrome. Br J Sports Med. 2013; 47(10):649-53.

Johnston CA, Wiley JP, Lindsay DM, et al. Iliopsoas bursitis and tendinitis. A review. Sports Med. 1998;25(4):271-83.

Larsson LG, Baum J. The syndrome of anserine bursitis: an overlooked diagnosis. Arthritis Rheum. 1985;28(9):1062-5.

Paluska SA. An overview of hip injuries in running. Sports Med. 2005;35(11):991-1014.

Swartout R, Compere EL. Ischiogluteal bursitis. The pain in the arse. JAMA. 1974;227(5):551-2.

Williams BS, Cohen SP. Greater trochanteric pain syndrome: a review of anatomy, diagnosis and treatment. Anesth Analg. 2009; 108(5):1662-70.

SECTION 10

Pediatric Pain

Miles Day

Management of Painful Procedures in Pediatric Patients

Mina MM

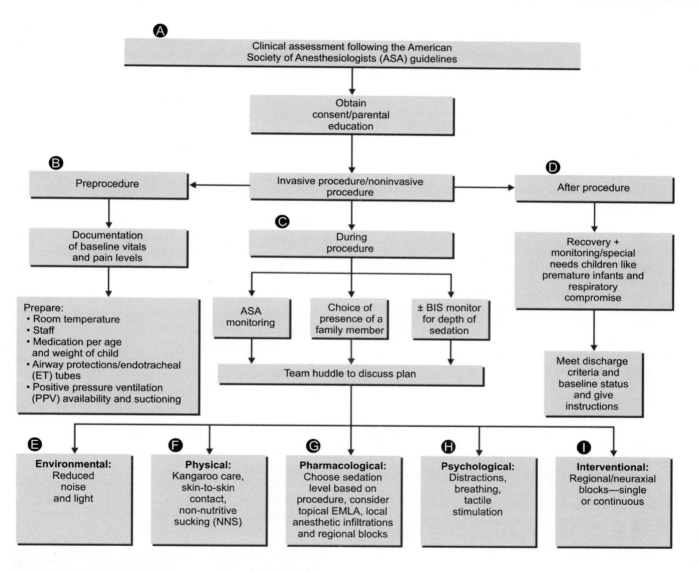

Although the field of pain management in children remains a gray area, there is still a need to eliminate pain in painful procedures. While it is impossible to remove all pain, unresolved pain can lead to short- and long-term negative consequences physically, psychologically, and emotionally. Therefore, it is important to assess the patient's pain before, during, and after painful procedures, with the goal being child's safety, while minimizing pain, obtund physiological responses, amnesia, control movement and return to baseline before discharge.

Ⓐ Procedural pain management starts by anticipation, selecting an approach tailored to procedural pain intensity, duration, coping means of child and family using a multimodal approach that meets the child's needs. The child and family should be educated regarding what to expect and methods to reduce stress and discomfort is essential and is completed in advance. Basic guidelines for all pediatric painful procedures: to avoid interrupting sleep, be planned far from mealtimes and other invasive procedures to allow time for recovery.

B Prior to the procedure, equipment and emergency medications are to be checked with availability of positive pressure ventilation, oxygen supply, suctioning, and airway equipment appropriate for the age of the child. Nothing-by-mouth (NPO) status should be tailored to each child. Parents should be educated regarding the procedure and informed consent obtained. In our practice, if appropriate, we allow a parent to attend the procedure. Examination of the child should be performed prior to the procedure, with the documentation of vitals throughout and after the procedure using Standard American Society of Anesthesiologists (ASA) monitors; adding a bispectral index (BIS) monitor is an option to evaluate depth of sedation.

C During procedures, the least painful method should be utilized, and the positioning/swaddling of the child should be taken into consideration. For noninvasive procedures, sedation and monitoring are sufficient but might require a general anesthetic; for invasive procedures like a bone marrow biopsy, analgesia is necessary. Full understanding of age-related changes in pharmacokinetics and pharmacodynamics should serve as a guide to treatment requiring regular assessments to titrate doses tailored to the responses of each child. Caution with newborns and premature infants having immature liver enzymes and reduced renal clearance leads to higher concentrations of medications and longer elimination half-lives, requiring less frequent dosing intervals. The diminished ventilatory responses to hypoxia and hypercapnia should be taken into consideration when administering opioids.

D Following the procedure, appropriate monitoring for recovery should be tailored to the child's age, comorbidities, prematurity, extent of procedure and depth of sedation, ensuring safe return to baseline and meeting discharge criteria if going home. Parents should be provided while providing the parents with instructions for alarming signs.

A multimodal approach should be used during the procedure: environmental, physical, pharmacological, psychological and interventional.

E *Environmental*: Recommendations in this category include minimizing the number of painful procedures, reducing environmental noise and light and keeping a calm and relaxed environment during the procedure.

F *Physical*: Strategies in this category include kangaroo care, which involves skin-to-skin contact and helps pediatric patients with the regulation of their heart rate and breathing. Another strategy in this category includes non-nutritive sucking (NNS) such as sucking on a thumb, a pacifier, or other object such as a blanket or toy. Other strategies include facilitated tucking (holding the child in a flexed position) and breastfeeding during painful procedures. In our facility, physicians are encouraged to carry smaller children to the procedure room with their favorite blanket and/or toy.

G *Pharmacological*: Delivery of medication should be administered with the least painful, most effective route: (1) 15–24% sucrose with or without neonatal sucking for acute single-event procedures with a topical anesthetic; (2) topical local anesthetics include EMLA cream for all ages, which needs to be applied at least 30 minutes to an hour before procedures and infiltrating site with buffered lidocaine; (3) benzodiazepines, such as short-acting midazolam, do not have analgesic properties but help with anxiety and muscle spasms; (4) oxygen and nitrous oxide mixtures can be used but should be calibrated with a minimum of 25% oxygen concentration, providing analgesia and sedation; (5) paracetamol and ketorolac for mild to moderate pain, no nonsteroidal anti-inflammatory drugs (NSAIDs) below 3 months of age; (6) opioids can be used with the goal of early and effective pain control tailored to response and side effects. Short-acting opioids are preferable, including fentanyl and remifentanil, which could be titrated or given as a continuous infusion; (7) ketamine has been used for dissociative sedation with profound analgesia and amnesia while protecting airway reflexes and spontaneous ventilation particularly in patients with respiratory compromise and hypotension; and (8) propofol infusions might need analgesics.

H *Psychological*: Cognitive behavioral methods using imagery and relaxation techniques provide pain relief done alone or accompanied by other modalities. Children between the ages of 2 months and 11 years will benefit from clinician-led distraction techniques. For children older than 3 years, child-led distractions and slow deep breathing or blowing in combination with psychological interventions are recommended. Any child over the age of 4 will get some relief from tactile stimulations such as rubbing or stroking the skin near the injection site with moderate intensity before and during an injection.

I *Interventional*: Regional and neuraxial blocks, single or continuous, as intercostal blocks and epidural catheters done with ultrasound guidance offer another tool for preemptive analgesia and postprocedural pain management.

Acknowledgments: For their great efforts in collecting and reviewing the research and data: Eman Mina, MD, Eirene Rophael, MBA, Marina Mina, Cyril Mina.

SUGGESTED READING

American Academy of Pediatrics Committee on Drugs: Guidelines for monitoring and management of pediatric patients during and after sedation for diagnostic and therapeutic procedures. Pediatrics. 1992;89:1110-5.

Lee GY, Yamada J, Kyololo O, et al. Pediatric clinical practice guidelines for acute procedural pain: a systematic review. Pediatrics. 2014;133:500-15.

CHAPTER 93

Chronic Benign Pain in Children

Mina MM

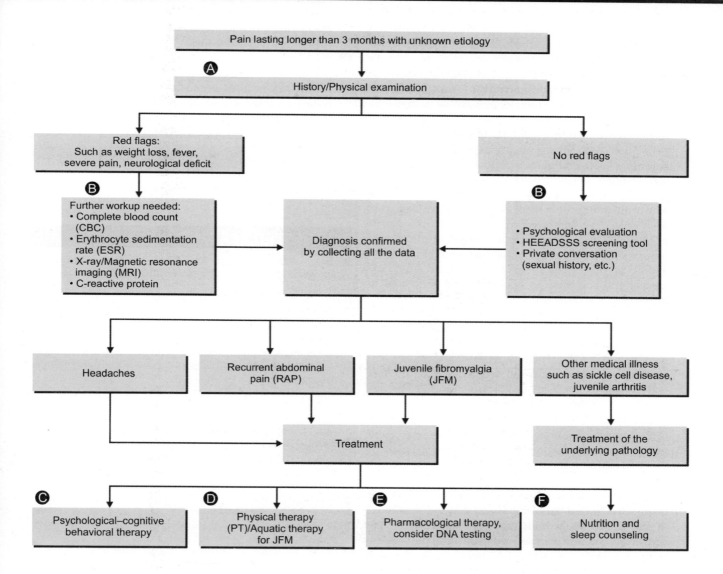

Pain lasting longer than 3 months with unknown etiology

Ⓐ History/Physical examination

Red flags:
Such as weight loss, fever, severe pain, neurological deficit

No red flags

Ⓑ Further workup needed:
- Complete blood count (CBC)
- Erythrocyte sedimentation rate (ESR)
- X-ray/Magnetic resonance imaging (MRI)
- C-reactive protein

Diagnosis confirmed by collecting all the data

Ⓑ
- Psychological evaluation
- HEEADSSS screening tool
- Private conversation (sexual history, etc.)

Headaches

Recurrent abdominal pain (RAP)

Juvenile fibromyalgia (JFM)

Other medical illness such as sickle cell disease, juvenile arthritis

Treatment

Treatment of the underlying pathology

Ⓒ Psychological–cognitive behavioral therapy

Ⓓ Physical therapy (PT)/Aquatic therapy for JFM

Ⓔ Pharmacological therapy, consider DNA testing

Ⓕ Nutrition and sleep counseling

Chronic benign pain (CBP) in children is a continuous or recurrent pain with unknown organic etiology persistent for more than 3 months. Prevalence of CBP in children and adolescents is rising; most common are headaches, recurrent abdominal pain (RAP), and juvenile fibromyalgia (JFM) compromising 15–20% of pediatric population. Migraines are the most common among headaches and they affect adolescents between the ages of 12 years and 17 years with occurrences at least 15 days per month with at least eight episodes and are most common in girls. RAP consists of weekly occurrences of abdominal pain for more than 2 months, severe enough to affect activities around 20% of school-age children using Rome III criteria. JFM, also known as juvenile primary fibromyalgia syndrome or JPFS, is present in 2–6% of school children, mostly adolescent females, with predominant symptoms of widespread pain lasting more than 3 months accompanied by fatigue, sleep disturbances, mood disturbances, somatic disorders, cognitive disorders with presence of painful "tender points" on examination.

Chronic pain also accompanies chronic illness such as juvenile arthritis, sickle cell disease, and cancer. A significant socioeconomic burden accompanies CBP in children reflected in direct costs involving multiple office visits with investigations and indirect costs involving loss of productivity of the child at school and parents taking time off work. Predisposing factors include the child's and parents' psychology while interactions at the school with teachers and peers might influence and sustain the pain.

A The evaluation of chronic pain in children is far more complex with paucity of evidence and standardized protocols for pain assessment and treatment; if not well treated, it will evolve into complicated physical and mental disorders later in adulthood. A comprehensive history and examination provide reassurance to the child and the family that their concerns and frustrations are taken seriously and compassionately with attention to social past medical history and all previous treatments and investigations.

B Appropriate assessment tools for pain should be used with attention to age, disability and cognitive level. Psychosocial history is essential in looking for factors contributing to perception, maintenance and reinforcement of pain by parents as well as school interactions like the HEEADSSS screening tool, which stands for Home, Education, Eating, Activities, Drugs, Sexuality, Suicide, and Safety. Private conversation regarding sexual history and psychological fears should be addressed without the child's parents' presence. Physical examination is required to rule out organic causes. Further workup with a normal examination and no alarming signs are not warranted and add to the anxiety and confusion as essential, only performed in presence of red flags. Red flags to be considered include sudden or severe symptoms, positional headaches, change of pattern, associated neurological symptoms and deficits, weight loss, fever, change of bowel habits, altered mental status and focal neurological deficits.

Diagnosis is best achieved by gathering all the data and consulting with all healthcare providers. In our experience, addressing the family empathetically with reassurances of treatment for identifiable causes and that CBP disorders are nonprogressive and not associated with serious complications facilitates the engagement of the child and family into the multidisciplinary program.

Treatment strategies include pharmacological and nonpharmacological techniques. Treatment goals should be directed toward pain control and prevention tailored to the child's needs with attention to quality of life addressing children with delayed maturity appropriately. Nonpharmacological strategies include psychological interventions, physical therapy, nutritional and sleep counseling.

C Psychological interventions rely mostly on cognitive behavioral therapy, relaxation techniques and biofeedback including family interventions.

D Physical therapy modalities enforcing participation with the school-based exercise program are crucial; aquatic therapy essential for JFM.

E Pharmacological therapy, although lacking evidence, includes nonopiate analgesics and adjuvant agents such as antiepileptic medications, gabapentin and pregabalin are used for JFM; antidepressants like duloxetine, fluoxetine, and escitalopram help in JFM and depression; muscle relaxants such as cyclobenzaprine have a role in headaches. The use of opiates should be avoided, but might have a role in juvenile rheumatoid arthritis, sickle cell disease and cancer pain.

F Counseling on proper nutrition and sleep hygiene is beneficial.

The prognosis of chronic pain is favorable, but there is the possibility of persisting pain. This should alert us to early recognition, diagnosis and intervention for the child and family to avoid long-term sequelae.

Acknowledgments: For their great efforts in collecting and reviewing the research and data:
Eman Mina, MD, Eirene Rophael, MBA, Marina Mina, Cyril Mina.

SUGGESTED READING

Drossman DA, Dumitrascu DL. Rome III: New standard for functional gastrointestinal disorders. J Gastrointestin Liver Dis. 2006;15(3):237-41.

Duarte MA, Penna FJ, Andrade EM, et al. Treatment of nonorganic recurrent abdominal pain: cognitive-behavioral family intervention. J Pediatr Gastroenterol Nutr. 2006;43(1):59-64.

Headache Classification Committee of the International Headache Society. Cephalalgia, 3rd edition. London, UK: Sage; 2013. pp. 629-808.

Hershey AD, Winner P, Kabbouche MA, et al. Headaches. Curr Opin Pediatr. 2007;19(6):663-9.

Hicks CL, von Baeyer CL, McGrath PJ. Online psychological treatment for pediatric recurrent pain: a randomized evaluation. J Pediatr Psychol. 2006;31(7):724-36.

Kashikar-Zuck S, Ting TV. Juvenile fibromyalgia: current status of research and future developments. Nat Rev Rheumatol. 2014; 10(2):89-96.

McGrath P. Pain in child health. Pain Res Manag. 2012;17(6):385.

Perquin CW, Hazebroek-Kampschreur AA, Hunfeld JA, et al. Pain in children and adolescents: a common experience. Pain. 2000; 87:51-8.

Sleed M, Eccleston C, Beecham J. The economic impact of chronic pain in adolescence: methodological considerations and a preliminary costs-of-illness study. Pain. 2005;119(1-3):183-90.

Vetter TR. A clinical profile of a cohort of patients referred to an anesthesiology-based pediatric chronic pain medicine program. Anesth Analg. 2008;106(3):786-94.

Cancer-Related Pain in Children

Driver LC, Spain TL, McAnally AA

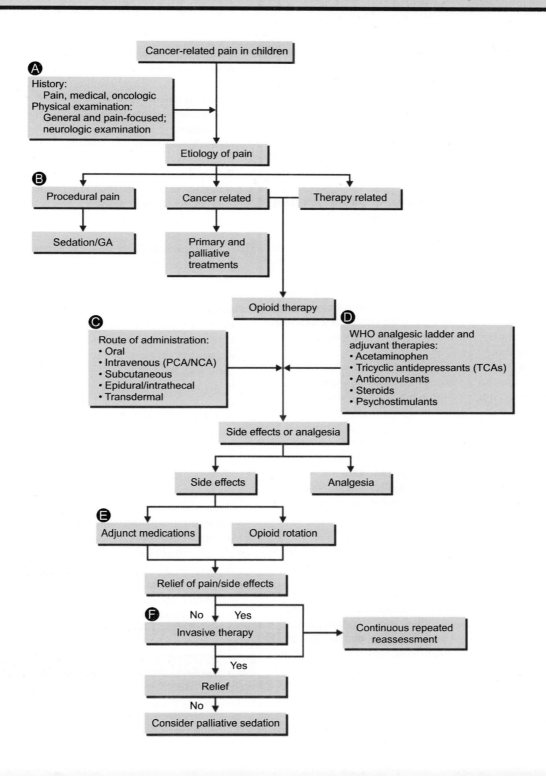

The challenge of caring for a child with a life-threatening illness such as cancer is that pain management is only one aspect of the care of the dyad for child and parents. Ideally, the management team constructs a care program centered on cure, simultaneously focusing on symptom management, and ultimately dealing with end-of-life issues in some cases. As with adults, pain can be caused by the cancer itself, which may involve visceral thoracic or abdominal pain, somatic pain caused by direct invasion of anatomic structures, and/or bone and joint pain due to primary hematologic or metastatic disease. When a tumor invades the peripheral or central nervous system, pain is often at issue. Moreover, the pain caused by the invasive diagnostic and therapeutic procedures used in cancer patients is seen more often in pediatric cancer patients and this diagnostic/treatment-related pain is most feared by children. Additional considerations include the recognition and management of nausea and vomiting, mucositis, nutritional status, utilization of hematopoietic growth factors, acute radiation side effects, management of central venous catheters, post-treatment immunizations, and palliative care.

A As for most types of pain, a thorough history is important, including both a medical and an oncologic history. An age and developmentally appropriate pain scale must be used. It is important not only to measure the pain using an appropriate tool but also to involve the parents and other caregivers when formulating the assessment by relying on their observations. The medical examination should include a neurologic evaluation, looking for clues about the nature of the process. Because cancer is a dynamic disease, regular reassessment of pain and collateral symptoms should be done.

B Procedure-related pain is amenable to appropriate sedation and/or anesthetic protocols. Cognitive and behavioral adjuncts are often included in these protocols. However, if pain is either disease- or treatment-related, a more traditional opioid pharmacologic approach is recommended. The three-step analgesic ladder of the World Health Organization, the National Comprehensive Cancer Network (NCCN) guidelines, and the National Cancer Institute all provide helpful information regarding pharmacologic management. Opioids are a cornerstone of pharmacotherapy, and dosing should generally be titrated to the point of providing pain relief or the development of recognized side effects. Remember to include palliative and potential curative anticancer therapy when considering a treatment plan.

C The appropriate route of administration depends on the interplay of the intensity of the pain and the availability of the various routes. The oral route should be used as a first-line approach for most pediatric patients when initiating therapy. When oral treatments are not appropriate, alternate techniques include subcutaneous, intermittent intravenous, patient-controlled analgesia (PCA), nurse/parent-controlled analgesia (NCA), continuous infusions, and transdermal routes of administration. As in adults, basal opioids should be administered to the pediatric patient on a regular schedule with the provision of breakthrough or rescue medications as needed.

D When titrating opioids to effect, it is important to reassess the adequacy of the pain relief or the development of side effects at regular intervals. If adequate relief is obtained, simply continuing opioid therapy with periods of reassessment is indicated. If side effects develop, appropriate adjunctive treatment is warranted. However, if pain relief is inadequate, dose escalation of at least 25–50% is indicated to achieve an adequate effect. If at this point relief is still inadequate despite dose escalation, or if it is difficult to manage unpleasant side effects despite appropriate therapy, it is important to switch or rotate opioids. When switching opioids, it is important to bear in mind the relative differences in opioid potency. Initial doses of new opioids should be 25–50% less than the estimated equivalent dose of the prior opioid to allow for incomplete cross-tolerance. Importantly, if rotation to methadone is planned, one must reduce the equianalgesic dose by 75% or more to avoid significant sedation. If the new regimen provides adequate relief and management of side effects, there should be continued reassessment guiding the continuation of opioid therapy.

E If opioid rotation and dose escalation are not providing adequate analgesia or relieving the side effects, one should consider invasive approaches. These might include spinal or epidural drug delivery or surgical or neuroablative procedures, depending on the nature of the tumor process and disease status. Unfortunately, a small percentage of patients still obtain no relief despite aggressive, invasive therapy. At this point, one should meet with the family to consider palliative sedation. This is an infrequently used treatment arm in pediatric cancer management because 90% of patients who experience pain find relief with opioids alone.

F During opioid therapy, one must anticipate, recognize, and treat opioid-related side effects. Adjunct medications can be beneficial in limiting the amount of opioid required and for diminishing opioid-related side effects. Corticosteroids can help with pain resulting from acute nerve compression, visceral distension, soft tissue infiltration, or increased intracranial pressure. Anticonvulsants may be beneficial when neuropathic pain is present. Tricyclic antidepressants also are beneficial for neuropathic pain, as well as to treat depression and help with insomnia. Psychostimulants, such as methylphenidate or dexamphetamine, are beneficial for combating the somnolence of opioid therapy. Neuroleptics may be beneficial when dealing with hallucinations during opioid therapy.

SUGGESTED READING

Agrawal AK, Feusner J. Supportive care of patients with cancer. In: Lanzkowsky P, Lipton JM, Fish JD (Eds). Lanzkowsky's Manual of Pediatric Hematology and Oncology, 6th edition. San Diego: Academic Press; 2016. pp. 620-55.

Baumbauer KM, Young EE, Starkweather AR, et al. Managing chronic pain in special populations with emphasis on pediatric, geriatric, and drug abuser populations. Med Clin North Am. 2016;100(1):183-97.

Bennett R, Givens D. Easing suffering for a child with intractable pain at the end of life. J Pediatr Health Care. 2011;25(3):180-5.

Mercadante S, Giarratano A. Pharmacological management of cancer pain in children. Crit Rev Oncol Hematol. 2014;91(1):93-7.

National Comprehensive Cancer Network, Inc. NCCN Guidelines Version 1. (2014). Adult cancer pain. [online] Available from *www.nccn.org/cancerpain.* [Accessed January, 2017].

PDQ® Supportive and Palliative Care Editorial Board, PDQ Cancer Center Pain, Bethesda, MD: National Cancer Institute. (2016). Cancer Pain (PDQ)–Patient Version. [online] Available from *http://www.cancer.gov/about-cancer/treatment/side-effects/ pain/pain-hp-pdq.* [Accessed January, 2017].

Rabbitts JA, Holley AL, Groenewald CB, et al. Association between widespread pain scores and functional impairment and health-related quality of life in clinical samples of children. J Pain. 2016;17(6):678-84.

Raslan AM, Burchiel KJ. Neurosurgical approaches to pain management. In: Benzon HT, Rathmell JP, Wu CL, Turk DC, Argoff CE, Hurley RW (Eds). Practical Management of Pain, 5th edition. Philadelphia: Mosby; 2014. pp. 328-34.

Rosenberg AR, Orellana L, Ullrich C, et al. Quality of life in children with advanced cancer: a report from the PediQUEST study. J Pain Symptom Manage. 2016;52(2):243-53.

Shah R, Sawardekar A, Suresh S. Continuous peripheral nerve blocks for pediatrics. Adv Anesth. 2012;30:61-73.

Stjernsward J, Colleau SM, Ventafridda V. The World Health Organization Cancer Pain and Palliative Care Program. Past, present and future. J Pain Symptom Manage. 1996;12:65-72.

CHAPTER 95

Complex Regional Pain Syndrome in Children

Mina MM

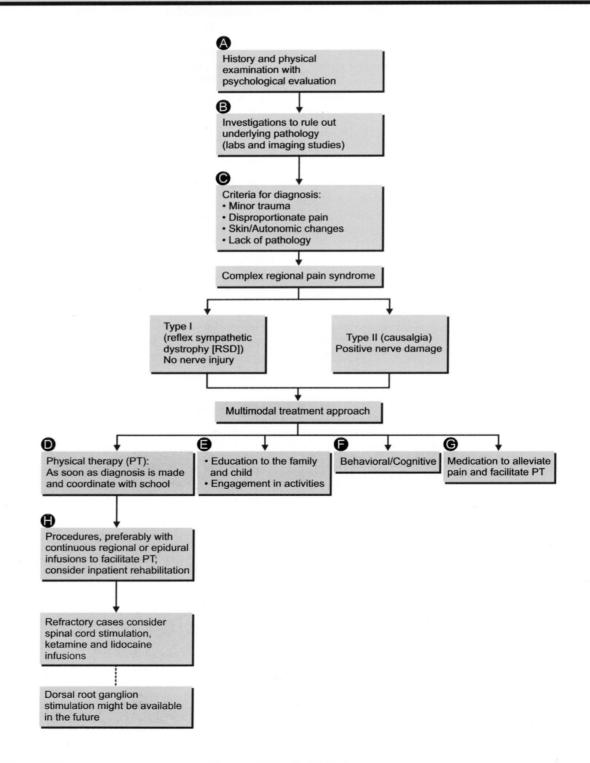

A History and physical examination with psychological evaluation

B Investigations to rule out underlying pathology (labs and imaging studies)

C Criteria for diagnosis:
• Minor trauma
• Disproportionate pain
• Skin/Autonomic changes
• Lack of pathology

Complex regional pain syndrome

Type I (reflex sympathetic dystrophy [RSD]) No nerve injury

Type II (causalgia) Positive nerve damage

Multimodal treatment approach

D Physical therapy (PT): As soon as diagnosis is made and coordinate with school

E • Education to the family and child
• Engagement in activities

F Behavioral/Cognitive

G Medication to alleviate pain and facilitate PT

H Procedures, preferably with continuous regional or epidural infusions to facilitate PT; consider inpatient rehabilitation

Refractory cases consider spinal cord stimulation, ketamine and lidocaine infusions

Dorsal root ganglion stimulation might be available in the future

Complex regional pain syndrome (CRPS) types I and II, formerly known as reflex sympathetic dystrophy (RSD) and causalgia respectively, are defined by the International Association for the Study of Pain (IASP) as amplified pain (1) occurring after blunt or minor injury, (2) disproportionate to the traumatic event, (3) with sensory, vasomotor and autonomic disturbances causing allodynia, hyperalgesia, and skin changes in temperature, color, appearance, and trophic changes, and (4) lacking pathology in the area affected. CRPS type II constitutes nerve injury while in type I there is no identifiable nerve injury.

Predisposing factors could be (1) psychological, (although the psychological factors may also be consequences) and (2) genetic as is more common with a positive family history. With the rise in prevalence of CRPS in children, knowledge of presentations in the pediatric population is key as differing from adults, with a higher female to male ratio, usually in late childhood and puberty, and more common in the lower extremity. When compared to adults, there is a higher difference in skin temperature, less limited range of motion, less hyperesthesia and tremors, and less paresis in the involved extremity. CRPS type II has roughly equal incidence in both boys and girls.

A Diagnosis is achieved with a detailed history including a social history. This is followed by a clinical examination of the affected site. Comparison to the contralateral extremity is important in the examination process, and the practitioner should note sensory disturbances including hyperalgesia and allodynia; motor impairment as loss of function, decreased range of movement, muscle spasms and atrophy; skin temperature differences (typically run colder in children) and color changes; and abnormal sweating such as hyperhidrosis. A psychological evaluation is also important in the pediatric population. "Red flags" should be excluded.

B Investigations and imaging studies (sedimentation rate, C-reactive protein and bone scans) are done to exclude underlying pathology in the presence of red flags. Other tests, such as quantitative sudomotor and thermography do not play a role but delay the onset of treatment, and can cause more anxiety in the child and the parents. Disease prevention using vitamin C has been used in adults but is not well established in children.

C If the diagnostic criteria (pain that is disproportionate to clinical presentation with one autonomic dysfunction sign such as lower skin temperature, cyanosis, edema or sweating) are fulfilled and the "red flags" (major trauma, local and systemic signs of inflammatory conditions, and tumors or soft tissue mass) are excluded, a diagnosis of CRPS can be made.

Treatment involves a multimodal approach using:

D Physical and occupational therapy modalities should be instituted early, and are the most important component. These modalities aim for restoration of function and include desensitization, hydrotherapy, and aerobic exercises. Activity can be facilitated by adequate pain relief using regional blocks for outpatient or inpatient therapy preferably with a continuous infusion to minimize repeated procedures.

E Educating the family and child regarding the child's diagnosis helps in bonding with the child and earns their trust which promotes physical activity in a hobby or a sport, i.e. baking and playing with dough for upper extremity and soccer or similar activity for the lower extremity. To encourage the child, we engage them into physical therapy while attending school.

F Behavioral and psychological therapies are geared toward the child and the parents. These include cognitive behavioral therapy, relaxation techniques, biofeedback, and family counseling for coping and avoidance of pain reinforcements. If significant psychological comorbidities are found, a child psychiatrist should be consulted. Consider nutritional counseling and sleep hygiene with continuation of academic achievements and physical accommodations at school.

G Pharmacological therapy involves topical medications like Lidoderm patches, capsaicin and compounding solutions. Systemic medications include: (1) antiepileptics such as gabapentin and pregabalin, (2) antidepressants such as amitriptyline can help with sleep, and (3) ketamine and lidocaine infusions, along with low doses of naltrexone, have been used in refractory cases. A transcutaneous electrical nerve stimulation (TENS) unit can also be tried.

H Pain-reducing procedures facilitate participation in a multidisciplinary program particularly with physical therapy. Regional and epidural blocks with or without continuous infusions using local anesthetics and clonidine are sometimes necessary. These can achieve a sympathetic and sensory blockade so that extensive inpatient physical therapy can be started. As an inpatient, the family can be educated with regards to the infusion and become comfortable managing the catheter as outpatient. This is preferable over repeated single blocks. Patients with intractable diseases might benefit from spinal cord stimulation to facilitate physical, occupational, and behavioral therapy. Dorsal root ganglia stimulation is being used in Europe but is not yet approved in the United States.

Acknowledgments: For their great efforts in collecting and reviewing the research and data:

Eman Mina, MD, Eirene Rophael, MBA, Marina Mina, Cyril Mina.

SUGGESTED READING

Bernstein BH, Singsen BH, Kent JT, et al. Reflex neurovascular dystrophy in childhood. J Pediatr. 1978;93(2):211-5.

de Rooij AM, de Mos M, Sturkenboom MC. Familial occurrence of complex regional pain syndrome. Eur J Pain. 2009;13(2):171-7.

Harden RN, Bruehl S, Stanton-Hicks M, et al. Proposed new diagnostic criteria for complex regional pain syndrome. Pain Med. 2007;8(4):326-31.

IASP Task Force on Taxonomy; Merskey H, Bogduk N. Classification of Chronic Pain Descriptions of Chronic Pain Syndromes and

Definitions of Pain Terms, 2nd edition. Seattle, WA: IASP Press; 1994.

Low AK, Ward K, Wines AP. Pediatric complex regional pain syndrome. J Pediatr Orthop. 2007;27:567-72.

Sherry DD, Wallace CA, Kelley C, et al. Short- and long-term outcomes of children with complex regional pain syndrome type I treated with exercise therapy. Clin J Pain. 1999;15:218-23.

Stanton-Hicks M. Plasticity of complex regional pain syndrome (CRPS) in children. Pain Med. 2010;11:1216-23.

Tan EC, Zijlstra B, Essink ML, et al. Complex regional pain syndrome type I in children. Acta Paediatr. 2008;97(7):875-9.

Wilder RT. Management of pediatric patients with complex regional pain syndrome. Clin J Pain. 2006;22:443-8.

SECTION 11

Pharmacology

Ameet Nagpal

Local Anesthetic Choice and Toxicity

Wolf J, Rubens A, Pino CA

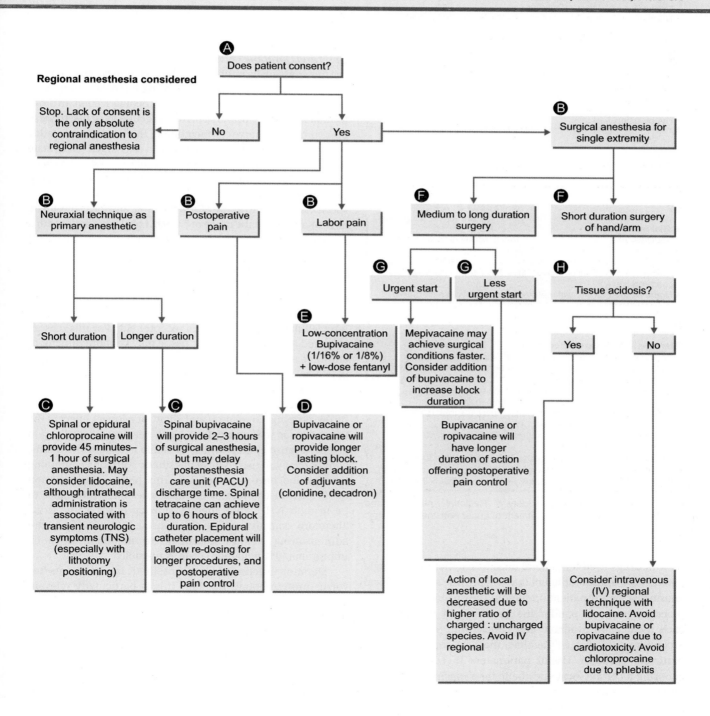

Recognition and management of local anesthetic systemic toxicity (LAST)

- Apply American Society of Anesthesiologists (ASA) standard monitors prior to performing regional technique (electrocardiogram [EKG], blood pressure [BP] cuff, pulse oximeter)
- Aspirate prior to injection, confirm absence of blood
- Utilize local anesthetic with epinephrine (1:200,000 or 5 μg/mL) mixture for intravascular marker
- Utilize incremental dosing of 5 mL, allowing for 30 seconds between doses

Patient's condition deteriorates→
- Altered mental status
- Seizure activity noted
- Arrhythmia develops
- Hypotension

Immediately abort procedure and initiate advanced cardiac life support

Initial management
- Ventilate with 100% oxygen, intubate if airway is compromised
- Treat seizure activity with benzodiazepines and/or propofol→ avoid propofol if cardiovascular instability is present
- Epinephrine in small doses for impending cardiovascular compromise
- Notify nearest facility with cardiopulmonary bypass capability

Management of cardiac collapse
- Initiate advanced cardiac life support (ACLS)
- Avoid vasopressin, calcium channel blockers or beta blockers
- Prepare 20% lipid emulsion→
  - Bolus. 1.5 mL/kg (~100 mL), followed by→
  - Infusion: 0.25 mL/kg/min (~18 mL/min in 70 kg patient)
  - Repeat bolus if no initial response, increase infusion to 0.5 mL/kg/min for persistent hypotension
  - Continue infusion for 10 minutes following return of cardiovascular stability
  - Recommended maximum dose is 10 mL/kg over 30 minutes
- If lipid emulsion therapy fails, immediate transport to facility with cardiopulmonary bypass capability→ continue ACLS throughout

Adapted from the American Society of Regional Anesthesia and Pain Medicine Checklist for Treatment of Local Anesthetic Systemic Toxicity.

As with drugs used for general anesthesia, there is no single perfect local anesthetic agent that will provide adequate local anesthesia for any patient undergoing any technique. Rather, practitioners must ponder the benefits and drawbacks of each medication available and choose one (or sometimes a combination) that will achieve the best conditions for a particular scenario. Useful parameters to consider when choosing a certain local anesthetic for a regional anesthesia application include time to onset, duration of action, mechanism of metabolism, and potential complications.

Structure and Metabolism: Structurally, local anesthetics are weak bases consisting of a lipophilic benzene ring connected to a hydrophilic amine group by either an ester or amide linkage. Therefore, local anesthetics are classified as either "esters" or "amides" based on their type of linkage structure. The clinical differences between amides and esters relates to metabolism. Amides are metabolized by enzyme-mediated N-dealkylation and hydroxylation in the liver. Esters, however, are degraded by pseudocholinesterase in the plasma (with the exception of cocaine which is degraded by esterases in the liver).

Onset and Duration: Local anesthetics temporarily impair nerve cell transmission by binding to sodium channels and inhibiting them from opening, thereby decreasing influx of sodium ions into a neuron and ultimately inhibiting depolarization. In order to initiate an effect, local anesthetic molecules must first traverse the hydrophobic nerve cell membrane. This occurs most readily when a molecule's amine group is in an uncharged (NH_2) state but at physiologic pH, local anesthetic molecules carry a positive charge (NH_3^+) on their amine group. The pH at which a drug in solution has an equal number of ionized and nonionized species is referred to as the pKa of the drug, and local anesthetic have pKa values in the range of 7.6–9.0. Local anesthetics with a pKa closer to physiologic pH are relatively less basic and have a higher percentage of unprotonated (uncharged or NH_2) drug at physiologic pH, which speeds onset of action.

While the NH_2 state will predispose the drug molecule to cross the cell membrane and confers a faster rate of onset, it is the NH_3^+ species that has a physiological effect at the intracellular sodium channel's receptor site. For this reason, inflamed and therefore acidic tissue may be more difficult to anesthetize than normal tissue that has a lower concentration of H^+ ion.

Epinephrine can be added to local anesthetic solution, and the localized vasoconstriction it induces may prevent uptake by the systemic circulation and allow for a longer effect at the target site, as well as a denser block per dose of medication given. Because epinephrine is unstable in alkaline solutions, commercially prepared local anesthetic solutions containing epinephrine have a pH of 4–5. This higher concentration of H^+ ion causes more of the local anesthetic molecules to be in their NH_3^+ state, thereby slowing onset of the drug. Therefore, consider adding epinephrine immediately before administering a local anesthetic to maintain as much unprotonated (uncharged) drug as possible.

Duration of action of a local anesthetic is related to its free versus protein-bound fraction. This is particularly relevant in infants, as they may demonstrate longer than expected duration of local anesthetic or even toxic effect due to low circulating plasma levels of alpha-1-acid glycoprotein.

Different types of nerve fibers demonstrate different responses to local anesthetic blockade. Typically, preganglionic sympathetic B-fibers require minimal local anesthetic doses to be blocked and, therefore, will lose their ability to transmit signals before other types of nerve fibers. Loss of sensation for pain and temperature (transmitted by A-delta fibers) requires a higher dose of local anesthetic, and finally loss of motor function as well as touch and proprioception sensations (transmitted by alpha fibers) requires the highest amount of local anesthetic. This differential in local anesthetic requirement for certain nerve fibers is demonstrated by the common clinical observation that sympathetic blockade often occurs 2–6 dermatomes beyond a given dermatomal level of sensory blockade, and motor impairment will occur at two fewer vertebral levels compared to sensory blockade.

A Local anesthetics are most commonly used in regional anesthesia procedures. First and foremost, consent is necessary for the procedure. If the patient does not consent, the procedure should not be performed.

B After consent is obtained, the reason for the use of local anesthetic should be identified. These reasons include postoperative pain, single extremity surgical anesthesia, labor pain, and/or neuraxial techniques.

C For neuraxial approaches, the practitioner should decide if the procedure will require a short duration or long duration blockade. Chloroprocaine and lidocaine are the best agents for short procedures, while bupivacaine and tetracaine are commonly used for longer procedures. Placement of an epidural catheter can allow for rapid "on and off" titration of medication which may be preferable.

D Bupivacaine or ropivacaine local anesthetic blocks for postoperative pain are most likely to give prolonged analgesia.

E In the case of labor pain, low dose bupivacaine mixed with fentanyl is the best choice for epidural analgesia as it relates to local anesthetic choice.

F For single extremity anesthesia and analgesia, the duration of the surgery must be known to determine which local anesthetic to use.

G Medium- and long-duration surgeries differ relative to the urgency of the start. In urgent cases, mepivacaine may be used, which allows for a quicker onset of blockage. Bupivacaine or ropivacaine can be added to the mepivacaine to prolong the block. For less urgent cases, bupivacaine or ropivacaine may be used in isolation so as to create the longest possible blockade.

H In shorter cases, the practitioner should identify whether tissue acidosis is present. If it is, intravenous regional anesthesia (IVRS) can be attempted, but the onset may be delayed due to the tissue acidosis. If there is no acidosis, then IVRS can safely be attempted with lidocaine. Bupivacaine and ropivacaine should be avoided due to the prolonged blockade and the possibility of cardiac toxicity (see **Table 1**).

Local Anesthetic Toxicity: While rarely observed, local anesthetics at sufficient plasma concentrations may result in significant systemic toxicity. Excessive plasma concentrations of the local anesthetics most commonly result from inadvertent intravascular injection of a large volume of the drug, typically during the performance of a peripheral nerve block. However, factors such as the particular local anesthetic used, dose, the site of injection, use of a vasoconstrictor and

patient weight also determine the likelihood and magnitude of systemic toxicity.

A Due to the potential devastating consequences of systemic toxicity, appropriate monitoring and prevention techniques are crucial to the administration of any significant dose of local anesthetics. These include use of repeated aspiration followed by intermittent dosing of the local anesthetic combined with epinephrine (5 µg/mL) to act as a vascular marker. Life-threatening effects of local anesthetic systemic toxicity are demonstrated in two organ systems in particular: (1) the central nervous system and (2) the cardiovascular system.

Central nervous system (CNS) toxicity is either due to the systemic absorption of local anesthetic until a toxic level accumulates or due to direct intravascular injection, with the degree of CNS toxicity-dependent on the plasma concentration of the offending local anesthetics. As plasma concentrations increase, the potential for CNS excitation and seizure increases concordantly. The potency of each local anesthetic is also directly proportional to the potential for toxicity. Potent, lipid-soluble local anesthetics, such as bupivacaine, display a higher degree of toxicity at lower concentrations compared to those that are less potent.

B As the plasma concentrations of local anesthetics progressively increase, the typical order of symptoms is: numbness around the mouth→facial tingling→restlessness→vertigo→tinnitus→slurred speech→tonic-clonic seizures. Seizure activity as a result of local anesthetic toxicity is best managed by CNS depressants, such as benzodiazepines for less severe reactions or propofol for an emergent situation not involving cardiovascular instability. Intubation is indicated if the patient is no longer able to protect their airway, or there is impending cardiovascular collapse.

While the cardiovascular system does display a higher degree of resistance to the toxic effects of local anesthetics, at clinically significant plasma concentrations, local anesthetics may demonstrate hypotensive and cardiac depressant effects. As local anesthetics bind and inhibit cardiac sodium ion channels, the conduction and pacemaker functions of the cardiac myocytes become impaired. Not all local anesthetics are equal in this regard, for example, the dose of bupivacaine required to produce cardiac collapse is roughly half that of lidocaine's. While prevention and avoidance of intravascular injection of local anesthetics is recommended first and foremost, adverse outcomes do occur.

C Treatment of cardiovascular instability and/or collapse as a result of local anesthetic toxicity is possible utilizing a lipid rescue technique after calling for help, appropriately managing the airway, and initiating emergency protocols to stabilize the patient.

D A recent study demonstrated improved cardiovascular recovery from bupivacaine toxicity in rats treated with intravenous lipid emulsion compared to saline or no treatment. The current recommended dosing algorithm published by the American Society of Regional Anesthesia

Table 1: Local anesthetics used for blocks

Local anesthetic	Infiltrative anesthesia	IV regional anesthesia	Topical anesthesia	Peripheral nerve blocks	Neuraxial blocks	Maximum dose* (mg/kg)
Amides **Long duration**						
Bupivacaine	0.25–0.5% Common	Not recommended		0.25–0.5% Common	Commonly used	2.5–3.5
Ropivacaine	0.25–0.5% Common	Not recommended		0.25–0.5% Common	Commonly used	2.5–3.5
Levobupivacaine	0.25–0.5% Common	Not recommended		0.25–0.5% Common	Commonly used	2.5–3.5
Etidocaine	Can be used	Has been successfully used No epinephrine		Motor block may outlast Sensory block Fast onset	Can be used Dense motor block Motor block may outlast Sensory block Fast onset	4.0–5.5
Intermediate duration						
Lidocaine	0.5–2.0% Common	3 mg/kg (40 cc of 0.5%) Preservative free No epinephrine Only LA FDA approved for IV regional anesthesia	2–4% topical or nebulized part of EMLA 5% ointment Lidoderm patch	1–2% Common	Can be used SAB-associated with syndrome of transient neurologic symptoms	7
Mepivacaine	0.5–2.0% Common	Has been used successfully		1–2% Common	Can be used SAB-associated with syndrome of transient neurologic symptoms	7
Short duration						
Prilocaine	Can be used	3 mg/kg (40 cc of 0.5%) Preservative free No epinephrine Methemoglobinemia	Part of EMLA Methemoglobinemia	Can be used Methemoglobinemia		8
Esters **Intermediate duration**						
Tetracaine	Can be used		1–2% Common	Can be used	Can be used	2
Short duration						
Chloroprocaine	Can be used	Not recommended because of thrombophlebitis	Poor choice	Can be used	Can be used epidurally and intrathecally Associated with syndrome of transient neurologic symptoms Preservatives, large doses, pH-related problems	12–15
Procaine	Can be used	Has been used successfully No epinephrine	Poor choice	Can be used	SAB-associated with syndrome of transient neurologic symptoms SAB-associated with N/V	10–14
Benzocaine			Mucosal application Subcutaneous application Methemoglobinemia			200 mg total

EMLA, eutectic mixture of local anesthetics; FDA, Food and Drug Administration; IV, intravenous; LA, local anesthetics; N/V, nausea and vomiting; SAB, subarachnoid block
*Higher doses with the use of 1:200,000 epinephrine. Clinically significant methemoglobinemia associated with prilocaine doses higher than 600 mg.

and Pain Medicine includes an intravenous (IV) bolus of 1.5 cc/kg of 20% lipid emulsion, followed by an infusion at 0.25 cc/kg/min for at least 10 minutes following return of hemodynamic stability. An additional bolus and increased infusion rate to 0.5 cc/kg/min is recommended if no response is seen to the initial attempt.

SUGGESTED READING

Barash PG, Cullen BF, Stoelting RK, et al. Clinical Anesthesia, 7th edition. Philadelphia: Lippincott Williams & Wilkins; 2013. pp. 572-66.

Fettiplace MR, Akpa BS, Ripper R, et al. Resuscitation with lipid emulsion: dose-dependent recovery from cardiac pharmacotoxicity requires a cardiotonic effect. Anesthesiology. 2014;120(4):915-25.

Miller RD, Pardo MC. Basics of Anesthesia, 6th edition. Philadelphia: Elsevier; 2011. pp. 136-8.

Neal JM, Bernards CM, Butterworth JF, et al. ASRA practice advisory on local anesthetic systemic toxicity. Reg Anesth Pain Med. 2010;35(2):152-61.

Stoelting RK. Pharmacology and Physiology in Anesthetic Practice, 3rd edition. Philadelphia: Lippincott-Raven; 1999. pp. 158-81.

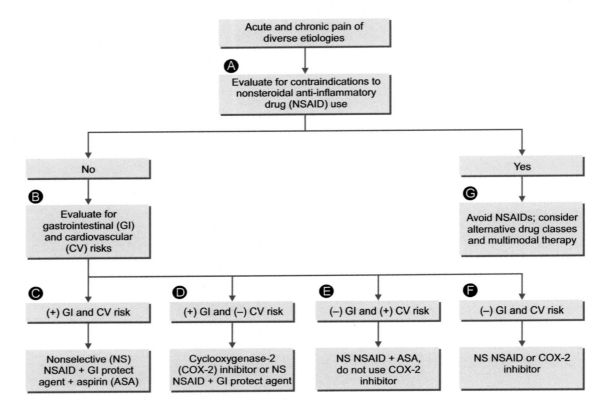

Arachidonic acid has been found to be the major source of prostaglandins. Phospholipase A2 converts phospholipid to arachidonic acid as it is released from the cell membrane. The cyclooxygenase (COX) enzyme catalyzes the formation of prostanoids from arachidonic acids. During inflammatory responses, prostaglandin E2 (PGE2) has been the most closely associated prostanoid, and it is for this reason, that PGE2 presence is often considered an indicator of local COX activity. Two COX isoforms, COX-1 and COX-2, have been identified. While COX-1 is detectable in most cells such as the gastrointestinal (GI) tract and platelets, COX-2 is mainly recognized during times of inflammation and at baseline in the brain and renal system.

During the selection process, clinicians must consider the pharmacokinetic profile of the drugs available. Specifically, absorption, distribution, and elimination will affect efficacy and tolerability. Although most nonsteroidal anti-inflammatory drugs (NSAIDs) are rapidly absorbed in their oral forms, the amount of drug absorption from the gastric tract is more important than the rate. Additionally, most members of this class of drugs are weak acids, maintain very good lipid solubility, and usually are highly bound to plasma proteins. While minor elimination occurs via the renal system, cytochrome P450-mediated oxidation and glucuronide conjugation by way of hepatic biotransformation remains the major route of elimination.

Aspirin irreversibly acetylates and inactivates both COX-1 and COX-2 while other drugs in this group are considered reversible inhibitors. Aspirin is converted to salicylates via first pass metabolism in the small intestine and liver. While the COX enzyme is reproduced by cells of the body, platelets lack this ability. Platelets remain inhibited for their entire lifetime.

Indomethacin provides good anti-inflammatory properties, but is limited by a high occurrence of adverse effects. It is used in many patients for arthritis symptoms but has fallen out of favor due to possible gastritis and renal dysfunction.

Ketorolac is efficacious for the treatment of postoperative pain. It is wholly bound to plasma proteins leading to a minimum volume of distribution and subsequent and extensive conjugation and excretion via the kidneys. Additionally, ketorolac is available as an oral formulation. Due to possible GI toxicity and operative site bleeding, it should not be used for more than 5 days.

Ibuprofen provides effective analgesia for arthritis patients at doses of 1200 mg/day and higher. However, when maximum recommended doses are reached, such as 3200 mg/day, adverse side effects such as nausea and dyspepsia become common. If patients are hypovolemic and hence have a low cardiac output, renal compromise is almost always expected with this drug. Likewise, naproxen is almost entirely excreted in the urine and, due to its long half-life, can be dosed twice daily. Consideration should be given to prolonged bleeding time due to platelet aggregation inhibition.

Meloxicam is one of the newer agents found to be beneficial in the treatment of osteoarthritis, rheumatoid arthritis, ankylosing spondylitis, and acute rheumatic pain. Due to its COX-2 selectivity, it has a better GI side effect profile than most other general NSAIDs. Although it is not recommended in patients with renal failure, its 20 hour half-life allows for once-daily dosing of both the 7.5 mg and 15 mg tablets. It has been safely administered with methotrexate, warfarin, furosemide, aspirin, and antacids.

Drugs in the class known as COX-2 inhibitors were developed specifically with the idea of reducing GI side effects such as dyspepsia, abdominal pain, gastric or duodenal ulcer, perforation, or bleeding. This class includes medications such as celecoxib, rofecoxib, and valdecoxib (The latter 2 are not available in the United States). An increased incidence of thrombotic cardiovascular events has been seen with NSAIDs and more commonly with the COX-2 inhibitors. While NSAIDs decrease thromboxane A2 (TXA2) and prostacyclin (PGI2) via suppression of COX-1 and COX-2, COX-2 inhibitors only affect a decrease in PGI2. It is the difference that is blamed for the rise in blood pressure, early development in atherosclerosis, exaggerated thrombotic response to plaque rupture, and incidence of myocardial infarction seen with long-term COX-2 inhibitor use.

When considering NSAID selection, the clinician is left to consider the clinical utility versus the adverse side effects. From a GI standpoint, certain risk factors have been identified. These risk factors include aspirin use, concomitant anticoagulant use, increased age (>60) and dose, previous GI bleed, and alcohol consumption. Additionally, as discussed earlier, aspirin irreversibly inhibits platelet activation via COX-1 inhibition. This in turn leads to a reduction in viable TXA2 thereby inhibiting platelet aggregation for 7–10 days. However, aspirin also suppresses COX-2, and thus PGI2, which explains the cardioprotection benefit. NSAID-induced renal toxicity is another concern when selecting appropriate therapy. Impaired regulation of renal blood flow is often to blame for this side effect. Patients susceptible to this include those over age 65, those with underlying kidney disease, those with volume depletion, and those with chronic diseases such as congestive heart failure (CHF), diabetes, and hypertension.

Lastly, there has been a concern for impaired bone healing in the perioperative period with NSAID use. There is a large body of data with studies showing conflicting results. Use of NSAIDs in the perioperative period has largely been left to each individual clinician.

Nonsteroidal anti-inflammatory drugs continue to play a pivotal role in treating both acute and chronic pain conditions. As they affect many organ systems of the body, a risk-benefit ratio with reliance on sound clinical judgment must be used in clinical decision making. Efforts should be made that utilize the most effective therapy at the lowest possible dose and for the shortest length of therapy.

Ⓐ Prescribers should refrain from using NSAIDs in patients with known active GI bleeding, ulcers, or hypersensitivity or allergies. Furthermore, patients with active renal failure or reduced or long standing chronic renal insufficiency, preexisting platelet defects or thrombocytopenia, and women who may be actively trying to conceive should avoid NSAIDs. Although NSAIDs are generally considered to be safe during pregnancy, during the conception period, they can block blastocyst implantation and should be stopped 6–8 weeks prior to term as NSAIDs can prolong gestation or labor, peripartum blood loss, and anemia.

Ⓑ Once relative and/or absolute contraindications have been reviewed, choice of NSAID therapy is largely guided by a patient's susceptibility to GI versus cardiovascular (CV) side effects. Multiple studies from the 1990s have shown morbidity and mortality data with high yearly hospitalizations and deaths from NSAID-related GI bleeding. Additionally, NSAIDs can induce hypertension, CHF, and cardiovascular events such as stroke or myocardial infarction.

Ⓒ In patients with both GI and CV risk factors and/or active conditions, the recommendation is to start them on a nonselective NSAID with GI protective agents such as a proton pump inhibitor (PPI), histamine H2 blocker, or misoprostol.

Ⓓ For patients with known GI disease but no CV considerations it would be appropriate to start them on a nonselective NSAID with GI protective agents or selective COX-2 inhibitors (celecoxib).

Ⓔ In patients presenting with a recent history of CV event or at high-risk, COX-2 inhibitors should be avoided. These patients should be maintained on nonselective NSAID therapy in combination with aspirin.

Ⓕ Patients with no GI or CV profile with increased risk or history can be started on either therapy with nonselective NSAIDs or COX-2 inhibitors. These patients are typically young and healthy and will tolerate minor adverse effects such as stomach upset, nausea, etc.

Ⓖ When patients are known to have relative or absolute contraindications to NSAID therapy, clinicians should consider treatment with alternative classes of medications. In many cases, patients may ultimately need to be evaluated and treated with a multimodal approach with medications, cognitive behavioral therapy, physical therapy, and interventional techniques.

SUGGESTED READING

Brian B, Buvanendran A. Nonsteroidal anti-inflammatory drugs, acetaminophen, and COX-2 inhibitors. In: Benzon H, Rathmell JP, Wu CL, Turk DC, Argoff CE, Hurley RW (Eds). Practical Management of Pain, 5th edition. Philadelphia: Elsevier; 2014. pp. 553-67.

FitzGerald GA. Cardiovascular pharmacology of nonselective nonsteroidal anti-inflammatory drugs and coxibs: clinical considerations. Am J Cardiol. 2002;89(6A):26D-32D.

Giuliano F, Warner TD. Origins of prostaglandin E2: involvements of cyclooxygenase (COX)-1 and COX-2 in human and rat systems. J Pharmacol Exp Ther. 2002;303(3):1001-6.

Hunter TS, Robinson C, Gerbino PP. Emerging evidence in NSAID pharmacology: important considerations for product selection. Am J Manag Care. 2015;21(7 Suppl):S139-47.

Silverstein FE, Faich G, Goldstein JL, et al. Gastrointestinal toxicity with celecoxib vs nonsteroidal anti-inflammatory drugs for osteoarthritis and rheumatoid arthritis: the CLASS study: A randomized controlled trial. Celecoxib Long-term Arthritis Safety Study. JAMA. 2000;284(10):1247-55.

CHAPTER 98

Corticosteroids

von Kriegenbergh KM, Day M

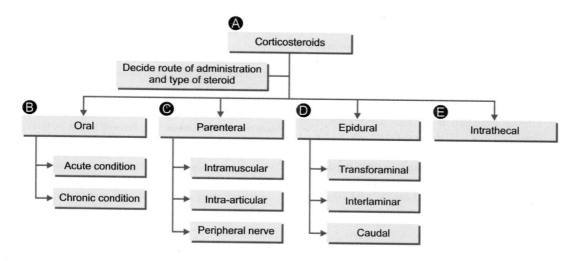

A *Corticosteroids:* Corticosteroids are used for anti-inflammatory and membrane stabilizing properties in the management of pain. Inhibition of the phospholipase A2 enzyme decreases the concentration of arachidonic acid metabolites—leukotrienes, thromboxanes, prostaglandins, and prostacyclins, ultimately leading to decreased inflammation. The short-lived membrane stabilizing effect on nociceptive C fibers prevent ectopic discharge from injured nerve segments and result in a transient break in efferent pain pathways.

B *Oral Steroids:* Oral steroids are used in the management of both acute and chronic inflammation and pain. Acute issues such as radiculopathy, arthritis, and herpes zoster, and chronic rheumatic and collagen disorders—rheumatoid arthritis, lupus erythematosus, and ankylosing spondylitis are treated with oral steroids.

Side effects of chronic oral steroid use include immunosuppression, gastric bleeding, fluid and electrolyte imbalances, musculoskeletal problems manifesting as osteoporosis and fractures, and endocrine disorders including cushingoid features and blood sugar derangements. Suppression of the pituitary-adrenal axis may require additional steroid replacement during periods of increased stress, like surgery. Depending on the dose and duration of oral steroid therapy, tapering of the dose may be necessary to avoid an adrenal crisis.

C *Parenteral Steroids:* Long-acting preparations such as methylprednisolone in a depot form (Depo-Medrol™), triamcinolone (Aristocort™ and Kenalog™) and beta-methasone (Celestone™) are commonly used. These long-acting preparations, usually in the form of a suspension, are combined with other compounds to increase solubility. Depo-Medrol™ precipitates when mixed with a local anesthetic or saline, while other steroids stay in the solution for a longer period and are more likely to provide uniform distribution when a large volume is injected. Dexamethasone (Decadron™) has been suggested by some groups as an alternative to particulate steroids for some procedures (transforaminal epidural steroid injections) given its nonparticulate nature.

Although the intravenous route is not commonly utilized for pain management, parenteral steroid preparations can be directly injected into muscles and joints to provide pain relief.

Intramuscular injection of steroid combined with a local anesthetic into trigger points can treat myofascial pain.

Intra-articular or bursae injection can be effective in treating joint pain not only of the shoulders, hips, and knees, but axial joint pain, i.e. facet joint and the sacroiliac joint, as well. Repeated injections into a joint can produce weakening of the underlying bone, therefore many clinicians limit the number of injections.

Injections of steroid and local anesthetic are also used for peripheral nerve blocks in cases where the physician believes there is an inflammatory component to pain in a particular nerve distribution, e.g. carpal tunnel, supraorbital neuralgia, saphenous neuralgia, etc.

D *Epidural Steroids:* Epidural steroid injection via the transforaminal, interlaminar or caudal approach is one of the most commonly performed interventions in pain management. Inflammation of the nerve root, spinal stenosis, and postlaminectomy syndrome are indications for epidural steroid injection with or without a local anesthetic. Patients with pain of different etiology including facet arthopathy, myofascial or sacroiliac joint pain are not likely to benefit from epidural steroid injection.

Long-acting steroids remain in the epidural space for up to 3 weeks. Therefore, repeated injections at shorter intervals can lead to systemic effects as listed earlier. Intra-arterial injection of methylprednisolone or triamcinolone into radicular arteries has produced spinal cord infarction and paralysis. Betamethasone has the smallest particulate size of the insoluble steroids and may be preferred for transforaminal epidural injections, where the risk of radicular arterial injection is greater. Dexamethasone, the only commercially available nonparticulate steroid, has also been suggested as a safer alternative and recent data demonstrates equianalgesia with particulate steroids. Doses of 40–120 mg (methylprednisolone and triamcinolone), 6–12 mg betamethasone, and 10–20 mg dexamethasone per injection are common.

E *Intrathecal Steroids:* Intrathecal steroid use remains controversial due to concerns about neurologic adverse events due to the presence or absence of preservatives and other compounds present in the long-acting preparations. However, there exists some data to support the use of intrathecal steroids in certain chronic pain conditions such as postherpetic neuralgia and complex regional pain syndrome.

SUGGESTED READING

Kim D, Brown, J. Efficacy and safety of lumbar epidural dexamethasone versus methylprednisolone in the treatment of lumbar radiculopathy: a comparison of soluble versus particulate steroids. Clin J Pain. 2011;27(6):518-22.

Lee DG, Cho YW, Jang SH, et al. Effectiveness of intra-articular steroid injection for atlanto-occipital joint pain. Pain Med. 2015; 16(6):1077-82.

Manchikanti L, Knezevic NN, Boswell MV, et al. Epidural Injections for Lumbar Radiculopathy and Spinal Stenosis: A Comparative Systematic Review and Meta-Analysis. Pain Physician. 2016; 19(3):E365-410.

Manchikanti L, Benyamin RM. Key safety considerations when administering epidural steroid injections. Pain Manag. 2015; 5(4):26172.

CHAPTER
99

Antidepressants

Day M, McClure BS

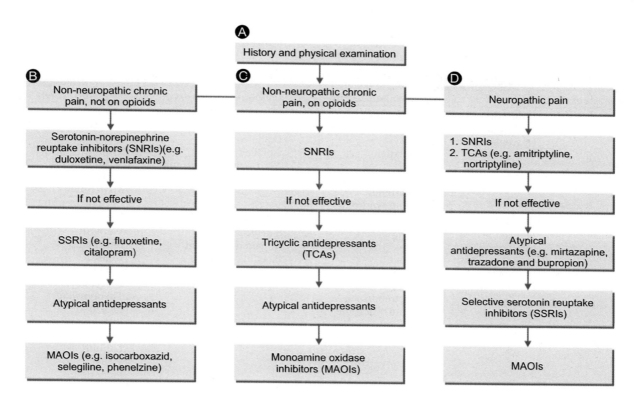

Depression is an extremely common comorbidity associated with chronic pain. It is estimated to occur in approximately 60% of chronic pain patients. Several theories surrounding this phenomenon have been hypothesized including the thought that depression precedes the chronic pain and another implying that depression is a result of the chronic pain.

Although depression and chronic pain are often comorbid, it is important to remember that they can also occur independent of each other. The physiologic pathways of depression are the most likely targets for pharmacotherapy aimed at treating chronic pain-associated depression. Both chronic pain and depression are mediated by the central neurotransmitters serotonin and norepinephrine, among others. Depression can lead to a decrease in the pain threshold, decrease physical and social activity, and increase in analgesic requirements. Additionally, medications used to treat chronic pain can also lead to medication-induced depression necessitating an evaluation for such interactions. These medications include but are not limited to opioids, corticosteroids, beta blockers, calcium channel blockers, anticonvulsants, benzodiazepines, muscle relaxants and

nonsteroidal anti-inflammatory drugs (NSAIDs). Tricyclic antidepressants (TCAs) have traditionally been used for the treatment of chronic pain, especially neuropathic pain. Selective serotonin reuptake inhibitors (SSRIs) provide less benefit, and selective serotonin-norepinephrine reuptake inhibitors (SNRIs) have been shown to be effective at treating chronic pain with and without depression. Additional agents also exist depending on the clinical scenario.

While antidepressant pharmacotherapy can aid the treatment of depression in patients with chronic pain, it is also useful in treating chronic pain in patients not experiencing depression. After a thorough evaluation of the patient with chronic pain has been performed, institution of antidepressant pharmacotherapy is one of the multiple modalities that should be considered. Introduction of antidepressants in the chronic pain population without depression has shown promising results in the reduction of pain scores, increases in physical activity and objective measures of quality of life. It has also been shown to decrease the analgesic requirement in that population and should thus be considered in spite of lack of depressive symptoms.

It should be noted that many classes of antidepressants including SNRIs, SSRIs and TCAs have been strongly associated with an increased risk of suicidality and should be used with extreme caution or avoided in high-risk populations.

A *History and Physical Examination:* There are many factors to consider when selecting an agent for antidepressant pharmacotherapy. Of the many antidepressant drugs available, none has been shown to be universally effective. Important factors to consider include past use and efficacy of a certain drug or class of drug, depressive symptoms if present, risk of suicidality, comorbidities, medication interactions and cost. Other patient-specific factors to consider include the type of pain being treated and the compliance of the patient. Many antidepressants require several weeks before the full effect of the medication can be felt and objectively assessed. The type of pain being treated is another major factor to consider when choosing an antidepressant as part of a patient's medication regimen. Flow chart serves as a guide for initiation and adjustment of antidepressant therapy. There are many different antidepressants to choose from when considering a drug regimen for chronic pain. **Table 1** lists the different classes and agents available as well as significant attributes of each.

Table 1: Different classes and agents available for antidepressant therapy

Antidepressant class	Agents	Significant side effects	Contraindications or cautions	Drug interactions
SNRIs	Duloxetine Venlafaxine Desvenlafaxine	Hypertension Anticholinergic effects Nausea Constipation Anorexia Fatigue Hyponatremia Serotonin syndrome	Heart disease Cirrhosis Diabetes Suicide risk Narrow angle glaucoma	MAOIs Cimetidine SSRIs TCAs St. John's Wort Tramadol Meperidine Cyclobenzaprine
SSRIs	Sertraline Fluoxetine Citalopram Escitalopram Paroxetine Fluvoxamine	Nausea Vomiting Diarrhea Insomnia Headache Agitation or anxiety Hyponatremia Serotonin syndrome	Cirrhosis Suicide risk Impaired cognition Bleeding disorders	MAOIs Warfarin Beta blockers Digoxin Cimetidine Diazepam Theophylline Linezolid St. John's Wort Tramadol Lithium TCAs Meperidine
TCAs	Amitriptyline Amoxapine Clomipramine Desipramine Doxepin Imipramine Nortriptyline Protriptyline Trimipramine	Sedation Anticholinergic effects Orthostatic hypotension Seizures Conduction abnormalities	Conduction abnormalities or recent MI Seizure disorder Hypothyroidism Cirrhosis Impaired cognition Suicide risk	MAOIs Drugs that prolong QT interval Anticholinergics Diphenhydramine Atropine
MAOIs	Isocarboxazid Phenelzine Selegiline Tranylcypromine	Severe hypertension Anticholinergic effects Postural hypotension	Cardiovascular disease Liver disease Endocrine disorders Seizure disorders Suicide risk	SSRIs SNRIs Bupropion Opioids Buspirone Sympathomimetics Reserpine Tryptophan Meperidine Dextromethorphan
Other or atypical	Mirtazapine Vortioxetine Trazodone Nefazodone Bupropion	Multiple	Multiple	Multiple

MAOIs, monoamine oxidase inhibitors; MI, myocardial infarction; SNRIs, serotonin-norepinephrine reuptake inhibitors; SSRIs, selective serotonin reuptake inhibitors; TCAs, tricyclic antidepressants

B Serotonin-norepinephrine reuptake inhibitor antidepressants are first-line therapy in treating non-neuropathic chronic pain in patients not on opiates. Prescribers should consider interactions with other medications especially serotonergic medications as well as sedating medications and use extreme caution with both as adverse effects can be permanent or even life-threatening. Dopaminergic effects caused by SNRIs should limit their use in patients with significant cardiac disease. Their use can also be limited by their effects on fasting glucose in diabetic patients and should be titrated slowly with careful observation of hemoglobin A1C levels in these patients.

Selective serotonin reuptake inhibitors are second-line therapy for patients with non-neuropathic chronic pain who are not on opiates. They can also be helpful in patients with neuropathic pain. SSRIs can also lead to serotonin syndrome and should be avoided with other serotonergic medications. They are less effective at treating chronic pain than SNRIs. They should be used with extreme caution when in combination with other antidepressants and avoided with concurrent SNRI therapy. They can inhibit the CYP450 pathway inhibiting the metabolism of a variety of medications, but of particular note in chronic pain patients, inhibit the metabolism of commonly prescribed opiates.

Atypical antidepressants exhibit limited use in chronic pain management but are sometimes implemented when other therapies fail. They can be considered in non-neuropathic chronic pain without opiates after SSRIs due to their side effects which can occasionally be used to a patient's advantage. For example, monoamine oxidase inhibitors (MAOIs) are considered last-line therapy for pain management in non-neuropathic chronic pain without opiate use secondary to their propensity for interactions with both medications and common foods that can be extremely dangerous, even life-threatening. They are known to be hepatotoxic, serotonergic, and can exhibit fatal interactions in some cases when used in combination with other antidepressants, meperidine, and various over-the-counter medications and some foods.

C Serotonin-norepinephrine reuptake inhibitor antidepressants are first-line therapy in treating non-neuropathic chronic pain in patients on opiates. Prescribers should consider interactions with other medications especially serotonergic medications as well as sedating medications and use extreme caution with both as adverse effects can be permanent or even life-threatening.

If SNRI antidepressants are ineffective or contra-indicated in certain patients, TCAs can be implemented as second-line therapy. Their side effect profiles and drug interactions are varied and extensive depending on the medication, but can often be tailored to the patients other comorbidities. Drowsiness, anticholinergic effects, dopaminergic and histaminergic side effects can limit their use. They should be avoided in postmyocardial infarction patients and with extreme caution in patients with extensive heart disease secondary to their arrhythmogenic effects.

As third-line therapy, atypical antidepressants exhibit limited use in chronic pain management but are sometimes implemented when other therapies fail. They can be considered in other chronic pain with opiates after SSRIs and TCAs have proven ineffective due to their side effect profile.

D Both SNRIs and TCAs are considered first-line therapy in treating neuropathic pain. Prescribers should consider interactions with other medications especially serotonergic medications as well as sedating medications and use extreme caution with both as adverse effects can be permanent or even life-threatening. Both can be sedating and are not typically used in combination due to this effect as well as synergistic dopaminergic effects as well. If SNRIs and TCAs are either contraindicated or ineffective, second-line therapy consists of atypical antidepressants, followed by SSRIs and MAOIs with careful consideration made for patient comorbidities and medication side effects.

SUGGESTED READING

Jackson KC, St Onge EL. Antidepressant pharmacotherapy: considerations for the pain clinician. Pain Pract. 2003;3(2): 135-43.

Jann MW, Slade JH. Antidepressant agents for the treatment of chronic pain and depression. Pharmacotherapy. 2007;27(11):1571-87.

Skljarevski V, Desaiah D, Liu-Seifert H, et al. Efficacy and safety of duloxetine in patients with chronic low back pain. Spine (Phila Pa 1976). 2010;35(13):E578-85.

CHAPTER
100

Anticonvulsants

Davies E, Souza S

Anticonvulsant therapy for neuropathic pain

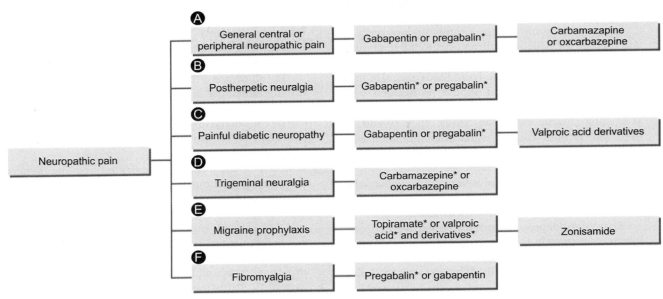

* FDA labeled indication

Anticonvulsants are a commonly used class of pharmacological agents used in the treatment of pain, specifically neuropathic pain. They are rarely used as monotherapy, but rather as adjuvant treatment in combination with other neuropathic and nociceptive targeting agents. There are multiple anticonvulsant agents that can be used for either central or peripheral neuropathic pain diagnoses, depending on their mechanism of action. Some anticonvulsants are first-line therapy for labeled indications, for example, carbamazepine for glossopharyngeal or trigeminal neuralgia (TGN). Others are used as first-line options for off-label indications, for instance the use of gabapentin for painful diabetic neuropathy (PDN) or neuropathic pain. Common pain diagnoses that may benefit from anticonvulsant therapy include postherpetic neuralgia (PHN), complex regional pain syndrome (CRPS), radiculopathies, painful human immunodeficiency virus (HIV)-associated neuropathies, central poststroke pain, spinal cord injury, phantom limb pain, and prevention or treatment of migraine headache.

The use of older anticonvulsant agents is very limited due to many drug-drug interactions and severe adverse effect profiles. Contemporary anticonvulsant agents have different mechanisms of action, fewer drug-drug interactions due to having less interaction with the cytochrome P450 enzyme system, and more tolerable side effect profiles, leading to increased use and patient tolerance. The majority of the anticonvulsant medications have a warning involving an increased risk of suicide ideation (0.43% of treated patients compared to 0.24% of patients receiving placebo), with risk observed as early as 1 week after initiation and continued through duration of therapy. All anticonvulsants should be carefully and slowly titrated up, and slowly weaned down to aid in the reduction of any withdrawal symptoms, unless safety concerns indicate otherwise.

Calcium Channel Blockers: Gabapentin and pregabalin are both calcium channel alpha 2 delta ($\alpha2\delta$) ligands and bind to the $\alpha2\delta$-1 and $\alpha2\delta$-2 subunits of presynaptic voltage-gated calcium channels, therefore reducing the calcium dependent release of neurotransmitters. The major difference between gabapentin and pregabalin is bioavailability. Pregabalin has more than 90% bioavailability between single doses of 25–300 mg. Gabapentin has a dose-dependent bioavailability, which decreases with each single dose. Both medications need to be dosed based on the patient's renal function. Common side effects of these two medications include sedation, dizziness, blurred vision, peripheral edema, and weight gain. Pregabalin is a controlled substance due to euphoric type side effects. Gabapentin has been reformulated into various long-acting formulations due to its bioavailability issues. Major advantages with these medications include a positive effect on sleep architecture by increasing slow wave and rapid eye movement (REM) sleep stages. Again, gabapentin and pregabalin have minimal concern for drug-drug interactions making them extremely advantageous in chronic pain patients who often take multiple medications for various ailments.

Gabapentin has been well-studied in neuropathic pain states, with Food and Drug Administration (FDA) labeled indications for PHN. Gabapentin is used frequently off-label for neuropathic pain, PDN, restless legs syndrome (RLS), fibromyalgia, and postoperative pain.

Pregabalin has FDA labeling for fibromyalgia, diabetes and spinal cord injury-associated neuropathic pain, PHN, and is used off-label for RLS.

Sodium Channel Blockers: Carbamazepine is a first generation anticonvulsant that functions by blocking voltage-gated sodium channels, reducing ectopic nerve discharges and stabilization of hyperexcited neural membranes. It is structurally related to tricyclic antidepressants, accounting for anticholinergic, muscle relaxant, antimanic, and antidepressive properties. It is first-line for TGN at doses of 200–1000 mg/day. Carbamazepine has a few drawbacks, including an adverse effect profile involving severe hematologic and metabolic effects that require monitoring of blood counts, liver enzymes, and serum levels, and lengthy drug-drug interaction profile due to induction of hepatic CYP450 enzyme and auto-induction of its own metabolism. Common adverse effects include ataxia, cognitive deficits, diplopia, and weight gain. Carbamazepine is rarely used off-label for neuropathic pain due to the aforementioned side effects. Oxcarbazepine is a second generation anticonvulsant, and a structural analog of carbamazepine. Oxcarbazepine has the same mechanism of action, but an improved safety profile in comparison to carbamazepine. Oxcarbazepine is used off-label for TGN and neuropathic pain diagnoses. It is typically tolerated better and less monitoring is required when compared to carbamazepine. Initial dose range is 150–300 mg at bedtime with increase of 150–300 mg per day every 2–5 days. Target range of 900–1800 mg per day in divided doses is optimal. Oxcarbazepine has the greatest incidence of adverse effects of the second generation anticonvulsants, with somnolence, ataxia, nystagmus, diplopia, visual abnormalities, and blood dyscrasias being most common. Oxcarbazepine is also a hepatic enzyme inducer, leading to numerous drug interactions, although to less of an extent than carbamazepine.

Topiramate is an anticonvulsant that has multiple mechanisms of action including prolongation of sodium channel blockade, gamma-aminobutyric acid (GABA) agonism, glutamate receptor antagonism, and weak inhibition of carbonic anhydrase. It is FDA approved for migraine prophylaxis and is used off-label for cluster headache prophylaxis, and neuropathic pain states. Currently, evidence for off-label use for neuropathic pain is not very robust. The initial dose ranges from 25 mg to 50 mg per day. Adverse reactions include paresthesia, drowsiness, dizziness, fatigue, memory and speech impairment, mood disorder, weight loss, anorexia, and diarrhea. The dose may need to be adjusted in renal failure.

Mixed Mechanism Agents: Valproic acid and divalproex sodium derivatives affect synthesis, re-uptake, and breakdown of GABA in selected brain regions. It also is a sodium and calcium channel blocker causing membrane stabilization and decreased neurotransmitter release, respectively. Valproic acid and divalproex sodium derivatives are thought to block N-methyl-D-aspartate (NMDA) receptors. Labeled indications (divalproex sodium) include migraine prophylaxis, and have evidence for off-label use for PDN and PHN. The use of valproic acid and derivatives has been limited by a high rate of adverse effects to include drowsiness, nausea, vomiting, diplopia, visual disturbances, abdominal pain, thrombocytopenia, tremor, and weakness. Valproic acid and derivatives have black box warnings for pancreatitis and hepatic failure and require regular monitoring of blood counts, liver enzymes, and drug levels.

Zonisamide is second generation anticonvulsant sulfonamide that may be useful for treatment of neuropathic pain. Zonisamide has several mechanisms of action, including stabilization of neuronal membranes and suppression of neuronal hypersynchronization through sodium and calcium channel blockade. Its off-label use is increasing for migraine prophylaxis. Most common side effects include somnolence, dizziness, and weight loss.

Additional anticonvulsants have been studied, but lack of strong evidence for efficacy in neuropathic pain diagnoses exists, despite similarities in mechanism of action with the agents listed earlier. These include levetiracetam, lacosamide, vigabatrin, lamotrigine, and phenytoin.

Selection of a particular anticonvulsant medication is usually a result of careful consideration of multiple factors including mechanism of action, proven efficacy, adverse effects, potential drug interactions, and cost. Mechanism of action of the agent used must be considered, especially when switching or adding anticonvulsant agents.

(A) In general central or peripheral nerve pain states, pregabalin and gabapentin should be first-line and second-line should be carbamazepine or oxcarbazepine.

(B) In PHN, gabapentin or pregabalin should be first-line treatment.

(C) In PDN, gabapentin or pregabalin should be first-line treatment and valproic acid or divalproex sodium should be second-line treatment or additive treatment to the calcium channel blocker.

(D) In TGN, carbamazepine or oxcarbazepine should be first-line treatment. Though it is not in the scope of this chapter, baclofen, a muscle relaxant, is also first-line treatment in TGN.

(E) With migraine prophylaxis, many medications are effective. For further details, see Chapter 62 Migraines. In terms of use of anticonvulsants, topiramate and valproic acid derivatives are considered first-line and zonisamide is considered second-line.

F Fibromyalgia patients should be offered pregabalin (on-label) or gabapentin (off-label) as first-line therapy. Other pharmacologic treatment options are primarily antidepressants (see Chapter 99 Antidepressants).

SUGGESTED READING

Birse F, Derry S, Moore RA. Phenytoin for neuropathic pain and fibromyalgia in adults. Cochrane Database Syst Rev. 2012; (5):CD009485.

Eisenberg E, River Y, Shifrin A, et al. Antiepileptic drugs in the treatment of neuropathic pain. Drugs. 2007;67(9):1265-89.

Hearn L, Derry S, Moore RA. Lacosamide for neuropathic pain and fibromyalgia in adults. Cochrane Database Syst Rev. 2012; (2):CD009318.

Lexi-Comp. Version 1.9.2. (2012). Gabapentin, Pregabalin, Ziconotide, Carbamazepine, Oxcarbazepine, Valproic Acid and derivatives, Topiramate, Zonisamide, Tiagabine, Levetiracetam, Lacosamide, and Vigabatrin Full Monographs. [online] Available from *online.lexi.com/lco/action/home.* [Accessed January, 2017].

Mendlik MT, Uritsky TJ. Treatment of Neuropathic Pain. Curr Treat Options Neurol. 2015;17(12):50.

Mohammadianinejad SE, Abbasi V, Sajedi SA, et al. Zonisamide versus topiramate in migraine prophylaxis: a double-blind randomized clinical trial. Clin Neuropharmacol. 2011;34(4): 174-7.

Wiffen PG, Derry S, Lunn MP, et al. Topiramate for neuropathic pain and fibromyalgia in adults. Cochrane Database Syst Rev. 2013; (8):CD008314.

Wiffen PG, Derry S, Moore RA, et al. Carbamazepine for chronic neuropathic pain and fibromyalgia in adults. Cochrane Database Syst Rev. 2014;(4):CD005451.

Wiffen PG, Derry S, Moore RA, et al. Levetiracetam for neuropathic pain in adults. Cochrane Database Syst Rev. 2014;(7):CD010943.

Wiffen PJ, Derry S, Moore RA. Lamotrigine for chronic neuropathic pain and fibromyalgia in adults. Cochrane Database Syst Rev. 2013;(12):CD006044.

CHAPTER 101

Antispasmodics and Antispasticity Pharmacology

Verduzco-Gutierrez M, Dragojlovic N

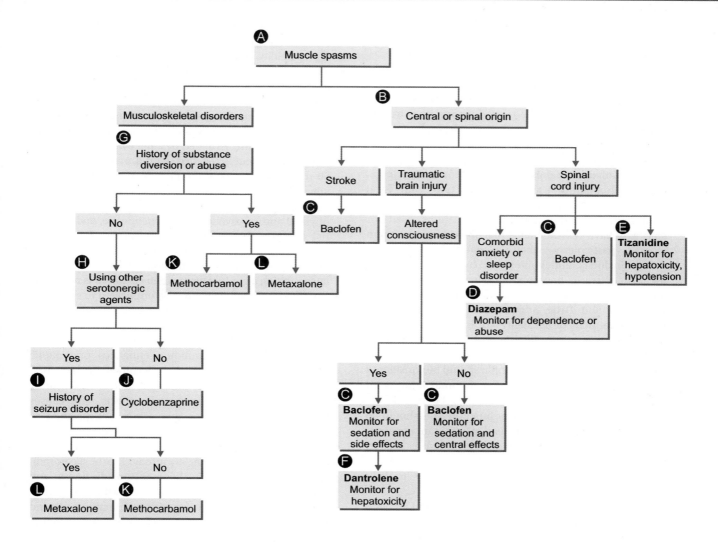

In the setting of musculoskeletal pain, numerous pathological processes are at work, including altered biomechanics, destructive arthritic processes, and inflammation to neural structures. Muscle spasms develop in an attempt to safeguard and protect these vital structures, worsening pain and impairing function even further than the initial injury.

Ⓐ When a practitioner considers using an antispasmodic agent, the first decision to be made is whether the use is for a musculoskeletal disorder or spasticity from central origin. In the setting of an upper motor neuron neurologic injury, like cerebral palsy, stroke, or spinal cord injury, spasticity can develop and limit strength and

range of motion and cause pain. In both of these patient populations, oral antispasmodics and antispasticity medications are used to effectively treat acute muscle spasms and spasticity, reducing pain and helping to restore function. Recent Cochrane reviews have validated the use of antispasmodic medications for the temporary relief of musculoskeletal pain; however, their chronic use is limited by central side effects, particularly dizziness and drowsiness. They should not be prescribed for over 6 weeks. There is also a growing body of research to suggest that these agents may suppress nociceptive inputs through the gamma-aminobutyric acid-A (GABA-A) system, or provide anxiolytic effects to ease patient discomfort, helping improve pain independent of their effect on muscle tone. Though never to be used alone as an analgesic, these agents are useful adjuncts to decrease muscle spasms or treat spasticity.

Antispasticity Agents:

B The decision of which antispasmodic to use in upper motor neuron spasticity patients is based upon the origin of their injury. Spasticity, as a component of the upper motor neuron syndrome, is defined as a velocity-dependent resistance to passive range of motion. Spastic muscles interfere with the functional use of limbs, limiting strength and range of motion, and can cause pain. When left untreated, muscle and joint contractures will develop, often rapidly and progressively. However, not all spasticity should be treated. Spasticity is treated when it becomes disabling, affecting a person's mobility, self-care, or activities of daily living. Oral medications for the management of spasticity are best reserved for those patients with a more global pattern of spastic hypertonia, but are frequently used in conjunction with focal treatments such a phenol neurolysis or intramuscular botulinum toxin injection. All medications used for spasticity have central effects that should be monitored closely, particularly when a patient's medication profile includes anticholinergics, hypnotics, or those for nociceptive or neuropathic pain, due to the risk of additive and untoward central effects. Oral medications with Food and Drug Administration (FDA) approval for the treatment of spasticity are limited to baclofen, diazepam, tizanidine, and dantrolene, which will be discussed here, as they are also the most efficacious and well tolerated. In all cases, baclofen should be considered first-line. In the event of a traumatic brain injury with altered consciousness, dantrolene can be prescribed, but frequent assessment of liver function tests should be made because dantrolene can lead to fulminant hepatitis. In the case of spinal cord injury, tizanidine is a good first-line choice in addition to baclofen, as is diazepam, especially in patient's with comorbid anxiety or sleep disorders.

C Baclofen is the most commonly used oral agent across a diverse set of patient populations. It is related structurally to GABA, and binds presynaptic GABA-B receptors in the cerebrum, brain stem, and dorsal horn of the spinal cord. This results in the reduction of gamma motor activity and inhibition of reflex pathways that normally promote spastic muscle contraction. Initial doses should begin at 15 mg/day, and titrated up every 2–3 days until desired therapeutic effect is reached, with maximal dosage of 80 mg/day. Due to its short half-life, TID dosing is required. Central side effects include decreased seizure threshold, drowsiness, sedation, memory impairment, or impaired attention; other adverse effects include motor weakness, ataxia, constipation, or urinary retention. The adverse central effects may be more pronounced in those with cerebral injuries or cognitive impairment, and are the primary limiting factor for dose escalation. The sudden withdrawal of baclofen is a life-threatening event and can result in seizures, hallucinations, rebound spasticity, autonomic instability, and death, and as such, the medication should be tapered off gradually. Despite these characteristics, it is generally well tolerated and clinicians should not be discouraged from its use.

D Diazepam is a sedative hypnotic from the class of benzodiazepines, and promotes the release of GABA from GABA-A neurons, resulting in presynaptic inhibition across the central neural axis. It is an effective treatment for spasticity, but is also used to treat anxiety and epilepsy. Due to its untoward effects on memory and alertness, it is generally avoided in patients with acute cerebral injuries. However, diazepam is well-established in the treatment of spasticity from multiple sclerosis and spinal cord injury. Initial doses are 4 mg nightly or 2 mg BID, and are escalated by 2 mg every 2–3 days until therapeutic effect is reached, with a maximal dosage of 60 mg/day. Physicians should monitor for the primary adverse effects of weakness, sedation, and impaired coordination. Furthermore, prolonged use can lead to physical and/or psychological dependence, and given its risk of abuse, patient selection is of utmost importance. As with baclofen, abrupt cessation can lead to withdrawal resulting in irritability, tremor, seizures, or death necessitating a gradual taper when cessation is required.

E Noradrenergic pathways are also implicated in spasticity, and tizanidine, a selective alpha-2-adrenergic agonist, is used to target these pathways and has demonstrated efficacy in the treatment of spasticity of both cerebral and spinal origins. Tizanidine enhances presynaptic inhibition of sensory afferents, resulting in decreased tone. Though related to clonidine, it has significantly less hypotensive and bradycardic effects, and causes less peripheral weakness than other antispasmodics. Recommended initial doses are 2–4 mg/day, usually at bedtime due to sedation, increasing dose and frequency as tolerated up to maximal 36 mg/day. The most common side effects are sedation, hypotension, dizziness, and dry mouth. Hepatotoxicity can be seen with chronic use, requiring regular monitoring of liver function tests and concomitant use with fluoroquinolone antibiotics should be avoided.

F Dantrolene is the only peripherally acting drug in this class of medications, impairing calcium release from sarcoplasmic reticulum in skeletal muscle. It has been used in traumatic brain injury and other cerebral causes given its lack of central effects, or as an adjunct in other cases. Recommended initial doses are 25 mg daily for 7 days, then increased to 25 mg three times a day, then increased weekly until the desired control of spasticity is reached, up to maximal 100 mg three times a day dosing. There is a significant risk of hepatotoxicity associated with this medication and is, therefore, contraindicated in active hepatic disease. Other risk factors include female gender, age less than 35 years old, doses greater than 400 mg daily, and polypharmacy. As with tizanidine, liver function tests should be monitored regularly while using this medication. When central effects are of significant concern, or when a systemic adjunct is desired, dantrolene is an effective spasmolytic.

Antispasmodic Agents: Antispasmodics for musculoskeletal pain are centrally acting and reserved to two classes, (1) benzodiazepines (e.g. diazepam, lorazepam), and (2) non-benzodiazepines. Non-benzodiazepine agents are amongst the more commonly used antispasmodics for musculo-skeletal pain, and include cyclobenzaprine, methocarbamol, metaxalone, and carisoprodol. Special interest will be given to carisoprodol. Carisoprodol is a synthetic propanediol dicarbamate that blocks interneuron activity in the spinal cord and reticular formation. Dosing is at 250–350 mg every 8 hours as needed, with close monitoring for central effects as with other agents in its class. It is the least commonly used owing to its risk for psychological and physical dependence. Unfortunately, it is also sought after by patients because of its enhancement of euphoria when combined with opiates. Most medical societies have stated opposition to this medication. The European Union's European Medicines Agency has determined that the risks of use of carisoprodol outweigh its benefits and it should not be used. For these reasons, carisoprodol is not utilized in our decision-making algorithm.

G Before deciding which antispasmodic to use for musculoskeletal pain, the practitioner must evaluate for a history of substance abuse. In those with a history of substance abuse or diversion, metaxalone and metho-carbamol have the lowest risk of abuse and should be considered first-line.

H In those patients without a history of substance abuse, further history should be taken to assess if the patient is already taking a serotonergic agent. If so, cyclobenzaprine should be avoided as it can cause serotonin syndrome when combined with other serotonergic substances.

I In patients without a history of substance abuse who are taking serotonergic agents, a determination must be made as to whether the patient has a history of a seizure disorder. Methocarbamol can lower the seizure threshold and should be avoided in those patients with a history of epilepsy.

J Cyclobenzaprine is structurally related to tricyclic antidepressants and acts on the brain stem to reduce somatic motor activity, with serotonergic and anticholinergic effects. It tends to be more sedating than the other members in its class, with other anticholinergic effects such as dry mouth, dizziness, or constipation. It is contraindicated when used in conjunction with monoamine oxidase (MAO) inhibitors due to the risk of

hyperpyretic crisis, seizures, and death. Initial dosing is recommended at 5 mg every 8 hours as needed, titrated up to 10 mg every 8 hours as needed. Long-acting formulations are available, but should be avoided in those with hepatic impairment.

K Methocarbamol is a centrally acting skeletal muscle relaxant in the carbamate class of compounds. It should be used with caution in those with seizures, and is poorly tolerated in the elderly and frail. Initial dosing begins at 1500 mg every 6 or 8 hours as needed, with target dosing of 3–4 g per day, and maximal daily dose of 8 g per day.

L Metaxalone is an oxazolidinone with centrally acting skeletal muscle relaxant properties, and is less sedating than other agents. However, its absorption is enhanced when taken with food, enhancing its more common adverse effects like headache, dizziness, and drowsiness. Initial dosing is recommended at 800 mg every 6 or 8 hours as needed. It should be dosed with caution in those with hepatic impairment, and serial monitoring of liver function studies should be performed during its use.

Muscle spasms associated with various musculoskeletal conditions undoubtedly contribute to pain and decreased function. In a Cochrane review studying the efficacy of skeletal muscle relaxants in low back pain, there was strong evidence that antispasmodics, when used in conjunction with analgesics or nonsteroidal anti-inflammatory drugs (NSAIDs), helped to improve and accelerate recovery. Patients with central neurologic injuries with more global spasticity patterns are at risk of further functional impairments and medical complications when their spasticity goes unmanaged. The medications discussed earlier are helpful in the management of these conditions, but need to be used cautiously and increased slowly, while monitoring for central and other drug-specific effects. Prescribers should tailor their use to each patient based on their individual goals and medical comorbidities.

SUGGESTED READING

Friedman BW, Dym AA, Davitt M, et al. Naproxen With Cyclobenzaprine, Oxycodone/Acetaminophen, or Placebo for Treating Acute Low Back Pain: A Randomized Clinical Trial. JAMA. 2015;314(15):1572-80.

Meythaler JM, Kowalski S. Pharmacologic management of spasticity: oral medications. In: Brashear A, Elovic E (Eds). Spasticity: Diagnosis and Management, 1st edition. New York: Demos Medical Publishing; 2010. pp. 199-227.

Richards BL, Whittle SL, Buchbinder R. Muscle relaxants for pain management in rheumatoid arthritis. Cochrane Database Syst Rev. 2012;1:CD008922.

van Tulder MW, Touray T, Furlan AD, et al. Muscle relaxants for non-specific low back pain. Cochrane Database Syst Rev. 2003;(2):CD004252.

Interventional Spasticity Management with Botulinum Toxin

Mimbella PC, Verduzco-Gutierrez M

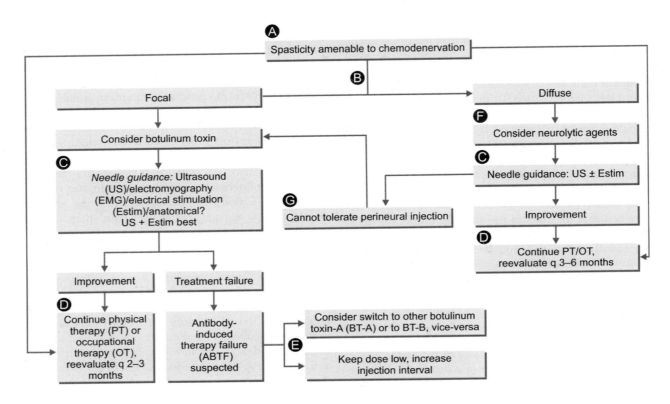

Botulinum toxin (BT) is a potent neuromuscular toxin produced by the *Clostridium botulinum* species. There are seven classified serotypes of BT labeled -A, -B, -C, -D, -E, -F, and -G of which only BT-A and BT-B are currently used in humans. BT disrupts the chemical transmission of electrical impulses to muscles at the neuromuscular junction resulting in muscle relaxation. There are various subtle differences between compounds that make one compound favorable over another depending on the clinical setting. There is comparable efficacy of each of the commercial available compounds in the treatment of spasticity **(Table 1)**.

The following are the various approved indications for BT injections: bladder dysfunction, chronic migraine, upper or lower limb spasticity, cervical dystonia, primary axillary hyperhidrosis, glabellar lines, blepharospasm, and strabismus. There are more than 60 uses of BT reported in the literature. Focal dystonias (not limited to the cervical musculature), tremors, tics, myoclonus, nystagmus, lumbago, myofascial pain syndromes, headaches, smooth muscle hyperactive disorders (e.g. detrusor sphincter dyssynergia,

achalasia cardia, Hirschsprung's disease), proctalgia fugax, and other hyperhidrosis disorders are among those uses not formally approved. The focus on this chapter will be spasticity. Prior to intervention, current clinical practice requires review of the patient's medications and allergies.

Ⓐ The diagnosis and etiology of the spasticity must be clearly delineated in conjunction with explicit documentation describing conservative management techniques that have already been attempted and have failed. Absolute contraindications for intervention are few. BT injection is contraindicated in patients who are hypersensitive to any BT preparation or any of the components in the formulation. Injection is contraindicated in the presence of infection or suspected infection at the proposed injection site. BT is labeled "Category C" by the Food and Drug Administration (FDA) in regards to pregnancy and nursing. This is considered precautionary more so than a direct recommendation as no developmental abnormalities have been observed thus far. A patient with a preexisting compromised respiratory status would

Table 1: Commercial available compounds for the treatment of spasticity

	Botox®	*Dysport®*	*Neuro or Myobloc®*	*Xeomin®*
Compound	Onabotulinum toxin A	Abobotulinum toxin A	Rimabotulinum toxin B	Incobotulinum toxin A
Manufacturer	Allergan Inc.	Ipsen Ltd.	Solstice Inc.	Merz Pharmaceuticals
Neurotoxin	BT-A	BT-A	BT-B	BT-A
SNARE target	SNAP-25	SNAP-25	VAMP	SNAP-25
Preparation	Powder	Powder	Ready-to-use	Powder
pH at injection	7.4	7.4	5.6	7.4
Storage	<8°C	<8°C	<8°C	<25°C
Shelf life	36 months	24 months	24 months	36 months
Excipients	Albumin or NaCl	Albumin or lactose	Albumin/ disodium/ NaCl/HCl	Albumin or sucrose
Specific bioactivity	60 MU–EV/ng	100 MU–EV/ng	5 MU–EV/ng	167 MU–EV/ng
Activity versus Botox	1	1/3	1/40	1

BT, botulinum toxin; HCl, hydrochloric acid; NaCl, sodium chloride; SNAP, soluble NSF attachment protein; SNARE, soluble NSF attachment protein receptor; VAMP, vesicle-associated membrane protein

be a relative contraindication to BT injection at or near any of the muscles contributing to respiratory function. Preexisting neuromuscular disorders and neuropathic disease such as amyotrophic lateral sclerosis (ALS), myasthenia gravis, or Lambert-Eaton syndrome are also at increased risk of profound effects from intervention with BT. Concomitant use of muscle relaxants and/or anticholinergic medications may potentiate botulinum effects. Aminoglycosides have also been found to potentiate the effects of BT.

B Once a patient's spasticity is deemed amenable to chemodenervation, history and physical examination should be used to determine whether the spasticity is focal or diffuse. Focal spasticity is defined as spasticity limited to muscles crossing 1–2 contiguous joints, and/or a clinical scenario in which all muscles involved can be covered with a recommended dose of toxin. Selection of the appropriate muscle targeting technique is required.

C The current techniques employed for targeting include anatomical landmarks, ultrasound guidance, electromyography (EMG), and/or neurostimulation. A combination, rather than any single technique, is recommended in practice. As previously noted, electrical stimulation may enhance uptake of the toxin and even potentially minimize the risk of diffusion of the toxin into adjacent tissues. Therefore, it may be most prudent to use ultrasound along with electrical stimulation during injection. These techniques require the expertise of an experienced clinician and ultrasonographer for proper employment.

D If the desired effect is obtained, physical modalities or therapies and follow-up in 2–3 months for reevaluation are recommended. The muscle relaxing effects of BT injection can be detectable as early as 2–3 days but

typically reach their maximal effects at 2 weeks. The effects can be expected to decline after 2.5 months. Repeat injections are rarely done prior to the 12 week mark.

E Uncommonly, treatment failure can eventually develop even in a patient who has been successfully treated several times with BT.

Antigenicity has been described in the literature. Because BT is made of foreign proteins, antibodies can essentially be formed against all of them. Antibody-induced therapy failure (ABTF) has been well-described in the literature in both the neurologic and cosmetic fields. There are two major controllable contributing factors to ABTF: (1) the dose applied during treatment and (2) the interval between repeat treatments. In clinical practice, ABTF may be an indication to change particular drug formulations in an effort to maximize the desired effect.

Another cause for treatment failure is spread of the toxin beyond the local site of injection. The symptoms will, therefore, be consistent with the mechanism of action of botulinum. This is most clinically significant in the management of cervical musculature spasticity and the patient should be advised to seek immediate medical attention should he/she develop problems with swallowing, speech, or respiration up to 2 weeks after intervention. Due to the potential effect of the dose, it is recommended to use the lowest effective dose of toxin to prevent any potential ABTF or spread past the local site.

F In the case of diffuse spasticity, defined as spasticity that exceeds safe BT dose coverage, a separate algorithm is recommended. This can occur with larger muscle groups. Neurolytic injections may then be considered for reduction in tone (see Chapter 105 Neurolytic Agents). We also recommend combined ultrasound and electrical stimulation when available for nerve targeting to ensure accurate lysis of the intended target.

G Oftentimes, patients cannot tolerate perineural injection with alcohol or phenol due to procedural pain, in which case the clinician may want to reconsider BT. The major advantage of neurolysis is that the duration of the nerve-signaling block is longer than with BT. There are two primary concerns with intramuscular neurolysis: (1) myonecrosis and (2) the fact that neurolysis is typically an "all or nothing" block. This does not lend well to reducing tone in different muscles to varying degrees. Botulinum allows the interventionist a greater degree of target specificity while preserving surrounding musculature in an effort to maximize a particular afflicted patient's function. Nevertheless, if the intended functional improvement is noted with phenol neurolysis we recommend continued physical modalities and return for reevaluation in 3–6 months.

As with all therapies targeting function, the multidisciplinary approach must be maintained. These interventions should be combined with physical modalities to maximize the benefit to the patient and the potential gains in function that may ultimately lead to an increased quality of life.

SUGGESTED READING

Allergan Pharmaceuticals. (2016). Botox Medication Guide. [online] Available from *www.allergan.com/miscellaneous-pages/allergan-pdf-files/botox_med_guide*. [Accessed January, 2017].

Dressler D. Pharmacology of botulinum toxin drugs. In: Brashear A, Mayer NH (Eds). Spasticity and Other Forms of Muscle Overactivity in the Upper Motor Neuron Syndrome: Etiology, Evaluation, Management, and the Role of Botulinum Toxin. New York: We Move; 2008.

Ipsen Biopharmaceuticals. (2016). Dysport Medication Guide. [online] Available from *www.dysport.com/pdfs/Dysport_Medication_Guide.pdf*. [Accessed January, 2017].

Lee SK. Antibody-induced failure of botulinum toxin type A therapy in a patient with masseteric hypertrophy. Dermatol Surg. 2007;33(1 Spec No.):S105-10.

Merz Pharmaceuticals. (2011). Xeomin Medication Guide. [online] Available from *www.fda.gov/downloads/drugs/drugsafety/ucm222360.pdf*. [Accessed January, 2017].

Solstice Neurosciences. (2009). Myobloc Medication Guide. [online] Available from *www.myobloc.com/myobloc/hcp/medguide/medguide.pdf*. [Accessed January, 2017].

Wiegand H, Erdmann G, Wellhöner HH. 125I-labelled botulinum A neurotoxin: pharmacokinetics in cats after intramuscular injection. Naunyn Schmiedebergs Ach Pharmacol. 1976;292(2):161-5.

Cannabis

Pangarkar SS, Leung E

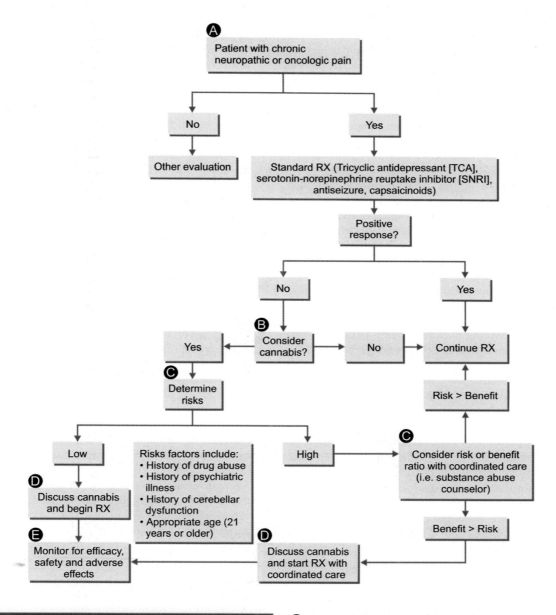

PREFACE

It is beyond the scope of this chapter to discuss the evolving legislation associated with cannabis for medical or recreational use. The rapid changes in classification may be a reflection of changing views in the medical community and lay public.

Ⓐ *Medical Indication:* Cannabis has garnered increased interest for its application in treating a variety of medical ailments and has been approved by the Food and Drug Administration (FDA) for chemotherapy-induced nausea and acquired immunodeficiency syndrome (AIDS)-associated weight loss. The potential utility of cannabis in the treatment of chronic pain is an emerging and controversial field. Randomized controlled trials evaluating the efficacy of cannabinoid therapy have shown positive outcomes in chronic neuropathic and oncologic pain; however, the scientific data is inconsistent and limited by variable dosing, small sample size, adverse effect and difficulty with blinding. In addition, there are currently no standards for quality, efficacy dosing or adverse effect monitoring. Given its limitations, there is no FDA approval of cannabis for the treatment of chronic pain. Nevertheless, as of April 2016, 23 states and Washington DC have legalized cannabis for medical use through voter driven initiatives, bypassing the FDA.

Ⓑ *Consideration of Cannabis and Mechanism of Action:* Medical cannabis refers to the use of an herbal cannabinoid drug derived from plants belonging to the *Cannabis* genus. The cannabis plant itself contains approximately six dozen different phytocannabinoids or plant-derived cannabinoids. These compounds are generally classified as terpenophenolics. The best-known natural analgesic cannabinoids are tetrahydrocannabinol (THC), cannabidiol (CBD) and cannabinol (CBN).

While not FDA approved, randomized controlled trials have shown positive outcomes in chronic neuropathic and oncologic pain. Medical cannabis can be considered as an adjuvant agent for patients with chronic neuropathic pain nonresponsive to standard treatment. Although still poorly understood, one mechanism by which cannabinoids are thought to produce analgesia is through partial agonism of endogenous cannabinoid receptors. These receptors have been found abundantly in the supraspinal, spinal and peripheral tissue that function in ascending and descending pain pathways. Additionally, phytocannabinoids without cannabinoid receptors 1 or 2 (CB1 or CB2) activity have shown the greatest effects at transient receptor potential vanilloid (TRPV) receptors, which may offer another mechanism of analgesia.

Ⓒ *Determining Risks:* Careful evaluation of risks and benefits should be performed prior to initiation of medical cannabis treatment. Patients should be above the age of 21, as regular smoking of cannabis is associated with altered brain development, poor educational outcome, cognitive impairment, and diminished life satisfaction and achievement in adolescents. Patients who have a history of drug abuse or are at risk for drug abuse should be carefully monitored if initiating medical cannabis given its psychoactive properties. In this population, consider coordinated care with other professionals such as a substance abuse counselor.

Other risks factors include history of drug abuse, history of psychiatric illness, and history of cerebellar dysfunction. In individuals with a history of existing psychotic disorders, cannabis is associated with increased symptoms and relapse. Recent evidence also demonstrates patients with existing posttraumatic stress disorder may experience worsening symptoms, increased violent behavior and increased alcohol use. Although the exact mechanism remains unknown, chronic cannabis exposure can potentially affect cerebellar function. Functional imaging studies have demonstrated differences in activation patterns between chronic exposure to cannabis and controls.

Ⓓ *Mechanism of Action and Administration of Cannabis:* Cannabis is generally administered either by inhalation, oral or topical routes. Inhalation of cannabis provides rapid onset of action, achieving maximum effect within 30 minutes and lasting 2–3 hours. Oral administration is subject to variable absorption depending on gastric contents and first pass liver metabolism. There is a slower onset (30 minutes to 2 hours), with a longer duration of action of 5–8 hours. There is limited available information on the biomechanics and bioavailability of topical application of cannabis.

In the plasma, about 95–99% of THC and CBD are bound to lipoproteins. THC is metabolized primarily by the liver through microsomal hydroxylation via the cytochrome P-450 isoenzyme CYP2C9 to its active metabolite 11-OH-THC and the isoenzyme CYP3A (including CYP3A4) to 8-B-hydroxyl-THC. 11-OH-THC is then further oxidized by CYP450 isoenzymes to its inactive form 11-nor-9-carboxy-THC (THC-COOH). This form conjugates with long-chain fatty acids and is the form THC is stored in tissue. CBD and CBN are metabolized similarly to THC. Elimination of THC occurs in several days; however, THC metabolites have been found in the urine of frequent cannabis smokers up to 80 days following their last consumption. Approximately 65–80% is eliminated in feces, 20–35% in urine and less than 5% as unchanged drug. Dosing adjustments in geriatric patients or those with renal or hepatic impairment have not been studied.

Medical cannabis is currently not FDA approved for the treatment of chronic pain; however, it is medicinally legal in 23 states and in Washington DC for physicians to recommend it. Cannabis is currently manufactured and marketed as dronabinol capsules (Marinol®), nabilone capsules (Cesamet®) and oromucosal spray nabiximols (Sativex®, currently undergoing FDA approval) **(Table 1)**. Alternative availability of cannabis includes herbal formulations, which can be inhaled (smoking or vaporization), ingested or inserted buccally. There are currently no accepted standards for dosing of cannabis for chronic pain.

Table 1: Manufacturers of cannabis		
Drug	*Trade name*	*Availability*
Dronabinol	Marinol®	2.5 mg, 5 mg and 10 mg PO
Nabilone	Cesamet®	1 mg PO
Nabiximols (undergoing FDA approval)	Sativex®	Buccal spray, 5.5 mL and 10 mL vials

FDA, Food and Drug Administration

E *Safety Monitoring and Adverse Effects:* Currently, there are no standardized guidelines for patient monitoring after initiation of medical cannabis. Approved formulations of cannabis are categorized by the FDA as controlled substances (Schedule II and Schedule III). Adverse effects of medical cannabis that are reported in the literature include dizziness, dry mouth, nausea, fatigue, somnolence, euphoria, depression, vomiting, diarrhea, disorientation, asthenia, drowsiness, anxiety, confusion, balance disorders, hallucinations, dyspnea, paranoia, psychosis, weakness, falls, hypotension, palpitations, tachycardia, infections, urinary retention, and seizures. These adverse effects place individuals at increased risk of injury secondary to motor incoordination and altered judgment.

There are currently no studies evaluating long-term adverse events of medical cannabis; however, there is evidence that the regular smoking of herbal cannabis can lead to addiction, increased risk of developing cancer, oral cavity disease, cardiovascular disease, chronic bronchitis, infertility, renal and urological disease, immunologic disease, cerebellar dysfunction and increase risk of chronic psychosis. In adolescents, regular smoking of cannabis is associated with altered brain development, poor educational outcome, cognitive impairment, diminished life satisfaction and achievement.

Other potential adverse effects and toxicity can be related potential contaminants in herbal cannabis. Due to the lack of public health infrastructure to monitor the quality of herbal cannabis, patients may be unknowingly exposed to contaminants such as molds and pesticides.

SUMMARY

There is promising medical literature suggesting that cannabis has a positive analgesic effect in the treatment of chronic pain; however, more studies are needed to determine safety, dosing and efficacy. As regulations governing cannabis change, clinicians should be familiar with common uses and adverse effects related to this drug. Systematic monitoring should be implemented to optimize patient safety and well-being.

SUGGESTED READING

Aggarwal SK, Pangarkar S, Carter GT, et al. Medical marijuana for failed back surgical syndrome: a viable option for pain control or an uncontrolled narcotic? PM R. 2014;6(4):363-72.

Aggarwal SK. Cannabinergic pain medicine: a concise clinical primer and survey of randomized-controlled trial results. Clin J Pain. 2013;29(2):162-71.

Bachhuber MA, Saloner B, Cunningham CO, et al. Medical cannabis laws and opioid analgesic overdose mortality in the United States, 1999-2010. JAMA Intern Med. 2014;174(10):1668-73.

Brady JE, Guohua Li. Trends in alcohol and other drugs detected in fatally injured drivers in the United States, 1999–2010. Am J Epidemiol. 2014;179(6):692-9.

Carter GT. The argument for medical marijuana for the treatment of chronic pain. Pain Med. 2013;14(6):800.

Cutando L, Busquets-Garcia A, Puighermanal E, et al. Microglial activation underlies cerebellar deficits produced by repeated cannabis exposure. J Clin Invest. 2013;123(7):2816-31.

Ganzer F, Bröning S, Kraft S, et al. Weighing the Evidence: A Systematic Review on Long-Term Neurocognitive Effects of Cannabis Use in Abstinent Adolescents and Adults. Neuropsychol Rev. 2016;26(2):186-222.

Gordon AJ, Conley JW, Gordon JM. Medical consequences of marijuana use: a review of current literature. Curr Psychiatry Rep. 2013;15(12):419.

Pierre JM. Cannabis, synthetic cannabinoids, and psychosis risk: What the evidence says. Curr Psychiatry. 2011;10(9):49-58.

Volkow ND, Baler RD, Compton WM, et al. Adverse health effects of marijuana use. N Engl J Med. 2014;370(23):2219-27.

Whiting PF, Wolff RF, Deshpande S, et al. Cannabinoids for Medical Use: A Systematic Review and Meta-analysis. JAMA. 2015;313(24):2456-73.

Wilkinson ST, Stefanovics E, Rosenheck RA. Marijuana use is associated with worse outcomes in symptom severity and violent behavior in patients with post-traumatic stress disorder. J Clin Psychiatry. 2015;76(9):1174-80.

CHAPTER 104

N-Methyl-D-Aspartate Antagonists

Mitchell B, Garza R III

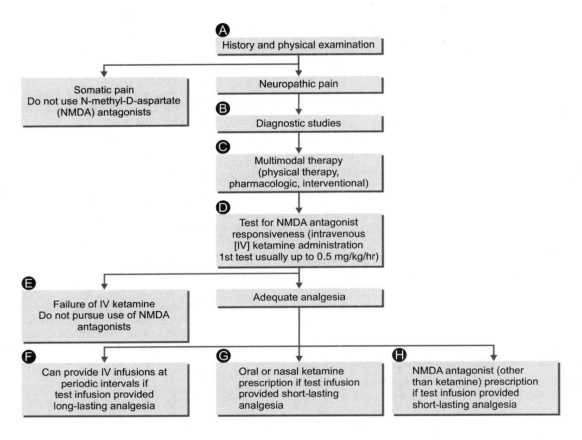

The ideal approach to chronic pain is the routine use of multimodal analgesic techniques that act on the central and peripheral nervous systems to improve pain control. In practice, patients are given some form of neuropathic pain medication with or without opioids but physicians are left with few alternatives when these options fail. With our increasing knowledge that opioids may potentially worsen patient outcomes but induce tolerance, hyperalgesia and addiction, it becomes necessary to explore other options to minimize the side effects and limitations from traditional analgesic techniques. Antagonists to the N-methyl-D-aspartate receptors (NMDARs) are an example of this targeted approach to pain management, particularly for pain that has been refractory to traditional modalities.

To understand the mechanism of the NMDA antagonist we will briefly discuss the role of the NMDAR as it relates to the pain mechanism. Pain is mediated via the unmyelinated C and small myelinated A-delta nociceptive fiber. The primary excitatory neurotransmitter released via the C fibers is glutamate and aspartate that acts at multiple subtype receptors to include the NMDAR. When exposed to inflammation, these receptors change their firing characteristics to become sensitized, decreasing the threshold and increasing the frequency of activation. Nociceptors that travel in the vicinity of these damaged nociceptors may also be affected.

NMADRs are ligand-gated ion receptors that become "activated" or open when glutamate and glycine bind to the receptor. The Ca^{2+} influx is crucial for the induction of the NMDA receptor-dependent long-term potentiation, which is thought to underlie neural plasticity, including the development of central sensitization. The activation of the NMDARs leads a Ca^{2+} or calmodulin-mediated activation of nitric oxide (NO) synthase, which plays a crucial role in nociception and neurotoxicity. By interfering with the development of the "wind-up" phenomenon and the generation of central sensitization, NMDAR antagonist produce antinociceptive effects attenuating symptoms of hyperalgesia, allodynia, and blocking and/or reversing opioid tolerance, theoretically improving the efficacy of opioids.

In the United States, there are several commercially available NMDAR antagonists to include ketamine, dextromethorphan, memantine, amantadine, and methadone. Each differs in their level of activity on the NMDAR, with ketamine as the most potent of the antagonists. The severity and frequency of side effects depend on affinity for the NMDAR. In adults, adverse effects are mainly central nervous system (CNS) side effects.

Ketamine: A non-competitive antagonist with potent anesthetic, analgesic and amnestic properties formulated as a racemic mixture of S (+) and R (-) isomers with the S isomer as the more potent general anesthetic and NMDA antagonist. Ketamine is also active at the opioid, norepinephrine, serotonin, and muscarinic cholinergic receptors; it acts by inhibiting serotonin and dopamine reuptake and inhibits voltage-gated Na^+ and K^+ channels. Other proposed mechanisms include activation of monoaminergic descending inhibitory pathway.

Amantidine: A non-competitive NMDA antagonist, which is used for the treatment of parkinsonism and as an antiviral against influenza. Clinical trials have shown mixed results in reducing postoperative pain and analgesic requirements. Randomized control trials (RCT) seem to suggest that the administration of amantadine intravenously is superior to oral but there are limited studies comparing the two.

Memantine: A non-competitive NMDA antagonist that is better tolerated compared to other antagonists with a safer side effect profile. Memantine is approved for the treatment of dementia in moderate to severe Alzheimer's disease. The efficacy of memantine for established (at least 12 month) chronic phantom limb pain was studied in a RCT but failed to demonstrate a reduction in chronic pain scores. In contrast, a more recent RCT with memantine 20–30 mg/dL initiated immediately after upper limb amputation demonstrated a nearly fourfold decrease in the incidence of phantom limb pain at 6 months from 38% to 10%.

Dextromethorphan: Commonly found in over-the-counter (OTC) cough medications, has shown to reduce pain by 30% compared to placebo in an RCT. Dextromethorphan is metabolized via CYP2D6 to the active metabolite dextrorphan, leading to variation in analgesia when comparing rates of metabolism.

Methadone: The racemic mixture of methadone demonstrates that the D- and L-isomer may bind to the NMDAR. The D-isomer is weak or inactive at the opioid receptor but is antinociceptive in neuropathic pain as antagonist at the NMDAR. Unfortunately, methadone is often challenging to use because of the variable half-life, QTc prolongation, and many drug interactions.

A N-methyl-D-aspartate antagonists as analgesics should only be used in patients with neuropathic pain. A complete history and physical examination should be performed and somatic and cancer pain patients should not be offered NMDA antagonists as therapy.

B Diagnostic studies should be performed to rule out ominous causes of neuropathic pain such as malignancy and infection.

C As with all chronic pain, a multimodal approach to management should be implemented. This should include physical therapy and nonpharmacologic therapy such as nerve blocks.

D If the patient fails the standard pharmacologic treatment options, the patient should be tested for NMDA antagonist responsiveness with an intravenous ketamine infusion.

E If the patient fails ketamine infusions, then NMDA antagonist therapy should not be utilized.

F If the patient improves with ketamine intravenously, for a prolonged period, then use of periodic continuous ketamine infusions is warranted.

G If the analgesia from the test infusion is profound but short-lasting, the patient may be given a prescription for oral or nasal ketamine. The bioavailability of ketamine through mucosa and the gastrointestinal system is poor, and therefore, these preparations may be less efficacious than the intravenous route.

H A second option in the event that the test infusion leads to appropriate but short-lived analgesia is treatment with one of the oral NMDA antagonists listed in the earlier part of this chapter.

SUGGESTED READING

Bennett GJ. Update on the neurophysiology of pain transmission and modulation: focus on the NMDA-receptor. J Pain Symptom Manage. 2000;19(1 Suppl):S2-6.

Carlsson KC, Hoem NO, Moberg ER, et al. Analgesic effect of dextromethorphan in neuropathic pain. Acta Anaesthesiol Scand. 2004;48(3):328-36.

Devor M. The pathophysiology of damaged peripheral nerves. In: Wall PD, Melzack R (Eds). Textbook of Pain, 3rd edition. Edinburgh: Churchill Livingstone; 1994. pp. 79-100.

Ebert B. Andersen S, Krogsgaard-Larsen P. Ketobemidone, methadone and pethidine are non-competitive N-methyl-D-aspartate (NMDA) antagonist in the rat cortex and spinal cord. Neurosci Lett. 1995;187(3):165-8.

Flockerzi V, Frohmann MA, Geppetti P, et al. Handbook of Experimental Pharmacology. Berlin Heidelberg: Springer-Verlag; 2004. pp. 313-33.

Hewitt DJ. The use of NMDA-receptor antagonists in the treatment of chronic pain. Clin J Pain. 2000;16(2 Suppl):S73-9.

Okon T. Ketamine: an introduction for the pain and palliative medicine physician. Pain Physician. 2007;10(3):493-500.

Schley M, Topfner S, Wiech K, et al. Continuous brachial plexus blockade in combination with the NMDA receptor antagonist memantine prevents phantom pain in acute traumatic upper limb amputees. Eur J Pain. 2007;11(3):299-308.

Sinner B, Graf BM. Ketamine. In: Schuttler J, Schwilden H (Eds). Modern Anesthetics: Handbook of Experimental Pharmacology. Berlin Heidelberg: Springer-Verlag; 2008. pp. 313-33.

Snijdelaar DG, Koren G, Katz J. Effects of perioperative oral amantadine on postoperative pain and morphine consumption in patients after radical prostatectomy: results of a preliminary study. Anesthesiology. 2004;100(1):134-41.

Neurolytic Blocks

Lopez EM, Davies E

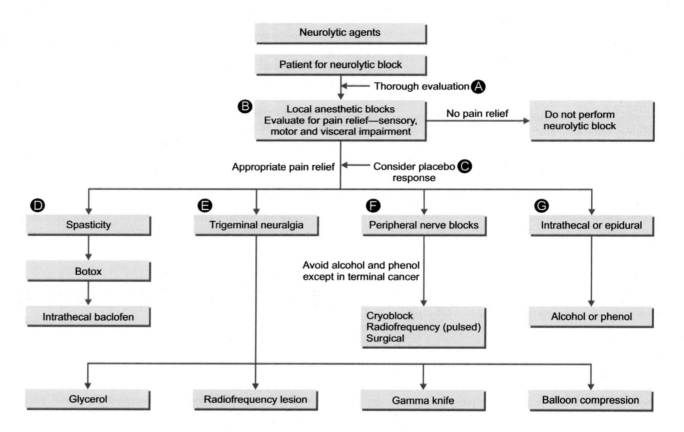

An increased understanding of pain mechanisms, the development of novel pharmacologic analgesics; and the widespread use of opioids, anticonvulsants, antidepressants, and other adjunctive analgesics has resulted in the reduction of neurolytic blocks over time. Chemical neurolysis is reserved for a small percentage of cancer patients via subarachnoid block (SAB) and sympathectomy with primarily two agents: (1) alcohol and (2) phenol. Neurolytic blocks (physical neurolysis) such as cryoneurolysis and radiofrequency (RF) lesioning are used today with increasing frequency, notably for solid tumors and facetogenic pain respectively. Surgical lesioning, particularly for sympathectomy, and stereotactic radiosurgery for trigeminal neuralgia are other physical techniques in use.

A A thorough history and physical examination should be undertaken by the physician prior to consideration of a neurolytic procedure. Specifically, the patient should have exhausted all other reasonable treatment options as neurolytic procedures are often irreversible. These procedures should be reserved for patients with pain due to malignancy, trigeminal neuralgia, spasticity, or pain conditions with well-known safety profiles (such as facetogenic pain).

B It should be routine to perform a diagnostic local anesthetic injection prior to performing a neurolytic block to ensure that the patient will benefit from the neurolysis. It should be noted that this step can be skipped in the case of refractory cancer pain, after discussion with the patient.

C If the patient responds well to the diagnostic injection, consideration should be made for the possibility of a placebo response before proceeding.

D *Spasticity:* In the event of spasticity, botulinum toxin injections and/or intrathecal baclofen can be utilized. For further details, see Chapter 41 Spasticity.

E In the case of trigeminal neuralgia, the neurolytic options include RF lesioning, glycerol neurolysis, and gamma knife radiosurgery. Balloon compressive neurolysis is another option which has fallen out of favor and will not be discussed in this chapter.

Glycerol is a mild neurolytic agent. 100% glycerol is used for neurolytic Gasserian rhizotomy. Conventional and pulsed RF techniques are also popular. There is no long-term data supporting one technique over the other; however, RF thermal lesioning has the highest complication rate, followed by glycerol rhizotomy and balloon compression (with the exclusion of sensory loss, an expected side effect) respectively.

Stereotactic radiosurgery (gamma knife radiosurgery) is a high-powered radiation therapy that allows specialized physicians to precisely deliver radiation to targeted areas with minimal to no damage of surrounding tissues. This modality can be used to treat not only intracranial lesions, but extracranial pathologies that cause chronic pain, including trigeminal neuralgia. In terms of complications, gamma knife radiosurgery has the lowest incidence of complications than any other neurolytic treatment option. One caveat is treatment effects that can take several months before they become clinically evident.

F Peripheral nerve neurolytic blocks can be accomplished using RF lesioning, pulsed RF neuromodulation, and/or cryoablation (See Chapter 136 Radiofrequency Ablation and Chapter 137 Pulsed Radiofrequency Neuromodulation). Cryoneurolysis involves neurodestruction by exposing nerves to extremely low temperatures via placement of a cryoprobe into the area. Modern machines contain a nerve stimulator function for localization or mapping of the site of intended effect. Two or three cycles consisting of 2 minute intervals are usually sufficient for the treatment of pain. In order to induce a prolonged conduction block, the nerve is frozen at -5° to -20°C causing axonal disintegration and breakdown of the myelin sheath. Although Wallerian degeneration occurs, the perineurium and epineurium remain intact, and regeneration is accurate and complete over time. Recovery of the lysed neuron depends on the rate of axonal regeneration (1–3 mm/day) and the distance of the cryolesion from the end organ. Pain due to small, well-localized conditions, for example ligaments, graft donor sites, peripheral nerves, cervical and lumbar facet joints, and radicular pain can be treated with cryoneurolysis.

G *Intrathecal and/or Epidural Neurolysis:* Chemical neurolysis is most useful in cancer pain, and prominently practiced for visceral and somatic pain in particular. Chemical neurolysis appears to be less effective for neuropathic pain. Intrathecal neurolysis has shown more useful for somatic pain, such as chest wall and peritoneum pain, as compared to visceral sources of pain, including pancreatic, gastric, and rectal sources. Chemical agents are also effective for neurolysis of the Gasserian ganglion for trigeminal neuralgia and the celiac plexus for

pancreatic cancer pain. More conservative treatments should be considered prior to consideration of neurolysis and significant pain relief with diagnostic small-volume local anesthetic blocks should be documented. Absolute contraindications for chemical neurolysis include coagulopathy and local infection of the area.

Ethyl alcohol is commercially available as an undiluted 100% solution and can be combined with local anesthetic. In contrast to phenol, it is hypobaric relative to cerebrospinal fluid, and has a specific gravity of less than 0.8. It produces a painful burning sensation on injection. A local anesthetic can be given prior to alcohol to minimize the burning, which may be useful for celiac plexus blocks. It exerts its nonselective degeneration effects via dehydration with sclerosis of nerve fibers and myelin sheaths leading to demyelination. The onset of neurolysis is immediate, with cerebrospinal fluid uptake ending within 30 minutes. After intrathecal injection, the patient should remain in the same position for 15–30 minutes. The full onset of effect is 3–5 days with variable duration.

Phenol is a neurolytic agent with local anesthetic properties. It is not commercially available, so it is typically prepared with contrast dyes, sterile water, saline or glycerin as a 4–10% solution. Due to the poor solubility of phenol in water, concentrations greater than 6.7% require the addition of glycerin, making it hyperbaric (specific gravity of 1.25). Phenol is directly neurotoxic and there is a direct relationship between concentration and extent of destruction. Concentrations less than 5% cause protein denaturation in axons and surrounding blood vessels. At concentrations more than 5%, phenol causes nonselective segmental demyelination and protein coagulation. Phenol injection produces an initial local anesthetic effect of warmth and numbness followed by nonselective destruction within 15 minutes. After intrathecal injection, the patient should remain in the same position for 30 minutes. The full effect is noted on the first day with the quality and extent of analgesia diminishing over the first 24 hours.

Overall, neurolytic agents can provide prolonged analgesia in many pain syndromes. Chemical agents offer predictable and reliable efficacy with a greater potential for complications since there is less control of the lesion in comparison to physical techniques. A thorough discussion of the potential risks and benefits of any neurolytic procedure should occur prior to proceeding and deciding the optimal treatment plan.

SUGGESTED READING

Byrd D, Mackey S. Pulsed radiofrequency for chronic pain. Curr Pain Headache Rep. 2008;12(1):37-41.

Cohen SP, Raja SN. Central and peripheral neurolysis. In: Benzon H, Raja SN, Fishman SM, Liu SS, Cohen SP (Eds). Essentials of Pain Medicine, 3rd edition. Philadelphia: Elsevier; 2011. pp. 531-7.

Evans PJ, Lloyd JW, Green CJ. Cryoanalgesia: the response to alterations in freeze cycle and temperature. Br J Anaesth. 1981;53(11):1121-7.

Kondziolka D, Lunsford LD, Flickinger JC. Stereotactic radiosurgery for the treatment of trigeminal neuralgia. Clin J Pain. 2002;18(1):42-7.

Leksell L. The stereotaxic method and radiosurgery of the brain. Acta Chir Scand. 1951;102(4):316-9.

Moller JE, Helweg-Larson J, Jacobson E. Histopathological lesions in the sciatic nerve of the rat following perineural application of phenol and alcohol solutions. Dan Med Bull. 1969;16(4):116-9.

Nathan PW, Sears TA, Smith MC. Effects of phenol solutions on the nerve roots of the cat: an electrophysiological and histological study. J Neurol Sci. 1965;2(1):7-29.

Rumsby MG, Finean JB. The action of organic solvents on the myelin sheath of peripheral nerve tissue. II. Short-chain aliphatic alcohols. J Neurochem. 1966;13(12):1509-11.

Saberski L, Fitzgerald J, Ahmad M. Cryoneurolysis and radiofrequency lesioning. In: Raj PP (Ed). Practical Management of Pain, 3rd edition. St. Louis: Mosby; 2000. pp. 753-67.

Sluijter ME, Mehta M. Treatment of chronic back and neck pain by percutaneous thermal lesions. In: Lipton S (Ed). Persistent Pain: Modern Methods of Treatment. London, England: Academic Press; 1981. pp. 141-79.

Tekin I, Mirzai H, Ok G, et al. A comparison of conventional and pulsed radiofrequency denervation in the treatment of chronic facet joint pain. Clin J Pain. 2007;23(6):524-9.

Umeda S, Arai T. Disulfiram-like reaction to moxalactam after celiac plexus alcohol block. Anesth Analg. 1985;64(3):377.

CHAPTER
106

Topical Agents

Davies E, Salas MM

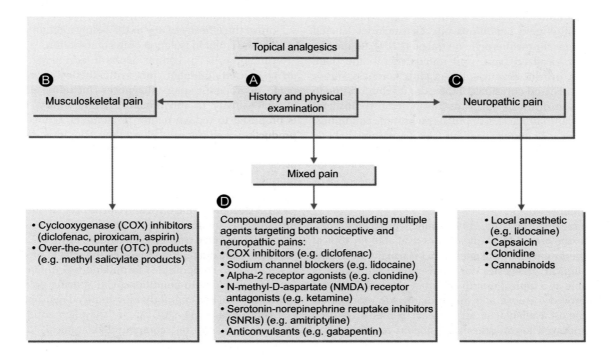

Topical analgesics

B Musculoskeletal pain

A History and physical examination

C Neuropathic pain

Mixed pain

- Cyclooxygenase (COX) inhibitors (diclofenac, piroxicam, aspirin)
- Over-the-counter (OTC) products (e.g. methyl salicylate products)

D Compounded preparations including multiple agents targeting both nociceptive and neuropathic pains:
- COX inhibitors (e.g. diclofenac)
- Sodium channel blockers (e.g. lidocaine)
- Alpha-2 receptor agonists (e.g. clonidine)
- N-methyl-D-aspartate (NMDA) receptor antagonists (e.g. ketamine)
- Serotonin-norepinephrine reuptake inhibitors (SNRIs) (e.g. amitriptyline)
- Anticonvulsants (e.g. gabapentin)

- Local anesthetic (e.g. lidocaine)
- Capsaicin
- Clonidine
- Cannabinoids

Topical analgesics including creams, lotions, gels, or patches, are one avenue for pain relief that are available both over-the-counter (OTC) for mild to moderate pain and can be prescribed for more severe pain conditions.

A A thorough history and physical examination should be undertaken to ensure that the patient is a candidate for topical medications. Often, topical analgesics are utilized for acute soft tissue injuries, neuropathic pain conditions, complex regional pain syndrome (CRPS), osteoarthritis, musculoskeletal injuries, migraines, and joint pain. Cost, absorption issues, application site reactions, and frequency of application are limitations of topical analgesics. However, topical analgesics are often used to reduce acute and chronic pain, and can help to reduce the amount of oral medications necessary to control chronic pain on a daily basis, making them very advantageous. Topical analgesics are particularly attractive due to low side effect profiles with reduced risk for abuse and addiction properties as compared to oral opioids.

B For musculoskeletal pain conditions, topical nonsteroidal anti-inflammatory drugs (NSAIDs) and several OTC agents are evidence-based options. Multiple NSAIDs are commercially available as topical products, and can

also be compounded into formulations for topical pain relief. NSAIDs inhibit prostaglandin, thromboxane, and/or prostaglandin synthesis through blockage of cyclooxygenase (COX) enzymes. NSAIDs are used for inflammatory pain including acute soft tissue injuries, knee pain, leg ulcers, and arthritic disorders. Diclofenac is available as a 1.3% topical patch and approved for acute pain due to minor strains, sprains, and contusions; a 1.5% solution approved for osteoarthritis pain of the knee, or 1% gel approved for osteoarthritis pain in joints amenable to topical therapy. Diclofenac topical formulations have proven clinical efficacy, with increased safety compared to oral formulations due to low systemic absorption. Ibuprofen is available for compounding into a topical cream (3–10%), as is ketoprofen (5–20%), piroxicam (0.5–1%), meloxicam (0.5–1%), flurbiprofen (10%) and mefenamic acid (1%).

Trolamine and methyl salicylate are both topical formulations that are available as combination OTC topical analgesics. Trolamine is combined with salicylic acid and is available as an OTC product ranging from 13–30% concentration in products like Icy Hot®, Thera-Gesic®, and Salonpas®. Adverse effects recorded for methyl salicylate products including toxicity, serious burns, and issues related to inhibition of platelet aggregation.

C In cases of neuropathic pain, topical local anesthetics and capsaicin have proven efficacy. Some local anesthetics function as non-selective sodium channel blockers, and when used topically can block the initiation and/or signal propagation of peripheral sensory afferents. Lidocaine is a widely used topical anesthetic agent available in many different formulations, including creams (2–5%), gels (0.2–5%), lotions (3%), ointments (5%), patches (4–5%), and solutions (2–4%). Lidocaine is typically used for neuropathic pain conditions but also includes labeled indications for postherpetic neuralgia (PHN), temporary relief of localized pain, oral mucus membrane pain, pruritus, pruritic eczemas, insect bites, soreness, minor burns, cuts, and abrasions of the skin, discomfort due to pruritus ani or anusitis, pruritus vulvae, hemorrhoids, anal fissures, and similar skin or mucus membrane conditions. Lidocaine is frequently used off-label for painful diabetic neuropathy (PDN) and allodynia. Lidocaine is often combined with other medications or local anesthetics for topical application, including the combination of 2.5% lidocaine and 2.5% prilocaine [eutectic mixture of local anesthetic (EMLA)].

Tetracaine, cocaine, benzocaine, prilocaine, and pramoxine are all local anesthetics available for topical use. This group of topical anesthetics is usually combined with topical analgesics for pain relief. Tetracaine is available as a topical mouth or throat solution (2%) and is approved for nose and throat diagnostic procedures. Cocaine is available as an external solution (4–10%) and approved for anesthesia of mucous membranes of oral, laryngeal, and nasal cavities as a C-II controlled substance. Pramoxine (1%) is available as a foam, lotion, or gel for minor skin irritation and/or hemorrhoidal itching.

Transient receptor potential vanilloid 1 (TRPV1) agonists are thought to reduce the pain signaling cascade by desensitization of the TRPV1 channel. The most well-known of the TRPV1 agonists is capsaicin. Capsaicin is available as a topical analgesic OTC creams, gel, lotion, and liquid as well as prescription strength patch (8%, Qutenza®). Capsaicin is approved for temporary treatment of minor pain associated with muscles and joints due to an acute injury, arthritic pain relief and PHN. Off-label uses include PDN, burning mouth syndrome, psoriasis and intractable pruritic pain, and oral mucositis. Adverse side effects include local erythema, pain, and burning sensation upon application. Zucapsaicin is another TRPV1 receptor agonist with similar properties to capsaicin, approved for osteoarthritic knee pain, not yet available in the United States (US).

Cannabinoid (CB1) receptors are present on sensory nerve endings in the periphery, dorsal spinal cord, and supraspinal brain regions important in pain signaling. CB2 receptors are observed on central and peripheral aspects of sensory neurons after nerve injury.

Tetrahydrocannabinol (27 mg/mL) and cannabidiol (25 mg/mL) are available as a combination buccal spray for spasticity or neuropathic pain associated with multiple sclerosis, or cancer pain and are available in Canada but not in the US.

D Mixed pain states are difficult to treat with topical analgesics, and the evidence for the use of many of the commonly used topical agents is lacking. These medications are commonly compounded into multiple agent creams or ointments with varying, anecdotal success. Randomized, controlled trials are needed to prove the efficacy of any of the below mentioned topical agents, either in isolation or in combination.

Clonidine is a central alpha-2 adrenergic receptor agonist used off-label for sympathetically maintained pain, neuropathic pain diagnoses including PDN, and hypersensitivity in inflammatory nerve injury. Clonidine is proposed to reduce neuron excitability, reduce cytokine production, and improve blood flow. Clonidine is available as a patch (0.1 mg/24 hr–0.3 mg/24 hr) that is applied once every 7 days or as a component of a compounded cream or ointment.

Ketamine is classified as an N-methyl-D-aspartate (NMDA) receptor antagonist and can be used in compounded formulations for topical applications. Ketamine has been reported to reverse central sensitization, lower the threshold for nerve transduction, and reduce the effects of substance P. Ketamine in compounded formulations is frequently used for neuropathic pain conditions, CRPS, acute pain, lumbar radicular pain, and chemotherapy-induced neuropathy.

Amitriptyline (1–5%) is a tricyclic antidepressant commonly used in compounded topical analgesics. Amitriptyline is used both topically and orally off-label for neuropathic pain conditions, PHN, PDN, postsurgical neuropathic pain, CRPS, chemotherapy-induced neuropathy, migraine prophylaxis, and musculoskeletal pain. Imipramine and doxepin are also serotonin-norepinephrine reuptake inhibitors that are used in combination compounded topical analgesics.

Gabapentin and pregabalin are calcium channel alpha-2 delta ($\alpha2\delta$) ligands and bind to the $\alpha2\delta$-1 and $\alpha2\delta$-2 subunits of presynaptic voltage-gated calcium channels, therefore reducing the calcium-dependent release of neurotransmitters. They are common anticonvulsants used in compounded creams for PHN, PDN, and neuropathic pain diagnoses.

SUGGESTED READING

Argoff CE. Topical analgesics in the management of acute and chronic pain. Mayo Clin Proc. 2013;88(2):195-205.

Lexi-Comp. Version 1.9.2. (2012). Diclofenac, clonidine, lidocaine, capsaicin, and ibuprofen Full Monographs. [online] Available from *www.online.lexi.com/lco/action/home*. [Accessed January, 2017].

Sawynok J. Topical analgesics for neuropathic pain: preclinical exploration, clinical validation, future development. Eur J Pain. 2014;18(4):465-81.

Regenerative Medicine

McCallin JP, Salas MM

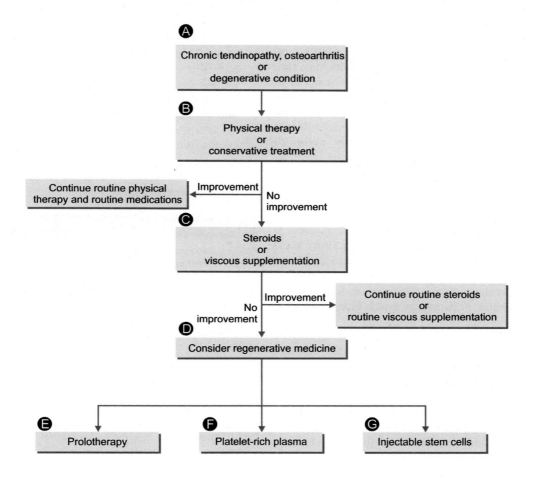

In the last 10–20 years, the field of regenerative medicine has gained more popularity as a possible treatment strategy for soft tissue and joint injuries and may be more advantageous for these particular types of chronic pain conditions. Two conditions with a large amount of evidence supporting the use of regenerative medicine are (1) chronic tendinopathies and (2) degenerative conditions involving cartilage and bone, specifically osteoarthritis.

Ⓐ Chronic tendinopathy is a distinct entity compared to tendonitis, which involves acute inflammation. Tendinopathy involves little to no signs of acute or chronic inflammation in pathologic patient specimens. Biologically, chronic tendinopathy has miniscule amounts of infiltration of inflammatory cells, but does include hypertrophy of fibroblasts, disorganization of collagen, hyperplasia of vasculature, and apoptosis, resulting in an impaired healing process. Here are regenerative medicine strategies currently available that should be considered in chronic tendinopathies, osteoarthritis or other degenerative conditions.

Ⓑ Initial conservative treatment for degenerative conditions typically involves medications for pain control and physical therapy. These treatments should be considered first prior to proceeding with interventional techniques.

Ⓒ If initial conservative treatments have failed, traditionally interventional techniques including injection of corticosteroid or viscous supplementation into large joints have been used with success in some patients. These interventional techniques should be considered prior to proceeding with regenerative medicine therapies.

Ⓓ Regenerative medicine should be considered when the earlier conservative treatment options have failed.

Regenerative medicine can be broken into three categories: (1) prolotherapy, (2) platelet-rich plasma (PRP) injections, and (3) stem cell therapy.

E Prolotherapy is a technique of injecting an irritant, typically a hyperosmolar dextrose solution into the area of pain. Historically, solutions containing varying concentrations of phenol, glycerin, and morrhuate sodium have been used, but hyperosmolar dextrose solutions are now accepted. One current theory behind the efficacy of prolotherapy is due to the spatially local injection of the irritant solution to the injury site, resulting in the migration of inflammatory mediators and simultaneous stimulation of growth factors, contributing to the initiation of the healing process (inflammation, proliferation, followed by remodeling). The majority of evidence supporting the use of prolotherapy is in chronic tendinopathy with the majority of literature supporting its use in Achilles tendinopathy and to a lesser degree chronic lateral epicondylitis. Unfortunately, there are no standards regarding the preparation of the injectate. This includes the specific irritant used, the concentration of the irritant, the number of injections, or the time between injections. Although clinical studies do not show robust results in all tendinopathies, there is evidence to support its use in degenerative conditions, specifically osteoarthritis of the knee and various finger joints. Thus, the development of a specific algorithm for prolotherapy recommendations is difficult and its limitations should be understood by the provider. Nevertheless, based on the available evidence, prolotherapy should be considered in refractory cases of chronic tendinopathy.

F Injection of PRP, a solution consisting of highly concentrated plasma that contains higher platelet concentration than the patients' baseline level, is also a regenerative therapy that can be considered in chronic tendinopathies. PRP solutions contain proteins, cytokines, and other biologic factors that affect the healing process. Preparation of PRP involves withdrawal of whole blood, addition of citrate to inhibit the clotting cascade, centrifugation steps to separate platelets from red blood cells and white blood cells, and finally the addition of a clotting factor to allow delivery. The majority of evidence for use of PRP in chronic tendinopathies is in cases of lateral epicondylitis and osteoarthritis of the knee. Limited evidence also recommends PRP in patellar tendinopathy, Achilles tendinopathy, lumbar discogenic pain, and in plantar fasciosis. PRP should be considered in refractory cases of tendinopathy. It should be noted that pain and function improvements seem pronounced after 12 months postprocedure. Intra-articular PRP improvements show a median duration of 9 months. Outcomes may be age-dependent, with significant improvement in younger aged patients with low degrees of degeneration.

G The use of injectable stem cells (SCs) in chronic pain caused by soft tissue and joint injuries remains controversial. Both mesenchymal stem cells (MSCs) and hematopoietic stem cells (HSCs) are utilized in regenerative medicine. There are multiple sources to derive SCs, and the use of embryonic, adult, and induced pluripotent SCs are available. MSCs are typically used in soft tissue injections and can be obtained from whole marrow aspirate, muscle biopsy, and adipose liposuction aspirate among other sources. Both autologous and allogeneic SCs can be utilized. Ethical and legal considerations should be taken depending on the source of the SCs utilized in the injected preparation. Unfortunately, chronic tendinopathy has limited human studies to support the use of SC technology. The majority of tendinopathy studies are in animal models and must be further validated in clinical studies. Although there are limited studies in clinical practice, an improvement in pain and function has been reported. Both osteoarthritis and degenerative disc disease have been the target for SC therapy, but again there is a paucity of human studies. With limited information and research available, recommendation guidelines for use of SCs in routine regenerative medicine practice is challenging. More research is necessary.

SUGGESTED READING

Bashir J, Sherman A, Lee H, et al. Mesenchymal stem cell therapies in the treatment of musculoskeletal diseases. PM R. 2014;6(1):61-9.

Berbrayer D, Fredericson M. Update on evidence-based treatments for plantar fasciopathy. PM R. 2014;6(2):159-69.

Centeno CJ. Clinical challenges and opportunities of mesenchymal stem cells in musculoskeletal medicine. PM R. 2014;6(1):70-7.

Chew KT, Leong D, Lin CY, et al. Comparison of autologous conditioned plasma injection, extracorporeal shockwave therapy, and conventional treatment for plantar fasciitis: a randomized trial. PM R. 2013;5(12):1035-43.

de Vos RJ, Windt J, Weir A. Strong evidence against platelet-rich plasma injections for chronic lateral epicondylar tendinopathy: a systematic review. Br J Sports Med. 2014;48(12):952-6.

Distel LM, Best TM. Prolotherapy: a clinical review of its role in treating chronic musculoskeletal pain. PM R. 2011;3(6 Suppl 1):S78-81.

Foster TE, Puskas BL, Mandelbaum BR, et al. Platelet-rich plasma: from basic science to clinical applications. Am J Sports Med. 2009;37(11):2259-72.

Gosens T, Peerbooms JC, van Laar W, et al. Ongoing positive effect of platelet-rich plasma versus corticosteroid injection in lateral epicondylitis: a double-blind randomized controlled trial with 2-year follow-up. Am J Sports Med. 2011;39(6):1200-8.

Kahlenberg CA, Knesek M, Terry MA. New Developments in the Use of Biologics and Other Modalities in the Management of Lateral Epicondylitis. BioMed Res Int. 2015;2015:439309.

Lai LP, Stitik TP, Foye PM, et al. Use of Platelet-Rich Plasma in Intra-Articular Knee Injections for Osteoarthritis: A Systematic Review. PM R. 2015;7(6):637-48.

Mautner K, Malanga GA, Smith J, et al. A call for a standard classification system for future biologic research: the rationale for new PRP nomenclature. PM R. 2015;7(4 Suppl):S53-9.

Mishra A, Collado H, Fredericson M. Platelet-rich plasma compared with corticosteroid injection for chronic lateral elbow tendinosis. PM R. 2009;1(4):366-70.

Mishra A, Pavelko T. Treatment of chronic elbow tendinosis with buffered platelet-rich plasma. Am J Sports Med. 2006;34(11): 1774-8.

Mishra AK, Skrepnik NV, Edwards SG, et al. Efficacy of platelet-rich plasma for chronic tennis elbow: a double-blind, prospective, multicenter, randomized controlled trial of 230 patients. Am J Sports Med. 2014;42(2):463-71.

Moraes VY, Lenza M, Tamaoki MJ, et al. Platelet-rich therapies for musculoskeletal soft tissue injuries. Cochrane Database Syst Rev. 2013;(12):CD010071.

Nguyen RT, Borg-Stein J, McInnis K. Applications of platelet-rich plasma in musculoskeletal and sports medicine: an evidence-based approach. PM R. 2011;3(3):226-50.

Oehme D, Goldschlager T, Ghosh P, et al. Cell-Based Therapies Used to Treat Lumbar Degenerative Disc Disease: A Systematic Review of Animal Studies and Human Clinical Trials. Stem Cells Int. 2015;2015:946031.

Oehme D, Goldschlager T, Rosenfeld JV, et al. The role of stem cell therapies in degenerative lumbar spine disease: a review. Neurosurg Rev. 2015;38(3):429-45.

Rabago D, Patterson JJ, Mundt M, et al. Dextrose prolotherapy for knee osteoarthritis: a randomized controlled trial. Ann Fam Med. 2013;11(3):229-37.

Sampson S, Botto-van Bemden A, Aufiero D. Stem cell therapies for treatment of cartilage and bone disorders: osteoarthritis, avascular necrosis, and non-union fractures. PM R. 2015;7(4 Suppl):S26-32.

Sanderson LM, Bryant A. Effectiveness and safety of prolotherapy injections for management of lower limb tendinopathy and fasciopathy: a systematic review. J Foot Ankle Res. 2015; 8:57.

Vora A, Borg-Stein J, Nguyen RT. Regenerative injection therapy for osteoarthritis: fundamental concepts and evidence-based review. PM R. 2012;4(5 Suppl):S104-9.

Opioid Pharmacology

Larry C Driver

CHAPTER
108

Opioids

Rana MV, Kusper TM

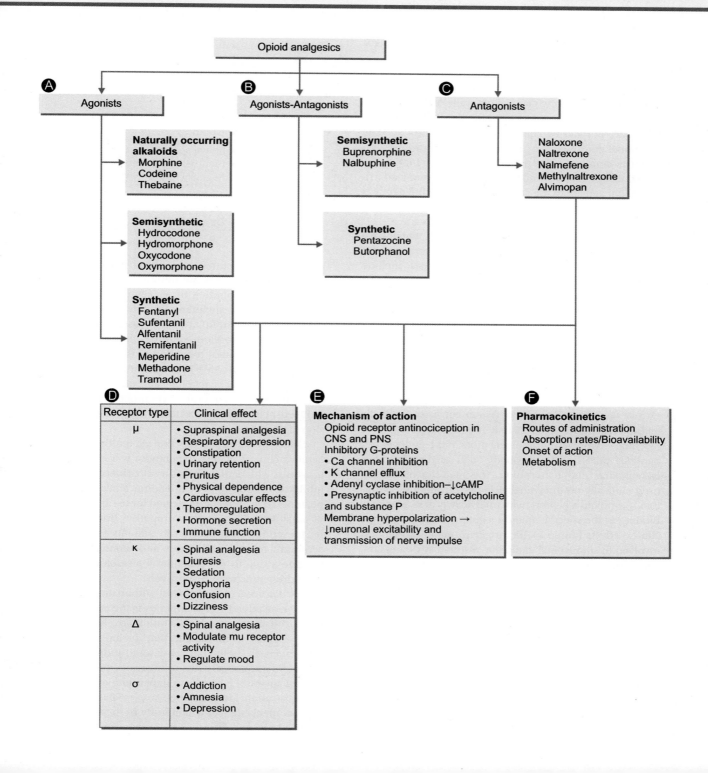

Opioid medications are an indispensable part of contemporary pain management. These drugs are extensively used to treat acute and chronic malignant and noncancer pain in inpatient and outpatient settings on a daily basis. Given their broad utilization in clinical practice, a thorough familiarity with opioid analgesics is of utmost importance. This chapter will provide a general overview of opioid medications, their classification systems, mechanisms of action, and common examples of opioids encountered in everyday practice.

Opioid Classification: Opioids are grouped, based upon their action at opioid receptors, into three separate categories: agonists, mixed agonists-antagonists, and antagonists.

Ⓐ Full opioid agonists bind and activate opioid receptors producing antinociception. Morphine, codeine, and thebaine belong to the class of naturally occurring alkaloids. Opioids are classified as synthetic or semisynthetic, which are derived by chemical modification of specific functional groups on the parent morphine molecule.

Ⓑ Agonists-antagonists (or partial agonists) also bind to the opioid receptors; however, this binding does not lead to a functional activity to the same degree as the full agonists (submaximal response). This category includes buprenorphine, nalbuphine, butorphanol, and pentazocine.

Ⓒ The last group consists of opioid antagonists, which have no intrinsic activity at the receptor site, and prevent opioid/receptor binding. Opioid antagonists include naloxone, naltrexone, nalmefene, methylnaltrexone, and alvimopan. When evaluating opioids, agents can have agonist activity at some receptors and antagonist/partial agonist activities at other receptors leading to clinical effect. For example, buprenorphine is a partial agonist at the μ-receptor and an antagonist at the κ-receptor. As an antagonist at the κ-receptor, buprenorphine would have less theoretical hallucinatory effect versus an agent that is a κ-agonist.

Ⓓ *Opioid Receptors:* The opioid system consists of specific types of receptors, which include mu (μ), kappa (κ), delta (Δ), and sigma (σ). These receptors bind endogenous peptides produced by the body such as β-endorphins, enkephalins, and dynorphins. The majority of opioids used clinically produce analgesia by activating predominantly μ-opioid receptors, with mild activity at κ-receptors. Binding to the specific opioid receptors produces unique clinical effects **(Table 1)**. Binding of μ-opioid receptors is involved in supraspinal analgesia, respiratory depression, constipation, urinary retention, pruritus, physical dependence, cardiovascular effects, thermoregulation, hormone secretion, and immune function. κ-receptors mediate spinal analgesia, diuresis, sedation, dysphoria, confusion, and dizziness. Delta-receptors mediate spinal analgesia, modulate μ-receptor activity, and regulate mood.

Ⓔ *Mechanism of Action:* Analgesia provided by the exogenous opioids results from stimulating opioid receptors with the nociceptive pathways present in the central nervous system and in the periphery. Specific areas containing nociceptive circuitry include the medulla locus coeruleus, periaqueductal gray area, the limbic, midbrain

Table 1: Opioid receptors	
Receptor type	*Clinical effect*
μ	• Supraspinal analgesia • Respiratory depression • Constipation • Urinary retention • Pruritus • Physical dependence • Cardiovascular effects • Thermoregulation • Hormone secretion • Immune function
κ	• Spinal analgesia • Diuresis • Sedation • Dysphoria • Confusion • Dizziness
Δ	• Spinal analgesia • Modulate μ-receptor activity • Regulate mood
σ	• Addiction • Amnesia • Depression

and cortical structures, and dorsal horn of the spinal cord. Opioid receptors are inhibitory G-proteins, which dissociate upon binding of an agonist resulting in the cascade of events, including inhibition of voltage-gated calcium channel, stimulation of potassium efflux through the rectifying potassium channels, inhibition of adenyl cyclase with resultant reduction of the cyclic adenosine monophosphate (cAMP) production, and inhibition of the presynaptic acetylcholine and substance P release. The end result is membrane hyperpolarization leading to reduced neuronal cell excitability and halted transmission of nerve impulses.

Select opioid agents function via multimechanisms to achieve clinical effects. Tapentadol is a centrally-acting μ-agonist with action also as a norepinephrine reuptake inhibitor. In addition to providing analgesia for acute postoperative pain, it is indicated for use in the treatment of patients with diabetic neuropathy. This agent should be prescribed with caution in patients taking selective serotonin reuptake inhibitors and monoamine oxidase inhibitors due to the potential for serotonin syndrome and adrenergic crisis, respectively.

Ⓕ *Opioid Pharmacokinetics:* Oral administration of immediate or sustained-release opioids is the most commonly employed route of administration in clinical practice. Other routes of administration include transdermal, transmucosal, sublingual, parenteral, and neuraxial (epidural and intrathecal). Absorption rates and bioavailability and speed of action vary depending on the routes of administration. Liver metabolism (first-pass metabolism) further affects the clinical efficacy of these medications. Certain opioid medications are metabolized in the liver by the uridine diphosphate glucuronosyltransferase (UGT) enzymes producing metabolites that might contribute to opioid toxicity. The addition of a glucuronic acid group to hydromorphone and morphine results in production of hydromorphone-3-glucuronide, morphine-6-glucuronide, and morphine-3-glucuronide.

SUGGESTED READING

Al-Hasani R, Bruchas MR. Molecular mechanisms of opioid receptor-dependent signaling and behavior. Anesthesiology. 2011;115(6):1363-81.

Chevlen E. Opioids: a review. Curr Pain Headache Rep. 2003;7(1): 15-23.

Khroyan TV, Wu J, Polgar WE, et al. BU08073 a buprenorphine analog with partial agonist activity at μ-receptors in vitro but long-lasting opioid antagonist activity in vivo in mice. Br J Pharmacol. 2015;172(2):668-80.

McDonald J, Lambert DG. Opioid receptors. Contin Edu Anaesth Crit Care Pain. 2005;5(1):22-5.

Pasternak GW. The pharmacology of mu analgesics: from patients to genes. Neuroscientist. 2001;7(3):220-31.

Vadivelu N, Timchenko A, Huang Y, et al. Tapentadol extended-release for treatment of chronic pain: a review. J Pain Res. 2011; 4:211-8.

CHAPTER
109

Opioid Toxicology

Kusper TM, Rana MV

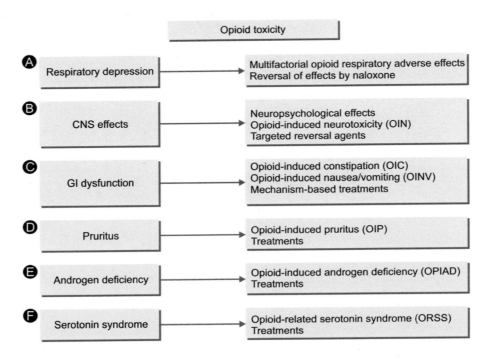

Opioid analgesics are associated with adverse effects posing health risks to patients when overused or misused. Some of the most important factors when evaluating the risk for opioid toxicity are daily opioid dose, history of opioid dependence, use of long-acting or extended-release opioids, comorbidities such as liver disease or lung disease, hospitalization 6 months prior to the toxicity or overdose event, and concomitant use of benzodiazepines and alcohol. A meta-analysis of randomized placebo-controlled studies reported that approximately 80% of patients had at least one adverse reaction from opioids, and that constipation (41%), nausea (32%), and somnolence (29%) are the most common adverse effects in patients with chronic noncancer pain taking opioid analgesics. While some side effects are more of a nuisance for those affected, others might pose immediate danger and result in increased morbidity and mortality. Naloxone, an opioid-receptor antagonist, is the agent used for the reversal of life-threatening adverse reactions, such as respiratory depression, and for opioid overdose. Additionally, multiple therapeutic options are available counteracting specific side effects **(Table 1)**. This chapter will describe common adverse reactions, proposed pathophysiology, and available reversal agents used for opioid toxicity.

A *Respiratory Depression:* One of the main and serious side effects associated with traditional and novel opioid analgesics is respiratory depression, resulting from the activation of the μ- and Δ-opioid receptors in the respiratory network. Binding of opioids to opioidergic receptors may potentially depress respiratory rate and depth, increase respiratory resistance, reduce pulmonary compliance, produce chest wall rigidity, and suppress responsiveness of the respiratory centers to CO_2 and hypoxia, and ultimately precipitate respiratory failure. The opioid-receptor antagonist naloxone is the main therapeutic option used to reverse respiratory depression. Loss of analgesic efficacy after naloxone administration has prompted the search for other non-opioid reversal options, such as serotonin-receptor agonists, AMPA-receptor modulators, and the antibiotic minocycline, which are all presently of limited clinical utility. Other documented consequences of opioid usage are central and obstructive sleep apnea, increased susceptibility to respiratory infections, opioid-induced pulmonary edema, acute lung injury (ALI), diffuse alveolar hemorrhage, and hypoxic respiratory failure. The pathophysiology of ALI and diffuse alveolar

Table 1: Opioid-induced adverse reactions, pathophysiology, and available treatments

Adverse effects of opioid medications		
Adverse reaction	*Mechanism*	*Management*
Nausea and vomiting	Direct stimulation of the chemoreceptor trigger zone (CTZ), increased vestibular sensitivity, and delayed gastric emptying	*Dopamine receptor antagonists:* • Prochlorperazine (5–10 mg PO; 5–10 mg IV; 25 mg rectally every 8 hours) • Metoclopramide (5–10 mg PO or IV every 6 hours) • Droperidol (0.625–2.5 mg every 3–4 hours) • Haloperidol (0.5–2 mg PO every 6 hours) • Promethazine (12.5–25 mg PO every 6 hours, 12.5–25 mg IV every 4–6 hours) *Serotonin (5-HT$_3$) receptor antagonist:* • Ondansetron (4 mg PO or IV 2–4 times per day)
Constipation	Increased transit time and decreased gastrointestinal motility, contraction of sphincters, and increased fluid absorption	*Peripheral opioid receptor antagonists:* • Naloxegol (12.5 or 25 mg PO once per day) • Methylnaltrexone (8–12 mg every other day) *Opioid receptor agonist/antagonist combination:* • Oxycodone and naloxone (maximum strength 40 mg/20 mg, taken orally every 12 hours) *Secretagogue chloride channel activator:* • Lubiprostone (24 µg PO twice daily)
Pruritus	Activation of the µ-opioid and serotonin (5-HT$_3$) receptors and histamine release by mast cells	*Antihistamines:* • Cetirizine 10 mg PO once a day • Diphenhydramine 25–50 mg PO every 4–6 hours • Loratadine 10 mg PO once a day • Hydroxyzine 25–100 mg PO at bedtime
Central nervous system effects	Direct toxic effects on neurons and inhibition of cholinergic activity	*Central nervous system stimulants:* • Caffeine (200 mg IV once daily) • Dextroamphetamine (2.5–15 mg PO 1–2 times a day) • Methylphenidate (2.5–5 mg PO twice daily) • Modafinil (100–200 mg orally once daily) *Acetylcholinesterase inhibitor:* • Donepezil (2.5–15 mg PO once daily) *Antipsychotics:* • Haloperidol (0.5–2 mg PO twice daily) • Quetiapine (25–50 mg PO twice daily) • Risperidone (0.25–1 mg PO twice daily)
Androgen deficiency	Inhibition of the hypothalamic-pituitary axis	*Testosterone replacement formulations:* • Intramuscular injections (75–100 mg weekly or 150–200 mg every 2 weeks) • Buccal tablets (30 mg tablet every 12 hours) • Patch 2.5 mg/24 hours or 5 mg/24 hours (once nightly) *DHEA supplements:* • 50 mg PO daily
Serotonin syndrome	Serotonin reuptake inhibition and increased release of intrasynaptic serotonin	*Serotonin receptor antagonists:* • Cyproheptadine (initial dose 4–8 mg orally; may be repeated in 2 hours; for a maximum of 32 mg in 24 hours) • Chlorpromazine (a dose of 50–100 mg)

hemorrhage is still poorly understood, but it is likely due to negative-pressure barotrauma and increased capillary permeability.

B *Central Nervous System Effects:* The neuropsychological effects due to opioid therapy are numerous, including sedation, cognitive decline, impaired concentration, memory deficits, psychomotor dysfunction, sleep disorders, delirium, and dementia. Another possible complication of opioid therapy is opioid-induced neurotoxicity (OIN), which is characterized by delirium, tremors, myoclonus, allodynia, and hallucinations. The most prevalent effects are memory deficits (73–81%), sleep disturbance (35–57%), fatigue (10%), and somnolence (7–13%). These effects are likely related to neurotoxic metabolites, which are generated by specific opioids, such as morphine, codeine, hydromorphone, fentanyl, and meperidine, and inhibition of cholinergic activity. Delirium and reduced cognition can be addressed with haloperidol, quetiapine, risperidone, or donepezil, while sedation might be improved with caffeine, dextroamphetamine, methylphenidate, or modafinil.

C *Gastrointestinal Dysfunction:* The results of the Bowel-Disease Questionnaire completed by chronic noncancer pain patients followed in a pain clinic and regularly taking opioids showed that 46.9% of patients reported constipation, 27% nausea, 9% vomiting, and 58.2% abdominal pain. Furthermore, higher prevalence was observed in those taking opioids for at least 2 years versus less than 6 months duration. Opioids stimulate enteric μ-opioid receptors, and thereby reduce gastric and intestinal motility, decrease gastric, biliary and pancreatic secretions, enhance fluid absorption from the bowels, and increase sphincteric tone, ultimately leading to constipation. Traditional remedies for opioid-induced constipation (OIC) include stimulants, stool softeners, laxatives, and enemas. Recent developments approved for OIC include opioid-receptor antagonists, opioid-receptor agonist/antagonist formulations, and chloride-channel activators. Opioid-induced nausea/vomiting (OINV) is produced through complex mechanisms involving distinct areas of the body. While delayed gastric emptying implicated in OIC contributes to OINV, other mechanisms involving direct stimulation of the chemoreceptor trigger zone (CTZ) in the medulla and vestibular apparatus also play a role. Though OINV appears to specifically result from the activation of μ- and Δ-opioid receptors, other receptors such as dopaminergic, serotonergic, histamine, acetylcholine, neurokinin-1, and cannabinoid receptor-1 are likely involved in the process as well. Consequently, OINV has been successfully treated with agents that block the corresponding receptors.

D *Pruritus:* Opioid-induced pruritus (OIP) occurs most commonly after neuraxial analgesia with the incidence ranging from 34.6% to 90%. The pathophysiology is still not completely understood. Possible mechanisms involve activation of the μ-opioid and serotonergic (5-HT$_3$) receptors in the dorsal horn and in the nucleus of the spinal tract of the trigeminal nerve in the medulla, and stimulation of mast cell degranulation with subsequent histamine release. Historically, several therapeutic options for treating pruritus have been explored, including antihistamines, serotonin-receptor antagonists, propofol, nonsteroidal anti-inflammatory drugs (NSAIDs), and naloxone. A recent review highlights nalbuphine, an opioid agonist-antagonist, as a promising treatment for this side effect. The findings reveal superior efficacy of nalbuphine when compared to diphenhydramine (83% vs 43%), propofol (83% vs 61%), and naloxone (25% vs 0%). The authors recommend nalbuphine as the first-line option for the treatment of pruritus, although mention that there is no established dosing regimen.

E *Androgen Deficiency:* Opioid-associated androgen deficiency (OPIAD), affecting both sexes, is a syndrome of inappropriately low levels of follicle stimulating hormone (FSH) and luteinizing hormone (LH), ultimately resulting in insufficient levels of sex hormones due to inhibition of the hypothalamic-pituitary axis by opioid medications. Clinical features include erectile dysfunction, decreased libido, testicular atrophy, decreased facial and body hair, menstrual abnormalities, hot flashes, depression, decreased muscle mass, osteoporosis, infertility, weight gain, and metabolic syndrome. Treatment of the

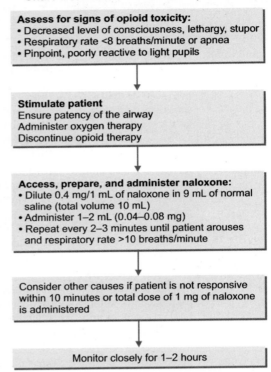

Chart 1: Naloxone treatment in opioid toxicity

Assess for signs of opioid toxicity:
- Decreased level of consciousness, lethargy, stupor
- Respiratory rate <8 breaths/minute or apnea
- Pinpoint, poorly reactive to light pupils

Stimulate patient
Ensure patency of the airway
Administer oxygen therapy
Discontinue opioid therapy

Access, prepare, and administer naloxone:
- Dilute 0.4 mg/1 mL of naloxone in 9 mL of normal saline (total volume 10 mL)
- Administer 1–2 mL (0.04–0.08 mg)
- Repeat every 2–3 minutes until patient arouses and respiratory rate >10 breaths/minute

Consider other causes if patient is not responsive within 10 minutes or total dose of 1 mg of naloxone is administered

Monitor closely for 1–2 hours

syndrome involves androgen replacement therapy (ART). Male patients treated with testosterone replacement exhibited increase in lean body mass and decrease in fat mass, and improved sex drive and overall quality of life. Women can be treated with DHEA supplements.

F *Serotonin Syndrome:* A toxidrome manifested by a triad of mental status changes, neuromuscular abnormalities, and autonomic instability, opioid-related serotonin syndrome (ORSS) may be seen in patients exposed to opioids while concomitantly taking serotonergic agents. Specific opioids implicated in the emergence of the syndrome include fentanyl, sufentanil, remifentanil, alfentanil, methadone, meperidine, and tramadol. Others, such as morphine, codeine, oxycodone, and buprenorphine do not precipitate the syndrome. Since antidepressants and antipsychotics are utilized as adjunctive treatment for various pain syndromes such as fibromyalgia, postherpetic neuralgia, painful diabetic neuropathy, a high index of suspicion is needed when patients present with agitation, anxiety, diaphoresis, hyperthermia, tremor, or other symptoms indicative of serotonin syndrome. Although the presentation resembles that of opioid withdrawal, the latter would be expected to occur in the context of opioid cessation or de-escalation, and patients would not exhibit hyperreflexia or myoclonus commonly seen with the syndrome. Mild to moderate cases usually resolve within 24–72 hours, and a majority of these cases resolve after stopping the opioid. The 5-HT serotonin-receptor antagonists, cyproheptadine, or chlorpromazine, might be used in moderate to severe cases **(Chart 1)**.

SUGGESTED READING

Basaria S, Travison TG, Alford D, et al. Effects of testosterone replacement in men with opioid-induced androgen deficiency: a randomized controlled trial. Pain. 2015;156(2):280-8.

Bijl D. The serotonin syndrome. Neth J Med. 2004;62(9):309-13.

Camilleri M. Opioid-induced constipation: challenges and therapeutic opportunities. Am J Gastroenterol. 2011;106(5):835-42; quiz 843.

Cole JB, Dunbar JF, McIntire SA, et al. Butyrfentanyl overdose resulting in diffuse alveolar hemorrhage. Pediatrics. 2015;135(3): e740-3.

Dahan A, Aarts L, Smith TW. Incidence, reversal, and prevention of opioid-induced respiratory depression. Anesthesiology. 2010;112(1):226-38.

Dhingra L, Ahmed E, Shin J, et al. Cognitive effects and sedation. Pain Med. 2015;16(Suppl 1):S37-43.

Dublin S, Walker RL, Gray SL, et al. Prescription opioids and risk of dementia or cognitive decline: A prospective cohort study. J Am Geriatr Soc. 2015;63(8):1519-26.

Gillman PK. Monoamine oxidase inhibitors, opioid analgesics and serotonin toxicity. Br J Anaesth. 2005;95(4):434-41.

Howlett C, Gonzalez R, Yerram P, et al. Use of naloxone for reversal of life-threatening opioid toxicity in cancer-related pain. J Oncol Pharm Pract. 2016;22(1):114-20.

Jannuzzi RG. Nalbuphine for treatment of opioid-induced pruritus: A systematic review of literature. Clin J Pain. 2016;32(1):87-93.

Jolley CJ, Bell J, Rafferty GF, et al. Understanding heroin overdose: A study of the acute respiratory depressant effects of injected pharmaceutical heroin. PLoS One. 2015;10(10):e0140995.

Kalso E, Edwards JE, Moore RA, et al. Opioids in chronic non-cancer pain: systematic review of efficacy and safety. Pain. 2004;112(3):372-80.

Koury KM, Tsui B, Gulur P. Incidence of serotonin syndrome in patients treated with fentanyl on serotonergic agents. Pain Physician. 2015;18(1):E27-30.

Kumar K, Singh SI. Neuraxial opioid-induced pruritus: An update. J Anaesthesiol Clin Pharmacol. 2013;29(3):303-7.

Lalley PM. Opioidergic and dopaminergic modulation of respiration. Respir Physiol Neurobiol. 2008;164(1-2):160-7.

Mao J, Gold MS, Backonja MM. Combination drug therapy for chronic pain: a call for more clinical studies. J Pain. 2011;12(2):157-66.

Nelson AD, Camilleri M. Chronic opioid-induced constipation in patients with nonmalignant pain: challenges and opportunities. Therap Adv Gastroenterol. 2015;8(4):206-20.

Pisani MA, Murphy TE, Araujo KL, et al. Factors associated with persistent delirium after intensive care unit admission in an older medical patient population. J Crit Care. 2010;25(3):540,e1-7.

Rajagopal A, Vassilopoulou-Sellin R, Palmer JL, et al. Symptomatic hypogonadism in male survivors of cancer with chronic exposure to opioids. Cancer. 2004;100(4):851-8.

Rastogi R, Swarm RA, Patel TA. Case scenario: opioid association with serotonin syndrome: implications to the practitioners. Anesthesiology. 2011;115(6):1291-8.

Smith HS, Elliott JA. Opioid-induced androgen deficiency (OPIAD). Pain Physician. 2012;15(3 Suppl):ES145-56.

Smith HS, Smith JM, Seidner P. Opioid-induced nausea and vomiting. Ann Palliat Med. 2012;1(2):121-9.

Swegle JM, Logemann C. Management of common opioid-induced adverse effects. Am Fam Physician. 2006;74(8):1347-54.

Tuteja AK, Biskupiak J, Stoddard GJ, et al. Opioid-induced bowel disorders and narcotic bowel syndrome in patients with chronic non-cancer pain. Neurogastroenterol Motil. 2010;22(4):424-30, e96.

Winegarden J, Carr DB, Bradshaw YS. Intravenous ketamine for rapid opioid dose reduction, reversal of opioid-induced neurotoxicity, and pain control in terminal care: Case report and literature review. Pain Med. 2016;17(4):644-9.

Yamanaka T, Sadikot RT. Opioid effect on lungs. Respirology. 2013;18(2):255-62.

Zedler B, Xie L, Wang L, et al. Risk factors for serious prescription opioid-related toxicity or overdose among Veterans Health Administration patients. Pain Med. 2014;15(11):1911-29.

CHAPTER 110

Opioid Withdrawal

Rana MV, Kusper TM

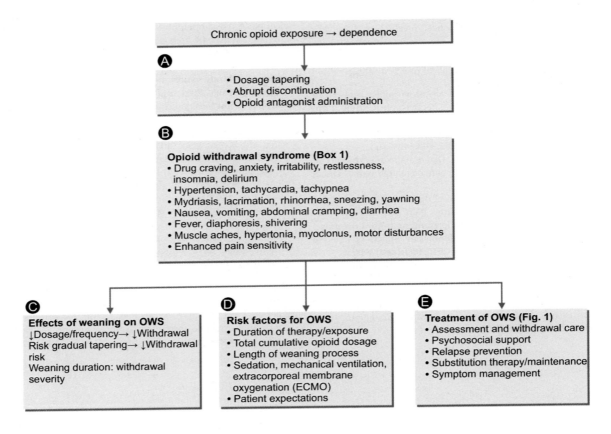

Chronic opioid exposure → dependence

Ⓐ
- Dosage tapering
- Abrupt discontinuation
- Opioid antagonist administration

Ⓑ

Opioid withdrawal syndrome (Box 1)
- Drug craving, anxiety, irritability, restlessness, insomnia, delirium
- Hypertension, tachycardia, tachypnea
- Mydriasis, lacrimation, rhinorrhea, sneezing, yawning
- Nausea, vomiting, abdominal cramping, diarrhea
- Fever, diaphoresis, shivering
- Muscle aches, hypertonia, myoclonus, motor disturbances
- Enhanced pain sensitivity

Ⓒ
Effects of weaning on OWS
↓Dosage/frequency→ ↓Withdrawal
Risk gradual tapering→ ↓Withdrawal risk
Weaning duration: withdrawal severity

Ⓓ
Risk factors for OWS
- Duration of therapy/exposure
- Total cumulative opioid dosage
- Length of weaning process
- Sedation, mechanical ventilation, extracorporeal membrane oxygenation (ECMO)
- Patient expectations

Ⓔ
Treatment of OWS (Fig. 1)
- Assessment and withdrawal care
- Psychosocial support
- Relapse prevention
- Substitution therapy/maintenance
- Symptom management

Ⓐ *Opioid Withdrawal Syndrome (OWS):* Chronic opioid exposure results in dependence represented by withdrawal syndrome after an abrupt discontinuation or tapering of the opioid therapy, or after the administration of an opioid antagonist.

Ⓑ Withdrawal syndrome is characterized by a constellation of constitutional symptoms, autonomic instability, thermoregulatory derangements, and other commonly reported signs and symptoms **(Box 1)**. In the pediatric population, the most common symptoms are diarrhea, vomiting, sweating, and fever. Reports indicate that opioid withdrawal occurred in 57% of neonates and 44% of children aged 2 weeks to 21 years after 5 days of continuous or scheduled opioid therapy in the intensive care unit (ICU).

Ⓒ *Effect of Weaning on the Withdrawal:* Much of the information on this subject comes from studies on pediatric patients treated with opioids in ICUs. Risk of withdrawal is reduced when patients are either weaned off opioids

or are given opioid doses less frequently. The literature indicates that the occurrence of withdrawal syndrome correlates with the speed of the opioid weaning process. Weaning strategies are instituted according to the duration of opioid exposure. One protocol involves a weaning duration of 5 days and 10 days for patients exposed to opioids for 7–14 days (short-term) and more than 14 days (long-term), respectively. In this case, withdrawal occurred in 20% of patients exposed to opioids for long-term, but overall the protocol reduced the weaning time without significant increases in withdrawal rates. It is possible that longer opioid exposure increases the risk of withdrawal, although the small sample size is insufficient to draw that conclusion. A similar study showed the withdrawal symptoms manifesting between days 4 through 7 in pediatric patients on continuous opioid therapy weaned with 5-day and 10-day therapies, without significant difference between the groups. Both of the above studies demonstrate a comparable effectiveness

Box 1: Signs and symptoms of opioid withdrawal

- Drug craving
- Irritability, anxiety, restlessness, insomnia
- Delirium
- Mydriasis
- Hypertension, tachycardia, tachypnea
- Lacrimation, rhinorrhea, sneezing
- Frequent yawning
- Enhanced pain sensitivity
- Nausea, vomiting
- Abdominal cramping, diarrhea
- Fever, diaphoresis, shivering
- Muscle aches, hypertonia, myoclonus
- Motor disturbances

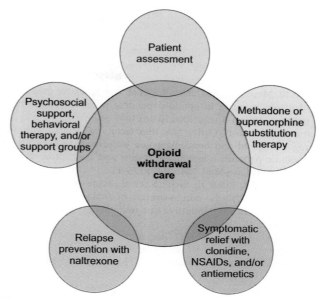

Fig. 1: Components of withdrawal care

with minimal risks between the two weaning approaches. In the outpatient setting, prescription opioid-dependent adults on 1–4-week buprenorphine tapers experienced more severe withdrawal after 1-week and 2-week tapering strategies 1 week after the last dose of buprenorphine, compared to the 4-week taper group. Based on this finding, it is reasonable to conclude that the severity of withdrawal is inversely related to the weaning duration.

D *Risk Factors:* Several risk factors predicting opiate withdrawal have been identified. Duration of opioid exposure, total opiate dose before weaning, length of the weaning process, and duration of mechanical ventilation, sedation, and of extracorporeal membrane oxygenation (ECMO) therapy are all predictors of withdrawal in the pediatric patients. Duration of therapy and cumulative opioid dose are the strongest predictors of the withdrawal syndrome. A total dose of more than 1.6 mg/kg or an ECMO therapy for more than 5 days increases the risk of neonatal abstinence syndrome (NAS). Opioid dose, duration of mechanical ventilation, use of neuromuscular blocking agents and propofol, and acute respiratory distress syndrome (ARDS) are all listed as potential predictors of withdrawal syndrome in the ICU adult population, and participants' expectations regarding withdrawal severity in the outpatient chronic opioid users.

E *Treatment:* The overarching goals in withdrawal management are gradual opioid weaning and reduction of withdrawal symptoms. Careful assessment of withdrawal signs must be done at regular intervals and therapy should be adjusted appropriately. Psychosocial support, withdrawal care, and relapse prevention are critical components of the withdrawal process **(Fig. 1)**. Switching to methadone or buprenorphine substitution therapy might be necessary to control withdrawal quickly and smoothly in order to prevent craving and deter relapse. Maintenance therapy with the μ-opioid-receptor antagonist naltrexone might provide some benefit in relapse prevention in opioid-addicted patients. Symptomatic care can be provided with the following pharmacological options.

Alpha$_2$-adrenergic agonist, clonidine, is well known for its benefits in reducing the symptoms due to uninhibited sympathetic excitation. Combination naltrexone-clonidine formulation demonstrates a superior efficacy in abolishing withdrawal symptoms compared to each of the medications used alone. Lofexidine is a well-tolerated and efficacious option for the treatment of withdrawal, currently approved in the United Kingdom.

Gabapentin, an antiepileptic medication that works at α_2-Δ calcium channels, when administered at a dose of 1,600 mg/day, effectively reduces the severity of some withdrawal symptoms, such as muscle tension, diarrhea, coldness, or even dysphoria and yawning.

Several novel options have emerged in recent years with documented efficacy in reduction of withdrawal symptomatology. Pramipexole, a dopamine receptor agonist, helps to attenuate the symptoms of restlessness; and 5-hydroxytryptophan (5-HTP), a serotonin precursor, was successfully used to ameliorate muscle spasms due to opioid withdrawal. Other alternative treatments include varenicline, a nicotinic receptor partial-agonist, and tetrodotoxin, a selective sodium-channels blocker, which also showed a promise in the treatment of withdrawal in clinical trials. Additionally, antiemetics, antidiarrheals, and nonsteroidal anti-inflammatory drugs (NSAIDs) are commonly utilized to treat nausea/vomiting, diarrhea, and muscle aches, respectively.

SUGGESTED READING

Adi Y, Juarez-Garcia A, Wang D, et al. Oral naltrexone as a treatment for relapse prevention in formerly opioid-dependent drug users: a systematic review and economic evaluation. Health Technol Assess. 2007;11(6):iii-iv, 1-85.

Anand KJ, Willson DF, Berger J, et al. Tolerance and withdrawal from prolonged opioid use in critically ill children. Pediatrics. 2010;125(5):e1208-25.

Arnold JH, Truog RD, Orav EJ, et al. Tolerance and dependence in neonates sedated with fentanyl during extracorporeal membrane oxygenation. Anesthesiology. 1990;73(6):1136-40.

Berens RJ, Meyer MT, Mikhailov TA, et al. A prospective evaluation of opioid weaning in opioid-dependent pediatric critical care patients. Anesth Analg. 2006;102(4):1045-50.

Best KM, Boullata JI, Curley MA. Risk factors associated with iatrogenic opioid and benzodiazepine withdrawal in critically ill pediatric patients: a systematic review and conceptual model. Pediatr Crit Care Med. 2015;16(2):175-83.

Cammarano WB, Pittet JF, Weitz S, et al. Acute withdrawal syndrome related to the administration of analgesic and sedative medications in adult intensive care unit patients. Crit Care Med. 1998;26(4):676-84.

Dais J, Khosia A, Doulatram G. The successful treatment of opioid withdrawal-induced refractory muscle spasms with 5-HTP in a patient intolerant to clonidine. Pain Physician. 2015;18(3):E417-20.

Dunn KE, Saulsgiver KA, Miller ME, et al. Characterizing opioid withdrawal during double-blind buprenorphine detoxification. Drug Alcohol Depend. 2015;151:47-55.

Fisher D, Grap MJ, Younger JB, et al. Opioid withdrawal signs and symptoms in children: frequency and determinants. Heart Lung. 2013;42(6):407-13.

Franck LS, Scoppettuolo LA, Wypij D, et al. Validity and generalizability of the Withdrawal Assessment Tool-1 (WAT-1) for monitoring iatrogenic withdrawal syndrome in pediatric patients. Pain. 2012;153(1):142-8.

Hooten WM, Warner DO. Varenicline for opioid withdrawal in patients with chronic pain: a randomized, single-blinded, placebo controlled pilot trial. Addict Behav. 2015;42:69-72.

Jin HS, Yum MS, Kim SL, et al. The efficacy of the COMFORT scale in assessing optimal sedation in critically ill children requiring mechanical ventilation. J Korean Med Sci. 2007;22(4):693-7.

Makhinson M, Gomez-Makhinson J. A successful treatment of buprenorphine withdrawal with the dopamine receptor agonist pramipexole. Am J Addict. 2014;23(5):475-7.

Mannelli P, Peindl K, Wu LT, et al. The combination very low-dose naltrexone-clonidine in the management of opioid withdrawal. Am J Drug Alcohol Abuse. 2012;38(3):200-5.

Robertson RC, Darsey E, Fortenberry JD, et al. Evaluation of an opiate-weaning protocol using methadone in pediatric intensive care unit patients. Pediatr Crit Care Med. 2000;1(2):119-23.

Salehi M, Kheirabadi GR, Maracy MR, et al. Importance of gabapentin dose in treatment of opioid withdrawal. J Clin Psychopharmacol. 2011;31(5):593-6.

Song H, Li J, Lu CL, et al. Tetrodotoxin alleviates acute heroin withdrawal syndrome: a multicentre, randomized, double-blind, placebo-controlled study. Clin Exp Pharmacol Physiol. 2011;38(8):510-4.

The National Alliance of Advocates for Buprenorphine Treatment. (2015). Dosing Guide for Optimal Management of Opioid Dependence. [online] NAABT website. Available from: *www.naabt.org/documents/Suboxone_Dosing_guide.pdf* [Accessed January, 2017].

Yu E, Miotto K, Akerele E, et al. A Phase 3 placebo-controlled, double-blind, multi-site trial of the alpha-2-adrenergic agonist, lofexidine, for opioid withdrawal. Drug Alcohol Depend. 2008;97(1-2):158-68.

CHAPTER 111

Opioid-Induced Hyperalgesia

Rana MV, Kusper TM

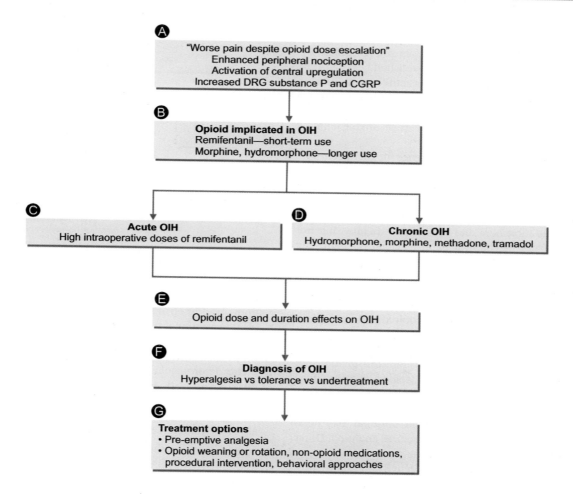

Ⓐ
"Worse pain despite opioid dose escalation"
Enhanced peripheral nociception
Activation of central upregulation
Increased DRG substance P and CGRP

Ⓑ
Opioid implicated in OIH
Remifentanil—short-term use
Morphine, hydromorphone—longer use

Ⓒ
Acute OIH
High intraoperative doses of remifentanil

Ⓓ
Chronic OIH
Hydromorphone, morphine, methadone, tramadol

Ⓔ
Opioid dose and duration effects on OIH

Ⓕ
Diagnosis of OIH
Hyperalgesia vs tolerance vs undertreatment

Ⓖ
Treatment options
• Pre-emptive analgesia
• Opioid weaning or rotation, non-opioid medications, procedural intervention, behavioral approaches

Ⓐ *Definition and Mechanism:* Opioid-induced hyperalgesia (OIH) refers to the phenomenon of increased pain sensitivity after exposure to opioid therapy. Clinically, the process manifests as pain intensification or emergence of a new pain with loss of analgesic benefits despite drug dose escalation. Distinct neuroanatomical sites and signaling systems have been implicated in OIH: (1) peripherally, enhanced nociception mediated by the glutamatergic system/N-methyl-D-aspartate (NMDA) excitatory neurotransmitters, (2) activation of descending signaling pathways arising from the rostral ventromedial medulla (RVM) resulting in upregulation of spinal dynorphin, and (3) enhanced production of nociceptive neurotransmitters substance P and calcitonin gene-related peptide (CGRP) within the dorsal root ganglia.

Incidence and Clinical Presentation: Although OIH has been well described in the literature, the incidence and prevalence of this phenomenon is not well known. The underreporting may be due to misdiagnosis. Clinically, the syndrome presents as a new onset of burning, diffuse, at times generalized pain, extending beyond the initial pain source. The pain may remain the same or worsen after dose escalation. Improvement occurs after dose reduction.

Ⓑ *Types of Opioids Implicated in OIH:* Remifentanil and morphine have been the most commonly implicated agents in the development of OIH. Most hyperalgesia appears to be related to the administration of short-acting medications (such as remifentanil) in the acute setting and to prolonged morphine or hydromorphone use. The literature concerning OIH and extended-release agents is rather sparse. Available reports on long-acting opioids include studies and case reports of methadone therapy in opioid-dependent and cancer patients. One study showed hyperalgesia to cold pain, but not to heat pain, after 1-month therapy with sustained-release morphine. A second study by Chu et al. failed to demonstrate a correlation between sustained-release morphine and OIH.

C *Acute OIH:* High intraoperative doses of remifentanil might lead to the emergence of acute OIH with higher pain scores and greater morphine requirements postoperatively in these patients. A systematic review and meta-analysis considered 27 randomized controlled trials on intraoperative opioid use published between 1994 and 2013. Analysis confirmed that remifentanil infusion results in postsurgical hyperalgesia for 24 hours, with the peak intensity at 1-hour after surgery, decreasing over the full 24 hours. Insufficient evidence exists linking fentanyl and sufentanil to OIH.

D *Chronic OIH:* There is mixed evidence for OIH in chronic pain patients on long-term (>4 weeks) opioid therapy. In one study, hyperalgesia to heat pain was shown in adults on chronic oral hydromorphone. Hyperalgesic effects were also shown for cold pressor pain in patients on chronic morphine and methadone therapy, but not for heat pain, mechanical pain, or electrical pain. The presence of OIH after chronic opioid therapy is also supported by anecdotal case reports of patients treated with morphine, methadone, and tramadol. Other studies failed to demonstrate differences in sensitivity to different pain stimuli between chronic opioid and non-opioid groups.

E *Dose and Treatment Duration versus OIH:* The documented studies that aimed to explore the relationship between opioid dosages and OIH yielded disparate findings. A positive correlation was found between greater doses and increased sensitivity to pain in patients on chronic opioid therapy. Treatment duration also positively correlated with the pain measures analyzed. Other studies failed to replicate these results.

F *Diagnosis:* Hyperalgesia is a subjective and highly individualized experience, leading to diagnostic challenges. No established clinical method or standard criteria exist for diagnosing OIH. Thorough evaluation is necessary to distinguish OIH from progression of the initial pain condition, tolerance in those on chronic therapy, and withdrawal in patients discontinuing therapy. One of the characteristics used to distinguish OIH from tolerance is a lack of pain reduction after opioid dose escalation. Prescribers must also consider the possibility that the preexisting pain might be undertreated.

G *Treatment Options:* Two general approaches are recognized for OIH treatment. First, perioperative "preemptive analgesia" is used to prevent an acute onset of hyperalgesia in the immediate postoperative period. Strategies include ketamine, propofol, magnesium sulfate, and nitrous oxide. The efficacy of ketamine in prevention of OIH has been demonstrated in both animal and human

Chart 1: Approach to diagnosis and treatment of opioid-induced hyperalgesia

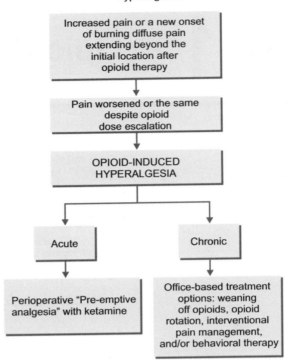

studies. The second approach entails office-based treatments including (1) weaning off opioids, (2) opioid rotation, (3) addition or switching to non-opioid medications, (4) interventional pain management, and (5) behavioral management. Adding or switching to opioid-sparing medications may reduce or eliminate opioid requirements. Pharmacological options include NMDA antagonists (ketamine or dextromethorphan), an opioid agonist with weak NMDA antagonism (methadone), partial opioid agonist and kappa antagonist (buprenorphine), and alpha-2 adrenergic agonist (clonidine) **(Chart 1)**.

Opioid Rotation: The process involves switching one opioid to another with the goal of reducing adverse reactions while maintaining adequate analgesia and treatment success. Equianalgesic dose tables are a standardized conversion guide, which provide estimates of relative potency among opioid medications. Therapy is titrated based upon the analgesic response to the medication and presence of side effects. One treatment approach involves converting patients to long-acting opioid therapy with several options of extended-release formulations available.

SUGGESTED READING

Angst MS, Koppert W, Pahl I, et al. Short-term infusion of the mu-opioid agonist remifentanil in humans causes hyperalgesia during withdrawal. Pain. 2003;106(1-2):49-57.

Angst MS. Intraoperative Use of Remifentanil for TIVA: Postoperative Pain, Acute Tolerance, and Opioid-Induced Hyperalgesia. J Cardiothorac Vasc Anesth. 2015;29(Suppl 1):S16-22.

Chen L, Sein M, Vo T, et al. Clinical interpretation of opioid tolerance versus opioid-induced hyperalgesia. J Opioid Manag. 2014;10(6):383-93.

Chu LF, Clark DJ, Angst MS. Opioid tolerance and hyperalgesia in chronic pain patients after one month of oral morphine therapy: a preliminary prospective study. J Pain. 2006;7(1):43-8.

Chu LF, D'Arcy N, Brady C, et al. Analgesic tolerance without demonstrable opioid-induced hyperalgesia: a double-blinded, randomized, placebo-controlled trial of sustained-release morphine for treatment of chronic nonradicular low-back pain. Pain. 2012;153(8):1583-92.

Cohen SP, Christo PJ, Wang S, et al. The effect of opioid dose and treatment duration on the perception of a painful standardized clinical stimulus. Reg Anesth Pain Med. 2008;33(3):199-206.

Davis MP, Shaiova LA, Angst MS. When opioids cause pain. J Clin Oncol. 2007;25(28):4497-8.

Doverty M, White JM, Somogyi AA, et al. Hyperalgesic responses in methadone maintenance patients. Pain. 2001;90(1-2):91-6.

Edwards RR, Wasan AD, Michna E, et al. Elevated pain sensitivity in chronic pain patients at risk for opioid misuse. J Pain. 2011;12(9):953-63.

Fine PG, Portenoy RK; Ad Hoc Expert Panel on Evidence Review and Guidelines for Opioid Rotation. Establishing "best practices" for opioid rotation: conclusions of an expert panel. J Pain Symptom Manage. 2009;38(3):418-25.

Fletcher D, Martinez V. Opioid-induced hyperalgesia in patients after surgery: a systematic review and a meta-analysis. Br J Anaesth. 2014;112(6):991-1004.

Gardell LR, King T, Ossipov MH, et al. Opioid receptor-mediated hyperalgesia and antinociceptive tolerance induced by sustained opiate delivery. Neurosci Lett. 2006;396(1):44-9.

Guignard B, Bossard AE, Coste C, et al. Acute opioid tolerance: intraoperative remifentanil increases postoperative pain and morphine requirement. Anesthesiology. 2000;93(2):409-17.

Hay JL, White JM, Bochner F, et al. Hyperalgesia in opioid-managed chronic pain and opioid-dependent patients. J Pain. 2009;10(3):316-22.

Hooten WM, Lamer TJ, Twyner C. Opioid-induced hyperalgesia in community-dwelling adults with chronic pain. Pain. 2015;156(6):1145-52.

Hooten WM, Sandroni P, Mantilla CB, et al. Associations between heat pain perception and pain severity among patients with chronic pain. Pain Med. 2010;11(10):1554-63.

Joly V, Richebe P, Guignard B, et al. Remifentanil-induced postoperative hyperalgesia and its prevention with small-dose ketamine. Anesthesiology. 2005;103(1):147-55.

Lee SH, Cho SY, Lee HG, et al. Tramadol induced paradoxical hyperalgesia. Pain Physician. 2013;16(1):41-4.

Mao J, Sung B, Ji RR, et al. Chronic morphine induces downregulation of spinal glutamate transporters: implications in morphine tolerance and abnormal pain sensitivity. J Neurosci. 2002;22(18):8312-23.

Ram KC, Eisenberg E, Haddad M, et al. Oral opioid use alters DNIC but not cold pain perception in patients with chronic pain - new perspective of opioid-induced hyperalgesia. Pain. 2008;139(2):431-8.

Reznikov I, Pud D, Eisenberg E. Oral opioid administration and hyperalgesia in patients with cancer or chronic nonmalignant pain. Br J Clin Pharmacol. 2005;60(3):311-8.

Sjogren P, Thunedborg LP, Christrup L, et al. Is development of hyperalgesia, allodynia and myoclonus related to morphine metabolism during long-term administration? Six case histories. Acta Anaesthesiol Scand. 1998;42(9):1070-5.

Suzan E, Eisenberg E, Treister R, et al. A negative correlation between hyperalgesia and analgesia in patients with chronic radicular pain: is hydromorphone therapy a double-edged sword? Pain Physician. 2013;16(1):65-76.

Wilson GR, Reisfield GM. Morphine hyperalgesia: a case report. Am J Hosp Palliat Care. 2003;20(6):459-61.

CHAPTER 112

Risk Evaluation and Mitigation Strategies for Opioids

Rana MV, Kusper TM

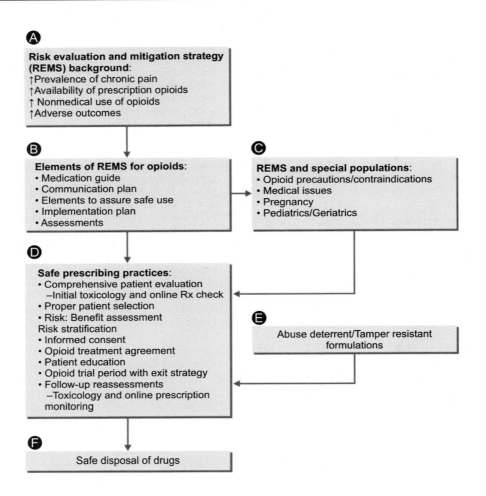

A Risk evaluation and mitigation strategy (REMS) background:
↑Prevalence of chronic pain
↑Availability of prescription opioids
↑ Nonmedical use of opioids
↑Adverse outcomes

B Elements of REMS for opioids:
• Medication guide
• Communication plan
• Elements to assure safe use
• Implementation plan
• Assessments

C REMS and special populations:
• Opioid precautions/contraindications
• Medical issues
• Pregnancy
• Pediatrics/Geriatrics

D Safe prescribing practices:
• Comprehensive patient evaluation
 —Initial toxicology and online Rx check
• Proper patient selection
• Risk: Benefit assessment
Risk stratification
• Informed consent
• Opioid treatment agreement
• Patient education
• Opioid trial period with exit strategy
• Follow-up reassessments
 —Toxicology and online prescription monitoring

E Abuse deterrent/Tamper resistant formulations

F Safe disposal of drugs

A *Opioid Risk Evaluation and Mitigation Strategies:* Extended-release/long-acting (ER/LA) opioids were prescribed to approximately 3.8 million patients annually between 2000 and 2009. The longer lasting agents provide steady-state analgesia to negotiate daily pain. Data collected in 2010 revealed that 35 million Americans, 12 years of age and older, used opioid therapy for nonmedical use at some point, compared to about 30 million users in 2002. Consequently, 343,000 emergency department visits involving nonmedical use of opioids occurred in 2009, with 14,800 deaths linked to opioid poisoning. Chronic pain promotes disability, lost productivity and diminished quality of life. Opioids have been a standard treatment for various types of chronic pain. According to the American Academy of Pain Medicine, chronic pain affects more Americans than diabetes, heart disease and cancer combined, with economic impact of at least $560–635 billion annually. Risk Evaluation and Mitigation Strategy (REMS) programs help to balance effective pain management and reduce problematic opioid use risks.

In 2011, the Food and Drug Administration (FDA) announced the REMS requirement for ER/LA opioids. Patient education and addiction risk, overdose and misuse represent the highlights of this program. REMS agents include morphine ER, hydromorphone ER, oxycodone, oxymorphone ER, tapentadol ER, morphine-naltrexone ER, methadone, fentanyl formulations, buprenorphine systems and naloxone (Suboxone).

B The REMS program for ER/LA opioids consists of the following five elements, although not all might be required:

1. *Medication Guide:* Distributed by the pharmacy, this patient information provides important information spotlighting the safe use of these drugs. Requirements include information applicable to all ER/LA formulations and product-specific content needed to assure safe and effective drug use.

2. *Communication Plan:* This information presents REMS prescriber protocols and implementation strategies on medication safety and risks.

3. *Elements to Assure Safe Use (ETASU):* This part highlights the FDA's requirement for a prescriber's education, training and/or special certification by accredited continuing medical education (CME) providers. The goal is risk mitigation associated with the prescribed product. Avoiding inappropriate prescribing practices such as early refills or writing ER/LA products to nonopioid-tolerant patients is key. Manufacturers are required to ensure access to training opportunities and provide education and/or materials necessary for effective counseling.

4. *Implementation Plan:* Monitoring and evaluation of the results of specific ETASUs contained in a REMS compromises this portion of the program. Compliance with certification requirements and adherence to prescribing, dispensing and distribution guidelines is presented. Aspects of the system include audits, and secure databases of prescribers, pharmacies, and other parties involved.

5. *Timetable for Submission of Assessments:* The FDA requires periodic REMS assessments to ensure that performance goals are met or require modification. The assessment includes an evaluation of the prescribers completing training programs, quality of educational materials, prescription pattern changes and medication utilization practices; along with patients' understanding of risk, and a drug-specific surveillance method to screen for signs of misuse coupled with intervention strategies when such signs are recognized.

C *Special Populations:* Opioid analgesics are contraindicated in patients with hypersensitivity to opioids, patients with a history of respiratory depression, patients with acute or severe asthma, and patients with paralytic ileus. Patients with kidney or liver disease require careful dosing of opioids, and care must be taken not to overestimate the dose when converting opioids using equianalgesic tables. Pregnant patients should be warned about the risk of neonatal opioid withdrawal syndrome, and appropriate treatment should be provided if this occurs. Oxycodone, hydrocodone, hydromorphone, morphine, and codeine have been found to increase the risk of fetal central nervous system (CNS) birth defects when used during the first trimester of pregnancy. Special consideration must be given to elderly and pediatric patients, as these two groups are at increased risk for overdose. Pain management in the elderly is challenging secondary to pharmacodynamic changes due to aging, concomitant comorbidities, and the likelihood of polypharmacy.

These factors make older patients vulnerable to adverse reactions from therapy. It is critical to appropriately assess pain, initiate and adjust dosage cautiously, and continuously evaluate for baseline status changes. Adjuvant therapy should be utilized when feasible. Pediatric pain management is equally challenging, although warnings and precautions for children do not differ from those for adult patients. Prescribers must closely supervise patients and parents during the use of opioid therapy in children. Recently, oxycodone ER has been approved by the FDA to manage severe pain in pediatric patients age 11 years and older. Currently, transdermal fentanyl patch and ER oxycodone are the only LA opioids with FDA-approved labeling for pediatric use. Patients should be educated on opioid storage away from children, with special safeguards to prevent accidental fatal ingestion. One review reported a 33% increase in the risk of future opioid misuse in children using opioids before the 12th grade. This finding highlights the importance of early intervention opioid prescription practices.

D *Safe Prescribing:* Safe prescribing begins with a thorough patient evaluation, including a detailed assessment of medical, surgical, and family history, a complete physical examination, use of appropriate testing, and a careful review of treatment records. Noting comorbidities precluding prescriptions along with prior surgical interventions that could lead to narcotic misuse is important. Knowledge of abuse history, addiction, or problematic opioid use, along with the presence of any psychosocial factors must be elucidated. Proper patient selection, assessment of benefit-to-harm ratio, risk stratification, recognition of aberrant behaviors, and ultimately prevention of life-threatening consequences, along with potential legal ramifications for the prescriber all need to be considered. Clinicians should obtain informed consent for opioid therapy and enter into an opioid treatment agreement with the patient. This entails continuous communication between the patient and the prescriber, providing patient education regarding treatment goals and expectations. Explaining possible adverse reactions and risks associated with the medications, along with exploring alternative treatment options are essential. Trial opioid therapy is initiated to determine the appropriate regimen. Modification occurs as progress is assessed. Doses should be individually titrated to decrease adverse reactions. ER/LA opioids should never be stopped abruptly since this might precipitate withdrawal symptoms. Point-of-care baseline and subsequent random urine drug testing is routinely done, followed by gas chromatography or mass spectrometry to help ensure drug compliance. Increased frequency of monitoring with heightened vigilance is required in patients on elevated doses and with higher risk strata.

E *Abuse Deterrent versus Resistant:* Several abuse-deterrent technologies target the expected route of inappropriate use. Available formulations are categorized into (1) physical/chemical barriers preventing medication tampering, release or extraction of active drug; (2) agonist-antagonist combinations, with the antagonist released when medication is improperly manipulated; (3) aversion formulations containing an irritant substance (capsaicin); (4) low-profile delivery systems, including depot injectable formulations and implants; (5) new agents and prodrugs which might require enzymatic conversion and/or specific receptor binding, leading to slower CNS penetration; and (6) combination formulations of the above.

F *Safe Disposal:* Safe storage and disposal of unused or expired drugs are key factors in harm reduction and prevention of opioid overdoses. Specific guidelines encourage and promote safe disposal practices. Community-based Drug Enforcement Administration (DEA)-authorized collection sites, "drop-boxes" or "take-back" events assist patients in convenient disposal of unneeded medications. Alternatively, medications can be disposed in the household trash by removing pills from their original container, mixing with dirt, kitty litter, used coffee grounds or other unpalatable substance in a sealed plastic bag, removing identifying information from the empty container prior to disposal. Many ER oral medications and sublingual, buccal and transdermal delivery systems can be safely disposed by flushing down the sink or toilet.

Websites for REMS Information

US Food and Drug Administration. (2007). Risk evaluation and mitigation strategies (REMS). [online] Available from *http://www.fda.gov/downloads/AboutFDA/Transparency/Basics/UCM 328784.pdf.* [Accessed January, 2017].

US Food and Drug Administration. (2015). Approved risk evaluation and mitigation strategies (REMS). [online] Available from *http://www.fda.gov/Drugs/DrugSafety/PostmarketDrugSafety InformationforPatientsandProviders/ucm111350.htm.* [Accessed January, 2017].

SUGGESTED READING

Chau DL, Walker V, Pai L, et al. Opiates and elderly: use and side effects. Clin Interv Aging. 2008;3(2):273-8.

Chou R, Fanciullo GJ, Fine PG, et al. Clinical guidelines for the use of chronic opioid therapy in chronic noncancer pain. J Pain. 2009;10(2):113-30.

Governale L. (2010). Outpatient prescription opioid utilization in the U.S., years 2000–2009. [online] Available from *http://www.fda.gov/downloads/AdvisoryCommittees/ CommitteesMeetingMaterials/Drugs/AnestheticAndLife SupportDrugsAdvisoryCommittee/UCM220950.pdf.* [Accessed January, 2017].

Gudin JA. The changing landscape of opioid prescribing: long-acting and extended-release opioid class-wide risk evaluation and mitigation strategy. Ther Clin Risk Manag. 2012;8:209-17.

Miech R, Johnston L, O'Malley PM, et al. Prescription opioids in adolescence and future opioid misuse. Pediatrics. 2015;136(5):e1169-77.

Nelson LS, Loh M, Perrone J. Assuring safety of inherently unsafe medications: the FDA risk evaluation and mitigation strategies. J Med Toxicol. 2014;10(2):165-72.

The American Academy of Pain Medicine. (2015). AAPM facts and figures on pain. [online] Available from *http://www.painmed. org/patientcenter/facts_on_pain.aspx#keyfindings.* [Accessed January, 2017].

US Food and Drug Administration. (2015). Abuse-deterrent opioids—evaluation and labeling. Guidance for industry. [online] Available from *http://www.fda.gov/downloads/drugs/guidance-complianceregulatoryinformation/guidances/ucm334743.pdf.* [Accessed January, 2017].

US Food and Drug Administration. (2015). CDER conversation: pediatric pain management options. [online] Available from *http://www.fda.gov/Drugs/NewsEvents/ucm456973.htm.* [Accessed January, 2017].

US Food and Drug Administration. (2015). Disposal of unused medicines: what you should know. [online] Available from *http://www.fda.gov/Drugs/ResourcesForYou/Consumers/ BuyingUsingMedicineSafely/EnsuringSafeUseofMedicine/ SafeDisposalofMedicines/ucm186187.htm.* [Accessed January, 2017].

US Food and Drug Administration. (2015). Extended-release (ER) and long-acting (LA) opioid analgesics risk evaluation and mitigation strategy (REMS). [online] Available from *http://www.fda.gov/downloads/Drugs/DrugSafety/Postmarket DrugSafetyInformationforPatientsandProviders/UCM311290. pdf.* [Accessed January, 2017].

US Food and Drug Administration. (2015). FDA blueprint for prescriber education for extended-release and long-acting opioid analgesics. [online] Available from *http://www.accessdata.fda. gov/drugsatfda_docs/rems/ERLA_opioids_2015.06.26_FDA_ Blueprint_for_Prescriber_Education_for_Extended-Release_ and_Long-Acting_Opioid_Analgesics.pdf.* [Accessed January, 2017].

US Food and Drug Administration. (2015). FDA drug safety communication: FDA has reviewed possible risks of pain medicine use during pregnancy. [online] Available from *http://www.fda.gov/ Drugs/DrugSafety/ucm429117.htm.* [Accessed January, 2017].

US Food and Drug Administration. (2015). Post-approval REMS notification. [online] *Available from http://www.fda.gov/down-loads/Drugs/DrugSafety/InformationbyDrugClass/UCM251595. pdf.* [Accessed January, 2017].

Willy ME, Graham DJ, Racoosin JA, et al. Candidate metrics for evaluating the impact of prescriber education on the safe use of extended-release/long-acting (ER/LA) opioid analgesics. Pain Med. 2014;15(9):1558-68.

CHAPTER
113

Weaning

Kusper TM, Rana MV

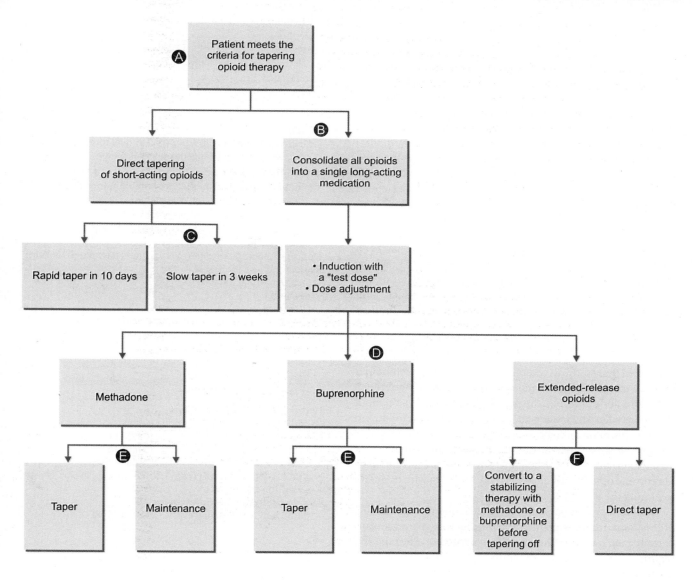

Opioid tolerance (decreased efficacy of the drug with exposure) and subsequent dependence associated with chronic opioid usage is a growing concern which necessitates safe and effective opioid tapering and weaning strategies. Safety concerns, inadequate analgesia, adverse effects, misuse and noncompliance are some of the reasons for tapering off opioids **(Table 1)**. A recent retrospective analysis and prospective chart review of 50 veterans on chronic opioid therapy demonstrated safe tapering to lower opioid doses without a corresponding increase in pain due to substitution with adjuvant therapy. Opioid tapering is largely an individualized process with the rate tailored to patient tolerability. Physician-patient collaboration holds paramount status for satisfactory results. Multiple treatment options are available with variable speed and rate of the taper **(Table 2)**.

Speed of Opioid Tapering: Most of the literature on detoxification strategies comes from the studies on opioid addiction, and the evidence concerning tapering regimens in chronic pain patients is sparse. A review of available clinical data

Table 1: Criteria for discontinuation of opioids

- Resolution of the pain state
- Adverse effects (sedation, drowsiness, mood changes, constipation, decline in memory and concentration, dry mouth, abdominal pain, nausea, sexual dysfunction, hyperalgesia)
- Inadequate therapeutic benefit despite dose escalation (tolerance)
- Safety concerns (physical dependence, addiction, abuse)
- Initiation of nonopioid agents or other therapeutic options (spinal cord stimulators)
- Planning of elective surgery
- Pain that is not responsive to opioids (neuropathic pain)
- Lack of improvement in quality of life and functional capacity
- Misuse and nonadherence to treatment regimen
- Violation of the opioid agreement
- Cost burden

Table 2: Available taper methods for long- and short-acting opioids

Tapers for long-acting opioids

- Methadone:
  - Decrease OD by 20–50% per day until 30 mg/day reached
  - Then decrease by 5 mg/day every 3–5 days to 10 mg/day
  - Then decrease by 2.5 mg/day every 3–5 days
- Morphine sustained-release (SR)/controlled-release (CR):
  Option A: Convert to methadone, approximately 20 mg daily (10 mg BID)
  - Then begin methadone taper, as tolerated
  Option B:
  - Decrease OD by 20–50% per day until 45 mg/day reached
  - Then decrease by 15 mg/day every 2–5 days
- Oxycodone CR:
  Option A: Convert to methadone, approximately 20 mg daily (10 mg BID)
  - Then begin methadone taper, as tolerated
  Option B:
  - Decrease OD by 20–50% per day until 30 mg/day reached
  - Then decrease by 10 mg/day every 2–5 days
- Buprenorphine:
  Reduction rate based on the daily maintenance dose
  - Above 16 mg: reduce by 4 mg every 1–2 weeks
  - 8–16 mg: reduce by 2–4 mg every 1–2 weeks
  - Below 8 mg: reduce by 2 mg every 1–2 weeks
- Fentanyl patch
  Option A: Decrease by 50% every 6 days (new patch on third day):
  - 50 µg/hour × 6 days, then 25 µg/hour × 6 days, then 12.5 µg/hour
  - Discontinue
  Option B: Decrease by 25 µg/hour (25%) every 15 days (new patch on third day, will use 1 box of 5 patches)
  - 75 µg/hour × 15 days, then 50 µg/hour × 15 days, then 25 µg/hour, then 12 µg/hour × 15 days
  - Discontinue

Tapers for short-acting opioids

- Hydrocodone/Acetaminophen
  Option A: Rapid taper (duration 10 days)
  - 1 tablet every 6 hours × 1 day (4/day), then
  - 1 tablet every 8 hours × 3 days (3/day), then
  - 1 tablet every 12 hours × 3 days (2/day), then
  - 1 tablet daily × 3 days (1/day), then
  - Discontinue
  Option B: Slow taper (duration 3 weeks)
  - Reduce by 1 tablet/day every 3 days until off

shows opioid tapering protocols of variable duration, from one day (ultra-rapid) to several weeks' duration (slow taper).

Ultra-rapid opioid detoxification under anesthesia serves to rapidly reverse opioid-dependence, designed to minimize the physical and emotional suffering commonly experienced during opioid withdrawal. It is performed in the hospital setting by the administration of naloxone, a μ-receptor antagonist. The α-adrenergic agonist, clonidine, is used for the treatment of the withdrawal symptoms. This approach has been studied in military burn patients on chronic opioid therapy and in opioid-addicted individuals with and without the presence of chronic pain. According to one study, this option provides absolute success in detoxification, as measured by the Clinical Institute Narcotic Assessment (CINA) scale withdrawal scores, which ultimately leads to better long-term outcomes. It also is an effective way of reducing opioid use, as illustrated by a study on veterans, who decreased their opioid use by 46% in a 12-month period. When compared to standard methadone tapering, the patients in the ultra-rapid taper showed greater abstinence rates at 1- and 2-month follow-up and less pronounced withdrawal symptoms. Taken together, the results show that ultra-rapid detoxification might be a viable alternative to traditional treatment strategies for eligible chronic opioid patients, especially for those with difficulty tolerating the withdrawal symptoms.

Fast and slow tapers have been described in the context of inpatient, multidisciplinary pain programs geared toward chronic pain patients. The effectiveness of the 7-day tapering regimen was examined in veterans with chronic pain admitted to a 3-week chronic pain rehabilitation program (CPRP). The opioid users demonstrated significant reduction in pain intensity and improvements in several outcome measures, such as activities of daily living (ADLs), coping skills, and sleep, among others.

Two studies show that opioids can be successfully withdrawn in chronic pain patients during a 3-week CPRP program. The patients reported high pain scores, depression and overall poor functioning on admission. A significant improvement in all pain score, depressive symptoms and functioning was noted at discharge and at 6-month follow-up. The utility

of this approach has again been tested in a group of consecutive chronic low back pain patients without a surgical intervention compared to those with a history of fusion and other spine surgery. About 84% of patients completed the program, and 78.6% of patients stopped using opioid medications. No data, however, is available on the long-term abstinence rates as this study focused on the immediate results of the program. A slow taper method lasting 8 weeks has been employed in the weaning of 11 codeine patients, with 50% reduction during the first 4 weeks of the treatment. Six out of 11 patients successfully completed the taper and 5 of those remained opioids-free at 3-month interval.

Rate of the Opioid Taper: Opioid taper practices vary greatly between different institutions. No single protocol is applicable to all patients and, frequently, a given strategy needs to be tailored to individual needs. For example, the process might be slowed down or halted in the event of intolerable withdrawal symptoms.

Ⓐ The first step in the tapering process is to establish patient's need for opioid weaning and confirm patient's readiness and commitment to the process.

Ⓑ Short-acting opioids can be weaned off either directly or converted to a single long-acting opioid medication and then tapered. If the decision is made to wean off from a long-acting opioid, the dose is adjusted accordingly based on the patient's response until an optimal dose is established and taper is begun once the patient is stabilized.

Ⓒ If the decision is made to wean off of short-acting opioids, it can be done rapidly over 10 days or a slow taper regimen spanned over a 3-week period.

Ⓓ In the event that long-acting opioid weaning is utilized, options include methadone, buprenorphine or other extended-release formulation. The first step in this pathway is to implement an induction "test dose", after which the patient is monitored for any signs of withdrawal or adverse reaction.

Ⓔ Depending on the individual response and needs, the patient may either be maintained long-term on methadone or buprenorphine, or the medications may be tapered down according to a specified schedule.

Ⓕ Extended-release opioids can either be converted to methadone or buprenorphine therapy before the taper or tapered off directly. A common practice is to reduce an opioid by 10% every 5–7 days until 30% of the original dose is reached, and then continue to reduce the remaining dose by 10%. Different taper rates are utilized for long- and short-acting opioids **(Table 2)**. Sometimes a maintenance treatment might be required in order to prevent withdrawal, suppress craving or hinder relapse into opioid use.

Risks Involved in a Taper: Acute withdrawal syndrome is one of the main immediate risks during the weaning process. Common symptoms include hypertension, tachycardia, tachypnea, mydriasis, anxiety, restlessness, diaphoresis, nausea, abdominal cramps and diarrhea. Duration of the withdrawal symptoms correlates with the duration of opioid treatment, the type of opioid, and the degree of dependence, but they reach their peak intensity within 36–72 hours postopioid cessation and then gradually decrease. The presence of psychiatric comorbidities such as anxiety and depression, increased pain intensity, and abstinence during the withdrawal process increase the risk of dropping-out from the therapy and relapsing into opioid use.

SUGGESTED READING

Berna C, Kulich RJ, Rathmell JP. Tapering long-term opioid therapy in chronic noncancer pain: evidence and recommendations for everyday practice. Mayo Clin Proc. 2015;90(6):828-42.

Crisostomo RA, Schmidt JE, Hooten WM, et al. Kerkvliet JL, Townsend CO, Bruce BK. Withdrawal of analgesic medication for chronic low-back pain patients: improvement in outcomes of multidisciplinary rehabilitation regardless of surgical history. Am J Phys Med Rehabil. 2008;87(7):527-36.

Department of Veterans Affairs (VA) and Department of Defense (DoD). (2010). Tapering and discontinuing opioids 2010 [cited 2015 6 Dec]. [online] Available from *http://www.healthquality.va.gov/guidelines/Pain/cot/OpioidTaperingFactSheet23May2013v1.pdf.* [Accessed January, 2017].

Farrell M. Opiate withdrawal. Addiction. 1994;89(11):1471-5.

Gold CG, Cullen DJ, Gonzales S, et al. Houtmeyers D, Dwyer MJ. Rapid- opioid detoxification during general anesthesia: a review of 20 patients. Anesthesiology. 1999;91(6):1639-47.

Group Health Cooperative. (2014). Chronic opioid therapy (COT) safety guideline for patients with chronic non-cancer pain 2014 [cited 2015 7 Dec]. [online] Available from *https://www.ghc.org/all-sites/guidelines/chronicOpioid.pdf.* [Accessed January, 2017].

Harden P, Ahmed S, Ang K, et al. Clinical implications of tapering chronic opioids in a veteran population. Pain Med. 2015;16(10):1975-81.

Heiwe S, Lonnquist I, Kallmen H. Potential risk factors associated with risk for drop-out and relapse during and following withdrawal of opioid prescription medication. Eur J Pain. 2011;15(9):966-70.

Krabbe PF, Koning JP, Heinen N, et al. Rapid detoxification from opioid dependence under general anaesthesia versus standard methadone tapering: abstinence rates and withdrawal distress experiences. Addict Biol. 2003;8(3):351-8.

Kral L, Jackson K, Uritsky T. (2015). A practical guide to tapering opioids 2015 [cited 2015 6 Dec]. [online] Available from *http://mhc.cpnp.org/doi/abs/10.9740/mhc.2015.05.102?journalCode=mhcl.* [Accessed January, 2017].

Kral L. (2006). Opioid tapering: safely discontinuing opioid analgesics 2006 [cited 2015 6 Dec]. [online] Available from *https://www.nhms.org/sites/default/files/Pdfs/Safely_Tapering_Opioids.pdf.* [Accessed January, 2017].

Levy B, Paulozzi L, Mack KA, et al. Jones CM. Trends in opioid analgesic-prescribing rates by specialty, U.S., 2007-2012. Am J Prev Med. 2015;49(3):409-13.

Maani CV, DeSocio PA, Jansen RK, Merrell JD, McGhee LL, Young A, et al. Use of ultra-rapid opioid detoxification in the treatment of US military burn casualties. J Trauma. 2011;71(1 Suppl):S114-9.

Murphy JL, Clark ME, Banou E. Opioid cessation and multidimensional outcomes after interdisciplinary chronic pain treatment. Clin J Pain. 2013;29(2):109-17.

Nilsen HK, Stiles TC, Landro NI, et al. Patients with problematic opioid use can be weaned from codeine without pain escalation. Acta Anaesthesiol Scand. 2010;54(5):571-9.

The National Alliance of Advocates for Buprenorphine Treatment. (2015). Dosing guide for optimal management of opioid dependence [cited 2015 14 Dec]. [online] Available from *http://www.naabt.org/documents/Suboxone_Dosing_guide.pdf.* [Accessed January, 2017].

Townsend CO, Kerkvliet JL, Bruce BK, Rome JD, Hooten WM, Luedtke CA, et al. A longitudinal study of the efficacy of a comprehensive pain rehabilitation program with opioid withdrawal: comparison of treatment outcomes based on opioid use status at admission. Pain. 2008;140(1):177-89.

Webster BS, Verma SK, Gatchel RJ. Relationship between early opioid prescribing for acute occupational low back pain and disability duration, medical costs, subsequent surgery and late opioid use. Spine (Phila Pa 1976). 2007;32(19):2127-32.

SECTION **13**

Noninterventional Therapeutic Modalities

Miles Day

Noninterventional Therapeutic Modalities

CHAPTER 114

Physical Therapy

Thakur S, DiTommaso C

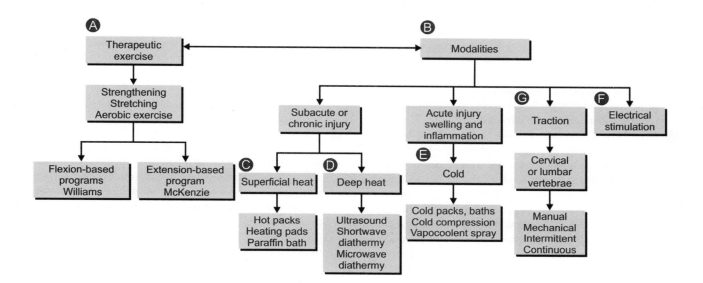

ROLE OF PHYSICAL THERAPY IN PAIN MANAGEMENT

Comprehensive physical therapy programs utilize exercise, adaptive equipment, and modalities for their therapeutic effects. The following is a brief description of commonly utilized therapeutic exercise methods and modalities, including indications and contraindications:

Ⓐ *Therapeutic Exercise:* Exercise and maintaining physical activity helps prevent disability in those with chronic pain. Formal physical therapy is particularly beneficial as it allows for a structured and set exercise regimen, rather than the ill-advised notion of "let pain be your guide." For those patients who express significant kinesiophobia, clinicians should reassure them that even small doses of physical activity can increase function and decrease pain. This observation is thought to be secondary to reduced anxiety and fear-avoidance behavior.

In low back pain, one goal of exercise is to strengthen and increase endurance of the muscles that support the spine (i.e. multifidi and transversus abdominus), as these muscles do not function well in those with low back pain. Also, motor retraining helps to treat deficits in the kinetic chain that often interfere with biomechanical efficiency, improving spinal alignment and posture.

Extension-based exercises based on the McKenzie method or mechanical diagnosis and therapy (MDT) are the most commonly utilized for low back pain. MDT divides the diagnosis of low back pain into three categories: (1) derangement, (2) dysfunction, and (3) postural syndromes. Each category presents with unique problems, and physical therapists assess symptomatic and mechanical responses to specific movements and postures.

Flexion-based programs, such as Williams flexion exercises (WFE), may be more appropriate for patients who have pain exacerbated by extension. For example, those with pathology related to the posterior elements of the spinal vertebrae like the facet joints and intervertebral foramen. The primary goal of WFE is to strengthen abdominal, gluteal, and hamstring muscles promoting balance between flexor and extensor postural muscles.

Ⓑ *Modalities:* The type of modality depends on whether the pain is acute, subacute, or chronic.

Ⓒ *Superficial Heat:* Heat is beneficial for many subacute and chronic conditions including muscle spasm, myofascial pain, low back pain, neck pain, postherpetic neuralgia, joint stiffness, arthritis, and chronic inflammation. It produces analgesia through increased blood flow, tissue distensibility and decreased muscle tone. It works synergistically with stretching and exercise, as heat increases tendon extensibility and collagenase activity. Excessive heat through prolonged exposure should be avoided, as temperatures greater than 113–122°F (45–50°C) may cause tissue damage.

Heat is commonly delivered via conduction, convection, or conversion. Conduction is most commonly used with the transfer of thermal energy between two objects directly in contact (hot packs, heating pads, paraffin baths). Fluidotherapy and whirlpool baths use convection or movement of heat through a medium (air or water). Superficial radiant heat (heating lamp) uses conversion as light energy is absorbed through the skin. Conversion is more commonly associated with deep heat modalities with greater tissue penetration, as in ultrasound and diathermy.

Heat is contraindicated with sensory impairment, vascular insufficiency, bleeding disorders, malignancy, and caution is needed with elderly or cognitively impaired patients, who may not be able to communicate or respond to pain appropriately. Even with sensate skin, prolonged use of superficial heat (>20 minutes) can cause temporary or permanent skin mottling.

D *Deep Heat:* Deep heat reaches tissue 3–5 cm below the skin by converting sound or electromagnetic energy into heat. It can be delivered via ultrasound, shortwave, and microwave diathermy to reach ligaments, bones, muscles, and joints. It increases the flexibility of collagen fibers.

Ultrasound works to produce heat as nonaudible sound waves (>20,000 Hz), that are absorbed by skin, fat, and muscle. The greatest amount of heat is produced at the bone-muscle-soft tissue interface. It has been used effectively to treat bursitis, tendinitis, degenerative arthritis and contractures (frozen shoulder, hip contractures). It is contraindicated in/near the following: eyes, reproductive organs, heart, brain, cervical ganglia, laminectomy sites, tumors, pacemakers, sites of infection, site of skeletal immaturity, prostheses with methyl methacrylate, arthroplasties.

Shortwave and microwave diathermy converts radiowave electromagnetic energy to thermal energy, providing heat over a larger area, at the depth of 4–5 cm. It is an ideal modality to treat various myalgias, muscle spasms with deep heating of large muscles. Contraindications are the same as for deep heat.

E *Cold:* Cold is generally beneficial for acute injuries as well as acute exacerbations of chronic injuries. It is used in acute traumatic injuries for reduction of edema and inflammation (24–48 hours postinjury). Also cold is used for acute myofascial pain and musculoskeletal conditions with joint inflammation including arthritis, bursitis, muscle strains and sprains. It is applied to the site of pain until numb or up to 20 minutes. Cold packs can decrease surface skin temperature by approximately 60°F (15°C) in about 10 minutes. Cool evaporation spray such as ethyl chloride or fluoromethane can be used for local anesthesia or in stretching exercises to treat myofascial and musculoskeletal pain. Cold compression units consist of pneumatic compression sleeves with circulating cool water approximately 45°F (7°C), used to treat acute musculoskeletal injuries or postoperatively to control edema. Cold can help treatment spasticity related to upper motor neuron syndrome, by decreasing the speed of nerve conduction and neuronal excitability.

Cold therapy is contraindicated in those with impaired sensation, impaired communication or cognition, hypersensitivity to cold (Raynaud's phenomenon, cyroglobulinemia), and should be used cautiously over superficial nerves (ulnar, peroneal nerves).

F *Electrical Stimulation:* Electrotherapy refers to the use of electricity to stimulate nerves or muscles through electrodes on the skin. Often referred to as e-stim, this modality increases range of motion and muscle contraction. It is hypothesized to reduce atrophy, increase strength, improve circulation, and decrease muscle spasms. It produces an analgesic effect by stimulating large type A myelinated nerve fibers, inhibiting ascending pain signals. For further information about the use of electrical stimulation in pain control, see Chapter 116 Transcutaneous Electrical Nerve Stimulation.

G *Traction:* Traction applies a force to the spinal vertebrae (cervical or lumbar) to provide joint distraction. It is achieved using manual techniques or through a pulley system or motorized device. It results in a reduction in the compression of nerve roots or stretching the adhesions in epineurium. It may provide analgesia, decrease muscle spasms, and inflammation. It is indicated for treating cervical and lumbar disc disease (degeneration or herniation), nerve root compression, muscle spasm, spinal osteoarthritis and joint hypomobility. Devices such as inversion tables may also be utilized, taking advantage of gravity which can provide distraction up to 40% of the patient's body weight. In manual traction, a therapist applies pressure in specific positions for separation of vertebra. In mechanical traction, patients wear a pelvic or cervical harness that is connected to a pulley or motorized system that provides traction force.

In the cervical spine, distraction of joints requires greater than 25 lbs usually within the 20–30° of neck flexion. This position allows for the opening of posterior elements (e.g. facet joints, intervertebral foramina) optimizing nerve root decompression. Intermittent traction is considered helpful in nerve root decompression and retraction of herniated disk material as it provides greater pull compared to continuous traction. Continuous traction is more effective for degenerative disk disease and muscle spasm. Contraindications for cervical traction include conditions of cervical ligamentous laxity and joint hypermobility, such as Ehlers-Danlos syndrome, rheumatoid arthritis, Down syndrome, known atlantoaxial subluxation, Marfan syndrome, and vertebrobasilar insufficiency.

In the lumbar spine, greater than 50 lbs is needed for separation of the posterior elements of the vertebrae and greater than 100 lbs for anterior separation. For lumbar traction, the patient is placed supine with hips and knees flexed to 90° to reduced lumbar lordosis and open intervertebral foramina. Total treatment duration is usually 20 minutes. Lumbar spine traction is contraindicated with cauda equina compression, hiatal hernia, peptic ulcer disease, aortic aneurysm and restrictive lung disease. Absolute contraindications to all traction therapies include infection of the spine, acute spinal injury or fractures, spinal cord compression, spinal malignancy, osteoporosis, uncontrolled hypertension and pregnancy.

SUGGESTED READING

Akyuz G, Kenis O. Physical therapy modalities and rehabilitation techniques in the management of neuropathic pain. Am J Phys Med Rehabil. 2014;93(3):253-9.

Barr KP, Harrast MA. Low back pain. In: Braddom RL (Ed). Physical Medicine and Rehabilitation, 4th edition. Philadelphia, PA: Saunders; 2011.

Brault JS, Parker R, Grogg BE. Manipulation, traction, massage. In: Braddom RL (Ed). Physical Medicine and Rehabilitation, 4th edition. Philadelphia, PA: Saunders; 2011.

Fann AV. The prevalence of postural asymmetry in people with and without chronic low back pain. Arch Phys Med Rehabil. 2002;83(12):1736-8.

Feine JS, Lund JP. An assessment of the efficacy of physical therapy and physical modalities for the control of chronic musculoskeletal pain. Pain. 1997;71(1):5-23.

Hayden JA, van Tulder MW, Tomlinson G. Systematic review: strategies for using exercise therapy to improve outcomes in chronic low back pain. Ann Intern Med. 2005;142(9):776-85.

Lee M, Song C, Jo Y, et al. The effects of core muscle release technique on lumbar spine deformation and low back pain. J Phys Ther Sci. 2015;27(5):1519-22.

Liddle SD, Baxter GD, Gracey JH. Exercise and chronic low back pain: what works? Pain. 2004;107(1-2):176-90.

Ljunggren AE, Weber H, Kogstad O, et al. Effect of exercise on sick leave due to low back pain. A randomized, comparative, long-term study. Spine (Phila Pa 1976). 1997;22(14):1610-6.

Razmjou H, Kramer JF, Yamada R. Intertester reliability of the McKenzie evaluation in assessing patients with mechanical low-back pain. J Orthop Sports Phys Ther. 2000;30(7):368-83; discussion 384-9.

Strax TE, Grabois M, Gonzalez P, et al. Physical modalities, therapeutic exercise, extended bedrest, and aging effects. In: Cuccurullo SJ (Ed). Physical Medicine and Rehabilitation Board Review, 3rd edition. New York, NY: Demos; 2015.

Werneke M, Hart DL. Centralization phenomenon as a prognostic factor for chronic low back pain and disability. Spine (Phila Pa 1976). 2001;26(7):758-64.

CHAPTER
115

Occupational Therapy

Thakur S, DiTommaso C

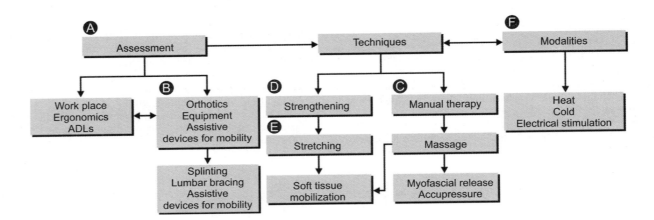

ROLE OF OCCUPATIONAL THERAPY IN PAIN MANAGEMENT

The occupational therapist (OT) plays an important role in multidisciplinary care with emphasis on patient education and training in functional activities. There are various techniques used by OT to optimize the function of patients suffering pain. There are a variety of manual therapy techniques and adaptive equipment that can be beneficial in the treatment of pain.

A *Assessment:* Occupational therapists evaluate the patient's ability to perform activities of daily living (ADLs), as well as work-related tasks. Observation of patients allows the identification of poor posture and body mechanics that may contribute to their pain. This is essential, as patients may be able to verbalize techniques to avoid painful positions/activities but may not be aware of their inability to follow these precautions. Additionally, more information regarding the patient's activity tolerance is gained. OTs are also valuable in the workplace, where they conduct ergonomic assessments. They identify and minimize factors that are injury risk factors, such as poorly designed tools, poor lighting, seating that encourages awkward postures, extreme temperatures and other sources of psychosocial or occupational stress. OT can also design prehire screenings to determine how suitable an individual is for a particular job.

B *Orthotics and Equipment:* Occupational therapists are experts in the application of orthosis, which is an external device that provides support and stability, thereby reducing pain and providing comfort to patients. For hand and wrist pain secondary to carpal tunnel syndrome, OT can fabricate or recommend an over-the-counter hand splint that positions the wrist between 0° and 30° of extension. The most commonly prescribed orthosis for low back pain is a lumbosacral corset; it works by reducing the load on the spine, reducing excessive lumbar lordosis and lateral bending. Patients must be reminded that lumbar bracing should not be worn around the clock and long-term use should be avoided due to the risk of weakening core muscles that support the trunk.

Occupational therapists can also provide training for individuals needing adaptive equipment for ambulation or ADLs. The proper use of assistive devices for ambulation (i.e. cane, walker, wheelchair) can be complex and OTs are able to instruct patients to minimize exacerbation of pain with mobility. For pain that limits performance of ADLs devices such shower chairs, shoe horns, modified jar openers, and nonslips mats are helpful.

C *Manual Therapy and Massage:* Massage works by applying pressure and stretching in a rhythmic pattern and results in improved vascular circulation, lymphatic drainage, breaks adhesions in muscles and mobilizes scars. It is also believed to decrease pain by the release of endogenous opiates. Myofascial release is a commonly used technique that applies light pressure along myofascial planes, stretching areas, specific areas of fascial or muscle tightness. Acupressure targets trigger or acupuncture points with finger pressure resulting in analgesia. In soft tissue mobilization, massage is performed with the patient in a stretched rather than relaxed position, with forceful massage that reduces contractures. Contraindications to manual therapy include acute infection or inflammatory conditions such as cellulitis, thrombophlebitis, gout flare, malignant lesions, nerve entrapment, deep venous thrombosis, varicose veins and therapeutic anticoagulation.

D *Strengthening:* Specific strengthening exercises are also frequently utilized. For example, combined cervical, shoulder, and scapulothoracic strengthening has been show to be beneficial for adults with neck pain.

E *Stretching:* Occupational therapists commonly use stretching and strengthening exercises in managing pain issues. All muscles, ligaments, tendons are mobile structures and limitations in motion of these structures can exacerbate pain. For example, decreased scapular mobility and tightness of the upper trapezius muscle can contribute to the development of neck and shoulder pain. Stretching exercises prescribed by OT target specific areas and teach patients safe and effective exercises that decrease pain and discomfort.

F *Modalities:* Occupational therapists use modalities similar to physical therapists (i.e. heat, cold, electrical stimulation). see Chapter 114 Physical Therapy.

GOALS OF TREATMENT

Occupational therapists attempt to educate patients in energy conservation and pacing techniques that can be implemented while performing ADLs, as well as work-related tasks. Further, treatment of faulty body mechanics and posture with specific methods are practiced. Patients also build strength through progressive repetitive tasks for specific activities, simulating work tasks, which also allow therapists to grade tolerance

to these tasks. Overall, OTs provide training to help patients become more independent and functional.

SUGGESTED READING

Al-Otaibi ST. Prevention of occupational back pain. J Family Community Med. 2015;22(2):73-7.

Andersen CH, Andersen LL, Zebis MK, et al. Effect of scapular function training on chronic pain in the neck/shoulder region: a randomized controlled trial. J Occup Rehabil. 2014;24(2):316-24.

Brault JS, Parker R, Grogg BE. Manipulation, traction, massage. In: Braddom RL (Ed). Physical Medicine and Rehabilitation, 4th edition. Philadelphia, PA: Saunders; 2011.

Gross A, Kay TM, Paquin JP, et al. Exercises for mechanical neck disorders. Cochrane Database Syst Rev. 2015;1:CD004250. [online] Available from *http://onlinelibrary.wiley.com/doi/10.1002/14651858.CD004250.pub5/abstract.* [Accessed January, 2017].

Smithline J. Low back pain. In: Pedretti LW (Ed). Occupational Therapy Practice Skills for Physical Dysfunction, 4th edition. St. Louis, MO: Mosby; 1996.

Stana L, Bouchez A, Fanello S, et al. Pain management: functional restoration for chronic low-back-pain clients. In: Söderback I (Ed). International Handbook of Occupational Therapy Interventions. New York, NY: Springer; 2009.

The American Occupational Therapy Association, Inc. (2004). Ergonomics. [online] Available from *http://www.aota.org/about-occupational-therapy/patients-clients/work/ergonomics.aspx.* [Accessed January, 2017].

Wolff MW, Weinik MM, Maitin IB. Bracing for low back pain. In: Cole AJ, Herring SA (Eds). The Low Back Pain Handbook, 2nd edition. Philadelphia, PA: Hanley and Belfus, Inc.; 2003.

Yanai K, Samuel M. Occupational therapy for chronic pain: a multidisciplinary approach in a pain relief unit of a general hospital. WFOT Bulletin. 2004;49(1):33-5.

CHAPTER 116

Transcutaneous Electrical Nerve Stimulation

Issa MA, DiTommaso C

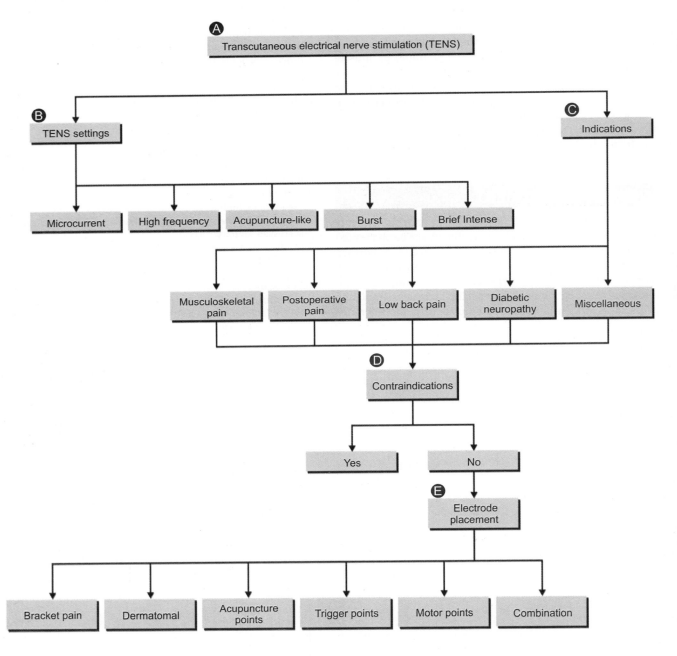

A *Introduction:* As a nonpharmacologic modality for treatment of pain, transcutaneous electrical nerve stimulation (TENS) can be used for a wide variety of acute and chronic conditions. TENS works by inhibiting C-fiber activity in the dorsal horn neurons through stimulation of large cutaneous A fibers. TENS may also access the body's endogenous opioids. The analgesia produced by some forms of TENS stimulation has been shown to be reversible by naloxone, an opioid antagonist, and by serotonin antagonists. TENS is safe and nonaddictive.

Device Characteristics: Modern TENS units are small, portable devices powered by a 9-volt battery. Most units have two channels, each controlling a pair of electrodes that are affixed to the body at the desired locations. The output of each channel is identical except for intensity-and can be altered by varying the stimulation parameters of the unit. Commercial units allow the clinician to alter intensity, pulse width, and pulse rate; and they may offer any or all such features as an automatic modulation mode, a dedicated burst or acupuncture mode, automatic timer, battery life indicator, and other stimulation or convenience options.

The TENS units produce a small electrical current ranging up to 120 mA, depending on the TENS unit selected. Most commercial devices automatically alter the voltage output to account for variations in skin resistance and produce a constant current. Depending on the unit, the pulse rate can be altered between 2 pulses/second and 200 pulses/second, and the pulse width can be varied from 9 μsec to 500 μsec. Most TENS units now offer a modulation setting that automatically alters pulse rate, pulse width, and intensity around previously selected parameters. This feature is said to diminish the body's tendency to accommodate to a constant stimulus. The waveform varies with the TENS unit selected and is generally not an adjustable parameter.

B *Settings:* Authorities differ in their recommendations of duration and frequency of stimulation during the day. Relief has been obtained experimentally with treatment ranging from 30 minutes twice a week to constant stimulation. Because TENS stimulation has a carryover effect, a treatment cycle that gives relief with scheduled on and off periods should be established. By avoiding constant use, it is theorized that accommodation to TENS may be delayed or prevented. Intermittent use may also slow or prevent depletion of endogenous pain-relieving substances accessed by TENS stimulation.

Transcutaneous electrical nerve stimulation devices are available in multiple stimulation modes:

Microcurrent TENS devices are being marketed that purport to use microamperage current to produce pain relief for conditions treated with traditional TENS. Numerous anecdotal claims are made for these devices, but no research exists at this time to validate their effectiveness.

High-frequency or conventional TENS is the stimulation mode most commonly used. It employs a pulse rate of 50–100 Hz and a short pulse width of 20–60 μsec. Treatment time may vary from 30 minutes to several hours per day at a perceptible, comfortable level of stimulation. Studies on a clinical pain population have shown that a subthreshold stimulus is also effective for initial TENS trials. Conventional TENS has been shown to be effective with a wide variety of conditions; it is the method of choice for use in acute or postsurgical situations and is a starting point for treating chronic pain conditions.

Acupuncture-like TENS, which may be more effective for chronic pain conditions, uses a low frequency (1–4 Hz) and wide pulse (150–250 μsec). Intensity is at a level that produces a strong, visible muscle contraction in the related myotome. Treatment time is 20–30 minutes once or twice a day. Analgesia takes longer to produce but is of longer duration than conventional TENS.

Burst TENS, this technique employs a series of 4–10 high-frequency pulses (70–100 Hz) delivered one to four times per second. Stimulation intensity is to the point of muscle contraction.

Brief intense TENS employs a high frequency (>100 Hz) and a wide pulse width (150–250 μsec) at the highest intensity the patient can tolerate for 1–15 minutes. It is hypothesized that this stimulus mode may disrupt the "pain memory" or act centrally in some other way.

C *Contraindications:* These include pregnancy and use over the carotid sinus area at the bifurcation of the common carotid artery as it may cause a rise in blood pressure, reflex vasodilation and decrease in the heart rate. Use of a cardiac pacemaker may not be an absolute contraindication as there are case reports of the safe cautious use of TENS with a pacemaker.

D *Indications and Efficacy:* Transcutaneous electrical nerve stimulation's role has been studied in multiple clinical trials which showed its effectiveness in controlling the pain experienced in a variety of acute and chronic conditions. TENS' immediate effectiveness in pain control has been shown to be up to 60–80% in some studies, but this falls off over time. At one year, estimates of TENS' effect on chronic conditions decrease to 25–30%.

MUSCULOSKELETAL PAIN

A study done by Law PP et al. comparing active TENS to placebo TENS showed a significant reduction in osteoarthritic knee pain and a subsequent increase in the maximum passive knee range of motion.

POSTOPERATIVE PAIN

Hamza MA et al. found that when TENS was utilized as an adjunct to a patient-controlled analgesic (PCA) pump, the postoperative opioid analgesic requirement after major gynecological surgeries decreased up to 53%. There was not only a decrease in the total opioid administration but also a reduction of the duration of PCA therapy.

LOW BACK PAIN

The effectiveness of TENS in low back pain is still controversial. The evidence-based review report published by the American Academy of Neurology (AAN) labeled TENS as an ineffective treatment for lower back pain. The review found conflicting evidence: two Class II studies showed modest benefit but were overshadowed by two Class I studies that showed no benefit.

DIABETIC PERIPHERAL NEUROPATHY

The evidence-based review report published by the AAN stated that TENS is probably effective in reducing pain from diabetic peripheral neuropathy based on two Class II studies. Kumar et al. evaluated the efficacy of TENS for chronic painful peripheral neuropathy in patients with type 2 diabetes and the study showed symptomatic improvement in 83% of patients who received electrotherapy.

MISCELLANEOUS

Transcutaneous electrical nerve stimulation has also been used effectively in other conditions like angina pectoris, dental pain, trigeminal neuralgia, and postherpetic neuralgia but with little empiric data.

E *Electrode Placement:* Successful electrode placement can be achieved using a number of methods shown by research to be effective. It is most common to place the electrodes on or bracketing the painful site. Electrodes may also be placed in the dermatome, myotome, or sclerotome in which the painful site is located. Specific sites in a region may be targeted (e.g. a trigger point), or placement may be on the anterior and posterior of the dermatome, as in the thoracic region.

Acupuncture points, trigger points, or motor points may also be effective stimulation sites. If pain with motion is a major difficulty, the clinician may try a series of electrode locations while the patient performs the offending action(s). Stimulus sites may be any combination of the points described above. This method can be time-consuming but is of great functional significance to the patient.

CONCLUSION

Successful use of TENS requires skill and perseverance on the part of the clinician and the patient. Initially, pain relief may require several hours or days of TENS application, as some individuals respond in a cumulative fashion. Long-term studies of patients who have used TENS successfully indicate that, for chronic conditions, optimum results with TENS are the question of individualizing the electrode type and placement, stimulation parameters, and stimulation time to the patient's requirements.

SUGGESTED READING

Barr JO, Nielsen DH, Soderberg GL. Transcutaneous electrical nerve stimulation characteristics for altering pain perception. Phys Ther. 1986;66:1515-21.

Barr JO. Transcutaneous electrical nerve stimulation for pain management. In: Nelson RM, Currier DP (Eds). Clinical Electrotherapy. Norwalk, CT: Appleton & Lange; 1991. pp. 261-316.

Berlant SR. Method of determining optimal stimulation sites for transcutaneous electrical nerve stimulation. Phys Ther. 1984;64:924-8.

Dubinsky RM, Miyasaki J. Assessment: efficacy of transcutaneous electric nerve stimulation in the treatment of pain in neurologic disorders (an evidence-based review): report of the Therapeutics and Technology Assessment Subcommittee of the American Academy of Neurology. Neurology. 2010;74(2):173-6.

Gersh MR, Wolf SL. Applications of transcutaneous electrical nerve stimulation in the management of patients with pain. Phys Ther. 1985;65:314-36.

Gersh MR. Microcurrent electrical stimulation: putting it in perspective. Clin Manage. 1989;9:51-4.

Hamza MA, White PF, Ahmed HE, et al. Effect of the frequency of transcutaneous electrical nerve stimulation on the postoperative opioid analgesic requirement and recovery profile. Anesthesiology. 1999;91(5):1232-8.

Johnson MI, Ashton CH, Thompson JW. An in-depth study of long-term users of transcutaneous electrical nerve stimulation (TENS): implications for clinical use of TENS. Pain. 1991;44:221-9.

Johnson MI, Ashton CH, Thompson JW. The consistency of pulse frequencies and pulse patterns of transcutaneous electrical nerve stimulation (TENS) used by chronic pain patients. Pain. 1991;44:231-4.

Lamm K. Optimal Placement Techniques for TENS: A Soft Tissue Approach. Tucson, AZ; 1986.

Law PP, Cheing GL. Optimal stimulation frequency of transcutaneous electrical nerve stimulation on people with knee osteoarthritis. J Rehabil Med. 2004;36(5):220-5.

Leo KC, Dostal WF, Bossen DG, et al. Effect of transcutaneous nerve stimulation characteristics on clinical pain. Phys Ther. 1986;66:200-5.

Nolan MF. Conductive differences in electrodes used with transcutaneous electrical nerve stimulators. Phys Ther. 1991;71:746-51.

Ottoson D, Lundeberg T. Pain Treatment by Transcutaneous Electrical Nerve Stimulation. New York: Springer-Verlag; 1988.

Shade SK. Use of transcutaneous electrical nerve stimulation for a patient with a cardiac pacemaker. Phys Ther. 1985;65:206-8.

Woolf CF, Thompson JW. Stimulation-induced analgesia: transcutaneous electrical nerve stimulation (TENS) and vibration. In: Wall PD, Melzack R (Eds). Textbook of Pain, 3rd edition. New York: Churchill Livingstone; 1994.

CHAPTER 117

Vocational Rehabilitation

McCallin JP, Kum-Nji G

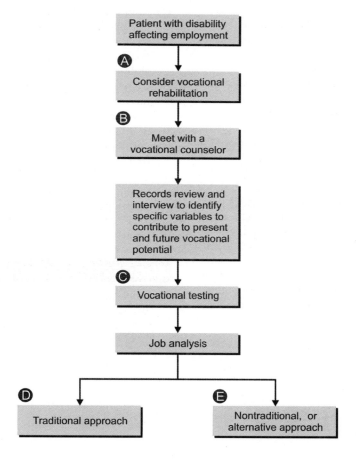

Disability in the United States is a complex, increasing socio-economic, and public health issue exacerbated by a drastic increase of disabled individuals unable to work. The Americans with Disabilities Act of 1990 defines a disability as a physical or mental impairment that substantially limits one or more major life activities. The World Health Organization defines *impairment* as any loss or abnormality of psychologic, physiologic, or anatomic structure or function. *Handicap* is defined as the disadvantage for a given individual resulting from an impairment or disability that limits or prevents the fulfillment of a role that is normal for that individual.

A There have been programs developed to address this issue in various ways, and one of these programs, which focuses primarily on returning disabled individuals to work, is vocational rehabilitation. Vocational rehabilitation is indicated in individuals with physical disabilities

to help engage in gainful employment. Vocational rehabilitation has been described as a four-phase sequence of events: (1) evaluation, (2) planning, (3) treatment, and finally (4) termination or placement. There are various approaches to vocational rehabilitation, including the traditional approach and the nontraditional approach. Nontraditional vocational rehabilitation programs include sheltered workshops, day programs, home-based programs, and employment programs.

B Traditional and nontraditional vocational rehabilitation both begin with the placement of a referral to a vocational rehabilitation counselor/expert by the person with the disability, a physician, or a social worker/case manager. The exact services provided by the rehabilitation counselor depend on the specifications of the referral, the source of funding, and regulatory requirements. These vocational experts begin with an initial evaluation, which consists of an interview and records review. The focus of this initial evaluation is to identify individual-specific variables that could contribute to present and future vocational potential. These variables include medical records that describe an individual's impairment and quantify work capacity, activities of daily living, avocational activities, behavioral health, cultural consideration, current financial resources, economic and earning history, education experience, household activities, medical functional capacity, language skills, military service experience, socioeconomic, and transportation resources. The hallmark of the planning stage of vocational rehabilitation is labor, market, research, and inquiry. Vocational counselors utilize multiple data sources, including government data sources, trade industry employment and wage statistics, and employment projections to help determine the patient's employability and placeability.

C If the patient is unable to return to his or her previous employment, vocational testing is recommended. There are numerous vocational tests, including Wechsler Adult Intelligence Scale-Revised, General Aptitude Test Battery, Differential Aptitude Test, and the Minnesota Multiphasic Personality Inventory. These tests assess various parameters, including the patient's intelligence, achievement, cognition, aptitudes, visual-spatial perception, eye-hand coordination, motor coordination, dexterity, interests, and work skills. Performance on vocational testing is used to group individuals into occupational categories listed in the Dictionary of Occupational Titles published by the Department of Labor. Once this has occurred, the requirements of potential job positions are determined by performing a job analysis.

D If the job position is considered appropriate, the patient may benefit from a training program for that position. This training can be done at a trade school, college, university, or on the job. Once training is complete, vocational goals are selected and utilized to determine whether a disabled individual is ready to return to work. This concludes the third phase of vocational rehabilitation unless further intervention is needed. The vocational expert then transitions to the final phase, which involves evaluating whether an individual meets hiring requirements of actual employers.

E Nontraditional or alternative approaches to vocational rehabilitation were developed because, historically, the traditional approach has not been very successful for various reasons—especially with individuals with severe disabilities. Sheltered workshops, day programs, and home-based programs provide job experience, but, by design, do not lead to gainful, integrated employment in a nonsheltered environment. This limitation led to the development of other nontraditional approaches, such as transitional and supported employment. Both provide job placement, training, and support services a person with disabilities may require upon return to competitive community employment. Traditional and supported employment programs have also been more effective because they provide additional services that may not be found in other vocational rehabilitation programs, such as job coaches.

SUGGESTED READING

Braddom R. Physical Medicine and Rehabilitation, 4th edition. Philadelphia: WB Saunders; 2011. pp. 1-10; 759-65.

Robinson R, Paquette S. Vocational rehabilitation process and work life. Phys Med Rehabil Clin N Am. 2013;24:521-38.

CHAPTER 118

Acupuncture

Zhang K, Ramamurthy S

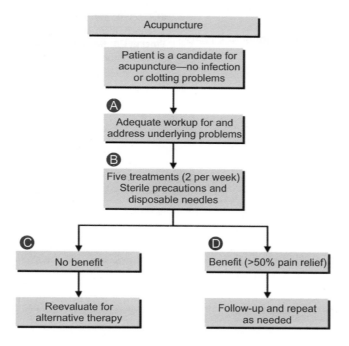

Acupuncture has its origin in ancient Chinese medicine and has been used to treat all types of the diseases. It is believed that energy chi flows through a complex system of meridians, and the imbalances in energy can be corrected through careful diagnosis and appropriate treatment by inserting needles in the acupuncture points located on these meridians. So far, scientific investigations have failed to demonstrate any anatomic or neurophysiologic evidence to support the claims of the classic acupuncture theories.

Despite innumerable animal and human studies, there is no consensus regarding the mechanisms, indications, number of treatments needed, number and location of needle placements, efficacy of acupuncture points versus nonacupuncture points, manual versus electrical stimulation, or evidence of long-term significant relief. Studies indicate that acupuncture, needling, or electrical stimulation of the trigger points are equally effective. There is a consensus that acupuncture is beneficial for headache and muscular back pain. Patients who believe in the effectiveness of acupuncture are more likely to benefit.

Acupuncture should be considered one of the modalities and not a complete system of treatment for management of pain.

Ⓐ A physician should consider acupuncture only after a thorough workup of the patient's problem. Other-

wise, an early diagnosis and treatment of serious illnesses can be missed. Knowledge of anatomy and sterile techniques is necessary for the administration of acupuncture.

ACUPUNCTURE PROCEDURE

Because of the lack of consensus, the following approach is utilized at our pain management center. Patients with bleeding and clotting disorders and patients with infection in the proposed area of needle insertion are excluded. Informed consent is obtained.

Ⓑ The patient is placed in a horizontal position to avoid vasovagal reactions. The skin is cleansed with alcohol, and 28- to 30-gauge disposable needles that are 2–4 cm long are inserted into the classic myofascial trigger points (We do not recommend the use of reusable needles). Approximately 15–20 needles are utilized per session. During needle insertions to the chest or neck, special precautions are taken to avoid pneumothorax. When placing needles close to the spine, care is taken to avoid inserting needles into the subarachnoid space or the spinal cord. Each needle is connected with an alligator clamp to a stimulator, and each pair of needles is stimulated at 4 Hz for 60 seconds using a current that produces maximum tolerable stimulation. Needles frequently oscillate with induced muscle contraction. In our experience, manual stimulation is more painful and induces significant histamine release around the needle site; we also occasionally find the needle more difficult to remove after utilizing rotational stimulation. At completion of stimulation, the needles are removed and the patient is allowed to rest before dressing. The initial course of treatment consists of five treatments over a period of 2 weeks. At this time, the patient is reevaluated.

C If no benefit has been obtained, the acupuncture is discontinued.

D If the patient receives greater than 50% pain relief, additional treatments can be scheduled as needed.

SUGGESTED READING

AMA 1981 Annual meeting report: acupuncture. J Tenn Med Assoc. 1981;75:202-4.

Lewith GT, Vincent C. On the evaluation of the clinical effects of acupuncture: a problem reassessed and the framework for future research. J Altern Complement Med. 1996;2:79-90; discussion 91-100.

Melzack R. Myofascial trigger points: relation to acupuncture and mechanism of pain. Arch Phys Med Rehabil. 1981;62:114-7.

Vincent CA, Richardson PH. The evaluation of therapeutic acupuncture: concepts and methods. Pain. 1986;24:1-13.

CHAPTER 119

Hypnosis, Biofeedback, and Meditation

Zhang K, Ramamurthy S

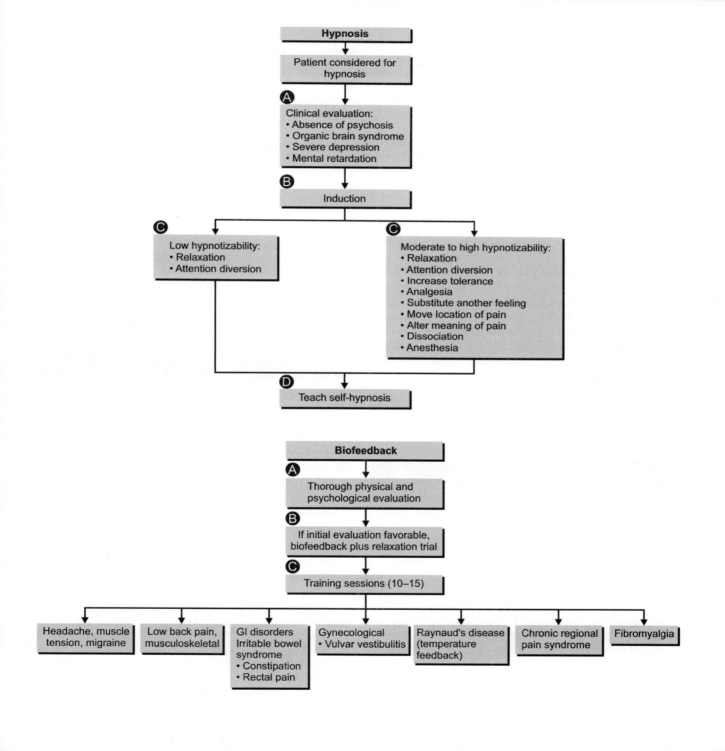

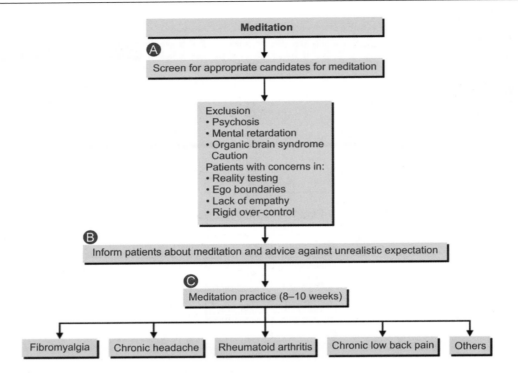

Meditation and hypnosis are two relaxation techniques used in chronic pain management, complementary to the conventional pharmacological and nonpharmacological therapies. In meditation, patients are asked to focus attention on objects, such as sound, own breath, an image (transcendental meditation), or a thought (mindfulness meditation), in order to achieve a state of relaxation, thus reducing conscious awareness of pain and distress. With hypnosis, patient is brought to a relaxation state under which the patient is susceptible to suggestions, and clinicians then make therapeutic suggestions. Growing bodies of convergent research in neurophysiology, i.e. electrophysiology and neuroimaging suggest that both processes implicate multiple brain structures and modulate various aspects of pain perception.

MEDITATION

In general, meditation is safe and can be applied to the patients with chronic pain of various etiologies. The evidence from a number of clinical trials suggest that meditation significantly improves patient's overall well-being in fibromyalgia, chronic headache, rheumatoid arthritis, and chronic low back pain.

A Before recommending meditation, a brief physical and psychological assessment may help to identify appropriate candidates. The patients with psychosis, organic brain syndrome, or mental retardation need to be excluded. It should be used with caution whenever there are concerns regarding reality testing, ego boundaries, lack of empathy, or rigid over-control.

B Patients should be well informed of the rationale of meditation for pain control and be advised not to have unrealistic expectation.

C A typical meditation course lasts 8 weeks with each session being less than 30 minutes, twice a day. Patients may be encouraged to self-practice after a few weeks of meditation under instruction.

HYPNOSIS

Hypnosis requires patients to engage in sustained or focused attention or concentration. When the ability to sustain focused attention is compromised, hypnosis provides little or no therapeutic value and may further frustrate the patient, diminishing motivation and compliance.

A An initial clinical evaluation should exclude the patients with psychosis, organic brain syndrome, mental retardation, or severe depression. The patients with significant depression should undergo antidepressant treatment before a trial of hypnosis.

B Patients are given a full explanation of hypnosis for pain control and then undergo a trial hypnotic induction to establish their susceptibility to hypnosis, i.e. low, moderate, or high hypnotizability, and to desensitize them to the procedure.

C Depending on their level of hypnotizability, the patient may choose to use this procedure for pain management. An audio recording of the procedure can help the patient practice hypnosis daily. Often patients can use self-hypnosis after repeated tape-recorded inductions.

D Some patients can learn self-hypnosis for pain control after a single trial of hypnosis. Repeated follow-up can reinforce the use of hypnosis to facilitate compliance and to modify the pain experience.

BIOFEEDBACK

Biofeedback is a technique that improves an individual's ability to voluntarily control physiologic activities by providing information back to the individual. The most common feedback given is regarding muscle tension using surface electromyography (EMG) electrodes or the skin temperature using a thermistor.

A The selection of candidates for biofeedback is typically preceded by an assessment process. In many cases, patients are selected for conservative treatment because more invasive approaches have failed or are deemed inappropriate. Psychological testing may be helpful in identifying patients with concentration difficulties secondary to depression, which may limit their capacity to participate in self-regulatory approaches to treatment. Patients with elevated scores on the Minnesota Multiphasic Personality Inventory (MMPI), hypochondriasis, and hysteria scales have been shown to experience poorer outcomes, and younger patients sometimes may have more favorable outcomes than older individuals. Patients with previously untreated depression should usually be referred for treatment of the mood disturbance before biofeedback training. Hypochondriacal trends are not a definitive contraindication to biofeedback treatment, but they may suggest a pattern of illness behavior or secondary gain that needs to be modified before a self-regulatory approach (such as biofeedback), has a reasonable chance for success.

B After a thorough evaluation of the chronic pain patient, biofeedback combined with relaxation can be used as the primary therapeutic modality in patients with muscle tension headache with high likelihood of benefit. The capacity of the patient to influence and control physiologic activity can be evaluated and monitored by assessing the ability of the patient to influence the physiologic activity prior to biofeedback and after the training session.

C 10–15 treatment sessions may be necessary to achieve useful level of control of pain and discomfort.

Biofeedback has proven to be most effective in managing muscle tension headache with a success rate of 45–60%. Success rate is further increased to 70–75% when biofeedback is combined with progressive relaxation techniques. Vascular headache such as migraine is less responsive whereas cluster headache is least likely to benefit from biofeedback. Biofeedback has also been used for various other painful conditions with variable reported success. Musculoskeletal low back pain and temporomandibular joint syndrome (myofascial pain dysfunction syndrome) are two major categories of chronic pain that are likely to benefit significantly with biofeedback training. Recent studies show that biofeedback relaxation reduces pain associated with continuous passive motion after total knee arthroplasty. Thermal biofeedback has been successfully utilized in the treatment of Raynaud's disease. Pain secondary to constipation has been treated with biofeedback both in children and in adults. Children appear to prefer temperature feedback. Irritable bowel syndrome, intractable rectal pain, vulvar vestibulitis and dyspareunia, fibromyalgia, and chronic regional pain syndrome have also been treated with biofeedback with varying results.

SUGGESTED READING

Arena JG, Blanchard EB. Biofeedback therapy for chronic pain disorders. In: Loeser JD, Butler SD, Chapman CR, Turk DC (Eds). Bonica's Management of Pain, 3rd edition. Baltimore: Lippincott Williams & Wilkins; 2001. pp. 1755-63.

Barber J. Rapid induction analgesia: a clinical report. Am J Clin Hypn. 1977;19:138.

Blanchard EB, Ahles TA. Biofeedback therapy. In: Bonica JJ (Ed). The Management of Pain, 2nd edition. Philadelphia: Lea & Febiger; 1990. p. 1722.

Crasilneck HB, Hall JA. Clinical Hypnosis: Principles and Applications. Orlando: Grune & Stratton; 1985.

De Benedittis G. Neural mechanisms of hypnosis and meditation. J Physiol Paris. 2015;109(4-6):152-64.

Eimer BN. Clinical applications of hypnosis for brief and efficient pain management psychotherapy. Am J Clin Hypn. 2000;43:17-40.

Greeson J, Eisenlohr-Moul T. Mindfulness-based stress reduction for chronic pain. In: Baer RA (Ed). Mindfulness-Based Treatment Approaches: Clinician's Guide to Evidence Base and Applications, 2nd edition. London: Academic Press; 2014.

Ouellette EA. Pain management and medical hypnosis. Instr Course Lect. 2000;49:541-3.

Wang TJ, Chang CF, Lou MF, et al. Biofeedback relaxation for pain associated with continuous passive motion in Taiwanese patients after total knee arthroplasty. Res Nurs Health. 2015;38(1):39-50.

Wolf SL, Nacht M, Kelly JL. EMG biofeedback training during dynamic movement for low back pain patients. Behav Ther. 1982;13:395-406.

Zeidan F, Martucci KT, Kraft RA, et al. Brain mechanisms supporting modulation of pain by mindfulness meditation. J Neurosci. 2011;31(14):5540-8.

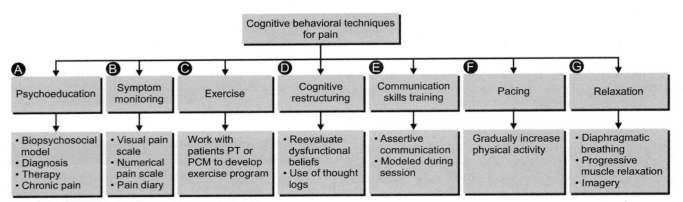

PT, physical therapist; PCM; primary care manager

Cognitive behavioral therapy (CBT) has been shown to be effective in the treatment of pain caused by disease states and musculoskeletal problems. The ultimate goals of CBT for pain management are to increase functional activities and to improve self-management of pain. CBT teaches the application of new skills through the use of homework and self-monitoring. There are many CBT techniques that can be particularly helpful in the treatment of pain.

Ⓐ *Psychoeducation:* In the case of pain management, psychoeducation refers to patient education regarding the biopsychosocial model, diagnoses, therapy, and chronic pain. As part of psychoeducation, a therapist will often describe the framework of treatment to the patient and explore patient expectations and responsibilities.

Ⓑ *Symptom Monitoring:* Symptom monitoring can take several different forms. Examples include visual and numerical pain rating scales or pain diaries. Visual or numerical pain rating scales can be used to monitor symptoms between sessions or as an outcome measure for treatment. A pain diary allows patients to record and monitor changes in experienced pain from day to day. This can be helpful for both patient and doctor to identify triggers, stressors, and patterns of pain.

Ⓒ *Exercise:* Psychologists should work in conjunction with the patient's physician or physical therapist to incorporate exercise into a pain patient's treatment plan. Due to fear avoidance, a patient may be hesitant to engage in physical activities. Patients suffering with chronic pain can become afraid that exercise may exacerbate a current injury or cause reinjury. Physical activity is necessary to keep muscles from becoming deconditioned. Deconditioning can lead to muscle weakness and atrophy. Exer-

cise helps to decrease muscle tension, stress, increase mood, and improve sleep. Exercise has the added benefit of encouraging weight loss which may decrease pain for individuals who are overweight.

Ⓓ *Cognitive Restructuring:* Cognitive restructuring allows the therapist and patient to examine thoughts/beliefs that lead to distressing consequences (such as decreases in mood) and helps to reevaluate dysfunctional beliefs that produce extremely negative reactions. Patients are often given a log to record stressful experiences, thoughts, beliefs, and emotions which are brought to the therapy session to discuss and evaluate.

Ⓔ *Communication Skills Training:* Patients are encouraged to replace aggressive and nonassertive communication with more appropriate responses. Communication skills are modeled and practiced during session and assigned as homework for further practice. These skills can be extremely helpful when interacting with coworkers, family, and physicians.

Ⓕ *Pacing:* Pain patients may overdo physical activities when they are not experiencing high levels of pain (e.g. cleaning the entire house). Unfortunately, as a result of overextending, pain is amplified and the patient may require extended time to recover. Pacing encourages pain patients to gradually increase the duration and intensity of activities over time to decrease pain.

Ⓖ *Relaxation:* As with exercise, relaxation techniques can be beneficial for pain patients in multiple ways. These techniques can reduce muscle tension, decrease anxiety, be a distraction from pain, and promote sleep. Different relaxation techniques can be taught based upon patient preference or level of disability. The type of relaxation used can be simple like diaphragmatic breathing for individuals with severe pain and disability to more involved techniques like progressive muscle relaxation.

While CBT has the most empirical support for the treatment of chronic pain, research has shown that acceptance and commitment therapy (ACT) has modest support as an empirical treatment for pain management. Rather than addressing dysfunctional thoughts as in CBT, ACT encourages the observation of thoughts and feelings without changing them. A focus of therapy is to assist patients to live according to their values and goals despite the presence of pain by teaching mindfulness and acceptance.

SUGGESTED READING

Keefe FJ. Cognitive behavioral therapy for managing pain. Clin Psychol. 1996;49(3):4-5.

Mundy E, DuHamel K, Montgomery G. The efficacy of behavioral interventions for cancer treatment-related side effects. Semin Clin Neuropsychiatry. 2003;8:253-75.

Turner J, Clancy S. Comparison of operant-behavioral and cognitive-behavioral group treatment for chronic low back pain. J Consult Clin Psychol. 1988;58:573-9.

Wetherell JL, Afari N, Rutledge T, et al. A randomized, controlled trial of acceptance and commitment therapy and cognitive-behavioral therapy for chronic pain. Pain. 2011;152(9):2098-107.

CHAPTER
121
Psychological Interventions

McGeary CA

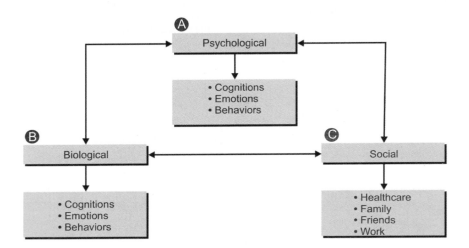

Effective pain management techniques are necessary due to the rising costs of pain-related healthcare. A comprehensive medical evaluation is needed for effective treatment. However, focus on the biomedical model alone is often insufficient to alleviate pain and a thorough psychological evaluation is also beneficial. To successfully manage pain, treatment should address biological, psychological, and social factors, as exemplified by the biopsychosocial model. This is often best accomplished through an interdisciplinary model of pain management. Interdisciplinary pain management encompasses a coordination of services in a comprehensive program with frequent communication among all healthcare professionals engaged in a patient's treatment. Current empirically supported pain management interventions tend to be based in cognitive behavioral therapy (CBT). The following interventions follow the biopsychosocial model of pain and are based on CBT techniques:

A *Biological:* From the biological standpoint, one of the most common psychological treatments to alleviate pain or the emotional turmoil that accompanies chronic pain is the prescription of antidepressants. Fortunately, there are also nonpharmacological methods to address biological factors that impact or are impacted by pain. Exercise should be part of the chronic pain sufferer's treatment plan once cleared for exercise by his/her physician. Exercise works against physical deconditioning which can complicate chronic pain. Exercise can also alleviate depression, stress, and anxiety related to pain. Chronic pain sufferers also often experience sleep disruption due to pain interfering with the sleep cycle. Medication may

be prescribed to improve sleep; however, CBT can also be used to manage sleep problems, by addressing sleep hygiene, sleep restriction, and challenging distorted thoughts regarding sleep.

B *Psychological:* Cognitive behavioral therapy is founded on the premise that our thoughts about a situation impact our emotions and behaviors. During CBT, patients are taught to examine the relationship between their thoughts and mood. Any unrealistic or dysfunctional thoughts regarding pain are modified in order to bring about changes in mood and behavior. The primary goals of CBT for pain management are to increase functional activities despite pain, to increase coping, to decrease pain catastrophizing, and to decrease fear avoidance. In turn, increasing activities, improving coping skills, decreasing pain catastrophizing and fear avoidance decreases depression and anxiety that is often present in pain patients. Some CBT techniques that are common for pain management include psychoeducation about pain, symptom monitoring, thought monitoring, pacing, relaxation, and problem-solving skills.

C *Social:* Social support to include family, friends, healthcare providers, and coworkers can impact the perception of pain. Individuals with chronic pain who describe high levels of social support report less distress and pain and social support is associated with overall better adjustment. Encouraging a patient to develop a positive social support network (if one does not already exist) can be a goal of treatment. Teaching communication skills to a patient to utilize with family, friends, healthcare providers and coworkers can help to build a social support network. Assigning homework assignments to engage others in meaningful social activities can also build social networks or improve existing ones.

SUGGESTED READING

Gatchel RJ, McGeary DD, McGeary CA, et al. Interdisciplinary chronic pain management: past, present, and future. Am Psychol. 2014;69(2):119-30.

López-Martínez A, Esteve-Zarazaga R, Ramírez-Maestre C. Perceived social support and coping responses are independent variables explaining pain adjustment among chronic pain patients. J Pain. 2008;9(4):373-9.

McGeary CA, Swanholm E, Gatchel RA. Pain management. In: Cautin RL, Lilienfeld SO (Eds). The Encyclopedia of Clinical Psychology. New York: Wiley-Blackwell; 2015.

Micó J, Ardid D, Berrocoso E, et al. Antidepressants and pain. Trends Pharmacol Sci. 2006;27(7):348-54.

Pigeon WR. Treatment of adult insomnia with cognitive-behavioral therapy. J Clin Psychol. 2010;66:1148-60.

chapter 122

Prosthetic Support: Management of Amputee-Related Pain

Benfield JA, Bushman TJ, Mugleston BJ

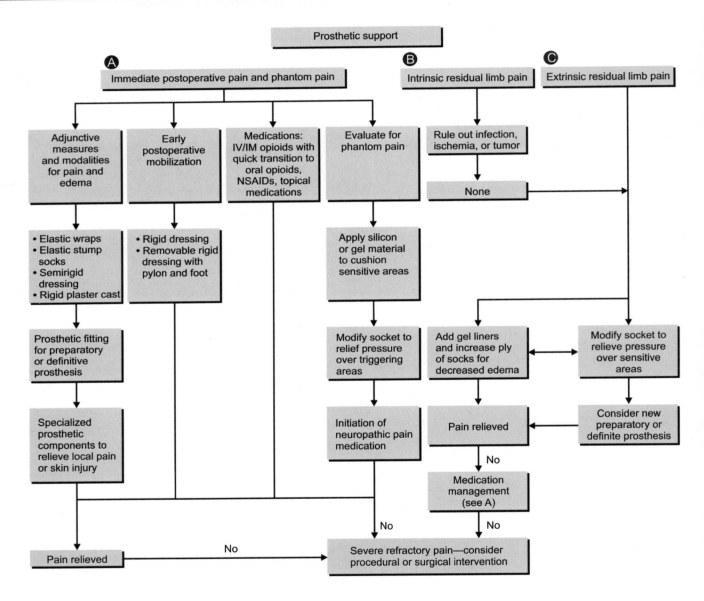

Amputee-related pain is categorized into postoperative, incisional, phantom, and persistent residual limb pain. Evaluation of amputee pain includes location, character, frequency, duration, and intensity of the pain. Treatments include oral medications, physical modalities, prosthetic modification, procedural and surgical interventions. Prosthetic appliances and support services play a dynamic role in management of amputee pain. These include facilitating wound healing,

controlling postoperative pain, restoring prior function, and managing persistent residual limb pain.

A *Postoperative and Phantom Pain:* Postoperative and phantom limb pain commonly follow amputation in up to 80% of amputees. It is characterized as burning, tingling, shooting, electric, cramping, or stabbing pain and generally improves in weeks to months. Effective treatment starts postoperatively with intravenous (IV)/intramuscular (IM), with transition to oral opioids in a few days. Treating postoperative pain reduces development of central nervous system-mediated and chronic pain. Opioids are appropriate initially, but transition to other treatment options, including desensitization techniques, antidepressants (tricyclic antidepressants [TCAs], serotonin-norepinephrine reuptake inhibitors [SNRIs]), anticonvulsants (gabapentin, pregabalin, topiramate), topical agents (capsaicin, lidocaine), and other non-pharmacologic modalities (stress-relaxation techniques, biofeedback, transcutaneous electrical nerve stimulation [TENS]) is encouraged. Additional pharmacologic options include gamma-aminobutyric acid (GABA) inhibitors, calcitonin, propranolol, and mexiletine. Procedural or surgical interventions, such as nerve or epidural blocks, steroid injections, radiofrequency ablation, and sympathectomy, are options for severe or refractory cases. Evaluation of prosthetic appliances including early consultation of a prosthetist significantly reduces postoperative pain by controlling edema and protecting the limb from external trauma. Use of removable elastic wraps, elastic socks/shrinkers, semirigid (Unna) dressings, prone positioning, leg board use with wheelchairs, and/or rigid plaster casting of the residual limb can be prescribed.

B *Intrinsic Residual Limb Pain:* Persistent residual limb pain occurs in up to 70% of lower limb amputees. Residual limb pain can be achy, sharp, throbbing, and burning and originating and affecting the terminal limb. Residual limb pain is classified as intrinsic or extrinsic, and treated with the same pharmacologic and nonpharmacologic modalities described above. Intrinsic residual limb pain is caused by underlying bony or soft tissues in the residual limb. Etiologies include neuromas, bony abnormalities, poor surgical technique, persistent ischemia, osteomyelitis or tumor recurrence. Neuroma-related pain is characterized by paroxysmal radiating pain and paresthesia usually in the distribution of the affected nerve. It may be precipitated by direct compression with manual palpation, socket pressure, percussion (Tinel's sign), or friction of nerves adjacent to scar tissue.

When prosthetic use exacerbates neuroma pain, incorporating gel socks or liners, flexible sockets, or socket modification to off-load and alleviate sensitive areas may be effective. Additional interventions can be used when minimal or no pain alleviation occurs with prosthetic modification and physical modalities. These include localized steroid/anesthetic injection, neuroma ablation with alcohol or phenol, radiofrequency ablation, cryoablation, or surgical excision. Bony overgrowth including heterotopic bone formation (heterotopic ossification) can occur in any amputee and is especially problematic in pediatric amputees. Excessive pressure over the abnor-

mal bone leads to localized pain and tenderness causing soft tissue injury to surrounding muscles, ligaments, tendons, bursa, and nerves. Initial management includes prosthetic socket modifications for improved pressure redistribution, addition of gels, liners and socks, and surgical revision in severe cases. Poor surgical technique is a known risk factor for a painful residual limb and includes incorrect shaping and beveling of cut bone ends, inadequate stabilization of soft tissues through myoplasty, myodesis, or inadequate soft tissue padding.

C *Extrinsic Residual Limb Pain:* Extrinsic residual limb pain is caused by a mismatch between the residual limb and the prosthesis because of poor socket fit or limb malalignment. Appropriate identification, fabrication, and integration of prosthetic components should optimize loading and shear forces placed on the residual limb helping to eliminate specific pains with prosthetic use. Most prosthetic sockets are designed for total contact with modifications to the socket shape to load weight tolerance tissues preferentially. The initial fit of a socket is inevitably compromised, as residual limb shape, volume, and muscle bulk change with time. Typically, amputees add socks over the residual limb to accommodate these changes. An inadequate fit occurs when weight-bearing loads shift to tissues with poor pressure tolerance, creating pain when standing or walking. Malalignment of components in lower limb prosthesis can create high or prolonged loading forces. Clinical manifestations of poor fit and excessive local tissue loading include persistent erythema following limb use, bursa development, proximal choking with distal edema formation, and skin breakdown. Ultimately, correction of an alignment problem or socket replacement is required.

CONCLUSION

Evaluation of amputee-related pain includes appropriate use of prosthetic appliances including early prosthetist consultation significantly reduces amputee-related pain by identifying the pain generator(s). Subsequent treatment with prosthetic modifications and services, physical modalities, oral medications, procedural and surgical interventions can decrease or alleviate pain with a hopeful increase in function.

SUGGESTED READING

Braddom RL. Physical Medicine and Rehabilitation, 4th edition. Philadelphia: Elsevier Health Sciences; 2010.

Cuccurullo S. Physical Medicine and Rehabilitation Board Review, 3rd edition. New York: Demos Medical Publishing; 2015.

Frontera WR, DeLisa JA. DeLisa's Physical Medicine and Rehabilitation: Principles and Practice, 5th edition. Philadelphia: Lippincott Williams & Wilkins; 2010.

SECTION **14**

Interventional Therapeutic Modalities

Larry C Driver

Interventional Therapeutic Modalities

CHAPTER
123

Epidurals

Adams CW, Day M

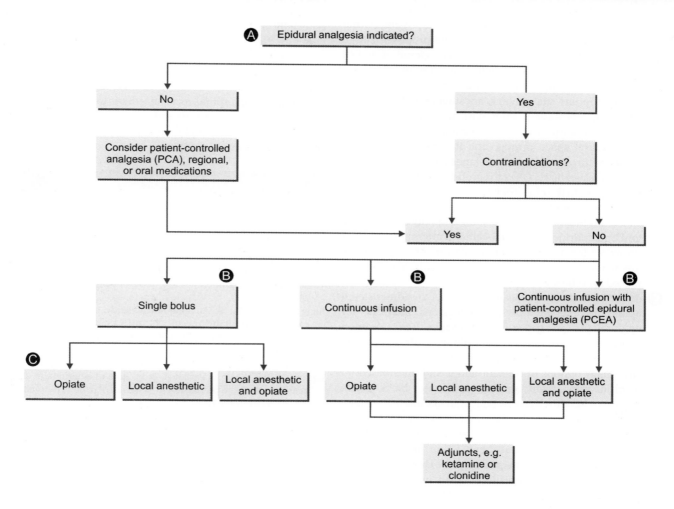

The epidural space is a common route for the administration of medications for analgesia, diagnosis of certain pain conditions, and procedural anesthesia. Medications are administered near the nerve roots responsible for the transmission of the signals intending to be blocked, i.e. sympathetic, sensory, or motor. Medication preparations are often isobaric and will follow gravity to affect other nearby levels. Medications from the epidural space have some vascular uptake as well as diffusion through the dura into nerve roots and the cerebrospinal fluid (CSF) to produce a wide range of effects.

Anatomy: The epidural space is a continuous compartment extending from the cranium to the sacrum containing fat, lymphatics, arteries, an extensive plexus of veins (Batson's plexus), connective tissue, spinal nerve roots, and ligaments. It extends around the dura mater circumferentially. For a midline approach, the path of the needle proceeds through skin and subcutaneous tissues, the supraspinous ligament, the interspinous ligament, and finally penetrates the ligamentum flavum to enter the epidural space. On a paramedian approach, the needle passes through skin, subcutaneous tissues, and the ligamentum flavum. Through either approach, accidental further advancement passes the dura mater, subdural space, arachnoid mater, and subarachnoid space. Paramedian placement incurs higher risk of intrathoracic or intra-abdominal placement.

A *Patient Selection:* Careful choice of patients is critical when performing epidural injections or infusions. Patient selection factors include the presence of anticoagulants or underlying coagulation defects, as epidural hematoma is a devastating potential complication. Patient anatomy is an important factor as several conditions may limit or prohibit epidural administration of medications. Previous spine procedures may have damaged, removed, or altered the epidural space. These procedures may cause loculations or other discontinuities in the epidural space that can limit or inhibit flow in the epidural space. Also body habitus or contractures can make placement or reaching the epidural space difficult or impossible. Other things to consider are infection at the proposed site of insertion, patient understanding and cooperation, as well as ability to tolerate an indwelling catheter for infusion.

B *Placement:* Epidural placement is performed by locating the appropriate site of entry, anesthetizing the skin and subcutaneous tissues, then passing a needle through the ligamentum flavum. Confirmation of entry into the epidural space through the ligamentum flavum is achieved through a loss of resistance technique including a loss of resistance (LOR) syringe, balloon or drip infusion techniques. In the obese or patients with altered anatomy, fluoroscopic guidance may be helpful. Once the epidural space has been reached, a test dose of a local anesthetic and epinephrine are administered to attempt to rule out intravascular or subarachnoid placement. Medications are then either directly injected or an epidural catheter is placed for infusion of medications.

C *Medications:* Many medications can safely be administered epidurally. Preparations of medications intended for epidural use are generally preservative free. Common medications are opioids (morphine, hydromorphone, fentanyl) and local anesthetics (bupivacaine, ropivacaine), with many options of concentrations and rates based on need for sympathetic, sensory, and motor block. Alpha agonists (clonidine) have recently gained some favors alone or in combination with other medications for procedural anesthesia. Epidural ketamine is another medication that has been investigated and been found to beneficial in some studies. Medications and adjuncts should be tailored to each patient and situation. When uncertain how a particular patient will respond the safest method is to start with the lowest concentration of medication and titrate up

to effect. This method also provides a glimpse at potential complications related to the increasing medication dosages.

Complications: Complications from epidural medication administration fall into two categories. The first are complications related to the placement or misplacement of the needle and/or catheter. These include misplacement into subdural, intrathecal, or intravascular locations. Bleeding and infection are always risks when penetrating the skin with a needle. There is also slight risk of causing pneumothorax especially in blind thoracic placement. If there is venous puncture there is risk of epidural hematoma which could be catastrophic. If the dura was punctured there is risk of CSF leak and headache. The second group of complications relates to the medications used. This includes complications such as hypotension, high spinal, local anesthetic toxicity, respiratory depression, nausea, pruritus and urinary retention. Even with these underlying risks, epidural injections and infusions are considered safe even in children.

SUGGESTED READING

Abd-Elsayed AA, Guirguis M, DeWood MS, et al. A Double-Blind Randomized Controlled Trial Comparing Epidural Clonidine vs Bupivacaine for Pain Control During and After Lower Abdominal Surgery. Ochsner J. 2015;15(2):133-42.

Jeon DG, Song JG, Kim SK, et al. Epidural hematoma after thoracic epidural analgesia in a patient treated with ketorolac, mefenamic acid, and naftazone: a case report. Korean J Anesthesiol. 2014;66(3):240-3.

Jiang H, Shi B, Xu S. An anatomical study of lumbar epidural catheterization. BMC Anesthesiol. 2015;15:94.

Kasanavesi RC, Gazula S, Pula R, et al. Safety of postoperative epidural analgesia in the paediatric population: A retrospective analysis. Indian J Anaesth. 2015;59(10):636-40.

Radvansky BM, Shah K, Parikh A, et al. Role of ketamine in acute postoperative pain management: a narrative review. Biomed Res Int. 2015;2015:749837.

Sawhney KY, Kundra S, Grewal A, et al. A Randomized Double Blinded Comparison of Epidural Infusion of Bupivacaine, Ropivacaine, Bupivacaine-Fentanyl, Ropivacaine-Fentanyl for Postoperative Pain Relief in Lower Limb Surgeries. J Clin Diagn Res. 2015;9(9):UC19-23.

Singhal S, Bala M, Kaur K. Identification of epidural space using loss of resistance syringe, infusion drip, and balloon technique: A comparative study. Saudi J Anaesth. 2014;8(Suppl 1):S41-5.

CHAPTER
124

Subarachnoid Block

Kraus GP, Lai TT

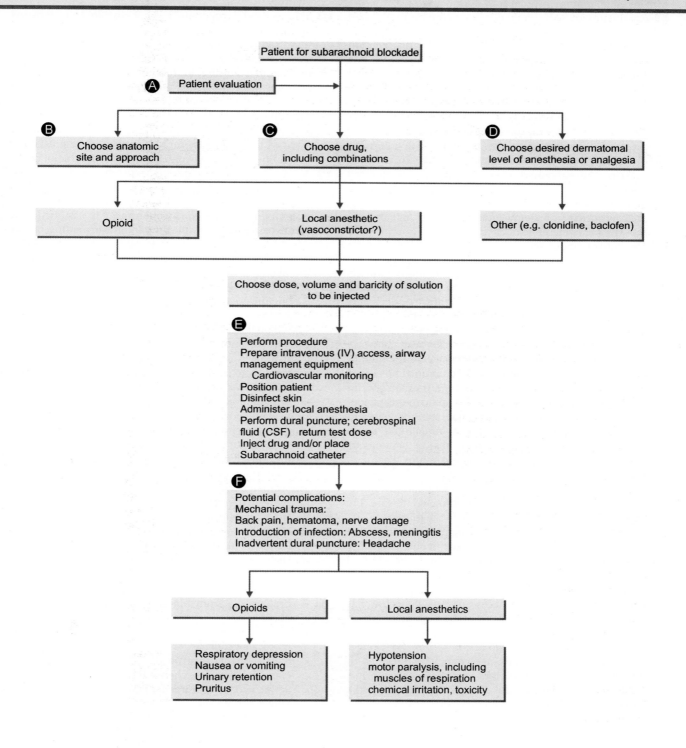

The subarachnoid space contains cerebrospinal fluid (CSF) that is contiguous with the intracranial CSF pathways and extends from the foramen magnum to the S2 spinal level in adults. Drugs injected into the CSF tend to have a rapid action due to direct contact on exposed nerve membranes of the spinal cord and nerve roots. Subarachnoid blocks (SAB) are used to treat various acute and chronic pain syndromes, for diagnostic purposes, and to treat muscular spasms associated with cerebral, motor, or spinal cord dysfunction.

Ⓐ Candidates for SAB should consent to the procedure and have stable neurologic function, normal clotting function, no evidence of systemic sepsis, and no inflammation or infection over the proposed site of injection. The American Society of Regional Anesthesia and Pain Medicine (ASRA) guidelines are available to minimize risk of epidural hematomas in patients that are taking anticoagulant or antiplatelet medications. Hypovolemic patients have an exaggerated hypotensive response to the sympathectomy caused by local anesthetics. Because of the risk of downward herniation of the brain, the dura must not be punctured when CSF pressure is elevated intracranially. Additional relative contraindications include severe valvular abnormalities, left ventricular outflow obstruction, demyelinating diseases, or concerns for sepsis or bacteremia.

Ⓑ The subarachnoid space can be entered with a needle anywhere along its path, but to prevent injury to the spinal cord, a site of entry caudal to the conus medullaris (L1-2 in adults or L2-3 in infants) is normally chosen. Surface anatomy can be used to identify Tuffier's line from the superior edges of the iliac crests. This line generally crosses L4 or the L4-L5 interspace. However, even experienced anesthesiologists have been shown to incorrectly identify the correct interspace. In the lumbar area, a midline approach is the most common and easiest to teach and perform. Because the spinous processes run nearly parallel to the long-axis of the spine in this region, a spinal needle placed into the interspinous ligament is directed perpendicularly. The subarachnoid space is accessed in the following order: skin, subcutaneous tissue, supraspinous ligament, interspinous ligament, ligamentum flavum, and then the dura and arachnoid mater prior to entering the subarachnoid space. Alternatively, the needle may be directed toward the midline from a position 1 cm lateral to the midline.

Ⓒ The choice and quantity of drug injected into the subarachnoid space are based on patient characteristics, the desired goal of the blockade, and the desired duration of the blockade. Any drug chosen should have a record of safety in the CSF and be free of preservative. For short surgical procedures, use of lidocaine has significantly decreased because of the high incidence of transient nerve root irritation syndrome. Preservative-free chloroprocaine is a good substitute. For longer procedures, one should use either tetracaine or bupivacaine. Vasoconstrictors (usually epinephrine, 1:200,000) can intensify the analgesia and prolong the blockade of most local anesthetics. The local anesthetic can be diluted with sterile water, preservative-free saline,

or preservative-free dextrose to make the specific gravity of the final solution less than, equal to, or greater than the specific gravity of CSF. In the case of hypobaric or hyperbaric solutions, some degree of control of the spread of the local anesthetic in the CSF can be attained by patient positioning. For isobaric solutions, the spread of the blockade is governed primarily by the number of molecules of local anesthetic injected, rather than the volume.

Ⓓ The required dermatomal level of any blockade depends on the level of the spinal cord at which the afferent pain impulses insert. For example, a blockade of somatic pain afferents may be affected by blockade of lower thoracic dermatomes during intra-abdominal surgery; visceral afferents passing through the celiac plexus and traveling along with the fibers of the sympathetic chain require a much higher level of blockade. Neurolytic agents for pain palliation can be injected into the subarachnoid space and directed toward the dorsal root ganglia while preserving motor fibers by using hypobaric or hyperbaric solutions.

Ⓔ Airway management devices must be at the bedside and readily accessible as well as established intravenous (IV) access before an SAB may be instituted. The skin overlying the proposed site of entrance is scrubbed with disinfectant solution while the patient is in a sitting, lateral decubitus, or prone position. Local anesthesia of the skin and subcutaneous area is achieved via infiltration, then the needle is advanced toward the dura with the bevel oriented parallel to the long-axis of the spine. As the dura is punctured, a distinct "pop" is often felt and CSF should return freely. Any heme should quickly clear, and there should be no paresthesias before or during the injection. After an injection of local anesthetic, the patient may be either turned immediately or left in the same position while the block is allowed to set. Vital signs should be taken every 5 minutes after injection of the local anesthetic, and the spread of anesthesia is closely monitored. For short surgical procedures, local anesthetics can be injected in a "one-shot" technique. For longer procedures and chronic pain therapy, a catheter may be passed through a larger needle and left in the subarachnoid space for intermittent or continuous injections of local anesthetic or opiates. The catheter may also be tunneled subcutaneously for longer term therapy.

Ⓕ Potential complications of SAB with local anesthetics include:
- Backache in up to 40% of patients
- Hypotension caused by sympathectomy
- Postdural puncture headache
- Nausea caused by unopposed vagal activity
- Bradycardia from blockade of cardiac sympathetic fibers
- Respiratory insufficiency due to hypotension or high motor blockade
- Spinal cord or nerve root damage due to mechanical or chemical irritation, chemical or bacterial meningitis
- Spinal and/or epidural hematoma and/or abscess.
  Subarachnoid opioids may cause the same complications as do epidural opioids.

SUGGESTED READING

Albright AL, Cervi A, Singletary J. Intrathecal baclofen for spasticity in cerebral palsy. JAMA. 1991;265(11):1418-22.

Bonnet F, Buisson VB, Francois Y, et al. Effects of oral and subarachnoid clonidine on spinal anesthesia with bupivacaine. Reg Anesth. 1990;15(4):211-4.

Cousins MJ, Cherry DA, Gourlay JK. Acute and chronic pain: use of spinal opioids. In: Cousins MJ, Bridenbaugh PO (Eds). Neural Blockade in Clinical Anesthesia and Management of Pain, 2nd edition. Philadelphia: Lippincott; 1987. pp. 955-1029.

Lee JA, Atkinson RS, Watt MJ. Sir Robert Macintosh's Lumbar Puncture and Spinal Analgesia: Intradural and Extradural, 5th edition. Edinburgh: Churchill Livingstone; 1985. p. 282.

Mulroy MF. Regional Anesthesia. Boston: Little Brown; 1989. p. 86.

Stienstra R, Greene NM. Factors affecting the subarachnoid spread of local anesthetic solutions. Reg Anesth. 1991;16(1): 1-6.

CHAPTER
125

Peripheral Nerve Blocks

Boies BT, Thome CM

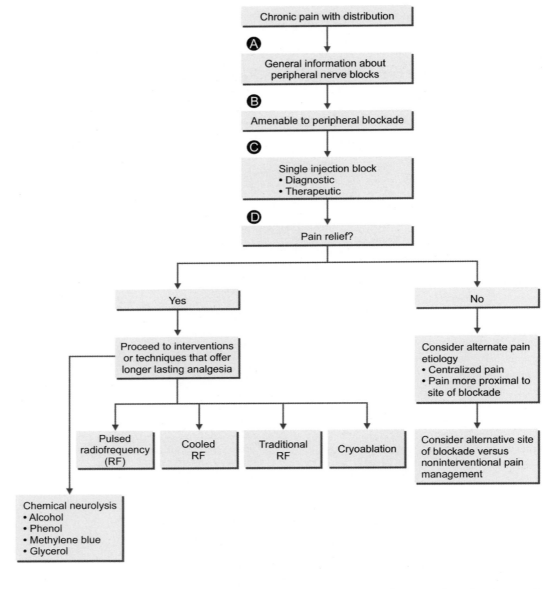

Peripheral nerve blocks have been used for many years to provide regional anesthesia for surgery and to treat acute and chronic pain. The goal of regional analgesia is to provide pain relief to a specific portion of the body, thus limiting systemic administration of analgesics and their associated adverse effects. When peripheral nerve blocks are combined with modalities such as continuous nerve block catheters, cryoablation, chemical neurolysis, and radiofrequency (RF)

ablation, prolonged targeted analgesia can be obtained. In addition to analgesia, peripheral nerve blocks can provide valuable diagnostic information. For example, a successful medial branch block with local anesthetic can indicate that an individual's pain is originating from the facet joint. The medial branches providing the sensory innervation to the corresponding facet joint can then be targeted with RF ablation or chemical neurolysis for long-term analgesia. This chapter provides a brief overview and introduction of peripheral nerve blocks and their application for chronic pain.

A Historically, techniques usually incorporated easily identifiable surface landmarks to take advantage of the most superficial locations of nerves to facilitate needle placement and limit complications. The advent of peripheral nerve stimulator (PNS) techniques increased the application, the success rate, and the ease of performing the blocks, as well as the safety of the procedures. Despite the benefits, there are still several limitations to PNS-guided blocks. For example, the motor response disappears after the injection of local anesthetic. Also, stimulation provides objective, but indirect, evidence of nerve location. PNS is primarily useful when a motor response is elicited, and motor response does not guarantee a successful block. PNS does not prevent intraneural or intravascular needle placement or medication administration. The use of ultrasound has drastically changed the application and reliability of peripheral nerve blocks. With ultrasound, the ability to observe the nerve location and the surrounding vascular, muscular, bony, and visceral structures allows for less dependence on variable external landmarks. Real-time visualization of needle movement and injectate administration allows for increased precision and safety with needle and medication placement. Combining ultrasound and PNS can be useful for patients with abnormal or difficult anatomy and in the setting where ultrasound image quality is limited.

B Common pain syndromes amenable to diagnosis and treatment via peripheral nerve blocks include peripheral neuralgias such as greater occipital, ilioinguinal, iliohypogastric, and meralgia paresthetica. Facial pain and headache can be treated by blockade of the various branches of the trigeminal nerve. Shoulder and hip joint pain may benefit from blockade of articular branches of peripheral nerves, as in the suprascapular nerve block for shoulder pain and in blocking of branches of the femoral and obturator nerves for hip pain. Intercostal nerve blocks are useful in the treatment of chest wall pain. The brachial plexus can be targeted at different locations for upper extremity analgesia, while the femoral and sciatic nerves can specifically be blocked for regional analgesia of the lower extremity. Medial branch blocks are used to provide analgesia for pain originating from the facet joints.

C Various local anesthetics can be used depending on the desired onset or duration of action. Awareness of the toxic dose for each local anesthetic is of paramount importance as the manifestation of local anesthetic toxicity is typically resistant to standard basic life support (BLS) or advanced cardiac life support (ACLS). Several different medications have been added to the local anesthetic to increase the duration, onset, or density of the peripheral nerve block. Common additives include epinephrine, sodium bicarbonate, steroids, opioids, and the alpha agonists including clonidine and dexmedetomidine. The additive's effect on the peripheral nerve block is variable on the medication class and the local anesthetic with which it is combined. When using additives, the side effects of the specific additive need to be considered in addition to the side effects of the local anesthetic.

D Continuous peripheral nerve infusions can be useful in the treatment of complex regional pain syndrome (CRPS) and phantom limb pain. One of the most common sites of continuous regional analgesia for chronic pain is the brachial plexus. Reliable analgesia can be obtained for the entire upper extremity via a single site of injection. Interscalene, supraclavicular, subclavian perivascular, infraclavicular, and axillary approaches have been described, with choice of technique usually based on the experience and familiarity of the operator. Intensive rehabilitation can be pursued during the period of analgesia if desired. Lower extremity plexus blocks, including anterior (femoral nerve) and posterior lumbar plexus blocks, and sciatic nerve blocks can also be used for CRPS and phantom pain.

Cryoablation is discussed in detail elsewhere in this book. When used for prolonged blockade of peripheral nerves, it can provide excellent analgesia with the potential for pursuing aggressive physical therapy. As this is an ablative procedure, it may cause significant numbness in the sensory distribution of the nerve or potential motor weakness.

Pulsed RF is also discussed elsewhere in this book. Its development has created a new option for providing long-term analgesia in the distribution of a peripheral nerve without destroying tissue or requiring equipment for continuous infusions.

SUGGESTED READING

Brummett CM, Williams BA. Additives to local anesthetics for peripheral nerve blockade. Int Anesthesiol Clin. 2011;49(4):104-16.

Chin KJ, Chan V. Ultrasound-guided peripheral nerve blockade. Curr Opin Anaesthesiol. 2008;21(5):624-31.

Gofeld M. Ultrasonography in pain medicine: a critical review. Pain Pract. 2008;8:226-40.

Hahn MB. Distribution of the trigeminal nerve. In: Hahn MB, McQuillan PM, Sheplock GJ (Eds). Regional Anesthesia: An Atlas of Anatomy and Techniques. St. Louis: Mosby; 1996. pp. 45-52.

Koscielniak-Nielsen ZJ. Ultrasound-guided peripheral nerve blocks: what are the benefits? Acta Anaesthesiol Scand. 2008;52(6):727-37.

Raj PP. Nerve blocks: continuous regional analgesia. In: Raj PP (Ed). Practical Management of Pain, 3rd edition. St. Louis: Mosby; 2000. pp. 710-20.

Saberski L, Fitzgerald J, Ahmad M. Cryoneurolysis and radiofrequency lesioning. In: Raj PP (Ed). Practical Management of Pain, 3rd edition. St. Louis: Mosby; 2000. pp. 753-67.

Sites BD, Spence BC, Gallagher J, et al. Regional anesthesia meets ultrasound: a specialty in transition. Acta Anaesthesiol Scand. 2008;52(4):456-66.

CHAPTER
126

Sympathetic Blocks

Lai TT, Lopez EM

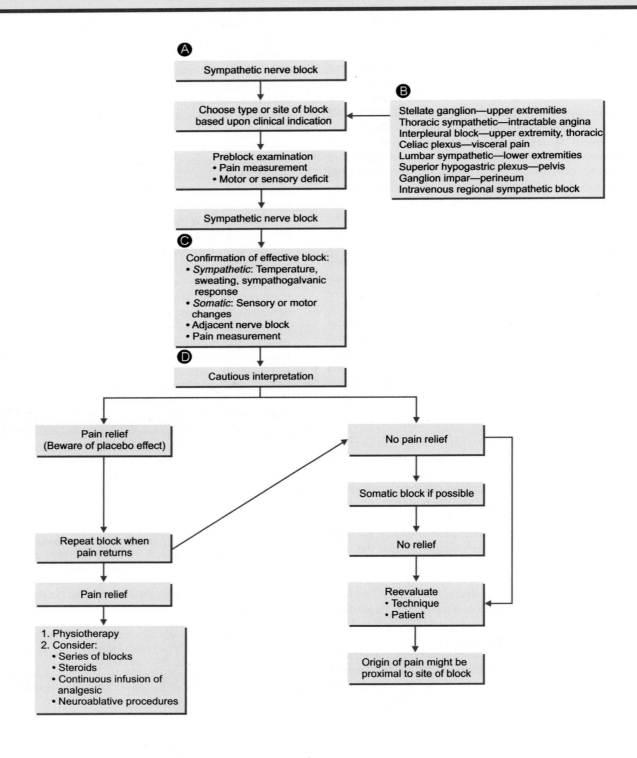

A Sympathetic nerve block

Choose type or site of block based upon clinical indication

B
Stellate ganglion—upper extremities
Thoracic sympathetic—intractable angina
Interpleural block—upper extremity, thoracic
Celiac plexus—visceral pain
Lumbar sympathetic—lower extremities
Superior hypogastric plexus—pelvis
Ganglion impar—perineum
Intravenous regional sympathetic block

Preblock examination
• Pain measurement
• Motor or sensory deficit

Sympathetic nerve block

C
Confirmation of effective block:
• *Sympathetic*: Temperature, sweating, sympathogalvanic response
• *Somatic*: Sensory or motor changes
• Adjacent nerve block
• Pain measurement

D
Cautious interpretation

Pain relief
(Beware of placebo effect)

No pain relief

Somatic block if possible

Repeat block when pain returns

No relief

Pain relief

Reevaluate
• Technique
• Patient

1. Physiotherapy
2. Consider:
   • Series of blocks
   • Steroids
   • Continuous infusion of analgesic
   • Neuroablative procedures

Origin of pain might be proximal to site of block

Substantial controversies still surround pain-relieving procedures that target the sympathetic nervous system. It is believed that sympathetic afferents may depolarize nociceptive afferent fibers at the site of nerve injury. It is also suggested that the cell bodies of sensory neurons in the dorsal root ganglion come under closer influence of sympathetic axons following nerve injury, so sympathetic activity may be capable of initiating or maintaining activity in sensory fibers. In either case, one of the main goals of sympathetic blocks is to determine how much a patient's pain is sympathetically mediated. However, even though patients may have a diagnosis of complex regional pain syndrome (CRPS) and what appears to be sympathetically-mediated pain, they may not be responsive to sympathetic blockade. Of note, sympathetically-mediated pain is defined as pain which responds to diagnostic sympathetic blocks with a 50% or more decrease in pain for the duration the anesthetic agent used.

(A) The list of indications for sympathetic blocks is long, and much of the evidence does not include randomized clinical trials. Common syndromes that are amenable to the use of sympathetic blocks include: CRPS, phantom limb pain, angina, and vascular insufficiency (i.e. Raynaud's syndrome, diabetes). The specific type of sympathetic block used depends on the location of pain.

(B) There are five commonly used sympathetic blocks: (1) stellate ganglion, (2) celiac plexus, (3) lumbar sympathetic, (4) superior hypogastric plexus, and (5) ganglion impar. It is important to understand general indications, basic anatomy and common complications for each sympathetic block.

1. Stellate ganglion block is indicated for head, neck, upper extremity and upper chest pain. The stellate ganglion is the confluence of the inferior cervical and first thoracic sympathetic ganglia. It is located between the C7-T1 vertebral levels, and injection is most often performed via a paratracheal approach. Chassaignac's tubercle (anterior tubercle of C6 transverse process) is one of the most common landmarks identified for stellate ganglion local anesthetic injection. Known complications include: pneumothorax, hoarseness (recurrent laryngeal nerve block), brachial plexus block (hemidiaphragm paralysis), hematoma, and subarachnoid or epidural block. Signs of successful blockade include Horner's syndrome (miosis, ptsosis enophthalmos, anhydrosis), nasal congestion, venodilation in ipsilateral upper extremity and increase in upper extremity temperature of at least 1.5°C.

2. Celiac plexus block is indicated for pain secondary to pancreatic cancer and other upper or middle intra-abdominal visceral malignancies. The celiac plexus is the confluence of multiple celiac ganglia and is located at the T12-L1 level just anterior to the aorta. This block is most often performed via the posterior approach (transcrural) under fluoroscopic guidance. Known complications or side effects include intravascular injection, orthostatic hypotension, diarrhea, retroperitoneal bleeding, mild kidney damage (hematuria), pneumothorax and rarely paraplegia (artery of Adamkiewicz injury). Successful blockade will usually provide almost immediate pain relief.

3. Lumbar sympathetic block is indicated for sympathetically-mediated pain in the lower extremities and pelvis. It is composed of four to five pairs of ganglia that are located at the T12-L4 levels along the anterolateral portion of the vertebral bodies bilaterally. This block is often performed via a posterior approach with the target being the anterolateral border of the vertebral bodies. A single needle injection technique is commonly employed at the L2 level, but a two needle injection technique at L2 and L4 can be performed if better caudal spread of local anesthetic is needed. Complications of this block include intravascular injection (local anesthetic toxicity), kidney injury (hematuria) and epidural/intrathecal/spinal nerve injection.

4. Superior hypogastric plexus block is indicated for pelvic viscera pain, which can cover sympathetically-mediated pain of the bladder, uterus, rectum, vagina and prostate. It is located at the anterolateral portion of the L5 vertebral bodies bilaterally and continues inferiorly to the sacrum. The injection technique used for this block mirrors an L5-S1 discography approach. Complications for this block include intravascular injection (in close proximity of the iliac vessels) and transient bladder and bowel dysfunction.

5. Ganglion impar (ganglion of Walther) block is indicated for visceral or sympathetically-mediated pain in the pelvis and perineum. It is the most caudal sympathetic ganglion (left and right ganglia fuse together) and is located just anterior to the sacrococcygeal junction. A common injection technique for this block is a midline approach through the sacrococcygeal ligament with medication injected just posterior to the rectum. Another approach is through the anococcygeal ligament with the needle advanced cephalad just anterior to the sacrum. Complications for this block include the potential for intravascular injection or rectal perforation with exposure of contaminants through the needle track resulting in abscess or fistula.

(C) Once a nerve block is performed, it is essential to confirm that the targeted nerve has been reached. It is also useful to know if an undesired block has occurred, such as blockade of an adjacent nerve. The postblock examination, at a minimum, should include assessment of temperature (a change of at least 1.5°C), sweating, and the sympathogalvanic response. Any sensory or motor change as well as a new pain measurement should be documented. The precision of sympathetic nerve blocks can be enhanced during their performance by techniques such as fluoroscopy with or without water-soluble contrast, sonography, or computed tomography guidance.

(D) Sympathetic denervation produces sudomotor, vasomotor, and ocular (stellate ganglion) changes. It leads to vasodilation, except in the trunk where vasoconstriction follows a segmental sympathetic block.

In practice, only pain relief of more than 50% should lead to a repeat block. As for any block, a result should be interpreted cautiously after a sympathetic block.

Overall, sympathetic blocks are performed to distinguish true sympathetic pain from other etiologies. Specifically, the objective is to interrupt nociceptive pathways and sympathetic vasomotor, sudomotor and visceromotor nerves, not sensory or motor nerves. This concept can be further clarified by recognizing subarachnoid and epidural blocks to provide sympathetic, sensory and motor blockade, but do not selectively differentiate sympathetically-mediated pain.

SUGGESTED READING

Buckley FP. Regional anesthesia with local anesthetic. In: Loeser JD, Butler SH, Chapman CR, Turk DC (Eds). Bonica's Management of Pain, 3rd edition. Philadelphia: Lippincott Williams & Wilkins; 2001.

Furman MB, Lee TS, Berkwits L. Atlas of Image-Guided Spinal Procedures. Philadelphia: Elsevier Saunders; 2013.

Hogan QH, Abram SE. Neural blockade for diagnosis and prognosis: a review. Anesthesiology. 1997;86(1):216-41.

Justins D, Siemaszko O. Rational use of neural blockade for the management of chronic pain. In: Giamberardino MA (Ed). Pain 2002: An Updated Review: Refresher Course Syllabus. Seattle: IASP Press; 2002.

Morgan GE, Mikhail MS, Murray MJ. Clinical Anesthesiology, 4th edition. New York: Langae Medical Books/McGraw-Hill; 2006.

Raja SN. Nerve blocks in the evaluation of chronic pain: a plea for caution in their use and interpretation. Anesthesiology. 1997;86:4-6.

Ramamurthy S, Winnie AP. Regional anesthetic techniques for pain relief. Semin Anesth. 1985;4:237.

Rathmell JP. Atlas of Image-Guided Intervention in Regional Anesthesia and Pain Medicine. Philadelphia: Wolters Kluwer/Lippincott Williams & Wilkins; 2011.

Cranial Nerve Blocks

Eckmann MS, Ramamurthy S

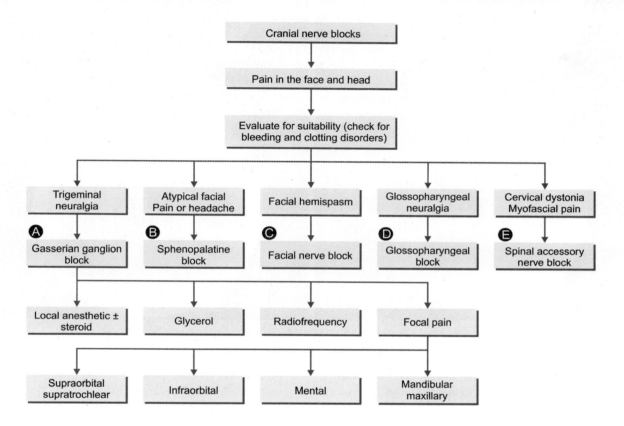

Cranial nerve blocks are utilized in the diagnosis and management of head and neck pain. While the usual precautions necessary for any local anesthetic injection are taken for these blocks, there are unique safety considerations. Arterial injection of a very small quantity of local anesthetic into a branch of the facial artery, or backflow into the middle meningeal or ophthalmic artery, can still produce seizure or blindness. By inference, embolic stroke is possible if bubbles or particles are injected intravascularly. Muscle anesthesia can produce impaired balance through loss of proprioception.

Dermatomal Distribution: Most of the face is supplied by the divisions of the trigeminal nerve. Skin over the lower part of the mandible and the lower part of the pinna of the ear is supplied by the branches of C2 (greater articular nerve). The posterior part of the top of the head is supplied by greater and lesser occipital nerves that arise from C2. The anterior two-thirds of the tongue is supplied by the lingual branch of the mandibular nerve. The posterior one-third of the tongue is supplied by the branches of the glossopharyngeal nerve.

The third, fourth, and sixth cranial nerves supply the muscles of the eye. The third cranial nerve carries sympathetic and parasympathetic fibers. These nerves are blocked during the retrobulbar block performed for ophthalmic surgery. The vagus and the cranial portion of the accessory nerve together innervate the mucosa and the muscles of the pharynx and the larynx. The spinal portion of the accessory nerve innervates the sternocleidomastoid and the trapezius muscles. Block of this nerve is useful during neck and shoulder surgery and in the management of cervical dystonia.

Ⓐ *Trigeminal Block:* The Gasserian ganglion can be blocked with local anesthetic and steroids to diagnose and stabilize trigeminal-mediated pain, while glycerol or radiofrequency techniques offer neurolytic options in the management of refractory trigeminal neuralgia. These procedures usually require a declined oblique fluoroscopic view (**Fig. 1**) or computerized tomography (CT) guidance to accurately access the foramen ovale and cavum trigeminale. The terminal branches such as

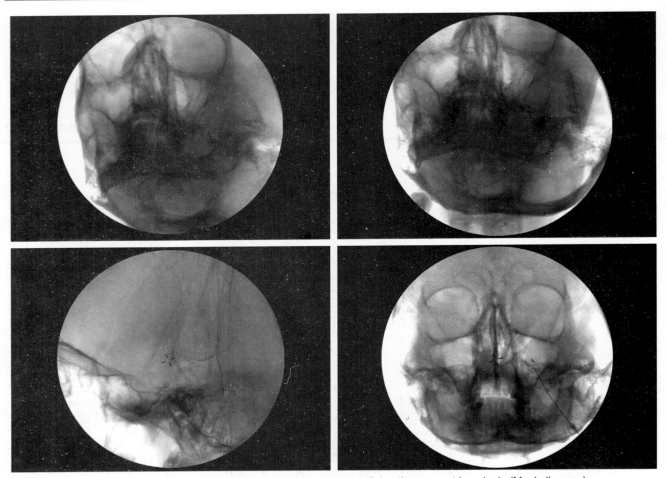

Fig. 1: Fluoroscopically-guided Gasserian ganglion block with contrast outlining the cavum trigeminale (Meckel's cave)

supraorbital, supratrochlear, infraorbital, and mental branches are blocked when pain distribution is very focal or there is history of local trauma; blind and ultrasound-guided techniques are sufficient. The mandibular nerve can be blocked in a variety of approaches (most commonly through the coronoid notch) near the foramen ovale and lateral pterygoid plate, either blindly or with fluoroscopic guidance, while the maxillary nerve can be blocked via the pterygomaxillary fissure in an infrazygomatic ultrasound window or with fluoroscopy **(Fig. 2)**. These nerves also can be blocked transorally and through the greater palatine foramen. The auriculotemporal nerve is blocked to relieve the pain originating from the temporo-mandibular joint.

B *Sphenopalatine Ganglion Block:* This ganglion can be blocked in three different ways. The most common method is to block it through the nose using local anesthetic-soaked cotton swabs through the nose and placing them in contact with the nasopharyngeal wall just posterior to the middle turbinate. Percutaneously the ganglion can be blocked through the coronoid notch and by directing the needle just anterior to the lateral pterygoid plate into the pterygomaxillary fissure. Transorally the needle is placed

through the greater palatine foramen and advancing that needle into the pterygopalatine fossa. Block of the sphenopalatine ganglion is useful in the treatment of atypical facial pain and persistent headache syndromes; it also can be a target for pulsed radiofrequency or electrical neuromodulation.

C *Facial Nerve Block:* This nerve can be blocked as it exits from the stylomastoid foramen. A needle is advanced along the anterior surface of the mastoid process connected to a nerve stimulator until contraction of the facial muscles is noted. Two to three milliliters of local anesthetic will produce a block. This nerve block is useful in patients who have hemifacial spasms.

D *Glossopharyngeal Nerve:* The 11th cranial nerve can be blocked transorally at the base of the posterior tonsillar pillar. Percutaneously the nerve can be blocked by advancing a needle just anterior to the mastoid process and redirecting the needle posteriorly after contacting the styloid process. The needle tip is very close to the carotid artery and the jugular vein. The vagus nerve is also blocked. This block is useful in the diagnosis of glossopharyngeal neuralgia. Fluoroscopy and/or ultrasound can assist in block placement.

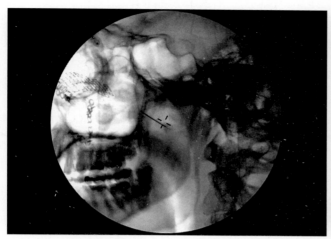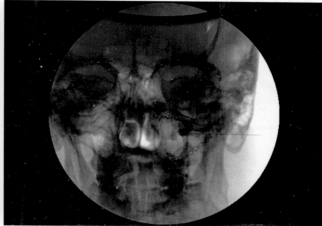

Fig. 2: Fluoroscopically-guided maxillary nerve block in a patient with prior facial trauma and fixation

E *Spinal Accessory Nerve:* This nerve is blocked by injecting 5 mL of local anesthetic into the proximal portion of the sternocleidomastoid muscle. This block can relieve myofascial pain and spasm in the trapezius muscle. It can also augment surgical conditions for awake shoulder surgery in combination with interscalene block.

SUGGESTED READING

Bedder MD, Lindsay D. Glossopharyngeal nerve block using ultrasound guidance: a case report of a new technique. Reg Anesth. 1989;14(6):304-7.

Elahi F, Reddy CG. Sphenopalatine ganglion electrical nerve stimulation implant for intractable facial pain. Pain Physician. 2015;18(3):E403-9.

Nader A, Kendall MC, De Oliveria GS, et al. Ultrasound-guided trigeminal nerve block via the pterygopalatine fossa: an effective treatment for trigeminal neuralgia and atypical facial pain. Pain Physician. 2013;16(5):E537-45.

Park HL, Lim SM, Kim TH, et al. Intractable hemifacial spasm treated by pulsed radiofrequency treatment. Korean J Pain. 2013; 26(1):62-4.

Ramamurthy S, Akkineni SR, Winnie AP. A simple technic for block of the spinal accessory nerve. Anesth Analg. 1978;57(5): 591-3.

Rosenberg M, Phero JC. Regional anesthesia and invasive techniques to manage head and neck pain. Otolaryngol Clin North Am. 2003;36(6):1201-19.

Uckan S, Cilasun U, Erkman O. Rare ocular and cutaneous complication of inferior alveolar nerve block. J Oral Maxillofac Surg. 2006;64(4):719-21.

CHAPTER 128

Intravenous Regional Analgesia

Naylor KJ, Anitescu M

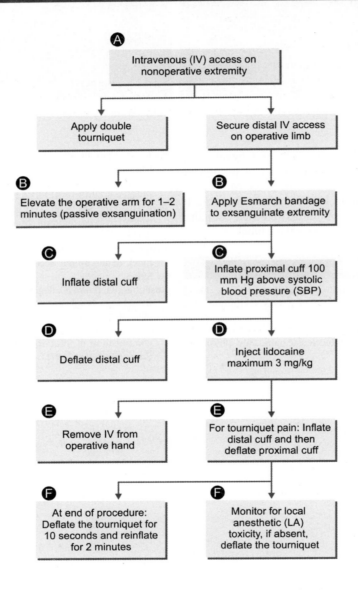

Intravenous regional analgesia (IVRA) was introduced by August Karl Gustav Bier in 1908, the father of regional anesthesia. It is now used for procedures on the extremities of less than 60 minutes duration and to treat complex regional pain syndrome (CRPS) and hyperhidrosis.

After IVRA fell out of popularity in anesthesia for almost 60 years, it was revived by Holmes in 1963 when the Bier block was once again reintroduced into clinical practice. Although effective as an anesthetic technique, IVRA to treat neuropathic pain in CRPS remained controversial. In CRPS, the sympathetic nervous system is dysfunctional, and sympatholytics given via IVRA have been tried as treatment. Bier blocks were therefore performed with local anesthetics, guanethidine (inhibitor of presynaptic release of norepinephrine), reserpine (inhibitor of norepinephrine synthesis and depletion of its stores), droperidol (alpha-adrenergic agonist), ketanserin (serotonin type 2 receptor antagonist), lidocaine and methylprednisolone. Studies compared results with IVRA to results with placebo and other techniques (stellate ganglion blocks or lumbar sympathetic blocks). Compared to placebo, lidocaine increased the duration of action of the regional block but did not modify the peak effect of sympathetic chain blocks.

To limit the systemic toxicity of local anesthetics, IVRA is performed after application of a tourniquet to the affected limb. To limit tourniquet pain, the technique is used for anesthesia in procedures lasting less than 1 hour. The local anesthetic commonly used in IVRA is lidocaine. Resuscitation equipment as well as immediate availability of lipid emulsion is mandatory.

During IVRA the local anesthetic is diffused via the vascular bed to the surrounding nerves. Tourniquet ischemia leading to hypothermia and acidosis enhances local anesthetic activity.

TECHNIQUE

A A double-cuffed tourniquet is used on the proximal part of the operative extremity. Two intravenous (IV) catheters are placed, one in the operative extremity to deliver the local anesthetic for the Bier block and another in the nonoperative extremity to deliver analgesic medications if needed for tourniquet pain or rescue medication in the event of complications from the procedure such as local anesthetic toxicity.

B Next the operative arm is exsanguinated. To do this, the physician raises the arm above the patient's head for 60 seconds and an Esmarch bandage is wrapped tightly around the extremity. If the blood left in the operative extremity dilutes the local anesthetic the block may be ineffective.

C The distal cuff is then inflated before the proximal cuff to 100 mm Hg above systolic blood pressure. Absence of an arterial pulse is confirmed before deflation of the distal cuff.

D Local anesthetic is injected slowly to a total dose of 3 mg/kg of 0.5% lidocaine without epinephrine (usually, 30 mL of 0.5% lidocaine for the upper extremity and 50 mg for lower extremity).

E Deflating the proximal cuff while inflating the distal cuff provides immediate relief of tourniquet pain and 15–30 minutes of additional analgesia.

F To avoid local anesthetic toxicity, the tourniquet is left inflated for a minimum of 20 minutes. Once the procedure is complete, the tourniquet is loosened in 10 second intervals and reinflated for 2 minutes.

Forearm tourniquets have been used with success for IVRA. In some studies, there was less pain than with traditional arm tourniquets and local anesthetic dose was reduced by 50% with equal effect.

In the treatment of CRPS, results with IVRA vary. Long-term relief has not been achieved, but IVRA is attempted when other modalities of treatment have not been successful.

POTENTIAL COMPLICATIONS AND SPECIAL CONSIDERATIONS

Contraindications to IVRA are Raynaud's disease, crush injuries, homozygous sickle cell disease, young age, skin infections on operative extremity, severe peripheral vascular disease, allergy to local anesthetic, severe hepatic insufficiency, atrioventricular shunts, and inadequate or unreliable tourniquets.

Complications associated with IVRA are: local anesthetic toxicity, hematoma, extremity engorgement, compartment syndrome, ecchymosis and hemorrhage.

Seizures have been reported with as little as 1.4 mg/kg of lidocaine, 4 mg/kg for prilocaine and 1.3 mg/kg of bupivacaine and with a tourniquet time up to 60 minutes. Cardiac arrest has resulted from 2.5 mg/kg of lidocaine and 1.6 mg/kg of bupivacaine.

ADJUNCTS TO BIER BLOCK

The addition of 1 mg of butorphanol to 3 mg/kg lidocaine prolonged the duration of postoperative analgesia and reduced narcotic consumption during the first 24 hours postoperatively compared to lidocaine alone.

Adding 50 µg/kg midazolam to 3 mg/kg lidocaine 2% diluted with saline to a total volume of 40 mL shortened onset time and prolonged sensory and motor recovery time. Intraoperative pain scores were lower and fentanyl use was less than by patients receiving plain lidocaine alone.

In a study of 24 patients, a single cuff tourniquet on the forearm resulted in less pain, narcotic use, and need for deep sedation compared to a single cuff tourniquet placed on the upper arm.

CONCLUSION

Intravenous regional blocks can be used as anesthetics in select cases. There is less support for such blocks in patients with sympathetically maintained neuropathic pain. In select chronic cases with refractory and severe pain, blocks should be carefully considered.

SUGGESTED READING

Bansal A, Gupta S, Sood D, et al. Bier's block using lignocaine and butorphanol. J Anaesthesiol Clin Pharmacol. 2011;27(4):465-9.

Barry LA, Balliana SA, Galeppi AC. Intravenous regional anesthesia (Bier block). Tech Reg Anesth Pain Manag. 2006;10(3):123-31.

Chiao FB, Chen J, Lesser JB, et al. Single-cuff forearm tourniquet in intravenous regional anaesthesia results in less pain and fewer sedation requirements than upper arm tourniquet. Br J Anaesth. 2013;111(2):271-5.

Defense and Veterans Center for Integrative Pain Management (DVCIPM). (2015). Bier Block. [online] Available from *www.dvcipm.org/files/maraa-book/chapt23.pdf*. [Accessed February, 2017].

dos Reis A. Eulogy to August Karl Gustav Bier on the 100th anniversary of intravenous regional block and the 110th anniversary of the spinal block. Rev Bras Anestesiol. 2008;58(4):409-24.

Guay J. Adverse events associated with intravenous regional anesthesia (Bier block): a systematic review of complications. J Clin Anesth. 2009;21(8):585-94.

Honarmand A, Safavi M, Nemati K, et al. The efficacy of different doses of Midazolam added to Lidocaine for upper extremity Bier block on the sensory and motor block characteristics and postoperative pain. J Res Pharm Pract. 2015;4(3):160-6.

Matt CM. Intravenous regional anaesthesia. Anaesth Intensive Care Med. 2007;8(4):137-9.

The New York School of Regional Anesthesia (NYSORA). (2013). Bier Block. [online] Available from *www.nysora.com/techniques/3071-bier-block.html*. [Accessed February, 2017].

Tran DQ, Duong S, Bertini P, et al. Treatment of complex regional pain syndrome: a review of the evidence. Can J Anaesth. 2010;57(2):149-66.

Vlassakov KV, Bhavani K. The forearm tourniquet Bier block. Logic and authority versus science and experience. Minerva Anestesiol. 2010;76(2):91-2.

CHAPTER 129

Intravenous Infusion Therapy in Chronic Pain States

Sudhakaran S, Anitescu M

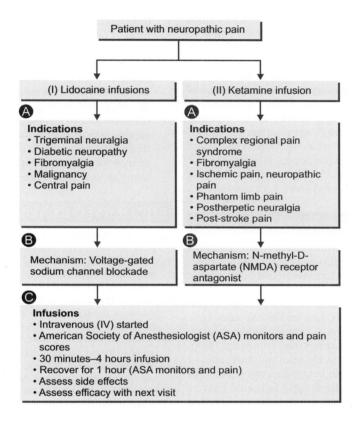

Intravenous infusion therapy is an effective treatment for pain syndromes such as fibromyalgia, neuropathic pain, phantom limb pain, and complex regional pain syndrome. Intravenous infusions are not a primary method for analgesia, but are adjunct therapy to minimize the severity of debilitating chronic pain states. There are currently no universal guidelines in place for intravenous (IV) infusions for chronic pain. We consider two anesthetic agents for infusion: (1) lidocaine and (2) ketamine.

LIDOCAINE

Ⓐ *History and Indications*: Lidocaine was the first amino-amide local anesthetic discovered and was first isolated by Nils Lofgren in 1943. IV lidocaine infusions gained popularity in the early 1960s with evidence that the infusion minimized opioid requirements after bowel surgery. By minimizing postoperative opioid requirements lidocaine improved the return of bowel function. Over the next 20 years, lidocaine usage decreased because of concerns about cardiac and neurologic toxicity. Other analgesics

were safer. In the 1980s, evidence mounted for use of lidocaine in patients with chronic pain.

Evidence exists today for the efficacy of lidocaine infusions in patients with trigeminal neuralgia, diabetic neuropathy, fibromyalgia, pain from malignancy and central pain.

Ⓑ *Mechanism*: Lidocaine's sodium channel blockade works in the peripheral and central nervous system. It affects nociceptors associated with the initiation and maintenance of hyperalgesia. Lidocaine inhibits generation of spontaneous impulses from the dorsal root ganglion and suppresses afferent spinal cord reflexes.

Ectopic discharge of injured nerves mediates neuropathic pain. Nerve injury and inflammation activate and proliferate voltage-gated sodium channels. In animal models, IV treatment with lidocaine suppressed spontaneous discharge. The plasma concentration of lidocaine required for analgesic effect is lower than the concentration to inhibit nerve conduction.

Ⓒ *Infusion Technique*: Since lidocaine is also an anti-arrhythmic medication, a baseline electrocardiogram

(ECG) is recommended in all patients considered for lidocaine infusion. Patients with electrocardiographic changes or electrolyte abnormalities are not given lidocaine infusions. Standard American Society of Anesthesiologist (ASA) monitors (blood pressure, heart rate, telemetry, pulse oximetry, capnography) are applied before infusion and monitored every 5 minutes for the duration of the infusion, usually 30 minutes. A small (22 or 24 gauge) IV catheter is placed. Dosing is usually initiated with a bolus before continuous infusion. A bolus dose is 1–2 mg/kg followed by an infusion of 2–4 mg/kg over 30 minutes. Pain scores are also monitored every 5 minutes during the infusion. Vital signs are monitored every 15 minutes for an additional 60 minutes after the infusion is stopped. Similarly, pain scores on numerical rating scale are solicited every 15 minutes. The patient is also assessed for signs and symptoms of toxicity. Some initial symptoms are tinnitus, circumoral numbness, changes in vision and dizziness. Toxicity can progress to tonic-clonic seizures, loss of consciousness and respiratory arrest. For safety, a lipid emulsion and resuscitation equipment should be readily available. Response to treatment is evaluated at a subsequent office visit. If effective (more than 50% pain relief), infusions can be repeated every 4–12 weeks.

KETAMINE

Ⓐ *History and Indications:* Ketamine is indicated for complex regional pain syndrome, fibromyalgia, ischemic pain, neuropathic pain, phantom limb pain and postherpetic neuralgia.

Developed in 1962, ketamine gained widespread use during the Vietnam War as a battlefield anesthetic because of its short half-life and hemodynamic stability. IV ketamine has analgesic properties in central pain, allodynia and hyperalgesia with minimal side effects. In patients with fibromyalgia, ketamine reduced central sensitization. In patients with chronic ischemic pain or with resting lower extremity pain, ketamine provided dose-dependent analgesia. An IV infusion of ketamine increased the pressure pain threshold and reduced hyperpathia in patients with phantom limb pain. It reduced allodynia and decreased hyperpathia in conditions of postherpetic neuralgia.

Ⓑ *Mechanism:* Ketamine has multiple effector sites including N-methyl-D-aspartate (NMDA) antagonism, weak agonism of the opioid receptor, sodium (Na) channel antagonism, calcium (Ca) channel antagonism, and inhibition of serotonin/dopamine/norepinephrine reuptake. Glutamate is an excitatory neurotransmitter in central pain pathways. It binds to NMDA and α-amino-3-hydroxy-5-methyl-4-isoxazolepropionic acid (AMPA) receptors to open multiple ionotropic channels. Ketamine mitigates chronic pain by antagonism of the NMDA receptor through prevention of central sensitization in the dorsal horn of the spinal cord. Ketamine infusions are particularly effective in NMDA receptor upregulation during the wind-up phenomenon of neuropathic pain in complex regional pain syndrome. Ketamine is not used in patients with increased intracranial pressure or history of psychoses.

Ⓒ *Infusion:* Patients are premedicated with 2 mg of IV midazolam to minimize the risk of psychomimetic side effects, with ondansetron to minimize nausea and with glycopyrrolate to prevent secretions. Standard ASA monitors (blood pressure, heart rate, telemetry, pulse oximetry, capnography) are applied and measured every 5 minutes during the infusions. IV infusion lasts for 30 minutes up to 4 hours, depending on the protocol. At our institution we initiate infusion at a dose of 0.2 mg/kg over 30 minutes. Monitoring of vital signs and pain scores is continued for an additional 60 minutes after the infusion is stopped. On subsequent visits, the dose can be titrated up to a maximum of 0.5–1 mg/kg in 0.2–0.4 mg/kg increments depending on the response to treatment. Patients are frequently assessed for side effects and adverse events. Common reactions are hypertension, sedation, dysphoria and hallucinations. If side effects are observed during the infusion, the intervention is discontinued to let the patient recover. The effect of the ketamine infusion is evaluated on subsequent clinic visits. If effective without side effects, infusions can be repeated every 4–12 weeks. Repeating ketamine infusions at shorter intervals may predispose the patient to tachyphylaxis.

SUGGESTED READING

Bartlett EE, Hutserani O. Xylocaine for the relief of postoperative pain. Anesth Analg. 1961;40:296-304.

Edwards WT, Habib F, Burney RG, et al. Intravenous lidocaine in the management of various chronic pain states: a review of 211 cases. Reg Anesth Pain Med. 1985;10(1):1-6.

Fanaee E, Anitescu M, Patil S. Sustained pain relief after lidocaine infusions for chronic pain syndromes: a retrospective analysis. Anesthesiology. 2010;113:A301.

Groudine SB, Fisher HA, Kaufman RP, et al. Intravenous lidocaine speeds the return of bowel function, decreases postoperative pain, and shortens hospital stay in patients undergoing radical retropubic prostatectomy. Anesth Analg. 1998;86(2):235-9.

Hocking G, Cousins MJ. Ketamine in chronic pain management: an evidence-based review. Anesth Analg. 2003;97(6):1730-9.

Koppert W, Weigand M, Neumann F, et al. Perioperative intravenous lidocaine has preventive effects on postoperative pain and morphine consumption after major abdominal surgery. Anesth Analg. 2004;98(4):1050-5.

Mao J, Chen LL. Systemic lidocaine for neuropathic pain relief. Pain. 2000;87(1):7-17.

Marmura MJ. Intravenous lidocaine and mexiletine in the management of trigeminal autonomic cephalalgias. Curr Pain Headache Rep. 2010;14(2):145-50.

Miyasaka M, Domino EF. Neural mechanisms of ketamine-induced anesthesia. Int J Neuropharmacol. 1968;7(6):557-73.

O'Connell NE, Wand BM, McAuley J, et al. Interventions for treating pain and disability in adults with complex regional pain syndrome. Cochrane Database Syst Rev. 2013;(4):CD009416.

Patil S, Anitescu M. Efficacy of outpatient ketamine infusions in refractory chronic pain syndromes: a 5-year retrospective analysis. Pain Med. 2012;13(2):263-9.

Rabben T, Skjelbred, P, Oye I. Prolonged analgesic effect of ketamine, an N-methyl-D-aspartate receptor inhibitor, in patients with chronic pain. J Pharmacol Exp Ther. 1999;289(2):1060-6.

Schwartzman RJ, Alexander GM, Grothusen JR, et al. Outpatient intravenous ketamine for the treatment of complex regional pain syndrome: a double-blind placebo controlled study. Pain. 2009;147(1-3):107-15.

Continuous Neural Block

Mitchell B, William JG

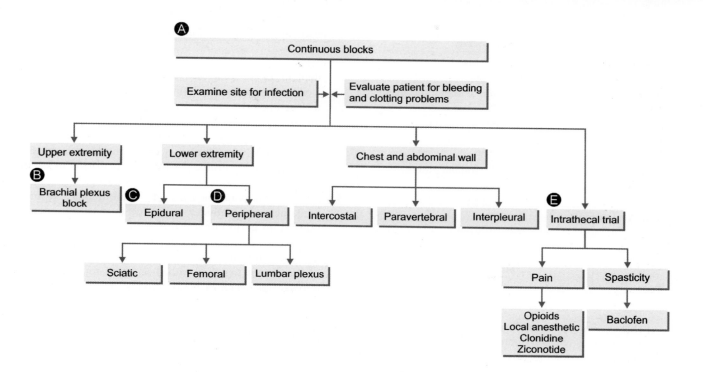

There has been significant improvement in technology and safety of continuous neural blockade. The availability of insulated Tuohy needles, stimulating catheters, nerve stimulators, fluoroscopy and ultrasound all have served to increase safety and accuracy of catheter placement. Ultrasound has emerged as an invaluable tool for nerve localization during regional anesthesia, improving safety, reducing procedure times, and improving patient satisfaction scores when compared to nerve stimulation. As with any interventional procedure, the patient must be evaluated for bleeding or clotting abnormalities prior to the procedure, which can be secondary to a disease process or pharmacotherapy. Additionally, the procedure site should be inspected carefully for any signs of infection. Some clinicians elect to utilize prophylactic antibiotics prior to the procedure to further minimize infection risk.

There are various models of convenient, portable infusion pumps that are available including battery-operated models and constant flow, balloon-type infusers.

A *Indications*: Typically, continuous peripheral nerve block is indicated for expected moderate to severe pain lasting longer than 24 hours. These procedures are commonly

used in the perioperative period; and, their use has been documented in the treatment of intractable hiccups, vasospasm of Raynaud's disease, peripheral embolism, chronic regional pain syndrome (CRPS), intractable phantom limb pain, terminal cancer, and trigeminal neuralgia. While a local anesthetic block can provide short-term, effective pain relief, placing a catheter can provide more long-term analgesia leading to longer interruption of the pain cycle and decreased opioid use (and thus adverse events). Additionally, a continuous nerve block may provide effective analgesia to optimize time spent in physical therapy. Based on the particular regional anesthetic field targeted, a variety of approaches can be utilized safely to provide sufficient analgesia **(Table 1)**. These techniques can also be employed with epidural and intrathecal trials with opioids, local anesthetics, or clonidine for analgesia as well as baclofen for spasticity.

B *Brachial Plexus Block*: Continuous interscalene, infra-clavicular, or axillary techniques can provide effective analgesia for upper extremity pain. These techniques are commonly utilized to provide prolonged, postoperative

Table 1: Catheter locations

Surgical site	Major approaches
Head	Mandibular and maxillary nerves
Shoulder and proximal humerus	Interscalene Cervical paravertebral Intersternocleidomastoid Supraclavicular
Elbow, forearm, and hand	Supraclavicular Infraclavicular Axillary Median nerve
Thorax and breast	Paravertebral Intercostal
Abdomen, iliac crest, and inguinal region	Transversus abdominis plane
Hip and thigh	Posterior lumbar plexus Femoral Parasacral
Knee and thigh	Posterior lumbar plexus Femoral Fascia iliaca
Leg, ankle, and foot	Parasacral Labat and Raj Subgluteal Popliteal Tibial nerve Femoral

Table 2: Common continuous infusion doses of epidural opioids

Analgesic	Continuous infusion dose/rate
Fentanyl	25–100 µg/hr
Sufentanil	10–20 µg/hr
Alfentanil	0.2 mg/hr
Morphine	0.1–1 mg/hr
Hydromorphone	0.1–0.2 mg/hr
Meperidine	10–60 mg/hr
Methadone	0.2–0.5 mg/hr

analgesia. Patients who have CRPS may also benefit significantly when the pain cycle is interrupted and analgesia is provided for physical therapy. After the initial block, a rate of 6–8 mL/hour of local anesthetic is usually sufficient to maintain analgesia.

C *Peripheral Nerve Blocks:* The continuous block of the femoral and/or sciatic nerves or lumbar plexus is commonly utilized for the management of lower extremity pain. A sciatic nerve catheter can be placed utilizing parasacral, lateral, and popliteal approaches. The femoral and lateral femoral cutaneous nerves are blocked using either 3-in-1 block or fascia iliaca approach. An infusion of a weak local anesthetic at a rate of 6–10 mL/hour is commonly used. Continuous intercostal, paravertebral, and intrapleural blocks are useful to provide analgesia over the chest and the abdominal wall.

D *Epidural Block:* Continuous epidural block is the most common technique used for the management of lower extremity, abdominal, and thoracic pain in the postoperative period. Thoracic epidural catheters are effective for management of thoracic and abdominal pain whereas lumbar catheters are effective for the management of lower extremity pain. With the catheter placed at the proper level, a 5–8 mL/hour rate of local anesthetic with an opioid provides excellent analgesia over a long period of time. The specific dose of the infusion will depend on the analgesic choice **(Table 2)**. This may also facilitate better participation with physical therapy during the postoperative period. The patient should be monitored for complications such as respiratory depression, muscle weakness, pressure sores (secondary to sensory loss), hypotension (secondary to sympathetic block), urinary retention, and pruritus. For hygienic reasons, the sacral epidural technique is not commonly utilized.

E *Spinal (Subarachnoid):* A continuous spinal (subarachnoid) catheter technique is most commonly utilized for an intrathecal trial with opioids or baclofen before considering the patient for permanent placement of an intrathecal infusion system. An appropriate dose of the opioid together with 3–5 mg of ropivacaine or bupivacaine over a 24-hour period is commonly utilized. A continuous trial with opioids or baclofen over 3–4 days seems to provide more useful information than single-shot, spinal opioid or baclofen. The patient should be monitored for complications such as respiratory depression or arrest, pruritus, sedation, nausea, vomiting, urinary retention, generalized muscle rigidity, seizure, myoclonus, hyperalgesia, and neurotoxicity. When compared to epidural administration, the intrathecal route has lower dose requirements and less systemic effects, however, it carries with it increased risk of neural injury, spinal headaches, and supraspinal distribution of medication.

SUGGESTED READING

Brookes J, Sondekoppam R, Armstrong K, et al. Comparative evaluation of the visibility and block characteristics of a stimulating needle and catheter vs an echogenic needle and catheter for sciatic nerve block with a low-frequency ultrasound probe. Br J Anaesth. 2015;115(6):912-9.

Hanna M, Ouanes J, Tomas V. Postoperative pain and other acute pain syndromes. In: Benzon H, Rathmell JP, Wu CL, Turk DC, Argoff CE, Hurley RW (Eds). Practical Management of Pain, 5th edition. Philadelphia: Elsevier Saunders; 2014. pp. 271-97.

Ilfeld B, Mariano E. Intrathecal opioid injections for postoperative pain. In: Benzon H, Raja SN, Fishman SM, Liu S, Cohen SP (Eds). Essentials of Pain Medicine, 3rd edition. Philadelphia: Elsevier Saunders; 2011. pp. 234-7.

Ilfeld BM. Continuous peripheral nerve blocks: a review of the published evidence. Anesth Analg. 2011;113(4):904-25.

Murphy J, Gelfand H, Wu C. Epidural opioids for postoperative pain. In: Benzon H, Raja SN, Fishman SM, Liu S, Cohen SP (Eds). Essentials of Pain Medicine, 3rd edition. Philadelphia: Elsevier Saunders; 2011. pp. 223-7.

Murphy J, Gelfand H, Wu C. Intrathecal opioid injections for postoperative pain. In: Benzon H, Raja SN, Fishman SM, Liu S, Cohen SP (Eds). Essentials of Pain Medicine, 3rd edition. Philadelphia: Elsevier Saunders; 2011. pp. 217-22.

Nanney A, Muro K, Levy R. Implanted drug delivery systems for the control of chronic pain. In: Benzon H, Raja SN, Fishman SM, Liu S, Cohen SP (Eds). Essentials of Pain Medicine, 3rd edition. Philadelphia: Elsevier Saunders; 2011. pp. 451-61.

Neal JM, Brull R, Horn JL, et al. The Second American Society of Regional Anesthesia and Pain Medicine Evidence-Based Medicine Assessment of Ultrasound-Guided Regional Anesthesia: Executive Summary. Reg Anesth Pain Med. 2016; 41(2):181-94.

CHAPTER 131

Intra-Articular Steroid Injections

Bartlett JJ, Goff BJ

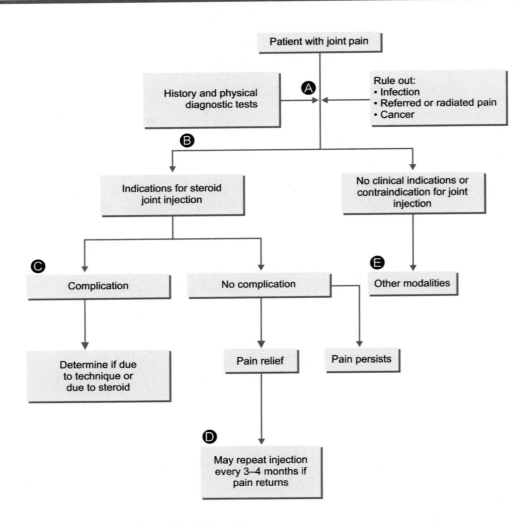

INDICATIONS FOR USE

Ⓐ Corticosteroid intra-articular joint injections have been used routinely to treat joint pain since the 1950s with demonstrated clinical efficacy in both inflammatory and noninflammatory arthritides. The use of steroid injections decreases inflammation and pain. This can speed recovery and enable the return to normal daily activities by decreasing pain sufficiently to allow a patient to begin a physical rehabilitation program that strengthens the musculature and alleviates future symptoms. Steroid injections may also be indicated when oral medications, including nonsteroidal anti-inflammatory drugs (NSAIDs) and other conservative therapies have failed, or are contraindicated. At that time, repeated intra-articular injections may provide episodic pain and symptom relief. Injections can be therapeutic or diagnostic or both. Patients may get immediate relief if a local anesthetic is added to the injection and the injection is correctly placed. The steroid begins to work after 1–2 days and reaches maximum effectiveness in 5–7 days. These injections may also help to determine the source of pain as articular or extra-articular. Additionally, patients may experience pain relief from other inflamed joints for a brief time.

PROPERTIES OF CORTICOSTEROIDS

Corticosteroids have glucocorticoid, anti-inflammatory, and mineralocorticoid activity. Steroids also produce immuno-suppressive effects in humans. The anti-inflammatory effects of steroids are produced by the inhibition of prostaglandin synthesis, collagenase formation, and granulation tissue formation. On a cellular level, steroids work at the nucleus by altering transcription in cells that contribute to inflammation such as lymphocytes, macrophages, and mast cells. Steroids reduce phagocytosis, lysosomal activity and the release of inflammatory mediators thereby reducing inflammatory pain and alleviating symptoms. Using intra-articular steroid injections provides the positive benefits of oral steroids while avoiding or reducing the majority of systemic effects such as skin thinning, peptic ulceration and increasing blood glucose because a significant portion of the steroid load remains in the joint.

CHOICE OF STEROID

Several corticosteroid agents are suitable for joint injections. Potency, onset, duration of action, and side effects should be considered before injection. **Table 1** provides details which may help to guide agent selection. The anti-inflammatory potency is relative to the potency of hydrocortisone and the dose depends on the size of the joint to be injected. Based on chemical structure alone, the duration of effect is usually inversely proportional to the solubility of the steroid. Few studies exist to delineate the efficacy of one agent over another. A 2014 study cited here evaluated the relative efficacy of various corticosteroids and found the use of triamcinolone hexacetonide may be favored over methylprednisolone for knee arthritis based on faster onset of action (level of evidence: 1B); in juvenile idiopathic arthritis patients for knee, wrist and ankle injections, there is evidence for using triamcinolone hexacetonide in favor of other corticosteroids based on longer duration of remission and possibly faster onset of action (level of evidence: 1B); and triamcinolone acetonide and methylprednisolone seem to be equally efficacious for knee and shoulder injections (level of evidence: 1B). In most cases, the choice of steroid is often driven by the personal preference of the provider.

LOCAL ANESTHETIC ADDITIVES

Amide-type local anesthetics are often combined with steroids for joint injections both as a diagnostic tool and to provide the patient with immediate relief of symptoms. Many clinicians believe that an immediate anesthetic response achieved by a local agent confirms proper placement while others feel this local agent dilutes potency of the steroid injection. Regardless, it is unclear whether this process has any impact on the effect of the steroid. Local anesthetics are postulated to provide relief through suppression of nociceptive discharge, blockade of the sympathetic reflex arc, blockade of axonal transport, blockade of sensitization, and anti-inflammatory effects. Bupivacaine is the most commonly used local anesthetic because it is more potent and has a longer duration of action than lidocaine. Ropivacaine, a newer amide local anesthetic, has similar potency but fewer cardiotoxic effects than bupivacaine. Ropivacaine has greater anesthetic potency and greater central nervous system toxicity than lidocaine. Additionally, ropivacaine appears to have less cytotoxicity than either which might make it the best option for cartilage-sparing effects inside joints. All of the local anesthetics can be used admixed with epinephrine to prolong their duration of action by up to 50%. It is imperative that the provider be aware of the maximum safe dose of a local anesthetic both with and without epinephrine. Contraindications to local anesthetic include hypersensitivity to any amide-type local anesthetic, rare anaphylactic allergy or delayed-type hypersensitivity to local anesthetics and local sepsis and coagulopathy are relative contraindications. For preparations with epinephrine, an additional relative contraindication includes patients also receiving monoamine oxidase inhibitors or tricyclic antidepressants due to possible severe prolonged hypertension.

CONTRAINDICATIONS

Contraindications to intra-articular joint injections include overlying soft tissue infection, bacteremia, articular instability, septic arthritis, avascular necrosis, osteonecrosis, neurotrophic joints, anatomic inaccessibility, known hypersensitivity to an intra-articular agent, unstable coagulopathy and patient refusal. Steroid injection in the Charcot joint provides short-term relief only. A surgical prosthetic joint is more prone

Table 1: Characteristics of corticosteroids

Characteristic	Methylprednisolone (Depo-Medrol)	Hydrocortisone (Cortisol)	Prednisolone (Hydeltra)	Triamcinolone (Aristospan)	Betamethasone (Celestone)
Anti-inflammatory potency	5	1	4	5	25
Salt retention property	0	2+	1+	0	0
Onset	Slow	Fast	Fast	Moderate	Fast
Duration of action	Intermediate	Short	Intermediate	Intermediate	Long
Plasma half-life (min)	180	90	200	300	300
Concentration (mg/mL)	40–80	50	20	20	6
Usual dose (mg)	10–40	25–100	10–40	5–20	1.5–6.0

0: no salt retention

to infection than a normal joint and, therefore, is a relative contraindication for steroid injection.

PERFORMING THE INJECTION

B The clinician performing the injection should have a thorough knowledge of the pharmacology of steroids, local anesthetics and a detailed knowledge of the anatomic basis of the procedure. Aseptic techniques should be respected at all times. Image guidance should be used for intra-articular steroid injections whenever possible due to the high rate of injections shown not to be intra-articular in cadaver sections after being performed without image guidance by experienced injectors. The site of injection under ultrasound guidance or fluoroscopic guidance should be selected by correlating computed tomographic or magnetic resonance imaging with clinical symptoms when appropriate. Correct needle positioning can be confirmed by fluoroscopic imaging and often the injection of a small amount of iodinated contrast material. The contrast fills the targeted space when positioned properly. Immediate pain relief following the procedure is diagnostic of a problem at the site of injection and predicts a successful action of the anesthetic and longer lasting relief from the steroid in 1–2 days.

A joint injection is done from the extensor surface where the synovium is closest to the skin. This minimizes the chance of injecting materials into arteries, veins, and nerves. A skin wheal may be raised with 1–2% lidocaine with or without bicarbonate. A 4 cm long 22–25 gauge needle is inserted through the skin and into the joint cavity. Aspiration prior to injection is necessary to avoid intravascular injection. Aspiration of synovial fluid confirms the position of the needle, although one may not always obtain fluid, as tissue may be resting against the bevel of the needle or there may not be enough joint fluid in a small joint to aspirate through such a long needle. The aspirated fluid should be checked for inflammatory components unless the fluid is clear and straw-colored. If an infection is suspected, the steroid joint injection is delayed until infection is ruled out. The injection should be resistance free and, once the medication is in place, the needle should be flushed with normal saline or local anesthetic.

COMPLICATIONS

C Complications associated with steroid injection into a joint are rare, but should be recognized. Possible complications include: infection, postinjection flare, atrophy of soft tissues including tendons, subcutaneous fat and skin with possible hypopigmentation and systemic toxicity. The infection rate is reported to be extremely low (0.005%) if strict aseptic technique is used. Postinjection inflammation typically lasts 4–12 hours and is treated with NSAIDs and ice. If the postinjection pain lasts longer than 1 day, the patient should be reevaluated for infection. Tissue atrophy is a significant concern when injecting a steroid into joints because of the proximity of the needle track to melanocytes. This can occur when the steroid leaks out of the joint through the needle track or if the injection is too shallow or outside the joint. Repeated injections into the same joint can result in calcification and subsequent rupture of the ligaments. Trauma to the articular cartilage is also a concern.

D Arbitrary rules of thumb are that large joints should be given an injection only three or four times per year or a maximum of 10 times total. Small joints should only be injected two or three times per year or a maximum of four times total. Other systemic effects include transient changes in blood glucose, hormonal suppression, fluid and electrolyte disturbances, gastrointestinal problems, dermatologic complications, and metabolic reactions.

E Of course, if joint injections are not clinically indicated, or are contraindicated, or if pain persists after adequate trial of intra-articular therapy, other modalities should be considered and utilized as indicated.

SUGGESTED READING

Garg N, Perry L, Deodhar A. Intra-articular and soft tissue injections, a systematic review of relative efficacy of various corticosteroids. Clin Rheumatol. 2014;33(12):1695-706.

Lavelle W, Lavelle ED, Lavelle L. Intra-articular injections. Med Clin North Am. 2007;91(2):241-50.

Lavelle W, Lavelle ED, Lavelle L. Intra-articular injections in interventional approaches to pain management. In: Smith H (Ed). Current Therapy in Pain Management, 1st edition. Philadelphia: Saunders; 2009. p. 591.

MacMahon PJ, Eustace SJ, Kavanagh EC. Injectable corticosteroid and local anesthetic preparations: a review for radiologists. Radiology. 2009;252(3):647-61.

Miller JC, Palmer WE, Goroll AH, et al. Anesthetic and steroid injections for musculoskeletal pain. J Am Coll Radiol. 2009;6(11):806-8.

Stephens MB, Beutler AI, O'Connor FG. Musculoskeletal injections: a review of the evidence. Am Fam Physician. 2008;78(8):971-6.

Wang DT, Dubois M, Tutton SM. Complications in musculoskeletal intervention: important considerations. Semin Intervent Radiol. 2015;32(2):163-73.

CHAPTER
132

Epidural Steroid Injections

Graff V, Pino CA

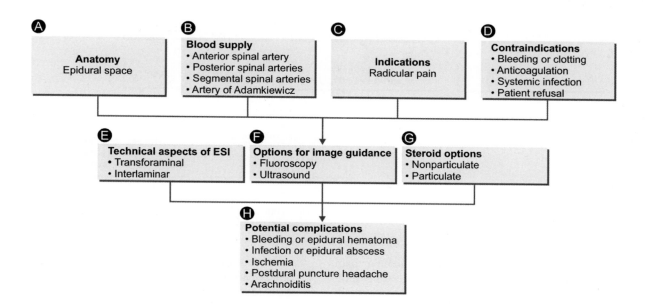

A   Anatomy
  Epidural space

B   **Blood supply**
- Anterior spinal artery
- Posterior spinal arteries
- Segmental spinal arteries
- Artery of Adamkiewicz

C   **Indications**
  Radicular pain

D   **Contraindications**
- Bleeding or clotting
- Anticoagulation
- Systemic infection
- Patient refusal

E   **Technical aspects of ESI**
- Transforaminal
- Interlaminar

F   **Options for image guidance**
- Fluoroscopy
- Ultrasound

G   **Steroid options**
- Nonparticulate
- Particulate

H   **Potential complications**
- Bleeding or epidural hematoma
- Infection or epidural abscess
- Ischemia
- Postdural puncture headache
- Arachnoiditis

A *Anatomy*: The epidural space is a potential space that surrounds the dura mater of the spinal cord and extends as a continuous space from the foramen magnum to the sacral hiatus. This space consists of fat, nerve roots, lymphatics, and an intricate venous plexus. Within the spinal canal and relative to the dura mater, the epidural space exists anteriorly, laterally, and posteriorly. The ligamentum flavum, a tough layer of connective tissue, overlies the posterior aspect of the epidural space within the spinal canal. The ligamentum flavum is an important layer for the purposes of pain interventions as one must go through this layer when accessing the epidural space via the midline or paramedian approach. The ligamentum flavum's thickness varies from the cervical, thoracic, lumbar, and sacral regions with the thickest portion in the lumbar region, and the thinnest in the cervical region. Geometrically, the ligamentum flavum is triangular in a cross-sectional view with the lateral edges being thinner than in the middle. Understanding this three-dimensional anatomy of the epidural space will guide the pain interventionalist to successfully access this space and administer medication for analgesic purposes.

B *Blood Supply*: One anterior spinal artery, two posterior spinal arteries, and segmental spinal arteries supply the spinal cord. The anterior spinal artery originates from the vertebral artery and the two posterior spinal arteries

originate from the inferior cerebellar artery. Numerous segmental spinal arteries originate from the intercostal and lumbar arteries, however, the most important of these branches is the artery of Adamkiewicz which is highly variable in location amongst individuals, existing somewhere between T7 and L4. Awareness of the location of vital arteries is always important in deciding the safest route of epidural steroid administration.

C *Indications for Epidural Steroid Injections*: Epidural steroid injections are commonly indicated for radicular pain caused either by mass effect or chemical irritation of the nerve roots. Mass effect can result from intervertebral disk displacement, bone spurs, or stenosis. Chemical inflammation by substances such as cytokines and prostaglandins typically cause radicular pain by irritating nerve roots that stem from the spinal cord. Frequently, this type of pain is distributed in a specific dermatomal pattern which can help localize what level the epidural injections should be administered.

D *Contraindications to Epidural Injections*: Bleeding or clotting disorders, anticoagulation, local and systemic infections, and patient refusal, are some of the common contraindications to epidural injections.

E *Access to the Epidural Space*: There are three routes to access the epidural space: (1) the interlaminar approach, (2) the transforaminal approach, and (3) the caudal approach. The interlaminar approach is appropriate

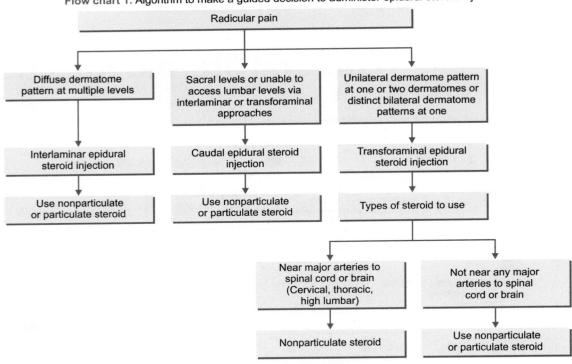

Flow chart 1: Algorithm to make a guided decision to administer epidural steroid injections

when there are several levels of diffuse radicular pain, whereas the transforaminal approach may be more appropriate when there are one or more specific nerve roots specifically causing the radicular pain, therefore, allowing a more concentrated dosage of steroid to be deposited adjacent to the inflamed nerve root. The caudal approach is appropriate when the source of pain is mostly from the sacral nerve roots or if it is difficult to access the lumbar nerve roots from the traditional interlaminar or transforaminal approaches.

For the interlaminar approach, the "loss of resistance" technique is most commonly used. The "hanging drop" technique, which relies on the existence of negative pressure within the epidural space, has been described to access the epidural space but it is not commonly used in interventional pain practice.

F *Use of Image Guidance*: Although interlaminar and caudal epidurals may be performed without the use of imaging, transforaminal epidurals cannot be accurately and safely placed without image guidance. Fluoroscopy, computed tomography (CT) and ultrasound have been used to perform epidural steroid injection, and most interventional pain medicine practitioners currently favor fluoroscopy.

G *Medications Used for Epidural Injections*: Steroids are commonly administered in the epidural space. Steroids can be considered broadly in two categories: (1) nonparticulate, and (2) particulate. The only nonparticulate steroid that is currently used is dexamethasone. Particulate steroids that are commonly used are betamethasone, triamcinolone (both smaller particulates), and methylprednisolone acetate (larger

particulate steroid). The decision to use nonparticulate versus particulate steroids depends on the location of the epidural injection and whether there is a major artery located adjacent to the epidural site that gives supply to vital structures such as the spinal cord or brain. If there is an artery supplying the spinal cord (i.e. radicular arteries such as the artery of Adamkiewicz) or brain (i.e. vertebral artery), then a nonparticulate steroid is highly recommended, as there is a risk of an embolic stroke occurring if a particulate steroid is used.

H *Complications of Epidural Steroid Injections*: Potential complications of epidural steroid injections include bleeding, infection, ischemia, osteoporosis or osteopenia secondary to steroid exposure, postdural puncture headaches, and arachnoiditis if the steroid is accidentally injected into the intrathecal space.

See **Flow chart 1** to help and guide the decision to administering an epidural steroid injection.

SUGGESTED READING

Breivik H. Local anesthetic blocks and epidurals. In: McMahon S, Koltzenburg M, Tracey I, Turk DC (Eds). Wall and Melzack's Textbook of Pain, 6th edition. Philadelphia: Elsevier Churchill Livingstone; 2013. pp. 529-37.

Brull R. Spinal, epidural, and caudal anesthesia. In: Miller RD, Eriksson LI, Fleisher LA, Wiener-Kronish JP, Cohen NH, Young WL (Eds). Miller's Anesthesia, 8th edition. Philadelphia: Elsevier Saunders; 2015. pp. 1684-8.

Patil M, Huntoon M. Interlaminar and transforaminal therapeutic epidural injections. In: Benzon H, Rathmell JP, Wu CL, Turk DC, Argoff CE, Hurley RW (Eds). Practical Management of Pain, 5th edition. Philadelphia: Elsevier; 2014. pp. 805-15.

CHAPTER
133

Medial Branch Blocks

Benedetti EM, Ellis SE

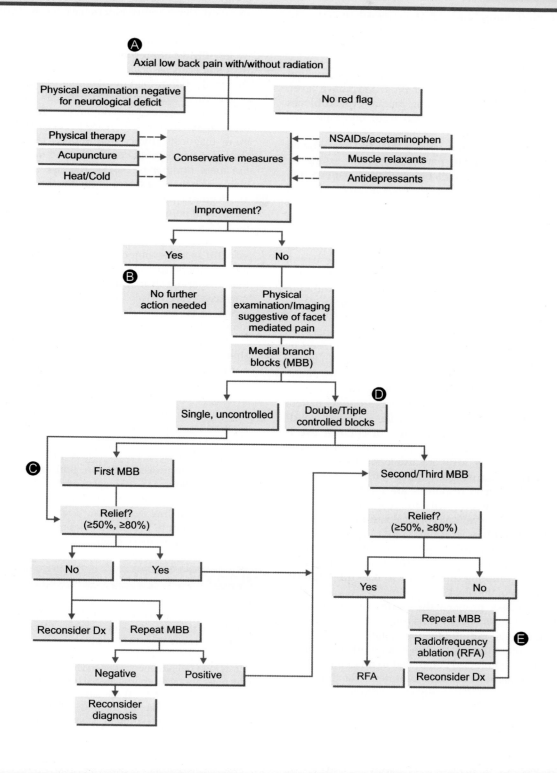

Ⓐ Low back pain (LBP) affects 80% of adults, has recurrence rates of 44% yearly and 85% lifetime, and has a prevalence of up to 84%. Its total annual costs are between $100 and $200 billion, and LBP is the second most common cause of disability in the U.S. Facet joints are the source of pain in 5–40% of patients with LBP and 36–67% of cervicalgia cases. Neck pain, on the other hand, has an estimated one year incidence of 10–21% and an annual prevalence of 30–50%.

The facet joints are paired structures that lie on the posterolateral aspect of the vertebrae. Innervation derives from the medial branch, which stems from the primary dorsal ramus of the spinal nerve. It is complex yet predictable, with each joint receiving dual innervation from contiguous medial branches at and above level. Consequently, when performing medial branch blocks (MBB) for the treatment of pain from one joint, two nerves must be blocked.

Facet-mediated pain is mainly axial and exacerbated by loading and motion, particularly spine extension. It can follow a pseudoradicular radiation pattern into the adjacent limb. Unfortunately, history, physical examination, and radiographic findings are not dependable methods for diagnosing facet disease as there are no uniform diagnostic criteria. Successful management can only occur if the etiology is correctly identified. This is more reliably made with the use of diagnostic MBB. The rationale lies in that, with the temporary blockade of the intended nerves, the duration of the pain relief should be concordant with the duration of action of the local anesthetic used.

Ⓑ Determination of whether an MBB is positive or negative is contingent on the variable criteria standard used by the practitioner and the subjective measure given by the patient. Designation of a block as "positive" relies on the pain relief cut-off (50%, 80%, and 100%). False-negative rates are up to 31% and are due to inappropriate patient selection, unrecognized intravascular injection, and/or poor technique. Hence, the use of contrast dye is advocated by some, and image guidance is encouraged by all. Unfortunately, MBB are also associated with high false-positive rates in the lumbar (40%) and cervical spine (63%). Placebo responses are the "uncontrolled" factors determining this, while the "controlled" culprit is the use of excessive volumes of local anesthetic. Volumes as small as 0.5 mL cover up to 6 cm^2 of tissue, allowing spread to adjacent non-targeted structures 2.28 times more frequently. This negatively affects the validity of the result; hence, limiting the volume to 0.25 mL improves the specificity of the block.

Ⓒ Some specialists propose the performance of single diagnostic blocks before moving forward to joint denervation via radiofrequency ablation (RFA). This approach argues that more stringent criteria (double- or triple-controlled blocks) could lead to missed diagnosis or to the denial of successful treatments for those who would have satisfied less rigorous criteria. Advocates for single blocks stand on the lack of cost-effectiveness of multiple blocks and on the fact that both procedures (MBB and RFA) have comparable complication rates.

Regrettably, the clinical role for uncontrolled blocks is limited, at best. Negative blocks have some predictive value, but a positive block, by itself, is considered nonspecific. Consequently, most argue that response to a single uncontrolled block is not valid given the unacceptably high false positive rate.

Ⓓ Hence, to increase the validity of these diagnostic injections, the use of double or triple controlled comparative blocks has been endorsed as the diagnostic standard. Comparative blocks have a sensitivity of 100% and a specificity of 65%. Some practitioners rigorously argue that comparative blocks are essential because, by identifying nonresponders early, one avoids further risks and costs associated with unnecessary procedures. One study determined though, that 64% of patients who receive two diagnostic blocks versus 39% who receive one block have a successful RFA outcome. This means that in order to obtain a 25% increase in successful RFAs, 100% more diagnostic interventions need to be performed. However, it is essential to understand that by increasing the mere number of blocks, the risk of false negative blocks also increases, further fueling the controversy.

Ⓔ The degree of possible success of an RFA as a function of the quantity of pain relief obtained from MBB has also come under scrutiny. Although some claim that when using more stringent pain relief criteria (≥80% vs ≥50%) after an MBB as a selection criteria, the RFA success rates are higher, others have shown that variables like publication bias, disparities in RFA technique, and patient selection may have played a role in the conclusions reached. There seems to be no correlation between the grade of relief after MBB and RFA outcomes.

To further complicate the issue, a study comparing sham, single, and double MBB concluded that using current reimbursement scales, proceeding to RFA without diagnostic blocks is probably the most cost-effective treatment paradigm, given that a significant number of patients with inadequate response to MBB or who do not undergo these diagnostic injections at all, still obtain good relief after an RFA.

Medial branch blocks seem to provide sustained pain relief, improved function, and employment status in some patients (14–16 weeks) and are used by some as therapeutic injections, even though no decrease in opioid consumption has been seen. The addition of steroids does not seem to prolong results and therefore have no significant role in these diagnostic injections.

SUGGESTED READING

Barnsley L, Lord S, Wallis B, et al. False-positive rates of cervical zygapophysial joint blocks. Clin J Pain. 1993;9(2):124-30.

Bogduk N. On the rational use of diagnostic blocks for spinal pain. Neurosurg Quart. 2009;19:88-100.

Cohen SP, Stojanovic MP, Crooks M, et al. Lumbar zygapophysial (facet) joint radiofrequency denervation success as a function of pain relief during diagnostic medial branch blocks: a multicenter analysis. Spine J. 2008;8(3):498-504.

Cohen SP, Williams KA, Kurihara C. Multicenter, randomized, comparative cost-effectiveness study comparing 0, 1, and 2 diagnostic medial branch (facet joint nerve) block treatment paradigms before lumbar facet radiofrequency denervation. Anesthesiology. 2010;113(2):395-405.

Dreyfuss P, Schwarzer AC, Lau P, et al. Specificity of lumbar medial branch and L5 dorsal ramus blocks. A computed tomography study. Spine (Phila Pa 1976). 1997;22(8):895-902.

Freburger JK, Holmes GM, Agans RP, et al. The rising prevalence of chronic low back pain. Arch Intern Med. 2009;169(3): 251-8.

Hogg-Johnson S, van der Velde G, Carroll LJ, et al. The burden and determinants of neck pain in the general population: results of the Bone and Joint Decade 2000-2010 Task Force on Neck Pain and Its Associated Disorders. Spine (Phila Pa 1976). 2008;33(4 Suppl):S39-51.

Manchikanti L, Singh V, Falco FJ, et al. Cervical medial branch blocks for chronic cervical facet joint pain: a randomized, double-blind, controlled trial with one-year follow-up. Spine (Phila Pa 1976). 2008;33(17):1813-20.

North RB, Kidd DH, Zahurak M, et al. Specificity of diagnostic nerve blocks: a prospective, randomized study of sciatica due to lumbosacral spine disease. Pain. 1996;65(1):77-85.

CHAPTER
134

Intradiscal Therapies

Benedetti EM, Feldman AT, Singh TSS

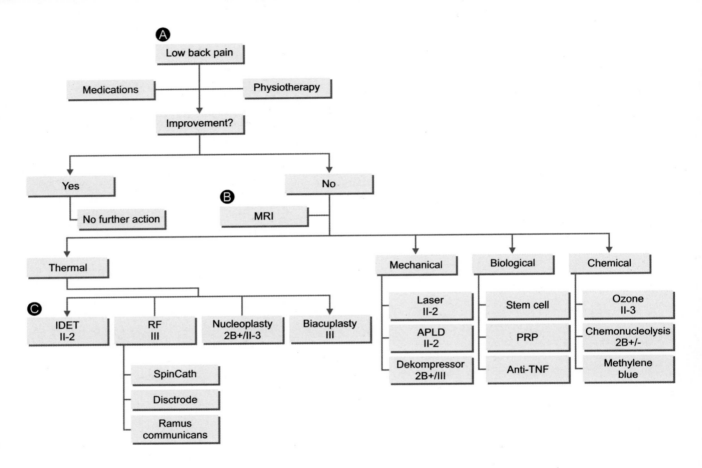

Ⓐ Low back pain is one of the most common causes of
doctor visits in the Western Hemisphere, affecting more
than 80% of adults, and costing the United States health
system up to 100 billion dollars yearly. Although typically
multifactorial, low back pain of discogenic origin due to
internal disc disruption (IDD) accounts for up to 42% of
low back pain cases reported. This term, recognized as an
independent pathologic clinical entity, is used to describe
the syndrome of back pain with pseudoradicular radiation
in a patient who has degenerative disc disease but no disc
herniation or segmental instability. Intradiscal therapies
are predominantly designed to treat discogenic back pain
secondary to IDD.

Ⓑ Magnetic resonance imaging can be helpful in identifying
the proton density of the disc, the presence of radial
fissures, and finally, the presence of a posterior annulus

high intensity zone (finding highly specific to correlate
with IDD). To further aid in the correct identification of the
disc as the painful source, the International Association
for the Study of Pain suggests the following findings
on provocative discography: concordant pain during
discography, annular disruption shown on computed
tomography (CT) after discography, and at least one
adjacent disc without concordant pain. The addition of
a post-discogram CT can improve the visualization of
the contrast spread providing a quantifiable measure of
the grade of disc disruption. Provocative discography
remains quite controversial given that its interpretation is
highly dependent on a patient's report of pain, therefore,
having a II-2 strength level of evidence.

Ⓒ Treatments for discogenic pain are of limited efficacy
and range from conservative measures like rehabilitative

strategies and polypharmacy to surgery. Surgical interbody fusion of the affected spinal segment as a treatment for IDD is most often indicated in patients when there is extensive disc height loss or structural instability. Caution must be exercised though when pursing the surgical option as outcomes on pain control are variable with relatively low success rates. The introduction of minimally invasive percutaneous treatments (thermal, mechanical, chemical, or biological) was indeed the logical intermediate step in the management of discogenic pain as an attempt to reduce unnecessary surgeries and decrease perioperative and postoperative morbidities. The most suitable choice of minimally interventional therapy should be made by an interdisciplinary team taking into account specific patient characteristics/desires, costs, availability, and interventionalist expertise.

Thermal procedures rely on the delivery of electrothermal energy to annular nociceptive fibers thought to contribute to discogenic pain as well as the eventual decrease of the nuclear volume during the healing process leading to reduction in the size of disc bulges. This category includes intradiscal electrothermal therapy (IDET), radiofrequency (DiscTrode, SpineCath, ramus communicans RF, etc.), biacuplasty, nucleoplasty, laser, and cryoablation. Mechanical procedures include Decompressor, Automated Percutaneous Lumbar Discectomy (APLD), and Percutaneous Lumbar Laser Disc Decompression. Biological procedures comprise the intradiscal injection of stem cells, plasma-rich protein, and anti-TNF (tumor necrosis factor), while chemical procedures include chymopapain chemonucleolysis, intradiscal ozone, and intradiscal methylene blue. These procedures are typically indicated for small, contained disc herniations and treatment is not recommended for more than two levels at one time.

Treatment failures may be due to a combination of variables, such as poor patient selection, lack of patient compliance, and technical incompetence. In addition, the majority of intradiscal procedures have a low level of evidence and long-term results are lacking. Restraint is again recommended when choosing the procedure balancing the technical ease and the low rate of complications versus the evidence and costs.

SUGGESTED READING

Chou R, Atlas M, Stanos S, et al. Nonsurgical interventional therapies for low back pain. Spine (Phila Pa 1976). 2009;34(10):1078-93.

Lu Y, Guzman JZ, Purmessur D, et al. Nonoperative management for discogenic back pain: a systematic review. Spine (Phila Pa 1976). 2014;39(16):1314-24.

Manchikanti L, Abdi S, Atluri S, et al. An update of comprehensive evidence-based guidelines for interventional techniques in chronic spinal pain. Part II: guidance and recommendations. Pain Physician. 2013;16(2 Suppl):S49-283.

Patel VB, Wasserman R, Imani F. Interventional Therapies for Chronic low Back Pain: A Focused Review (Efficacy and Outcomes). Anesth Pain Med. 2015;5(4):e29716.

CHAPTER 135

Vertebral Augmentation

Warner C, Beall DP

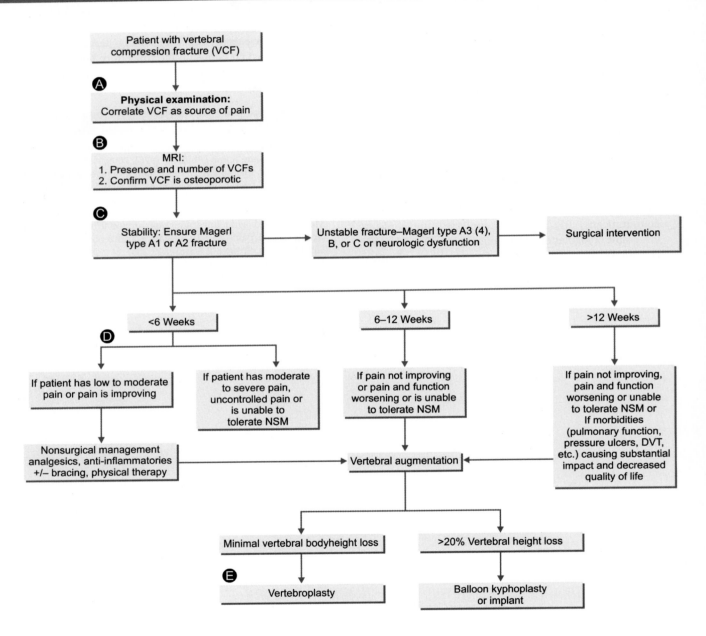

Vertebral compression fractures (VCFs) are the most common osteoporotic fractures. In the U.S., there are 1.5 million VCFs that occur annually and worldwide there is a vertebral fracture every 22 seconds. Overall, 25% of women over the age of 65 years and 40% of women over the age of 80 years will have a VCF. Following a VCF, there is a 23% increase in one-

year mortality and patients not treated for their VCFs have been found to have a 40% lower survival after 8 years than age-matched controls. An important consideration given the mortality risk for patients with VCFs is that the mortality has been shown to be decreased as much as 55% for those patients who are undergoing vertebral augmentation (VA), and the morbidity associated with these fractures can also be significantly reduced in patients. The morphologic severity of VCFs can be graded based on the percentage of compression: Grade 1—20 to 25% height reduction (10–20% vertebral area decrease), Grade 2—25 to 40% (20–40% area decrease), and Grade 3—more than 40% height or area reduction. However, the degree of compression has no relationship to the amount of adverse clinical symptoms produced by the VCF and compression fractures of less than 20% may still be painful, debilitating and benefit from the appropriate management.

Ⓐ A detailed history and physical examination are essential to the diagnosis of a symptomatic VCF. There are many different pain generators in the spine including degenerative disc disease, facet arthropathy, spinal canal, or neural foraminal stenosis; and the characteristics of fracture pain must be separated from the pain produced by other spine pathology. The closed fist percussion sign demonstrates a sensitivity of 87.5% and a specificity of 90% for correlating pain to the VCF. The examination is performed by percussing the spine with a closed fist along the length of the spine. The sign is positive when the patient complains of a sharp, sudden, fracture pain when percussed over the level of the fracture. The supine sign has a sensitivity of 81.25% and a specificity of 93.33%. The patient is asked to lie supine on the examination table (or magnetic resonance imaging [MRI] scanner) with only one pillow. If the patient cannot lie flat due to severe pain the sign is considered positive.

Ⓑ Osteoporotic VCFs may be differentiated from malignant or metastatic fractures based on their MRI appearance. MRI findings suggestive of acute osteoporotic VCFs are as follows: low-signal-intensity lines on T1- and T2-weighted images, spared normal bone marrow signal of the vertebral body, retropulsion of a posterior bone fragment, and the presence of multiple compression fractures. MRI findings suggestive of metastatic compression fractures are as follows: a convex posterior border of the vertebral body, abnormal signal intensity of the pedicle or posterior element, an epidural mass, an encasing epidural mass, a focal paraspinal mass, and other spinal metastases. Utilizing these criteria to distinguish between metastatic and acute osteoporotic compression fractures, the sensitivity, specificity, and accuracy is 100%, 93%, and 95%, respectively. The presence of osseous edema on short TI inversion recovery (STIR) images was not useful in delineating metastatic versus osteoporotic fractures, but may be useful in identifying more acute/subacute VCFs or symptomatic VCFs.

Ⓒ The stability of the fracture must also be assessed based on imaging and examination. Any evidence of neurologic compromise (weakness, saddle anesthesia, bowel/bladder dysfunction, etc.) should immediately undergo surgical evaluation. The Magerl classification system can also be utilized to evaluate the stability of VCFs. Magerl A1 and A2 type fractures are considered stable and do not require surgical fixation. These fractures are endplate compression, wedge compression, or simple coronal/sagittal split fractures. Magerl A3, B, and C type fractures are generally considered unstable and require surgical evaluation.

Ⓓ *Nonsurgical management (NSM) versus VA:* The initial step is delineating an approximate fracture age-based predominantly on pain history. The RAND criteria divides fracture age as less than 6 weeks, 6–12 weeks, and more than 12 weeks. If a fracture is less than 6 weeks old, the patient has low to moderate pain (VAS < 5), and/or pain is improving, then a trial of NSM is warranted. Management includes analgesics and anti-inflammatories with or without physical therapy or bracing. Bracing has been shown to be equivocal in some studies for improving pain or changing VCF height, but has been shown to improve trunk muscle strength, decrease pain, and improve VB height in one other evaluation comparing bracing with medical treatment with calcium, vitamin D, and a bisphosphonate medication. If pain is debilitating or not improving then VA has demonstrated a three times greater acute pain relief that is sustained, four times improvement in quality of life, and 5 fewer days in hospital. Patients treated with VA also demonstrate significantly higher survival rates at 4 years, 60.8% compared to 50.0% for NSM (p < 0.001). At 6–12 weeks if there is persistent pain, decreased quality of life (QOL) or activities of daily living (ADLs) then virtually all of these patients should proceed to VA. Treating chronic vertebral fractures remains somewhat controversial but it has been shown that 87% of patients with symptomatic VCFs older than 1 year demonstrated significant clinical benefit regardless of marrow edema on MRI. Additionally, symptomatic VCFs that were treated at nearly 2 years (mean 23.4 months) demonstrated significant pain relief, improved function, and QOL. Although edema on fluid sensitive MRI images is predictive of significant pain decrease when patients are treated with VA, the lack of increased signal does not mean a lack of reduction in pain as patients with painful VCFs still improve at least moderately with treatment.

Ⓔ *Vertebroplasty (VP) versus Balloon Kyphoplasty (BKP) or VA with implant:* Compression fractures with persistent pain and minimal vertebral height loss are candidates for vertebroplasty. However, VCFs with greater than 20% compression should undergo BKP or VA with an intrabody implant as height restoration helps to restore the normal curvature of the spine and has clinical benefit. Kyphoplasty increases vertebral height restoration more than 4.5 times over positioning with VP. BKP also demonstrates statistically significantly higher survival rate of 62.8% compared to the 57.3% survival rate with VP. Adjusted life expectancy is 115% greater for BKP and 44% greater for VP compared to NSM.

SUGGESTED READING

Anselmetti GC, Bernard J, Blattert T, et al. Criteria for the appropriate treatment of osteoporotic vertebral compression fractures. Pain Physician. 2013;16(5):E519-30.

Baaj AA, Downes K, Vaccaro AR, et al. Trends in the treatment of lumbar spine fractures in the United States: a socioeconomics perspective: clinical article. J Neurosurg Spine. 2011;15(4):367-70.

Barr JD, Barr MS, Lemley TJ, et al. Percutaneous vertebroplasty for pain relief and spinal stabilization. Spine (Phila Pa 1976). 2000;25(8):923-8.

Black DM, Cummings SR, Karpf DB, et al. Randomised trial of effect of alendronate on risk of fracture in women with existing vertebral fractures Fracture Intervention Trial Research Group. Lancet. 1996;348(9041):1535-41.

Bozkurt M, Kahilogullari G, Ozdemir M, et al. Comparative analysis of vertebroplasty and kyphoplasty for osteoporotic vertebral compression fractures. Asian Spine J. 2014;8(1):27-34.

Brown DB, Glaiberman CB, Gilula LA, et al. Correlation between preprocedural MRI findings and clinical outcomes in the treatment of chronic symptomatic vertebral compression fractures with percutaneous vertebroplasty. AJR Am J Roentgenol. 2005;184(6):1951-5.

Cauley JA, Thompson DE, Ensrud KC, et al. Risk of mortality following clinical fractures. Osteoporos Int. 2000;11(7):556-61.

Edidin AA, Ong KL, Lau E, et al. Morbidity and mortality after vertebral fractures: comparison of vertebral augmentation and nonoperative management in the medicare population. Spine (Phila Pa 1976). 2015;40(15):1228-41.

Edidin AA, Ong KL, Lau E, et al. Mortality risk for operated and nonoperated vertebral fracture patients in the medicare population. J Bone Miner Res. 2011;26(7):1617-26.

Genant HK, Wu CY, van Kuijk C, et al. Vertebral fracture assessment using a semiquantitative technique. J Bone Miner Res. 1993; 8(9):1137-48.

Jung HS, Jee WH, McCauley TR, et al. Discrimination of metastatic from acute osteoporotic compression spinal fractures with MR imaging. Radiographics. 2003;23(1):179-87.

Langdon J, Way A, Heaton S, et al. Vertebral compression fractures--new clinical signs to aid diagnosis. Ann R Coll Surg Engl. 2010;92(2):163-6.

Magerl F, Aebi M, Gertzbein SD, et al. A comprehensive classification of thoracic and lumbar injuries. Eur Spine J. 1994;3(4):184-201.

Pfeifer M, Begerow B, Minne HW. Effects of a new spinal orthosis on posture, trunk strength, and quality of life in women with postmenopausal osteoporosis: a randomized trial. Am J Phys Med Rehabil. 2004;83(3):177-86.

Shindle MK, Gardner MJ, Koob J, et al. Vertebral height restoration in osteoporotic compression fractures: kyphoplasty balloon tamp is superior to postural correction alone. Osteoporos Int. 2006;17(12):1815-9.

Tanigawa N, Komemushi A, Kariya S, et al. Percutaneous vertebroplasty: relationship between vertebral body bone marrow edema pattern on MR images and initial clinical response. Radiology. 2006;239(1):195-200.

Wardlaw D, Cummings SR, Van Meirhaeghe J, et al. Efficacy and safety of balloon kyphoplasty compared with non-surgical care for vertebral compression fracture (FREE): a randomised controlled trial. Lancet. 2009;373(9668):1016-24.

Radiofrequency Ablation

Eckmann MS

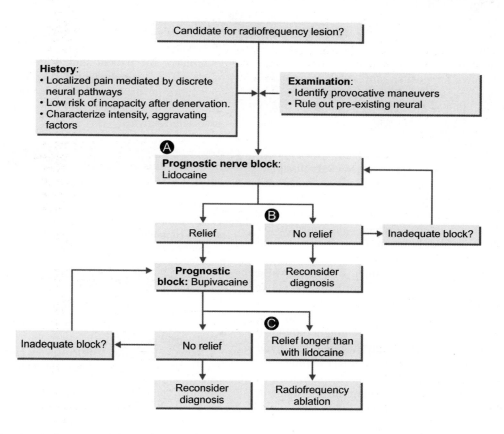

Therapeutic neurolysis may be accomplished by chemical, thermal, or physical means. Neurolysis is commonly used in the management of chronic pain as a method to produce intermediate- to long-term denervation of painful joints or soft tissues (including neural tissue, e.g. neuromas). Modern radiofrequency (RF) generators and cannulas induce frictional heating from electrical ionic oscillation, precisely heating a zone of tissue above 45°C, past which irreversible cell damage occurs. Diverse cannula options with straight, curved, and multitined electrically active tips are available to produce different lesion sizes and shapes. Grounding pads are applied to form a continuous circuit between the patient and RF generator for creation of monopolar lesions; bipolar lesions are created between dual cannulas. Continuous temperature monitoring and closed loop power adjustment by control software leads to consistent lesion size and avoidance of unintended damage to surrounding tissue. Nerve stimulating functionality can inform the operator of proximity to the target nerve, and importantly, adequate distance from unintended neural targets (usually those with motor function). Impedance monitors detect electric circuit malfunctions (shorts or noncontinuity), and may signal close proximity to bone (high impedance) or blood vessels (low impedance).

Radiofrequency ablation is well suited to small neural targets that can be identified by radiologic (x-ray, computed tomography scan, ultrasound, etc.) and/or functional (electrical stimulation) means. Such targets include sympathetic and dorsal root ganglia, the gasserian ganglion, and medial branches of the posterior primary rami of spinal nerves (for zygapophyseal joint denervation). Larger peripheral nerves are often not considered candidates for ablation, as the resulting sensory and motor dysfunction could disable the patient. However, they may be considered in special situations (terminal cancer pain, amputation neuroma, etc.).

Radiofrequency thermal lesions are produced by exciting ions within a field of alternating electric current at 500,000 Hz. Because current density decreases rapidly with distance from the electrode tip, the volume of the lesion is limited. The determinants of lesion size are electrode size, tissue conductivity (water content), adjacent tissues (bone, blood vessels, etc.), and RF generator output. Tissue charring/boiling places an upward limit on power and lesion size. Heating tissue to 80°C for 60 seconds creates a near maximal lesion, although in clinical conditions lesions may grow slightly more through 160 seconds. Bipolar lesions can continue to grow together over the 10-minute mark, depending on intertip distance. Cooled RF uses a double hulled probe through which a contained water source is circulated; this allows for greater power delivery without charring and, therefore, a larger lesion overall. Preinjection with electrically conductive fluid can increase lesion size. A clinical effect may also be possible, without heating the tissue significantly, using pulsed RF energy, possibly due to near destructive thermal effects and electrical field cellular effects. The inactive period between pulses allows heat to dissipate, minimizing procedural discomfort and tissue injury and possibly reducing the likelihood of postoperative neuralgia. It is speculated that the high-energy field or current density can produce sustained interruption of pain transmission without affecting large-fiber function. Limited clinical data supporting sustained outcomes are available.

A *Prognostic Block:* Prior to performing RF ablation of a target nerve, the physician should confirm that it is either generating or transmitting noxious stimuli. After selecting a potential target, a prognostic nerve block is performed. The physician should use nerve stimulation or radiologic reference points (or both) to identify the target, so a small volume of local anesthetic (0.5 mL or less) can produce a complete block. This small volume approximates the size of an RF lesion and prevents spread of the anesthetic to adjacent nerves. If the patient responds favorably to the prognostic injection, he or she may be a candidate for RF ablation.

B *Nerve Block Interpretations:* To maximize the predictive value of a positive prognostic nerve block, the physician may perform additional blocks with other local anesthetics. It is helpful to examine the patient before and after each block using provocative maneuvers that would ordinarily cause pain. Technical nerve block success should be confirmed with sensory and motor examination to rule out false positives and negatives. Patients whose response durations are inconsistent with the agents injected may be placebo responders. The prognostic value of a prolonged response to nerve block has not been well assessed in the literature, however, such responders could theoretically be managed with nerve blocks alone.

C *Decision to Proceed with Neurolysis:* The quality of the initial analgesic response should be documented; over 80% pain relief is a reasonable standard to proceed with neurolysis. The patient should identify an activity that normally produces the pain and keep a record of activity and pain intensity for at least a day after each block. He or she should note the exact time of pain recurrence and the associated activity.

SUGGESTED READING

Barnsley L, Lord S, Bogduk N. Comparative local anaesthetic blocks in the diagnosis of cervical zygapophysial joint pain. Pain. 1993;55(1):99-106.

Cohen SP, Hurley RW, Buckenmaier CC 3rd, et al. Randomized placebo-controlled study evaluating lateral branch radio-frequency denervation for sacroiliac joint pain. Anesthesiology. 2008;109(2):279-88.

Eckmann MS, Martinez MA, Lindauer S, et al. Radiofrequency ablation near the bone-muscle interface alters soft tissue lesion dimensions. Reg Anesth Pain Med. 2015;40(3):270-5.

Lord SM, Barnsley L, Wallis BJ, et al. Percutaneous radio-frequency neurotomy for chronic cervical zygapophysial-joint pain. N Engl J Med. 1996;335(23):1721-6.

Nath S, Nath CA, Pettersson K. Percutaneous lumbar zygapophysial (Facet) joint neurotomy using radiofrequency current, in the management of chronic low back pain: a randomized double-blind trial. Spine (Phila Pa 1976). 2008;33(12):1291-7.

Provenzano DA, Watson TW, Somers DL. The interaction between the composition of preinjected fluids and duration of radiofrequency on lesion size. Reg Anesth Pain Med. 2015;40(2):112-24.

Schwarzer AC, Aprill CN, Derby R, et al. The false-positive rate of uncontrolled diagnostic blocks of the lumbar zygapophysial joints. Pain. 1994;58(2):195-200.

Sluijter ME, van Kleef M. Characteristics and mode of action of RF lesions. Curr Rev Pain. 1998;2:143.

CHAPTER 137

Pulsed Radiofrequency Neuromodulation

Eckmann MS

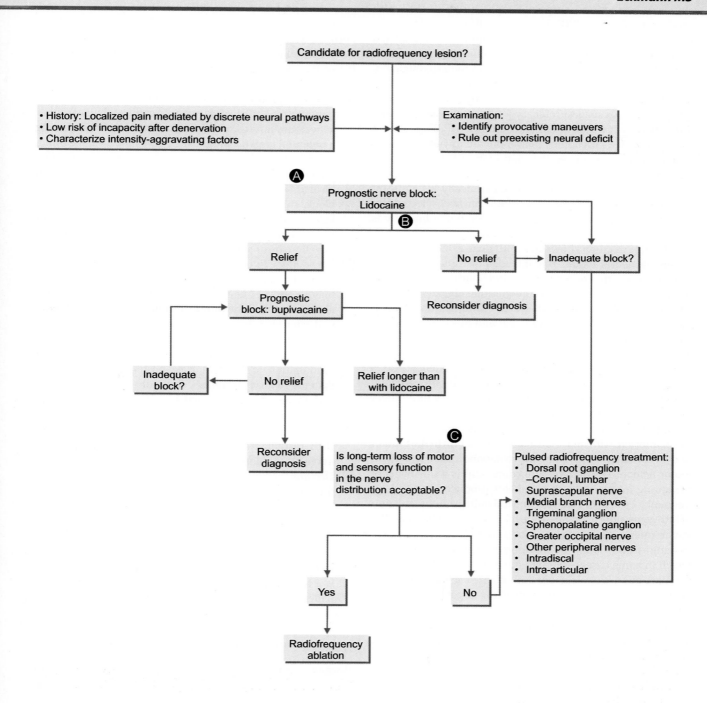

Pulsed radiofrequency (PRF) "ablation" is a modified mode of delivering RF energy to neural and peripheral tissues. For further technical details of RF ablation (RFA), refer to Chapter 136 (Radiofrequency Ablation). Radiofrequency energy is cycled on and off in a square wave function (usually at 2 Hz), which leads to far less tissue heating than continuous RF. It is considered to be a neuromodulatory procedure with minimal or no tissue denaturation; however, PRF can be applied in sufficient strength to surpass temperatures of 45°C with modern equipment. PRF is applied with contemporary RF equipment as an alternate mode, using the same insulated cannulas and probes. Evidence has accumulated particularly in the last 10 years for the role of PRF in neuropathic pain, axial spine-related pain, and large joint pain; however, more randomized, controlled, prospective study is needed. High-quality evidence suggests efficacy for cervical radicular pain. The relatively low risk of complication from PRF compared to truly ablative procedures makes the therapy attractive for treating chronic pain. While continuous RF is extensively used to ablate nerves with pure sensory function or where loss of motor function is considered clinically insignificant (multifidi, intercostal muscles), PRF can be selected for nerves with greater motor function since nerve integrity is maintained.

Preclinical study shows that PRF does exhibit biological effects on neural tissue. This includes disruption of microtubules and microfilaments, mitochondrial membrane morphologic change, myelin configuration change, c-fos and ATF-3 expression, TNF-α/IL-1β/IL-6 attenuation. Animal pain models show reduction in heat and mechanical hyperalgesia when PRF is applied to the dorsal root ganglion (DRG) for at least 120 seconds. Some of these changes may be due to the influence of high voltage and low-frequency pulses of electrical field which can suppress spinal cord synaptic transmission. Some changes may be due to very focal direct denaturation of tissue near the needle tip.

Although radiofrequency energy is selected purposefully to not interfere with neuromuscular conduction in the human body, PRF can produce some nerve depolarization leading to motor response during the procedure. This is a side effect of the strong intermittent electric fields produced by the low-frequency cycling of PRF and upward voltage autoregulation of PRF generators to compensate for less efficient heating. The low-frequency (2 Hz) cycling produces direct current voltage signatures not present in continuous RF, leading to muscle twitch in some cases. Although the exact clinical role of this depolarization is unclear, our authors use such a response as an indicator of excellent proximity to the target nerve (if it has mixed motor and sensory function).

The best temperature and duration settings of PRF for clinical use have yet to be determined, but now it is suggested that at least 4–8 minutes of total treatment time can improve outcomes. While standard commercial settings start with 42°C and 120 seconds, our authors have found in our practice that 8–10 minutes are preferred. For trigeminal ganglion, sphenopalatine ganglion, or greater occipital nerve procedures, our predominant experience is using

PRF at 48–50°; sensory function has been preserved in these cases. Masseter twitch is seen during trigeminal ganglion treatment, and voltages as high as 75 mV can be achieved. Pulse width, pulse frequency, and maximal voltage may have to be modified in generator settings to reach these higher temperatures. Mild-to-moderate sedation may be required. Patients are recommended by our authors to remain on their antineuropathic pain medication for 1 month after the procedure and then wean off, even if the pain is resolved, predominantly to avoid relapse and to help reestablish normal sleep patterns. Of note, conventional RF is known to be efficacious as well for refractory trigeminal neuralgia. If hemifacial swelling is noted after the procedure, a cold compress can be applied in the recovery room.

A *Prognostic Block:* Prior to performing RFA or PRF of a target nerve, the physician should confirm that it is either generating or transmitting noxious stimuli. After selecting a potential target, a prognostic nerve block is performed. The physician should use nerve stimulation and imaging reference points to identify the target, so a small volume of local anesthetic (0.5 mL or less) can produce a complete block. This small volume approximates the size of an RF lesion and prevents spread of the anesthetic to adjacent nerves. If the patient responds favorably to the prognostic injection, he or she may be a candidate for RF ablation.

B *Nerve Block Interpretations:* To maximize the predictive value of a positive prognostic nerve block, the physician may perform additional blocks with other local anesthetics. It is helpful to examine the patient before and after each block using provocative maneuvers that would ordinarily cause pain. Technical nerve block success should be confirmed with sensory and motor examination to rule out false positives and negatives. Patients whose response durations are inconsistent with the agents injected may be placebo responders; the prognostic value of a prolonged response to nerve block has not been well assessed in the literature, however, such responders could theoretically be managed with nerve blocks alone.

C *Decision to Proceed with Neurolysis:* If the target nerve transmits clinically important sensory and/or motor function, PRF can be considered as an alternative to RFA. This is particularly true for treatment of the DRG, where spinal nerve destruction would usually have unwanted consequences. The quality of the initial analgesic response should be documented; over 80% pain relief is a reasonable standard to proceed with treatment. The patient should identify an activity that normally produces the pain and keep a record of activity and pain intensity for at least a day after each block. He or she should note the exact time of pain recurrence and the associated activity.

SUGGESTED READING

Chua NH, Vissers KC, Sluijter ME. Pulsed radiofrequency treatment in interventional pain management: mechanisms and potential indications-a review. Acta Neurochir (Wien). 2011;153(4):763-71.

Malik K, Benzon HT. Pulsed radiofrequency: a critical review of its efficacy. Anaesth Intensive Care. 2007;35(6):863-73.

Thapa D, Ahuja V, Dass C, et al. Management of refractory trigeminal neuralgia using extended duration pulsed radiofrequency application. Pain Physician. 2015;18(3):E433-5.

Van Boxem K, de Meij N, Patijn J, et al. Predictive Factors for Successful Outcome of Pulsed Radiofrequency Treatment in Patients with Intractable Lumbosacral Radicular Pain. Pain Med. 2016;17(7):1233-40.

Van Boxem K, Huntoon M, Van Zundert J, et al. Pulsed radiofrequency: a review of the basic science as applied to the pathophysiology of radicular pain: a call for clinical translation. Reg Anesth Pain Med. 2014;39(2):149-59.

Van Zundert J, Patijn J, Kessels A, et al. Pulsed radiofrequency adjacent to the cervical dorsal root ganglion in chronic cervical radicular pain: a double blind sham controlled randomized clinical trial. Pain. 2007;127(1-2):173-82.

Vigneri S, Sindaco G, Gallo G, et al. Effectiveness of pulsed radiofrequency with multifunctional epidural electrode in chronic lumbosacral radicular pain with neuropathic features. Pain Physician. 2014;17(6):477-86.

CHAPTER
138

Intrathecal Therapy

Jones DT, Eckmann MS

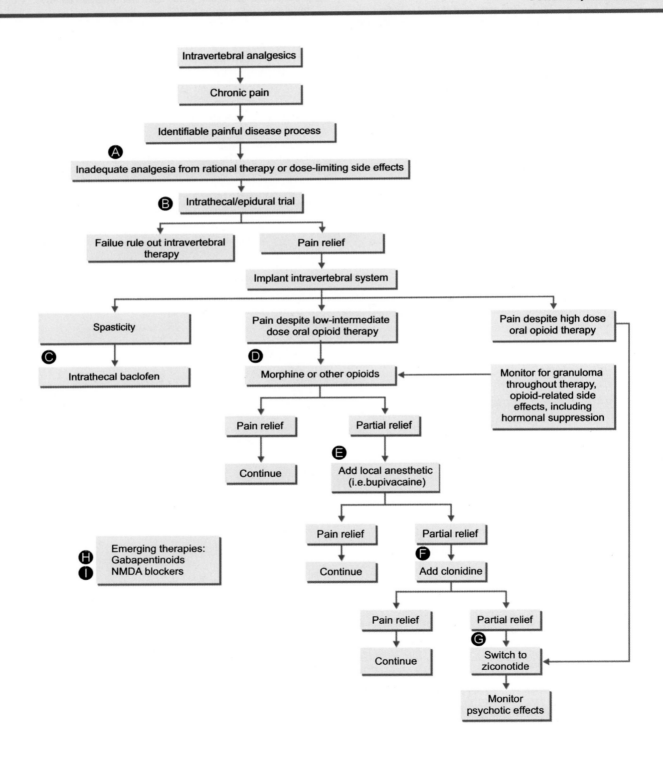

Drug delivery to the epidural and intrathecal space can provide relief of both acute and chronic pain. Various classes of medications can be used differentially to target chronic nociceptive or neuropathic pain. Food and Drug Administration (FDA) approved medications for pain treatment for intrathecal drug delivery devices are morphine and ziconotide currently.

A Intrathecal drug delivery devices should only be considered if the patient has a well-identified pain pathology, but other less invasive rational therapies are ineffective or have dose side effects.

B *Intrathecal/Epidural Trial:* Candidate medications can be trialed to confirm efficacy prior to implantation of a permanent infusion device. Trials may be conducted with a single injection in the outpatient setting or continuous infusion in the hospital setting. Trialing may be skipped in a patient who is terminally ill. The usual intrathecal trial dose for morphine is 0.1–0.5 mg/day; ziconotide is 0.5–2.4 µg/day.

C *Baclofen:* Baclofen, a γ-aminobutyric acid A (GABA-A) receptor agonist, has antihyperalgesic effects in patients with neuropathic pain. It is FDA approved for the treatment of spasticity of both cerebral and spinal origin (e.g. spinal cord injury and cerebral palsy). Central nervous system (CNS) side effects (sedation) tend to be minimized with intrathecal administration. Abrupt cessation of baclofen therapy may lead to significant withdrawal, which manifests as pruritus, return of deep tendon reflexes, fever, altered mental status, muscle rigidity, and may progress to end-organ damage and death. Treatment of baclofen withdrawal involves administration of oral or intrathecal baclofen, benzodiazepines, cyproheptadine, and/or dantrolene.

D *Opioids:* Opioids remain important in neuraxial analgesia; they are of most effective for nociceptive pain but can be used for neuropathic pain. Morphine is considered first-line therapy. The lipid solubility of opioids determines onset and duration of action, metabolism, and CNS side effects. Morphine has a low lipid solubility, slower onset, and longer duration of action but a greater spread in the cerebrospinal fluid (CSF). Fentanyl and sufentanil (highly lipophilic) conversely have a more limited spread. Intrathecal meperidine has been associated with CNS complications. Dosing varies greatly between patients. Morphine oral to epidural dose equivalence is 30:1; oral to intrathecal is 300:1.

Side effects include generalized pruritus, constipation, sedation, and confusion. Patients may also suffer from peripheral edema and hypogonadotropic hypogonadism. Possible catheter-tip granulomas, which come from the arachnoid layer of the meninges, warrant vigilant reevaluation. Higher doses/concentrations of medication (except fentanyl) and longer therapy duration increase the risk of granuloma formation. The first symptoms are a decreased effectiveness of therapy or changes in the characteristics of the pain, but may progress to neurologic compromise. Diagnosis is made by magnetic resonance imaging (MRI) with gadolinium contrast or computed tomography (CT)/myelogram. Granulomas may resolve spontaneously with cessation of the causative drug, but sometimes the catheter and granuloma must be neurosurgically removed.

E *Local Anesthetics:* Since Augustus Bier's discovery of the effectiveness of intrathecal cocaine in 1899, local anesthetics have remained in use for neuraxial routes of pain relief. Tachyphylaxis limits their utility for chronic administration, however, they are useful adjuvants for combination therapy as a second-line agent. Although bupivacaine is most frequently used, ropivacaine may offer lower cardiotoxicity and less motor blockade. Other less commonly used local anesthetics include lidocaine, levobupivacaine, tetracaine, and mepivacaine. Side effects may include sensory or motor changes at the level of administration, urinary retention, sedation, hypotension, and bradycardia.

F *Alpha-2 Agonists:* The α-2 adrenergic agonist clonidine has shown to be effective in neuraxial analgesia for both neuropathic and nociceptive pain, again as an adjuvant therapy. Clonidine works via its effects on both presynaptic and postsynaptic α-2 receptors in the spinal cord, and potentially by immunomodulation. Side effects include hypotension, bradycardia, and sedation. Dexmedetomidine, also an α-2 agonist, may have demyelinating effects.

G *Ziconotide:* Ziconotide, a noncompetitive N-type calcium channel blocker, has shown efficacy in treating malignant as well as nonmalignant chronic pain and should be considered first-line therapy for intrathecal treatment of chronic pain. Common side effects include pain, confusion, hallucinations, and nausea. Of note, ziconotide may have significant psychiatric side effects, including increased suicidality, cognitive impairment, and psychosis.

H *Gabapentinoids:* Gabapentin and pregabalin, via their binding to the α-2/δ-1 subunit of voltage-gated calcium channels, inhibit release of excitatory neurotransmitters, are frequently used orally in patients with chronic pain. When gabapentin is used for neuraxial analgesia, it may have an effect similar to epidural steroids, although some studies have found no benefit.

I *N-methyl-D-aspartate (NMDA) Antagonists:* Ketamine, a noncompetitive inhibitor of the NMDA receptor, has also been used for neuraxial analgesia. The S (+)-enantiomer has been used for acute perioperative analgesia, and may contribute to the relief of phantom limb pain and chronic neuropathic pain. When given intrathecally for extended periods, however, there has been concern that it may lead to spinal cord damage. Methadone, another NMDA antagonist, has been described for epidural use, but there are concerns regarding intrathecal methadone causing spinal cord toxicity.

SUGGESTED READING

Abdi S, Datta S, Trescot AM, et al. Epidural steroids in the management of chronic spinal pain: a systematic review. Pain Physician. 2007;10(1):185-212.

Cohen SP, Hanling S, Bicket MC, et al. Epidural steroid injections compared with gabapentin for lumbosacral radicular pain: multicenter randomized double blind comparative efficacy study. BMJ. 2015;350:h1748.

Deer T, Prager J, Panchal S, et al. Polyanalgesic Consensus Conference 2012: Recommendations for the Management of Pain by Intrathecal (Intraspinal) Drug Delivery: Report of an Interdisciplinary Expert Panel. Neuromodulation. 2012;15(5):436-66.

Deer TR, Prager J, Levy R, et al. Polyanalgesic Consensus Conference 2012: consensus on diagnosis, detection, and treatment of catheter-tip granulomas (inflammatory masses). Neuromodulation. 2012;15(5):483-96.

Duraclon (clonidine hydrochloride). Llinois: Bioniche Pharma USA LLC.

Meythaler J, Roper J, Brunner R. Cyproheptadine for intrathecal baclofen withdrawal. Arch Phys Med Rehabil. 2003;84(5):638-42.

Rathmell JP, Benzon HT, Dreyfuss P, et al. Safeguards to prevent neurologic complications after epidural steroid injections: consensus opinions from a multidisciplinary working group and national organizations. Anesthesiology. 2015;122(5):974-84.

Rauck R, Coffey RJ, Schultz DM, et al. Intrathecal gabapentin to treat chronic intractable noncancer pain. Anesthesiology. 2013;119(3):675-86.

Vranken JH, Troost D, de Haan P, et al. Severe toxic damage to the rabbit spinal cord after intrathecal administration of preservative-free S (+)-ketamine. Anesthesiology. 2006;105(4):813-8.

CHAPTER
139

Spinal Cord Stimulation

Pang EK, Pangarkar SS

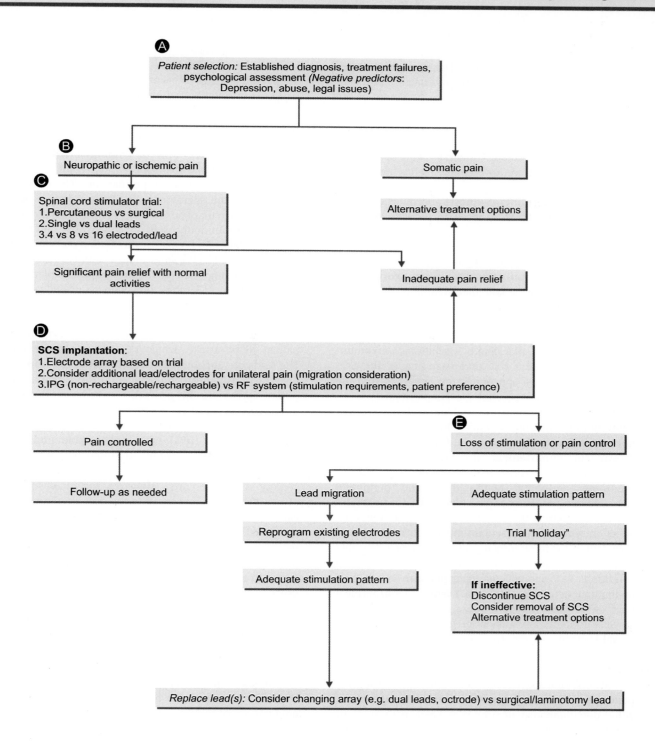

Ⓐ *Patient selection:* Established diagnosis, treatment failures, psychological assessment *(Negative predictors*: Depression, abuse, legal issues)

Ⓑ Neuropathic or ischemic pain

Somatic pain

Ⓒ Spinal cord stimulator trial:
1. Percutaneous vs surgical
2. Single vs dual leads
3. 4 vs 8 vs 16 electroded/lead

Alternative treatment options

Significant pain relief with normal activities

Inadequate pain relief

Ⓓ **SCS implantation**:
1. Electrode array based on trial
2. Consider additional lead/electrodes for unilateral pain (migration consideration)
3. IPG (non-rechargeable/rechargeable) vs RF system (stimulation requirements, patient preference)

Pain controlled

Ⓔ Loss of stimulation or pain control

Follow-up as needed

Lead migration

Adequate stimulation pattern

Reprogram existing electrodes

Trial "holiday"

Adequate stimulation pattern

If ineffective:
Discontinue SCS
Consider removal of SCS
Alternative treatment options

Replace lead(s): Consider changing array (e.g. dual leads, octrode) vs surgical/laminotomy lead

Spinal cord stimulation (SCS) is a reversible adjunctive treatment for chronic neuropathic pain. Successful SCS implantation can assist in decreasing pain, reducing medication use, and increasing function. The exact mechanism of SCS is unclear. The gate theory provides a partial explanation: SCS gives a direct stimulation of the large sensory fibers in the dorsal columns "closing the gate" and preventing the smaller pain fibers from entering the dorsal horn. The full mechanism of action is likely more complex, with proposed mechanisms including neurochemical changes that reduce dorsal horn neuronal hyperexcitability, supraspinal effects, and sympathetic effects (peripheral vasodilation). The cathode (negative pole) causes depolarization of the neuron, leading to an action potential that is propagated along the nerve. Close proximity of the anode to the cathode, as with all SCS multielectrode leads, allows a narrow, targeted stimulation field. The success of SCS has continuously improved since its inception. In addition to the advances in technology, materials, and design, the most important aspect of improved outcome has been better patient selection.

Ⓐ Careful patient selection is of utmost importance. Essential negative predictors for SCS success include inadequately treated depression or other psychiatric disorders, nonorganic or questionable etiologies of pain, ongoing drug or alcohol abuse, and ongoing legal issues related to the painful condition. After establishing a correct pain diagnosis and ensuring adequate treatment modalities, including injections, medications, and physical and psychological therapies have been considered, SCS may be used as a treatment option. A thorough psychological assessment by a mental health specialist is paramount to ensure the patient has understanding of the SCS treatment objectives, appropriate expectations, and the absence of significant psychological impairment.

Ⓑ Spinal cord stimulation works well for two broad types of pain: neuropathic and ischemic. Nociceptive pain does not respond as well as ischemic. Conditions that have shown pain improvement with SCS include complex regional pain syndrome (CRPS), failed back surgery syndrome, peripheral neuropathies, and peripheral ischemia and refractory angina. Using SCS for treatment of ischemic pain is more common in Europe due to its effect on sympathetic vascular tone and increased blood flow. Other less frequently used therapies include direct peripheral nerve or nerve root stimulation for such conditions as occipital neuralgia, migraine headaches, ilioinguinal neuralgia, interstitial cystitis, sacral/perineal pain of various etiologies. There are contraindications for SCS implantation such as pregnancy, severe central spinal stenosis, progressive spine instability, and severe cognitive impairment impeding ability to operate device.

Ⓒ The SCS trial is performed by placing stimulating leads into the epidural space (cervical level for upper extremity pain and low thoracic level for lower extremity pain), either percutaneously or surgically. Leads with 4-, 8-, or 16-electrode arrays may be used. Dual leads may be used

in an attempt to treat bilateral or midline pain as well as to correct for lead migration. The patient must be awake if sedation is utilized to ensure proper coverage. After selecting the type of electrode to cover the area, there are three adjustable parameters to fine-tune the stimulation: pulse width, frequency, and amplitude. The pulse width (100–400 ms) is the duration of a pulse. The frequency is typically set between 20 Hz and 120 Hz, but now can be up to 10 kHz with one manufacturer. Literature suggests this high-frequency stimulation removes SCS-induced paresthesia. The amplitude affects the intensity of individual pulse and can be under voltage or current control. The trial should last from 4 days to 7 days while the patient engages in his or her usual painful activities. However, during the trial, patient should avoid activities that cause lead migration such as raising arms over heads, bending, twisting, stretching, or lifting more than 5 lb. If the patient reports that the pain is reduced significantly (e.g. 50% or more), with or without a reduction in medications, the trial is considered successful.

Ⓓ After a successful trial, a permanent SCS system is implanted in the operating room. There are two types of leads used: percutaneous or surgical leads. Percutaneous leads (more commonly used) are less invasive, but have a higher tendency for breakage or migration that could lead to reoperation. Placing surgical leads reduces risk of lead breakage and migration but requires surgical implantation via laminotomy or laminectomy with associated possible surgical complications. Traditionally, the patient is awake to ensure adequate, appropriate stimulation paresthesias. However, one emerging device does not require the patient to be awake, which shortens procedure time. The leads are anchored and connected to extensions (if necessary), which are tunneled into the subcutaneous pocket containing the generator or receiver. There are three types of pulse generator power sources available: radiofrequency (RF) system and two subsets of implanted pulse generators (IPG) with rechargeable and non-rechargeable batteries. For the RF system with implanted receiver and external battery, no battery replacement surgery is ever required. However, the inconvenience of wearing an antenna taped to the skin interfering with activities of daily living may make it less desirable for patients. IPG systems with an internal battery, although requiring replacement surgery, are usually preferred by the patient. Non-rechargeable batteries can last from 1 year to as long as 5 years, depending on frequency of usage and intensity; whereas, rechargeable batteries can last 5–9 years. Automatic on/off cycling of the IPG can be programmed to prolong battery life. The patient can turn the unit on and off and adjust the amplitude, frequency, and pulse width up to the preset limits. Following implantation, the patient should avoid activities (strenuous bending, twisting, lifting, etc.) that might cause lead migration until the leads become fibrosed in the epidural space within 4–12 weeks (some advocate soft collars or corsets as "reminders"). The patient should be warned that the stimulation intensity may change with different positions, even after the fibrosis is complete, and that they should not drive or operate heavy machinery while the stimulator is turned on.

E Loss of adequate stimulation, pain control, or both requires intervention. Lead migration or breakage is the most common complication. Reprogramming may restore adequate stimulation with migrated leads. If reprogramming is unsuccessful or the leads are nonfunctioning, new leads can be placed. Extensions can break and generators/receivers can malfunction, requiring surgical replacement. "Tolerance" can also develop; epidural fibrosis may cause insulation of the electrodes and loss of stimulation, or neural plasticity may result in loss of pain control despite continued appropriate stimulation paresthesia. For the latter, the provider may consider a stimulation "holiday" to see if adequate pain control can be restored. Otherwise, removal of the system is warranted. Superficial infection is a potential complication that may be managed with oral antibiotics. To minimize this, prophylactic intraoperative antibiotics are often used in conjunction with postoperative oral antibiotics. These risks should be discussed with the patient *before* the trial and/or implantation.

SUGGESTED READING

Barolat G. Current status of epidural spinal cord stimulation. Neurosurg Q. 1995;5:98-124.

Burchiel KJ, Anderson VC, Wilson BJ, et al. Prognostic factors of spinal cord stimulation for chronic back and leg pain. Neurosurgery. 1995;36(6):1101-11.

DeJongste MJ. Spinal cord stimulation for ischemic heart disease. Neurol Res. 2000;22(3):293-8.

Jacobs MJ, Jörning PJ, Joshi SR, et al. Epidural spinal cord electrical stimulation improves microvascular blood flow in severe limb ischemia. Ann Surg. 1988;207(2):179-83.

Kapural L, Yu C, Doust MW, et al. Novel 10-kHz high-frequency therapy (HF10 therapy) is superior to traditional low-frequency spinal cord stimulation for the treatment of chronic back and leg pain. Anesthesiology. 2015;123(4):851-60.

Kumar K, Toth C, Nath RK, et al. Epidural spinal cord stimulation for treatment of chronic pain: some predictors of success; a 15-year experience. Surg Neurol. 1998;50(2):110-20.

North RB, Roark GL. Spinal cord stimulation for chronic pain. Neurosurg Clin North Am. 1995;6(1):145-55.

North RB, Wetzel FT. Spinal cord stimulation for chronic pain of spinal origin: a valuable long-term solution. Spine (Phila Pa 1976). 2002;27(22):2584-91.

Oakley JC, Prager JP. Spinal cord stimulation: mechanisms of action. Spine (Phila Pa 1976). 2002;27(22):2574-83.

Peripheral Nerve Stimulation

Pangarkar SS

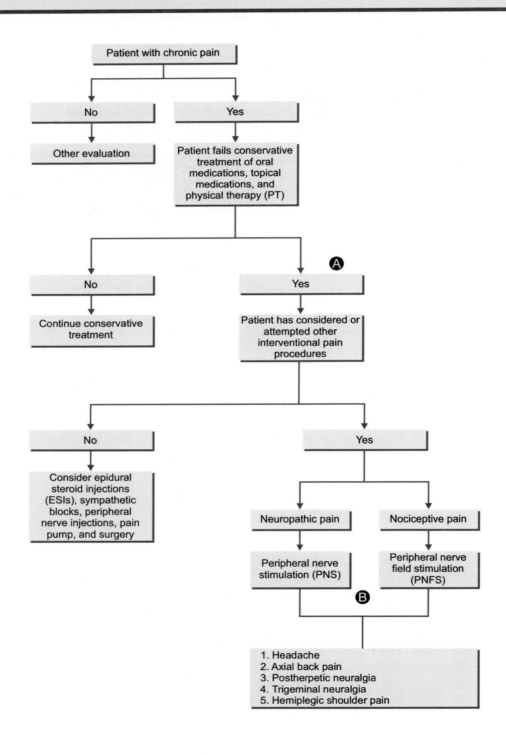

Shortly after Melzack and Wall published the gate control theory in 1965, interest in the field of electrical neurostimulation to treat neuropathic pain began to unfold. Peripheral nerve stimulation (PNS) has evolved from technology associated with spinal cord stimulation (SCS). The concept of PNS is similar to utilization of SCS; however, the electrical leads are placed near the peripheral nerve as opposed to inside the epidural space. If a specific peripheral nerve is targeted, the term PNS applies. However, if an area of pain is targeted, such as treatment of axial back pain, the reference term peripheral nerve field stimulation (PNFS) is used.

There are two basic types of electrical stimulation leads: (1) a cylindrical lead, which can be placed percutaneously, and (2) a relatively large paddle lead, which requires an incision to be made in the skin. For percutaneous lead placement, a Tuohy needle is inserted near the site of interest and fluoroscopy is used to properly guide the lead. Once the lead is fully inserted, intraoperative testing is performed to assess the correct positioning. The leads are attached to a low voltage pulse generator and an electrical current is applied to create paresthesias without muscle contraction. As with SCS, there is usually a trial time in which the generator is external to the body. If the trial is successful, the generator may be surgically implanted and the leads anchored to fascia or periosteum to prevent migration or displacement. A site is then chosen for the generator to be placed, such as in the gluteal region, abdominal wall or infraclavicular area. The electrodes or extension cables are then tunneled to the site of the generator. The electrical stimulation is then programmed to deliver intermittent or continuous current.

The exact mechanism of action for pain relief with PNS remains unclear. Possibilities range from the gate control theory to modulation of local blood flow in the involved painful area. PNFS can provide pain relief in patients with both neuropathic and nociceptive pain. It is believed to exert its effect on nociceptive pain by the current that passes through the mechanoreceptors. In recent years, PNS has been used to treat various ailments including peripheral neuropathy, headaches, back pain and shoulder hemiplegia.

A If a patient fails conservative approaches with oral and/or topical medications, and physical treatment modalities, and, has also considered or tried indicated interventional pain procedures, then possible next steps may include PNS or PNFS strategies.

B 1. For treatment of headaches, PNS leads may be applied to the supraorbital, frontal, occipital, or high cervical regions. In order to address occipital pain, subcutaneous electrode leads may be placed adjacent to the posterior cervical spine at the C1-C2 region. The exact mechanism in which PNS helps with headaches is not well understood. It is theorized that it may alter cerebral blood flow, thereby modifying thalamic activation. While using positive emission tomography, Magis et al. demonstrated that occipital nerve stimulation may restore balance to antinociceptive pathways. Efficacy of PNS for the treatment of headaches is somewhat limited given the quality of the trials and number of participants; however, current research is promising.

2. Peripheral nerve field stimulation has shown benefit in patients with chronic axial back pain by effectively stimulating lumbar and sacral nerve fibers directly in the painful areas. Treatment of axial back pain with PNFS is commonly accomplished by placing the electrode leads superficially and stimulating the terminal nerve fibers and dermal pain receptors. Kloimstein et al. performed implantation of PNFS in 105 patients with axial back pain and performed follow-up at 1, 3 and 6 months after implantation. Not only was pain and quality of life improved, medication utilization was reduced.

3. Peripheral nerve field stimulation has been used as a treatment for postherpetic neuralgia (PHN). Upadhyay et al. published a case study in which a middle-aged male who experienced severe intractable PHN pain refractory to oral pharmacological treatment was treated with PNFS. The PHN was located in the left supraorbital region, and therefore PNFS was utilized by placing leads subcutaneously from the left temporal region into his left supraorbital region, resulting in complete pain relief and the ability to taper and discontinue oral medications. A similar case report was also published in which an elderly female with intractable PHN involving her right shoulder and upper posterior chest wall that had failed oral medications was treated with PNFS, eventually resulting in her being able to taper off of all her oral pain medications while also reporting an improvement in sleep.

4. Peripheral nerve field stimulation treatment in the setting of trigeminal neuropathic pain (TNP) has also shown promising results. Recently, a report was published in which 10 patients with facial pain chiefly related to TNP were treated with PNFS. The mean symptom duration was approximately 10.5 years, and all participants had failed prior medical, interventional, and surgical treatments. PNFS leads were placed in a trajectory along the painful areas. Visual analog scale scores were reportedly markedly improved with the treatment; with preoperative average pain intensity 9.3 and postoperative scores of 0.75.

5. Peripheral nerve stimulation has been investigated as a possible treatment for hemiplegic shoulder pain (HSP). Studies have been conducted which entailed placement of percutaneous leads in the region of the shoulder in order to stimulate the surrounding peripheral nerves. Wilson et al. conducted a pilot randomized control trial to investigate the initial efficacy of short-term single lead PNS for the treatment of chronic HSP in which participants in the treatment group received a single lead inserted into the deltoid so that visible contraction of the middle and posterior deltoid muscles could be seen. Although the power of

the study was limited, the treatment group appeared to show a statistically significant improvement in HSP over the physical therapy group.

The overall complication rate of PNS is low compared to more invasive surgical options. This is felt to be from the small incision size, low infection rates, little bleeding risk, and limited scarring. Complications tend to be related to lead fractures, lead erosion or migration, equipment failure, and infection with possible associated sepsis.

In summary, PNS or PNFS has shown promising results over the last couple of decades for the treatment of chronic neuropathic and nociceptive pain. Barriers for increasing usage of peripheral stimulation include lack of knowledge and awareness of its potential use among both patients and healthcare personnel. Further research and clinical studies will hopefully advance knowledge and acceptance of utilizing PNS or PNFS as an alternative option for the treatment of chronic pain.

Peripheral nerve stimulation or peripheral nerve field stimulation may be considered in treating some of the conditions discussed earlier after the failure of physical therapy, pharmacotherapy, peripheral nerve injections, or surgeries. With the trial option, PNS or PNFS may be less invasive but not necessarily more effective than surgical options.

SUGGESTED READING

Abd-Elsayed AA, Grandhi R, Sachdeva H. Effective management of trigeminal neuralgia by neurostimulation. Ochsner J. 2015; 15(2):193-5.

Amin S, Buvanendran A, Park KS, et al. Peripheral nerve stimulator for the treatment of supraorbital neuralgia: a retrospective case series. Cephalalgia. 2008;28(4):355-9.

Cosman ER, Cosman ER. Electric and thermal field effects in tissue around radiofrequency electrodes. Pain Med. 2005;6(6):405-24.

Hann S, Sharan A. Dual occipital and supraorbital nerve stimulation for chronic migraine: a single-center experience, review of literature, and surgical considerations. Neurosurg Focus. 2013;35(3):E9.

Jasper JF, Hayek SM. Implanted occipital nerve stimulators. Pain Physician. 2008;11(2):187-200.

Klein J, Sandi-Gahun S, Schackert G, et al. Peripheral nerve field stimulation for trigeminal neuralgia, trigeminal neuropathic pain, and persistent idiopathic facial pain. Cephalalgia. 2016; 36(5):445-53.

Kloimstein H, Likar R, Kern M, et al. Peripheral nerve field stimulation (PNFS) in chronic low back pain: a prospective multicenter study. Neuromodulation. 2014;17(2):180-7.

Lee PB, Horazeck C, Nahm FS, et al. Peripheral Nerve Stimulation for the Treatment of Chronic Intractable Headaches: Long-term Efficacy and Safety Study. Pain Physician. 2015;18(5):505-16.

Magis D, Bruno MA, Fumal A, et al. Central modulation in cluster headache patients treated with occipital nerve stimulation: an FDG-PET study. BMC Neurol. 2011;11:25.

Matharu MS, Bartsch T, Ward N, et al. Central neuromodulation in chronic migraine patients with suboccipital stimulators: a PET study. Brain. 2004;127(Pt 1):220-30.

McRoberts WP, Wolkowitz R, Meyer DJ, et al. Peripheral nerve field stimulation for the management of localized chronic intractable back pain: results from a randomized controlled study. Neuromodulation. 2013;16(6):565-74.

Melzack R, Wall PD. Pain mechanisms: a new theory. Science. 1965;150(3699):971-9.

Reverberi C, Dario A, Barolat G. Spinal cord stimulation (SCS) in conjunction with peripheral nerve field stimulation (PNfS) for the treatment of complex pain in failed back surgery syndrome (FBSS). Neuromodulation. 2013;16(1):78-82.

Slavin KV. Peripheral nerve stimulation for neuropathic pain. Neurotherapeutics. 2008;5(1):100-6.

Upadhyay SP, Rana SP, Mishra S, et al. Successful treatment of an intractable postherpetic neuralgia (PHN) using peripheral nerve field stimulation (PNFS). Am J Hosp Palliat Care. 2010;27(1): 59-62.

Verrills P, Rose R, Mitchell B, et al. Peripheral nerve field stimulation for chronic headache: 60 cases and long-term follow-up. Neuromodulation. 2014;17(1):54-9.

Verrills P, Russo M. Peripheral nerve stimulation for back pain. Prog Neurol Surg. 2015;29:127-38.

Wilson RD, Bennett ME, Lechman TE, et al. Single-lead percutaneous peripheral nerve stimulation for the treatment of hemiplegic shoulder pain: a case report. Arch Phys Med Rehabil. 2011;92(5):837-40.

Wilson RD, Gunzler DD, Bennett ME, et al. Peripheral nerve stimulation compared with usual care for pain relief of hemiplegic shoulder pain: a randomized controlled trial. Am J Phys Med Rehabil. 2014;93(1):17-28.

Yakovlev AE, Peterson AT. Peripheral nerve stimulation in treatment of intractable postherpetic neuralgia. Neuromodulation. 2007; 10(4):373-5.

Yu DT, Chae J, Walker ME, et al. Intramuscular neuromuscular electric stimulation for poststroke shoulder pain: a multicenter randomized clinical trial. Arch Phys Med Rehabil. 2004;85(5):695-704.

CHAPTER 141

Neurosurgical Procedures for Pain

Bartanusz V

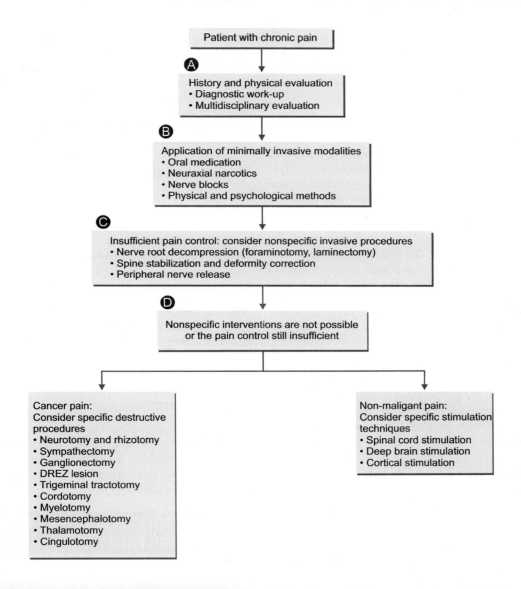

Patient with chronic pain

Ⓐ

History and physical evaluation
• Diagnostic work-up
• Multidisciplinary evaluation

Ⓑ

Application of minimally invasive modalities
• Oral medication
• Neuraxial narcotics
• Nerve blocks
• Physical and psychological methods

Ⓒ

Insufficient pain control: consider nonspecific invasive procedures
• Nerve root decompression (foraminotomy, laminectomy)
• Spine stabilization and deformity correction
• Peripheral nerve release

Ⓓ

Nonspecific interventions are not possible
or the pain control still insufficient

Cancer pain:
Consider specific destructive procedures
• Neurotomy and rhizotomy
• Sympathectomy
• Ganglionectomy
• DREZ lesion
• Trigeminal tractotomy
• Cordotomy
• Myelotomy
• Mesencephalotomy
• Thalamotomy
• Cingulotomy

Non-maligant pain:
Consider specific stimulation techniques
• Spinal cord stimulation
• Deep brain stimulation
• Cortical stimulation

INTRODUCTION

Neurosurgical procedures for pain can be *nonspecific* or *specific*. The former are not specifically designed to address pain, although the improvement of pain is one of the surgical goals. *Nonspecific* procedures include nerve root decompressions by laminectomy, hemilaminectomy, or foraminotomy, releasing peripheral nerve entrapments, stabilization of an unstable spine, and correcting major spine deformities with instrumentation. *Specific* procedures are exclusively designed to address intractable pain and include destructive procedures and central electrical stimulations. Indications for specific procedures are twofold: (1) cancer pain, and (2) chronic nonmalignant pain. Cancer pain is typically nociceptive, and the duration of the intractable pain period is shorter than in nonmalignant pain, which is the reason ablative procedures may be preferably indicated in the management of intractable cancer pain.

NEURODESTRUCTIVE PROCEDURES FOR CANCER PAIN

Destructive procedures for intractable pain management aim to interrupt the afferent nociceptive pathway starting at the periphery (neurotomy, sympathectomy, ganglionectomy, rhizotomy) through central nociceptive pathways (dorsal root entry zone [DREZ] lesion, cordotomy, myelotomy, trigeminal tractotomy, mesencephalotomy, thalamotomy) up to cortical integrative structures (cingulotomy). Despite the fact that destructive neurosurgical techniques have a long history, their efficacy has not been established based on contemporary standards of evidence-based medicine. Fortunately, advances in pharmacotherapy and neuraxial delivery have significantly decreased the need for these procedures.

Neurotomy and Rhizotomy

The results of neurotomy, aiming to interrupt peripheral nociceptive input, have been overall disappointing. Rhizotomy (sectioning dorsal rootlets at different segments of the neuraxis) has multiple indications including trigeminal neuralgia, atypical facial pain, cervical and lumbar facet joint pain, sphenopalatine neuralgia, and cancer pain in various locations.

Sympathectomy

Neurolytic celiac plexus block is the most common form of sympathectomy for visceral (e.g. pancreatic) cancer pain. Other interventions include surgical cervicothoracic (stellate) ganglion or lumbar sympathetic chain ablation, coagulation, or chemical (phenol, alcohol) destruction.

Ganglionectomy

C2 ganglionectomy for occipital neuralgia is the most frequent indication for this procedure, followed by chronic lumbosacral pain, and intractable chest pain (thoracotomy, herpes). Sphenopalatine ganglionectomy for cluster headache is also reported.

Dorsal Root Entry Zone Lesion

The central portion of dorsal rootlets, Lissauer's propriospinal fibers, and the dorsal layers of the posterior horn gray matter form the DREZ. Deafferentation pain due to brachial plexus avulsion and neuropathic pain after spinal cord injury are the most frequent indications for DREZ lesioning. Some cancer pain indications include Pancoast tumor, breast cancer, giant cell tumor of sacrum, and uterine cancer-related pain.

Trigeminal Tractotomy

Facial cancer pain, postherpetic facial pain, trigeminal neuralgia, idiopathic vagoglossopharyngeal neuralgia, and geniculate neuralgia are indications for this procedure.

Cordotomy

Sectioning of the spinothalamic pathway in the anterolateral spinal cord is the most extensively applied and studied procedure for both cancer and nonmalignant pain. Overall, cordotomy provides less satisfactory pain relief for non-malignant indications, and in long-term follow-up, it was complicated by unpleasant dysesthesias.

Myelotomy

Commissural myelotomy targets the ventral crossing of spinothalamic and spinoreticular fibers resulting in band anesthesia in the involved segments. *Extralemniscal myelotomy* is not intended to interrupt segmental decussating fibers, but rather the ascending nonspecific polysynaptic pathway at the dorsal cervicomedullary junction. In general, outcomes with myelotomy were reported less satisfactory than with cordotomy except for midline visceral cancer pain (cervical, pancreatic, and gastric cancers).

Mesencephalotomy

This procedure or its variant—*pontine tractotomy*—target the spinothalamic tract in the brainstem. Cancer pain, thalamic syndrome, and postherpetic trigeminal neuralgia are the most common indications. Due to serious complications these procedures have been essentially abandoned.

Thalamotomy

Targeting the centromedian, medial thalamic, or pulvinar nuclei, these lesions produce unreliable results in the long-term, and are often accompanied by psychiatric complications. Therefore, chronic nonmalignant pain patients are poor candidates for this procedure.

Cingulotomy

Although in the majority of cases lesioning the anterior part of the cingulate gyrus has been performed to treat psychiatric disorders, indications for this procedure also include intractable phantom limb pain, psychogenic pain, poststroke pain, and cancer pain.

STIMULATION TECHNIQUES FOR NONCANCER PAIN

As opposed to destructive procedures, electrical stimulation of central nervous structures is gaining popularity, especially in chronic nonmalignant pain therapy.

Spinal Cord Stimulation

Epidural stimulation of posterior spinal cord columns is widely used for neuropathic pain and a recent review of randomized controlled trials confirmed its effectiveness in lumbar failed back surgery syndrome.

Deep Brain Stimulation

Stimulation of thalamic nuclei, internal capsule, and periaqueductal gray matter has been used for intractable pain. A combination of unilateral stimulation of the ventral caudal thalamic nucleus and bilateral cingulotomy has been successfully used in the therapy of poststroke pain.

Cortical Stimulation

Invasive epidural motor cortex stimulation, repetitive transcranial magnetic stimulation (rTMS), and transcranial direct current stimulation (tDCS) are the most recently evaluated targets for chronic neuropathic pain therapy.

SUMMARY AND DECISIONAL ALGORITHM

A A thorough history, physical examination and diagnostic workup are important in patient selection. Multidisciplinary evaluation with special attention to psychological factors, drug-seeking behavior, and secondary gain factors is important.

B Noninvasive modalities and nonsurgical approaches including physiotherapy, pharmacotherapy, nerve blocks, and psychological methods should be given an adequate trial before considering surgical approaches.

C Nonspecific surgical procedures addressing radicular pain, peripheral nerve compression, or mechanical pain from spinal deformity and instability should be tried before considering ablative surgeries or neurostimulation techniques.

D Specific neurosurgical destructive procedures or stimulation techniques are indicated only if satisfactory pain control still cannot be achieved.

The advanced neurodestructive or neuromodulation approaches described earlier may provide further pain treatment options in challenging clinical scenarios.

SUGGESTED READING

Cetas JS, Saedi T, Burchiel KJ. Destructive procedures for the treatment of nonmalignant pain: a structured literature review. J Neurosurg. 2008;109(3):389-404.

Gadgil N, Viswanathan A. DREZotomy in the treatment of cancer pain: a review. Stereotact Funct Neurosurg. 2012;90(6): 356-60.

Grider JS, Manchikanti L, Carayannopulos A, et al. Effectiveness of Spinal Cord Stimulation in Chronic Spinal Pain: A Systematic Review. Pain Physician. 2016;19(1):E33-54.

Lefaucheur JP. Cortical neurostimulation for neuropathic pain: state of the art and perspectives. Pain. 2016;157(Suppl 1):S81-9.

Raslan AM, Cetas JS, McCartney S, et al. Destructive procedures for control of cancer pain: the case for cordotomy. J Neurosurg. 2011;114(1):155-70.

Sharma M, Naik V, Deogaonkar M. Emerging applications of deep brain stimulation. J Neurosurg Sci. 2016;60(2):242-55.

Brian T Boies

CHAPTER
142

Pain Management Ethics

Driver LC

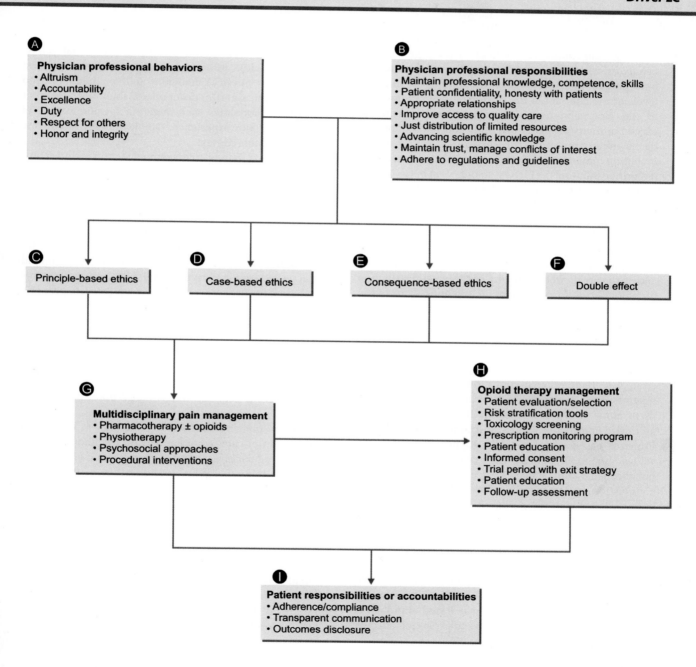

The ethical practice of pain medicine is consistent with the ethical practice of medicine in general—seeking to help patients by relieving pain and suffering from various collateral symptoms while trying to cure underlying disease or facilitate recovery from injury or surgery. The American Medical Association (AMA) has stated that "the social commitment of the physician is to relieve the suffering." Western cultural values hold that "no one should suffer" and patients expect "understanding and care" from their physician who should respect them as an individual and recognize patient autonomy in decision-making. We treat pain to improve clinical outcomes and enhance the patient's quality of life. We treat pain to increase patient satisfaction with care, and to meet regulatory standards of healthcare governing agencies. And, we treat pain because that is what we do as virtuous, moral and ethical physicians. William Osler said, "the practice of medicine is an art, not a trade; a calling, not a business, a calling in which your heart will be exercised equally with your head." This chapter will provide an overview of key aspects of ethical multidisciplinary pain management, with focus upon opioid therapy, particularly for non-cancer chronic pain.

A The physician should adhere to and exhibit *professional behaviors,* including—*altruism*: looking out for the best interests of patients; *accountability:* fulfilling the multiple levels of the contract of the doctor–patient relationship, to the profession and society; *excellence:* striving to exceed ordinary expectations; *duty:* freely accepting and displaying a commitment to service; *respect for others:* including patients, staff, colleagues, etc.; *honor and integrity:* exhibiting the highest standards of behavior and refusing to violate personal and professional codes.

B The physician should obey multiple *professional responsibilities,* including commitments to maintaining professional knowledge, competence and skills, honesty with patients and patient confidentiality, maintaining appropriate relations with patients and others, improving access to care as well as quality of care, just distribution of limited resources, advancing scientific knowledge, maintaining trust by managing conflicts of interest (at multiple levels), adhering to the various national and state regulations and guidelines.

Several approaches to ethical decision-making offer converging rationales to support our therapeutic strategies. Their relative contributions to our thinking may vary with evolving clinical scenarios, since none of them alone is always sufficient. These approaches are grounded in principles, cases, and consequences.

C Principle-based ethics consider guiding principles and values, including patient autonomy, nonmaleficence, beneficence, and social justice, along with trust, compassion, and truth telling. A decision is ethical if it is in accordance with the pertinent principles and values. Principle-based ethics can be helpful in framing ethical issues and questions in their proper context.

D Case-based ethics consider prior similar case scenarios, their treatment decisions, and outcomes as evidence in favor of or opposition to approaches considered for the current situation. A decision is ethical if it is concordant with ethical precedent cases. A case-based approach is meaningful for defining the particularities of specific clinical scenarios.

E Consequence-based ethics hinges upon the outcomes of decisions. A decision is ethical if the outcomes are beneficial to the patient and no harm is incurred. Benefits must outweigh burdens or harms, assuming that the ends are achieved by proper means.

F The doctrine of double-effect applies and is either overtly or implicitly considered when making clinical decisions about the use of opioid analgesic therapy—in situations where it is impossible to avoid all harmful effects or consequences of one's actions. A prescriber's intention to relieve pain (the good effect) outweighs the potential harm such as respiratory depression (the bad effect) that may come from opioids. The good must outweigh the harm.

G Pain management should be carried out via a multi-disciplinary treatment approach, including procedural interventions, pharmacotherapy, psychosocial-behavioral strategies, integrative-complementary-alternative approaches, physical medicine and rehabilitation and related physical and/or occupational therapies, and other treatment modalities each targeting specific aspects of the overall pain experience. Opioid therapy is but one modality in this context.

H Ethical opioid therapy management should include comprehensive patient evaluation, proper patient selection, relative risk management using risk stratification tools (opioid risk tool [ORT], screener and opioid assessment for patients with pain [SOAPP], etc.), toxicology screening, review of the state electronic prescription monitoring program, patient education, informed consent for opioid therapy along with a treatment agreement, opioid trial period with exit strategy, and follow-up assessments including further screening and review (see Chapter 112: Risk Evaluation and Mitigation Strategies for Opioids). Ongoing opioid treatment necessitates regular follow-up visits for patient evaluation, indicated toxicology assessment, review of e-PMP data, side effects management, indicated dosage adjustments and adjuvant agents. And, full documentation of the care includes the earlier along with evolving treatment plans based upon patient outcomes.

I Patient responsibilities include adherence to the agreed upon plan of care, compliance with treatments as prescribed, regular transparent communication of treatment effects and side effects, and reporting therapeutic benefits or unintended consequences of therapy. Patients should be accountable for their responsibilities in their care. Factored into every dynamic pain management assessment and plan will be consideration of patient age, gender, race or ethnicity, cultural and religious issues, socioeconomic factors, and individual features.

Finally, strongly recommended for review are Ballantyne and Fleisher's *Ethical Issues in Opioid Prescribing for Chronic Pain* along with Cohen and Jangro's *A Clinical Ethics Approach to Opioid Treatment of Chronic Noncancer Pain*, the source for the following "Six-step Ethical Decision Making for Opioid Treatment":

1. Establish the patient's pain narrative, including personal impact within contextual and psychosocial factors, functionality, collateral symptoms and comorbidities, helpful and problematic behaviors.

2. Identify relevant pain pathophysiology and pain generators in order to guide therapy that is rational and targeted to the extent possible.

3. Based upon thorough evaluation, establish individual and collaborative goals that are specific, meaningful, and personal; and that focus on quality of life.

4. Periodically reassess patient outcomes and progress, and adjust the plan of care accordingly.

5. Review accomplished goals and establish the patient's next goals; and, consider honing unachieved goals into doable tasks.

6. Intermittent comprehensive appraisal of the patient's outcomes and progress on the prescribed treatment plan that facilitates clarification of diagnosis and refinements or alterations of therapeutic strategies.

SUGGESTED READING

American Medical Association (AMA). (2016). Code of Medical Ethics. [online] Available from *www.ama-assn.org/about-us/code-medical-ethics*. [Accessed February, 2017].

Ballantyne JC, Fleisher LA. Ethical issues in opioid prescribing for chronic pain. Pain. 2010;148(3):365-7.

Beauchamp TL, Childress JF. Principles of Biomedical Ethics, 7th edition. Oxford: Oxford University Press; 2013.

Cohen MJ, Jangro WC. A Clinical Ethics Approach to Opioid Treatment of Chronic Noncancer Pain. AMA J Ethics. 2015;17(6): 521-9.

Robins LS, Braddock CH, Fryer-Edwards KA. Using the American Board of Internal Medicine's "Elements of Professionalism" for undergraduate ethics education. Acad Med. 2002;77(6):523-31.

Surbone A, Baider L. Personal values and cultural diversity. J Med Pers. 2013;11:11-8.

CHAPTER 143

Imaging Use During Interventional Procedures

Levin JE, Huynh L, Kennedy DJ

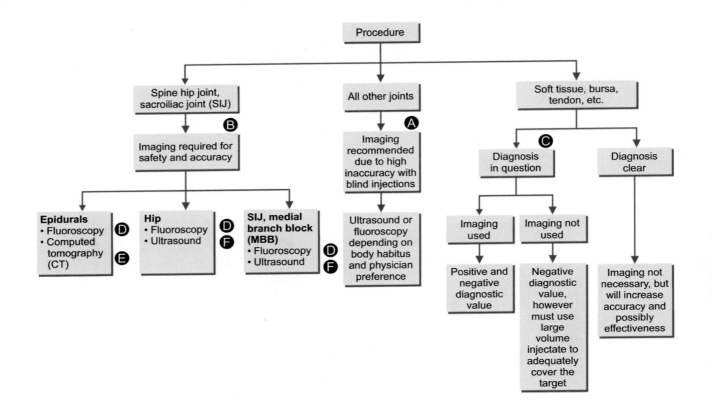

Historically, musculoskeletal injections have been done without image guidance (aka blind). With the advent of image guidance via computed tomography (CT), fluoroscopy, and ultrasound (US), practitioners now must decide when imaging is needed or required. The use of imaging is predicated on the ability to safely and accurately perform a procedure. Additionally, the necessity of image guidance is partially dependent on the anatomic target and the utility of the diagnostic component of the injection. The main disadvantages of using image guidance include added cost and radiation exposure with CT or fluoroscopic guidance. Conversely, image guidance has several advantages.

A The first advantage to utilizing imaging is that it clearly increases accuracy, as studies have repeatedly shown blind injections to be inaccurate. Blind injections have been shown to miss as high as 88% for the sacroiliac (SI) joint, 73% for the glenohumeral joint, 71% for the subacromial bursa, 57% for intra-articular knee joint injections, and 49% for intra-articular hip joint injections.

Surprisingly, even non-image-guided greater trochanter injections are often inaccurate. Fifty-five percent of these seemingly simple injections fail to result in a bursagram when subsequently confirmed with contrast dye under fluoroscopy, while 22% fail to even contact the greater trochanter. While accuracy rates of hip, knee, and shoulder injections are considerably better in other studies not cited earlier, the highest reported accuracy rate for intra-articular SI joint injections is only 78%. In the spine, interlaminar epidural injections done without image guidance have a failure rate (needle placement outside the epidural space) as high as 30%, whereas caudal epidural injections done without image guidance have a failure rate as high as 52%. While most studies that evaluated the accuracy of non-image-guided epidural injections simply assessed needle placement within the epidural space, one study assessed more relevant information—appropriate dye flow to the site of pathology. Despite being more accurate than most other studies in placing needles in the epidural space, this study showed a 74% failure rate in regards to dye flow reaching the intended pathologic structure. Given these high inaccuracy rates, image guidance is recommended for all spine and intra-articular procedures.

B The second advantage to image guidance is that it may enhance the procedural safety for some high-risk procedures. Due to the complexity of the spine and the risk of significant morbidity from adverse events, imaging is recommended for all procedures targeting the spine or SI joint.

C Another advantage to image guidance is that with the enhanced accuracy, additional diagnostic information can be obtained. For diagnostic procedures, image guidance is generally required to rule out a structure as a pain generator. If a non-image-guided injection fails to provide symptomatic relief, it is unclear whether or not the lack of relief was due to the treated structure not being the source of the pain, or if the procedure was simply technically unsuccessful. With a large volume of anesthetic in soft tissue injections, this negative response may be overcome, as the large volume of anesthetic should reach the targeted tissue. Simply injecting a larger volume of anesthetic may not work for intra-articular injections if the needle is not accurately placed. However, with image guidance, both positive and negative diagnostic value is added, although placebo rates of up to 40% should be considered when interpreting positive responses. Additionally, if image guidance is used and the patient does not achieve relief, then it can be stated with a higher degree of confidence that the treated structure is not the source of the patient's pain. Therefore, if the diagnosis is in question, image guidance should be considered.

When image guidance is required, fluoroscopy, CT, or US, each of which has its advantages and disadvantages, can provide this guidance.

D Fluoroscopy has traditionally been the most commonly used method for image guidance. The greatest advantage to fluoroscopy is that it is the only imaging modality that allows the physician to view contrast dye injection inside the spinal canal in real-time. Since the majority of devastating complications from interventional spine procedures occur when particulate steroids are injected into radiculomedullary arteries that feed the spinal cord, the identification of these feeder arteries is vital for performing these procedures safely. Live fluoroscopy has been shown to be more effective in identifying vascular dye patterns than static fluoroscopic images, and is likely the only way to accurately identify these potentially dangerous situations. Therefore, fluoroscopic guidance is the safest method for performing interventional spine procedures. The primary disadvantage of fluoroscopy is the equipment requirements and the resources needed to perform fluoroscopically-guided injections. This includes the fluoroscopy machine itself and a procedure suite with knowledgeable and licensed staff who can operate the equipment. Additionally, fluoroscopy exposes patients and staff to ionizing radiation. However, when available, fluoroscopy can be used both efficiently and safely to perform most procedures.

E Computed tomography guidance is another modality that has been used for many years in the performance of interventional spine and peripheral joint injections. CT guidance provides better bony visualization than fluoroscopy and can demonstrate the location of large vessels. Its use may be indicated in certain situations, such as extremely challenging anatomy, or morbidly obese patients in whom fluoroscopic visualization is limited. CT, however, does not allow real-time contrast visualization, and therefore, can fail to identify the potentially catastrophic complication of needle placement within a radiculomedullary artery during an epidural steroid injection. Also, the equipment and personnel requirements for CT are even greater than that of fluoroscopy, and the radiation dose to the patient is substantially higher.

F Ultrasound is the most recent imaging modality to be used for interventional procedures. It has the advantages of being small and portable enough to be used in the treatment room of a typical office. Also, no ionizing radiation is used. While US has become more universally accepted as a modality that can accurately guide joint and soft tissue injections, its use in interventional spine procedures is still debated. Large vessels can be seen and avoided with US guidance, and medication can be injected under live visualization. However, US does not allow for the visualization of live contrast dye during spine procedures that is required to ensure needle placement outside of a radiculomedullary artery. Therefore, it is not as safe as fluoroscopy in preventing a catastrophic complication during an epidural steroid injection. Although some practitioners have adopted US use for some spine procedures such as medial branch blocks and SI joint injections, most do not recommend using it for epidural steroid injections.

SUGGESTED READING

Cohen SP, Narvaez JC, Lebovits AH, et al. Corticosteroid injections for trochanteric bursitis: is fluoroscopy necessary? A pilot study. Br J Anaesth. 2005;94(1):100-6.

Diraçoğlu D, Alptekin K, Dikici F, et al. Evaluation of needle positioning during blind intra-articular hip injections for osteoarthritis: fluoroscopy versus arthrography. Arch Phys Med Rehabil. 2009;90(12):2112-5.

Eustace JA, Brophy DP, Gibney RP, et al. Comparison of the accuracy of steroid placement with clinical outcome in patients with shoulder symptoms. Ann Rheum Dis. 1997;56(1):59-63.

Fredman B, Nun MB, Zohar E, et al. Epidural steroids for treating "failed back surgery syndrome": is fluoroscopy really necessary? Anesth Analg. 1999;88(2):367-72.

Hansen HC. Is fluoroscopy necessary for sacroiliac joint injections? Pain Physician. 2003;6(2):155-8.

Renfrew DL, Moore TE, Kathol MH, et al. Correct placement of epidural steroid injections: fluoroscopic guidance and contrast administration. AJNR Am J Neuroradiol. 1991;12(5):1003-7.

Rosenberg JM, Quint TJ, de Rosayro AM. Computerized tomographic localization of clinically-guided sacroiliac joint injections. Clin J Pain. 2000;16(1):18-21.

Sethi PM, Kingston S, Elattrache N. Accuracy of anterior intra-articular injection of the glenohumeral joint. Arthroscopy. 2005; 21(1):77-80.

Smuck M, Fuller BJ, Chiodo A, et al. Accuracy of intermittent fluoroscopy to detect intravascular injection during trans-foraminal epidural injections. Spine (Phila Pa 1976). 2008;33(7): E205-10.

White AH, Derby R, Wynne G. Epidural injections for the diagnosis and treatment of low-back pain. Spine (Phila Pa 1976). 1980; 5(1):78-86.

Wind WM, Smolinski RJ. Reliability of common knee injection sites with low-volume injections. J Arthroplasty. 2004;19(7):858-61.

Radiographic Contrast Media

Eckmann MS

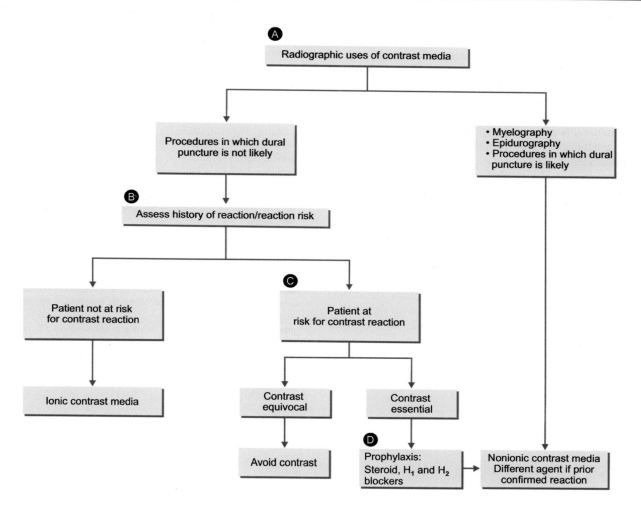

Contrast agents are useful for many pain management procedures requiring fluoroscopic assistance. They help to visualize location of the needle tip, the spread of the substance injected, and target structures. Radiographic contrast media are generally iodinated with the exception of gadolinium-based contrast agents (GBCAs) like Optimark (gadoversetamide). Two types of contrast agent are commonly used. The ionic contrast agents have high osmolarity and include Renografin (diatrizoate) and Conray (iothalamate). The nonionic agents have low osmolarity and include Isovue (iopamidol) and Omnipaque (iohexol).

A *Background:* In general, ionic contrast agents are neurotoxic, and therefore, not recommended for myelography, epidurography, or any other procedures

in which dural puncture is likely (e.g. epidural injection, facet joint injection, selective nerve blocks, discography). Nonionic agents are approved for those procedures and for intrathecal use. Nonionic contrast agents are more expensive. There is growing evidence that GBCAs accumulate in neural tissue with repeated exposure, however the clinical impact is still unclear.

B *History Relevant to Contrast Media:* Adverse reactions to contrast media include nausea, vomiting, pruritus, dyspnea, bronchospasm, anaphylactic reaction, and cardiac arrest. Severe reactions have an incidence of 0.02–0.5%. The incidence of these reactions is increased in individuals with known sensitivities (asthma, multiple food and drug allergies, prior reaction to contrast media), and may reach as high as 7–17% in sensitized individuals. Shellfish allergy does not confer a specifically increased risk over other food allergies. Contrast agents should be used with caution in patients with poor renal function and paraproteinemias.

C *Confirming Need and Role of Contrast:* Contrast is recommended for fluoroscopically-guided procedures for two primary reasons. Firstly, the interventional practitioner can confirm the absence of unintended injection, such as into the intravascular or intrathecal spaces during epidural or paravertebral procedures. Additionally, positive confirmation that the injection enters or surrounds the intended target can be obtained. This is pertinent to diagnostic procedures as interpretation depends on the premise that the intended nerve or structure has been blocked. Digital subtraction angiography (DSA) can augment information in both instances, suppressing static image signals to highlight changing signals (e.g. highlighting a faint wisp of vascular extravasation, or outlining contrast entry of the cavum trigeminale during Gasserian ganglion block where there is significant bony signal). DSA does have limitations, however, and comes at the expense of increased radiation exposure. If diagnostic information is not required from a specific procedure, and the anatomic area and agent for injection are considered to be extremely low-risk for complication from aberrant injection, the practitioner may elect to avoid contrast completely in a patient with high-risk for contrast reaction. Injections performed without contrast should be performed away from blood supply that can reach the spinal cord and use small amounts of local anesthetic agent.

D *Risk Reduction:* Patients at risk for allergic reactions to contrast agents should receive prophylactic treatment including steroids or H_1- and H_2-blockers (or both) before the exposure. In any case, the pain practitioner and staff should be knowledgeable about resuscitation and be prepared to manage adverse reactions that occur during pain management procedures. Patients with prior reaction to an ionic contrast agent or nonionic agent should be additionally switched to an alternative low-osmolar nonionic contrast agent if available.

SUGGESTED READING

Abe S, Fukuda H, Tobe K, et al. Protective effect against repeat adverse reactions to iodinated contrast medium: Premedication vs. changing the contrast medium. Eur Radiol. 2016;26(7):2148-54.

Curry NS, Schabel SI, Reiheld CT, et al. Fatal reactions to intravenous nonionic contrast material. Radiology. 1991;178(2):361-2.

Cusmano J. Premedication regimen eases contrast reaction. Diagn Imaging. 1992;181:185-6.

Greenberger PA, Patterson R. The prevention of immediate generalized reactions to radiocontrast media in high-risk patients. J Allergy Clin Immunol. 1991;87(4):867-72.

Lawrence V, Matthai W, Hartmaier S. Comparative safety of high-osmolality and low-osmolality radiographic contrast agents. Report of a multidisciplinary working group. Invest Radiol. 1992; 27(1):2-28.

Nagpal AS, Chang-Chien GC, Benfield JA, et al. Digital subtraction angiography use during epidural steroid injections does not reliably distinguish artery from vein. Pain Physician. 2016;19(4): 255-66.

Schabelman E, Witting M. The relationship of radiocontrast, iodine, and seafood allergies: a medical myth exposed. J Emerg Med. 2010;39(5):701-7.

Stojanov D, Aracki-Trenkic A, Benedeto-Stojanov D. Gadolinium deposition within the dentate nucleus and globus pallidus after repeated administrations of gadolinium-based contrast agents-current status. Neuroradiology. 2016;58(5):433-41.

CHAPTER 145

Controversial Therapies

Nagpal A, Eckmann MS, Ramamurthy S

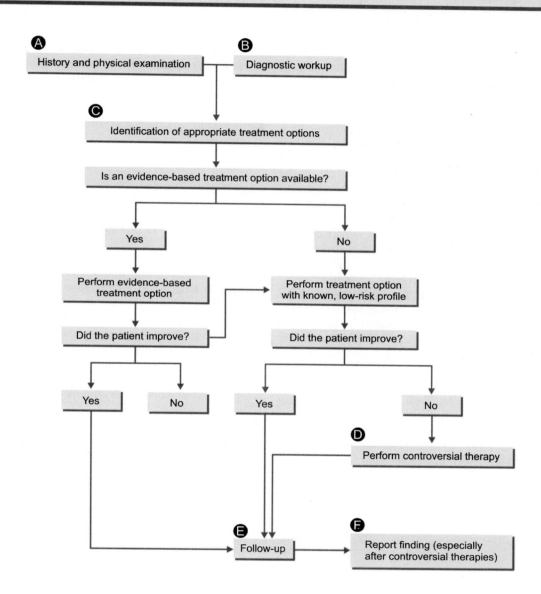

Pain management as a field represents an interesting dichotomy in that pain has been treated by physicians and healers since the dawn of mankind, yet as a field of independent study it has only existed for several decades. Many treatment options discussed in this book, such as cannabis and opioids, have been utilized for the treatment of painful medical conditions for centuries. The interventional procedures discussed in this book have been used, at best, for just one century and in some cases, for less than 10 years.

Because of the relative novelty of the field of pain medicine, burgeoning therapy options are constantly emerging. These treatment options are not necessarily interventional in nature. Pharmacological treatment options include oral, mucosal, transdermal, and infusion-based, all of which are perpetually being introduced to the market by pharmaceutical companies and independent research by physicians and scientists. The discerning physician will be able to evaluate the utility of these controversial therapies as they arise and determine whether they are beneficial to their patient on an individual basis.

Ⓐ *History and Physical Examination:* As always, the first step in management of the chronic pain patient is performing a thorough history and physical examination which will aid in diagnosis. This topic is discussed in the other sections of this text.

Ⓑ *Diagnostic Workup:* As referenced in several sections of this text, there are a multitude of diagnostic modalities that can be used to identify a particular condition. These range from imaging modalities such as radiographs, magnetic resonance imaging (MRI), and computed tomography (CT) scans to diagnostic injections such as nerve blocks and provocative discography.

Ⓒ *Identification of Appropriate Treatment:* Based upon the findings of the patient's history and physical examination and diagnostic workup, the physician should develop a treatment algorithm. It is best for the physician to first treat the patient with evidence-based options if at all possible. If evidence-based treatment does not exist or the patient has failed evidence-based options, the physician should then elect to treat the patient with therapy that has been in use for a long period of time with a known and tolerable risk profile. If evidence-based options and known risk profile treatments have failed or are not valid choices for an individual patient, the physician should then consider a controversial therapy.

Ⓓ *Performance of Controversial Therapy:* If the physician has chosen to use a controversial therapy in the treatment of their patient, they must firstly explain to the patient that the treatment is controversial, and the reason why it is so. This is almost always because the procedure is novel and poorly studied. Recent examples of this type of treatment include: oral or intravenous methylcobalamin for trigeminal neuralgia, ketamine and/or lidocaine infusions for complex regional pain syndrome, pulsed radiofrequency neuromodulation of peripheral nerves for neuropathic pain, intradiscal electrothermal annuloplasty (IDET) for lumbar discogenic pain, and minimally invasive laminar decompression (MILD) for spinal stenosis due to ligamentum flavum hypertrophy. The physician should then perform a detailed informed content with the patient which includes the theoretical risks to the procedure or treatment and the potential benefits. One of the risks that should be emphasized is the potential for a previously unrecognized adverse outcome since the therapy at hand may not be studied in enough patients to demonstrate all of its risks.

Ⓔ *Follow-up:* When a physician has elected to utilize a controversial therapy to treat a patient's painful medical condition, he or she should follow-up very closely with that individual patient. This follow-up is necessary to determine if the patient developed any known or unknown adverse effects and to establish the degree of analgesia and functional gains that the patient has had (if any). This should be done with all therapies prescribed to a patient (physical, interventional, pharmacological, or psychological) but is particularly important with controversial therapies because of the potential for unknown outcomes.

Ⓕ *Reporting Findings:* It is certainly not necessary for all physicians to report their findings after the utilization of novel treatment options. Yet, if an unknown outcome is found, the conscientious practitioner would report the finding so that others would be aware of this outcome—good or bad—and can then appropriately inform their patient population of the discovery during the informed consent process. Additionally, overutilization of healthcare, and specifically pain management procedures, has become a huge burden on the costs of healthcare in the United States. The prescriptions of opioids have led to the so-called "opioid epidemic," an international and growing phenomenon which has led to addiction to opioid medications in millions of people across the globe. If a controversial treatment is found to be efficacious in the practice of individuals of groups, it is paramount that this information be disseminated in order to both avail the treatment option to our patients and to continue to protect the specialty of pain medicine with superior evidence.

SUGGESTED READING

Ling W, Mooney L, Hillhouse M. Prescription opioid abuse, pain and addiction: clinical issues and implications. Drug Alcohol Rev. 2011;30(3):300-5.

Manchikanti L, Helm Ii S, Singh V, et al. Accountable interventional pain management: a collaboration among practitioners, patients, payers, and government. Pain Physician. 2013;16(6):E635-70.

INDEX

Page numbers followed by *b* refer to box, *f* refer to figure, and *t* refer to table